HANDBOOK OF
CENTRAL AUDITORY PROCESSING DISORDER

Volume II
Comprehensive Intervention

Second Edition

HANDBOOK OF CENTRAL AUDITORY PROCESSING DISORDER

Volume II
Comprehensive Intervention

Second Edition

Gail D. Chermak, PhD
Editor

Frank E. Musiek, PhD
Editor

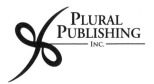

PLURAL
PUBLISHING
— INC. —

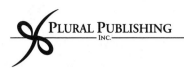

5521 Ruffin Road
San Diego, CA 92123

e-mail: info@pluralpublishing.com
Website: http://www.pluralpublishing.com

Typeset in 10½/13 Garamond by Flanagan's Publishing Services, Inc.
Printed in the United States of America by McNaughton & Gunn, Inc.

Library of Congress Cataloging-in-Publication Data

Handbook of central auditory processing disorder / Frank E. Musiek, editor,
Gail D. Chermak, editor.—Second edition.
    p. ; cm.
  Includes bibliographical references and index.
  ISBN-13: 978-1-59756-561-5 (v. 1 : alk. paper)
  ISBN-10: 1-59756-561-X (v. 1 : alk. paper)
  ISBN-13: 978-1-59756-562-2 (v. 2 : alk. paper)
  I. Musiek, Frank E., editor of compilation. II. Chermak, Gail D., editor of
compilation.
  [DNLM: 1. Language Development Disorders—diagnosis. WL 340.2]
  RC394.W63
  617.8—dc23
                                                      2013027153

CONTENTS

SECTION IV: CASE STUDIES 617

SECTION V: FUTURE DIRECTIONS 647

FOREWORD

Having the honor of writing a foreword for an important contribution to scientific literature also carries responsibility. The book you are holding in your hands is too scientific, too well considered, too unbiased, to preface it with a foreword that does not, like the contents of the book, acknowledge the diverse range of attitudes and opinions pertaining to our knowledge of central auditory processing and its associated disorders. It is likely that most professionals trained in neuroscience, audiology, speech-language pathology, and neuropsychology, and thus educated about the central auditory system, have an appreciation of its complexities. Despite the well deserved fascination with this intricate structure, however, not every audiologist or neuroscientist understands, or even believes in, central auditory processing disorders. It is not so much that they do not believe that central auditory processing disorder (CAPD) exists as an entity, it is that they do not believe it can be accurately diagnosed and subsequently treated. Much of this skepticism lies in the uneven nature and quality of the information and research that has been disseminated in the past, which has consequently led to both diagnosis and misdiagnosis of overlapping disorders and has created a plethora of treatments, some successful, some questionable, and some absurdly embellished. CAPD is not limited to any age group. But it can be so frustrating and difficult to endure, both for patients suffering from it and for their loved ones,

that placebos and exaggerated media claims of understandably hopeful clinicians and researchers have endured. The necessity for evidence-based research leading to better diagnosis and therapy has thus never been more important, both to expose less than accurate information and to advance the true science.

In this remarkable two-volume second edition of the *Handbook of Central Auditory Processing Disorder*, Frank Musiek and Gail Chermak, two of the most respected authorities in this field, provide the most thorough description of central auditory processing available, analyzing not only the anatomy, but the complex physiology that allows human beings to harness the power and proficiency of this amazing auditory function. Along the way, they explain the numerous ways this power can be diminished, dispel myths associated with central processing dysfunction, and demonstrate, through evidence-based research, the efficacy (and challenges) of diagnosis and treatment of these disorders.

The contributing authors in both volumes are a veritable Who's Who of the scientists and clinicians most responsible for our current state of knowledge of central auditory processing. Drs. Musiek and Chermak have thoughtfully organized the material in a logical manner, beginning with auditory neuroscience, fundamentals of diagnostics, the evaluation of central auditory processes (employing both behavioral and electrophysiologic measures), differential diagnosis, illustrated concepts with case studies, and future directions. And that's only in Volume 1! Volume 2 focuses and analyzes comprehensive intervention, including the foundations of therapies, many of which incorporate state-of-the-art computerized techniques. Consistent with Volume 1, these concepts are illustrated with case studies. All this is followed by another discussion about future directions.

The information contained in this work is applicable for clinical populations of all ages. Moreover, the multidisciplinary perspectives that are presented incorporate opinions relevant for audiologists, speech-language pathologists, physicians, neuroscientists, neuropsychologists, and researchers. I consider this body of work to be essential reading for any serious researcher or clinician interested in central auditory processing, and I believe it should be required reading for students of the science. Critics and skeptics alike need to study this book.

Robert W. Sweetow, PhD
San Francisco, California
July 12, 2013

PREFACE

Central auditory processing disorder (CAPD) is a deficit in neural processing of auditory stimuli that is not due to higher-order language, cognitive, or related factors, yet CAPD may lead to or be associated with difficulties in higher-order language, learning, cognitive, and communication functions. The comorbidity of CAPD with a range of language, learning, and communication disorders is the result of brain organization, about which we have learned much in recent years. The perspectives contained in the second edition of our two-volume Handbook reflect continuing advances in auditory neuroscience and cognitive science since a group of Italian otolaryngologists led by Ettore Bocca recognized that pure tone audiometry was insufficient for detecting central auditory lesions. This led them to develop a battery of *sensitized speech tests* to diagnose disorders of the central auditory nervous system. Through their clinical studies over a span of 20 years, they increased our understanding of the relationship between the site and extent of lesion and the nature and severity of auditory dysfunction, including the now well known *contralateral effect* in which temporal lobe lesions show a deficit in the ear contralateral to the lesion. Indeed, many of the tests in use today bear considerable resemblance to those developed by these physicians. Some 40 years later, then President George H. Bush proclaimed the 1990s the "Decade of the Brain." Since that proclamation, we have witnessed great strides in basic and clinical research in neuroscience

and cognitive science with considerable impact on the diagnosis and treatment of CAPD.

Perhaps a watershed event, leading clinicians and scientists from around the world convened in Boston, Massachusetts, in March 2012 at the first global conference on CAPD (held in conjunction with the annual convention of the American Academy of Audiology). Presenters and over 250 attendees shared knowledge, perspectives, and practices, which exposed areas of agreement, as well as differences. This conference sealed a commitment from all to seek greater opportunities for collaborative research and exchange. Indeed, the multidisciplinary efforts of thousands of scientists and health care professionals have led to greater insights regarding the nature of CAPD, brain organization and function, and directions for more accurate diagnosis and efficacious and effective interventions. With the recognition that neuroplastic changes in the brain underlie learning and rehabilitation and that significant neural reorganization can occur in response to injury or learning even in mature nervous systems, there is every reason to embrace an aggressive and optimistic approach to intervention knowing that behavioral interventions that appropriately stimulate plastic neural tissues should lead to positive change.

The complexity and heterogeneity of CAPD, combined with the heterogeneity of learning and related disorders, challenge scientists and clinicians as they attempt to understand and differentially diagnose individuals with listening deficits, language comprehension problems, attention deficits, learning disabilities, and other related behavioral, emotional, and social difficulties. This Handbook offers the most up-to-date and comprehensive coverage of the auditory neuroscience and the clinical science needed to accurately diagnose, assess, and treat the auditory and related deficits of individuals with CAPD. As in the first edition, the second edition of the Handbook melds science and practice, providing comprehensive coverage of the field of CAPD in children, adults, and older adults, involving the range of developmental (i.e., neurobiological) and acquired origins (i.e., aging and neurological diseases, disorders, and insults, including neurodegenerative diseases). Both volumes include many new chapters, new contributing authors (including international scientists and clinicians), and varied perspectives, and all chapters appearing in the first edition have been revised. Volume 1 provides an expanded section (four new chapters) on auditory neuroscience, new chapters and/or authors discussing diagnostic principles and procedures and multidisciplinary assessment, a chapter of case studies, and two chapters projecting future directions for the field. Volume 2, which concentrates on multidisciplinary rehabilitation and professional issues, contains nine new chapters, including one focused on the efficacy of auditory training, another on school policies, processes, and services, one providing a retrospective of the evolution of research and clinical practices in CAPD, three new chapters on specific treatment approaches, a chapter of case studies, and two chapters reflecting on the current issues requiring additional research and consensus as we consider the future opportunities for even greater treatment effectiveness and efficacy.

The Handbook is intended to serve three primary audiences. The contributing authors have written a comprehensive set of manuals for clinicians, primarily audiologists, speech-language pathologists, and psychologists, and other related health care professionals. The Handbook also should serve as a reference source for a range of clinical scientists engaged in research related to audition and speech perception. Finally, we hope our Handbook can serve graduate students in the classroom and in support of their clinical experiences.

The approaches and recommendations offered in this Handbook are not intended to serve as a sole source of guidance for the differential diagnosis and intervention of individuals with CAPD. Rather, the views and methods of the 47 authors contributing to the Handbook are designed to assist the clinician by providing a framework for decision making and implementing diagnostic and treatment strategies. They are not intended to replace clinical judgment or to establish a protocol for all individuals with CAPD. Individual differences and circumstances, including the presence of comorbid conditions, require flexibility and adaptation.

Notwithstanding considerable scientific, technological, and clinical strides forward, we still have much more to learn. As was the case when our first edition was published in 2007, continued research is needed to resolve certain longstanding questions, and address the new questions that arise continually as new knowledge begets new questions. Collaboration between clinicians and scientists—combining the clinician's firsthand knowledge of clinical needs with the researcher's expertise in the scientific method—provides a powerful approach to asking the right questions and obtaining enduring answers. Indeed, the contributing authors to the Handbook reflect this very collaboration between scientists and clinicians. Only through continued collaboration can we truly generate innovative approaches to questions and problems and accelerate the pace of discovery. In so doing, we will continue to advance our understanding of the central auditory nervous system and its intersections with cognitive and language domains that lead to the complex and heterogeneous clinical profiles of CAPD. It is imperative to seize the momentum that has taken us to our current level of understanding and clinical practice, as described in the Handbook. To ensure that we are able to deliver the best clinical services to our patients and their families, we as individuals and the professional organizations that represent us must remain engaged in developing strategic responses to and preparing for the rapidly changing health care landscape, changes that will focus on value-based service delivery and the convergence of patient-centered outcomes and cost-effectiveness.

In closing, we hope to contribute to enhanced *patient-reported* outcomes and the improved overall quality of the lives of individuals with CAPD, their families, and their communities with the knowledge and practices shared in this second edition of the Handbook.

Gail D. Chermak
Frank E. Musiek

ACKNOWLEDGMENTS

We offer our sincere appreciation to each of our chapter authors and the Plural team who have stood by us and worked hard to see this project through.

F. E. M and G. D. C

ABOUT THE EDITORS

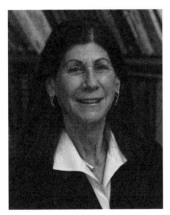

Gail D. Chermak, PhD

Gail D. Chermak is an internationally recognized authority on central auditory processing disorder (CAPD). She has published extensively and lectured around the world on differential diagnosis and treatment of CAPD. Dr. Chermak is professor of audiology and chair of the Department of Speech and Hearing Sciences at Washington State University. She is the recipient of numerous honors and awards, including the American Academy of Audiology's (AAA) Distinguished Achievement Award and the "Book of the Year Award" for the *Handbook of (Central) Auditory Processing Disorder* Vols. I and II (with Frank Musiek coeditor). She is a Fellow of the American Speech-Language-Hearing Association (ASHA) and is included in several major American and international biographical listings. She has served on a number of editorial boards and national professional committees and task forces, including the 2010 AAA task force which published evidence-based clinical practice guidelines for CAPD. She has authored over 100 articles and book chapters, and authored or edited 6 books.

Frank E. Musiek is Professor and Director of Auditory Research, Department of Speech, Language and Hearing Sciences and Professor of Otolaryngology, School of Medicine, University of Connecticut. He is the 2007 recipient of the American Academy of Audiology (AAA) James Jerger Career Award for Research in Audiology, the 2010 recipient of "The Honors of the American Speech-Language-Hearing Association for his contributions to Audiology and Auditory Neuroscience," and recipient of the "Book of the Year Award" for the *2007 Handbook of (Central) Auditory Processing Disorder*, Vols. I and II (with Gail Chermak coeditor). He has published over 200 articles and book chapters in the areas of auditory evoked potentials, central auditory disorders, neuroaudiology, and auditory neuroanatomy and has authored or edited 9 books. He has served on numerous national and international committees, editorial boards, and task forces, including chairing the 2010 AAA task force for clinical practice guidelines for central auditory processing disorder.

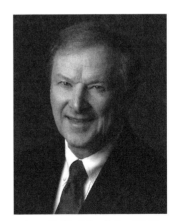

Frank E. Musiek, PhD

CONTRIBUTORS

Doris-Eva Bamiou, MD, MSc, PhD
Consultant in Neuro-otology
National Hospital for Neurology and
    Neurosurery
Department of Health HEFCE Clinical
    Senior Lecturer
Course Director
MScin Audiovestibular Medicine
University College London Ear Institute
London, United Kingdom
Chapter 16

Anuradha R. Bantwal, MSc
Lecturer
Department of Audiology
Ali Yavar Jung National Institute for the
    Hearing Handicapped
Kishenchand Marg
Bandra Reclamation (West)
Mumbai, India
Chapter 6

Jane A. Baran, PhD
Professor and Chair
Department of Communication Disorders
University of Massachusetts Amherst
Amherst, MA
Chapter14

Teri James Bellis, PhD
Professor and Chair
Department of Communication
    Sciences and Disorders
Director
Speech-Language-Hearing Clinics
Adjunct Professor
Basic Biomedical Sciences
Sanford School of Medicine
University of South Dakota
Vermillion, SD
Chapters 1, 3, and 22

Cassandra Billiet, AuD
Clinical Audiologist
Oakdale Ear, Nose and Throat Clinic
Maple Grove, MN
Chapter 21

Sharon Cameron, PhD
Senior Research Scientist
National Acoustic Laboratories
Chatswood, Australia
Chapter 8

Gail D. Chermak, PhD
Professor and Chair
Department of Speech and Hearing
    Sciences
Washington State University
Spokane, WA
Chapters 1, 3, 7, 10, 22, and 23

Harvey Dillon, PhD
Director of Research
National Acoustic Laboratories
Adjunct Professor
Department of Linguistics
Macquarie University
Chatswood, Australia
Chapter 8

M. Patrick Feeney, PhD
Director
National Center for Rehabilitative
    Auditory Research
Veterans Affairs Medical Center
Professor Provisional
Department of Otolaryngology, Head
    and Neck Surgery
Oregon Health and Science
    University
Portland, OR
Chapter 15

Jeanane M. Ferre, PhD
Audiologist
Private Practice
Oak Park, IL
Chapters 13 and 20

Carol Flexer, PhD
Distinguished Professor Emeritus,
    Audiology
The University of Akron
Akron, OH
Chapter 12

Donna Geffner, PhD
Professor and Director
Graduate Programs in Speech-Language
    Pathology
St. John's University Doctoral Program
Long Island Audiology Consortium
    Program
Speech and Hearing Center
Flushing, New York
Chapter 17

James W. Hall III, PhD
Extraordinary Professor
University of Pretoria
Pretoria, South Africa
Chapter 6

Lindsay Heath, PhD
Post-doctoral Neuropsychology Fellow
Geisel School of Medicine at Dartmouth
Department of Psychiatry
Lebanon, NH
Chapter 18

Annette E. Hurley, PhD
Associate Professor
Department of Communication
    Disorders
Louisiana State University Health
    Sciences Center
New Orleans, LA
Chapter 21

Vivian Iliadou, MD, PhD
Assistant Professor of Psychoacoustics
Aristotle University of Thessaloniki

Medical School
Thessoloniki, Greece
Chapter 16

Ella Inglebret, PhD
Associate Professor
Department of Speech and Hearing
    Sciences
Washington State University
Spokane, WA
Chapter 2

Warren D. Keller, PhD
Independent Practice
East Amherst Psychology Group
Buffalo, NY
Chapter 19

Dawn Konrad-Martin, PhD
Investigator
National Center for Rehabilitative
    Auditory Research
Veterans Affairs Medical Center
Associate Professor
Department of Otolaryngology, Head
    and Neck Surgery
Oregon Health and Science University
Portland, OR
Chapter 15

M. Samantha Lewis, PhD
Investigator
National Center for Rehabilitative
    Auditory Research
Veterans Affairs Medical Center
Assistant Professor
Department of Otolaryngology, Head
    and Neck Surgery
Oregon Health and Science University
Portland, OR
Chapter 15

Georgina T. F. Lynch, MS
Clinical Assistant Professor
Department of Speech and Hearing
    Sciences
Washington State University
Spokane, WA
Chapter 5

A.C. Maerlender, PhD
Assistant Professor
Director
Pediatric Neuropsychological Services
Neuropsychology and Brain Imaging Lab
Department of Psychiatry
Geisel School of Medicine at Dartmouth
Lebanon, NH
Chapter 18

Frank E. Musiek, PhD
Director of Auditory Research
Professor of Audiology
Department of Speech, Language and
    Hearing Sciences
Professor of Otolaryngology
Department of Surgery
School of Medicine
University of Connecticut
Storrs, CT
Chapter 1, 3, 7, 9, 22, and 23

Jane T. Pimentel, PhD
Associate Professor
Department of Communication
    Disorders
Eastern Washington University
Spokane, WA
Chapter 2

Cynthia M. Richburg, PhD
Associate Professor of Audiology
Indiana University of Pennsylvania
Indiana, PA
Chapter 5

Gabrielle Saunders, PhD
Associate Director
National Center for Rehabilitative
    Auditory Research
Veterans Affairs Medical Center
Associate Professor
Department of Otolaryngology, Head
    and Neck Surgery

Oregon Health and Science University
Portland, OR
Chapter 15

Deborah Ross-Swain, EdD
Clinical Director
The Swain Center
Santa Rosa, CA
Chapter 17

Jacek Smurzynski, PhD
Associate Professor
Department of Audiology and Speech-
    Language Pathology
East Tennessee State University
Johnson City, TN
Chapter 4

Linda M. Thibodeau, PhD
Professor
Coordinator of Pediatric Aural
    Habilitation
Advanced Hearing Research Center
Callier Center for Communication
    Disorders
University of Texas at Dallas
Dallas, Texas
Chapter 11

Kim L. Tillery, PhD
Professor and Chair
Department of Communication
    Disorders and Sciences
State University of New York at
    Fredonia
Fredonia, NY
Chapter 19

Jeffrey Weihing, PhD
Assistant Professor
Division of Communicative Disorders
University of Louisville
Louisville, KY
Chapters 3, 7, 9, and 22

*To my brother Steven and my dear friend Ruth, whose unwavering
support and love have grounded me throughout my life.*

To my sister, Luann, my original source of inspiration.

*To Frank Musiek, my esteemed colleague and dear friend,
with whom I have enjoyed the most stimulating, productive,
and enduring collaboration of my career.*

And to my children, Isaac and Alina, who compel me to expand my boundaries.

—Gail D. Chermak

*I would like to thank my wife Sheila for all her tolerance, support, and
thoughtfulness while I was working on this book. She always "looks after me"
so I can finish the task at hand. A hearty thanks to my sons Erik and Justin, my
daughter in law Amy and my three granddaughters, Emma, Anna Kate and Ella
Claire who serve as a source of immense pride and motivation to me every day.*

*I want to extend a profound thanks and admiration to my colleague and
dear friend Gail Chermak who I have worked with on so many projects.
Her work ethic, foresight and knowledge have been and continue to be
truly amazing to me. Gail has helped me (and many of our contributors)
through many tough spots on this second edition with her sage advice.*

*Finally, I want to mention Linda Guenette, audiologist superb, who passed
away this past spring. Over the years, Linda and I saw many cases of CAPD
together and she strongly supported efforts to advance our knowledge of the
central auditory system. She was a dear friend to me and many others.*

—Frank E. Musiek

SECTION 1

Foundations

CHAPTER 1

NEUROBIOLOGY, COGNITIVE SCIENCE, AND INTERVENTION

GAIL D. CHERMAK, TERI JAMES BELLIS, and
FRANK E. MUSIEK

A new understanding of how the brain is organized and how neuroplastic changes in the brain underlie learning has emerged over the last two decades. In this chapter, we highlight the implications of major findings in neuroscience and cognitive science for intervention. These findings help to explain the frequent comorbidity of central auditory processing disorder (CAPD) and related attention, language, and learning deficits; they undergird intervention methods and strategies that harness the brain's potential to *remodel* itself through learning; and they provide a framework for the development of subprofiles of CAPD based on patterns or clusters of functional symptoms, central auditory test findings, and associated neurophysiologic bases. These subprofiles lead to more customized, deficit-focused, and therefore more effective intervention.

Definition and Nature of Central Auditory Processing Disorder

CAPD is a deficit in the perceptual (i.e., neural) processing of acoustic stimuli in the central nervous system and the neurobiologic activity that underlies those processes and gives rise to the auditory evoked potentials (AAA, 2010; ASHA, 2005a, b) The perceptual deficits in CAPD manifest as abnormal neurophysiologic representation of stimuli primarily (if not solely) in the auditory modality. By definition, these perceptual deficits may co-occur with, but are *not the result of*, dysfunction in other modalities (AAA, 2010; ASHA, 2005a, 2005b). Comorbidity of CAPD with dysfunction in other modalities may occur due to shared neuroanatomical substrates or common etiological factors, or may be the result of nonrelated co-occurrence. However, CAPD itself is a disorder of the central auditory nervous system (CANS).

CAPD manifests behaviorally as poor performance in one or more of the following auditory behaviors: localization/lateralization, auditory discrimination, auditory pattern recognition, temporal processing (e.g., temporal integration, temporal discrimination, temporal ordering, temporal masking), and performance with competing or degraded acoustic signals (AAA, 2010; ASHA, 2005a, b). Although these processing difficulties cannot be attributed to higher order language, cognitive, or related supramodal (i.e., pansensory) dysfunction, CAPD may lead to or be associated with difficulties in higher order language, learning, and communication function (AAA, 2010; ASHA, 2005a, 2005b; Bellis, 2002c, 2003; Bellis & Ferre, 1999; Billiet & Bellis, 2011; Chermak & Musiek, 1997). A number of abilities, including phonological awareness, attention to and memory for auditory information, auditory synthesis, and auditory comprehension and interpretation, likely are dependent on or associated with intact central auditory function; however, these abilities are considered higher order cognitive/communicative and/or language-related functions and, therefore, are not included in the definition of CAPD (AAA, 2010; ASHA, 2005a). Notwithstanding the potential for modulation of auditory perceptual input by concurrent stimulation from other sensory modalities and/or top-down influences (Bellis, 2002a, 2003; Cacace & McFarland, 2005; Chermak & Musiek, 1997), CAPD is considered a *primarily* modality-specific perceptual dysfunction that cannot be attributed to peripheral hearing loss or to higher order, global cognitive, supramodal attention or memory, language-based, or related disorders (Musiek, Bellis, & Chermak, 2005). The nonmodular organization of the brain (discussed below) precludes defining CAPD as an *exclusively* modality-specific perceptual dysfunction. Indeed, it would be inappropriate to apply the label of CAPD to listening difficulties exhibited by individuals with higher order, global, multimodal, or supramodal disorders *unless* a comorbid deficit in the CANS can be demonstrated (ASHA, 2005a; Musiek et al., 2005). Through the use of diagnostic tests that have been shown to be sensitive to CANS dysfunction, along with additional multidisciplinary information, CAPD often is distinguishable from higher order, more global, pansensory or supramodal disorders of attention, cognition, and related function (ASHA, 2005a; Bellis, 2002a, 2003; Bellis, Billiet, & Ross, 2011; Bellis & Ferre, 1999; Chermak, 2004; Chermak & Musiek, 1997; Musiek et al., 2005). The reader is referred to Volume 1 of this handbook for discussion of differential diagnosis of CAPD.

Prevalence and Etiology

Prevalence estimates of CAPD in school-age children range from 2% to 5% (Bamiou, Musiek, & Luxon, 2001; Chermak & Musiek, 1997), with males presenting CAPD twice as often as females (Palfery & Duff, 2007). Estimates of CAPD in older adults range from 23% to 76% (Cooper & Gates, 1991; Golding, Carter, Mitchell, & Hood, 2004; Stach, Spretnjak, & Jerger, 1990).

In the majority of children with CAPD, the underlying etiology of the disorder cannot be determined definitively; however, it is suspected that abnormal neurophysiologic representation of auditory stimuli is to blame. Children with CAPD and learning problems in the absence of an identifiable underlying neuropathology most likely present some benign, diffuse neuroanatomic issues (e.g., ectopias, polymicrogyri) underlying their auditory problems or maturational delay due to slower course of myelination (or auditory deprivation) (Chermak & Musiek, 2011). Although neurologic disorder, insult, or abnormality underlies CAPD in children much less frequently (Musiek, Baran, & Pinheiro, 1994), interest has increased recently in acquired pathologies of the CANS in children (and adults), including: seizure disorders (e.g., Landau-Kleffner), neoplasms, neurodegenerative processes, traumatic brain injury, cerebrovascular accidents, metabolic disorders, and genetic disorders, across a variety of sites of lesion at all levels of the CANS (Chermak & Musiek, 2011). Depending on the individual, the abnormal neurophysiologic representation of auditory stimuli may involve inefficient interhemispheric transfer of auditory information and/or lack of appropriate hemispheric lateralization, atypical hemispheric asymmetries, imprecise synchrony of neural firing, or a host of other factors (Jerger et al., 2002; Kraus, McGee, Carrell, Zecker, Nicol, & Koch, 1996; Moncrieff, Jerger, Wambacq, Greenwald, & Black, 2004). See Chapters 4 and 8 in Volume 1 of the Handbook for discussion of neuroanatomic abnormalities, neurological disorders, and neuromaturational delays underlying CAPD in children.

The central auditory processing deficits of adults may be acquired or may reflect unresolved central auditory dysfunction that was present, but perhaps undiagnosed, since childhood. These deficits may result from accumulated damage or deterioration to the CANS due to neurological (including neurodegenerative) diseases, disorders or insults, and they may or may not involve fairly circumscribed and identifiable lesions of the CANS (Baran & Musiek, 1991; Musiek & Gollegly, 1988; Musiek, Gollegly, Lamb, & Lamb, 1990). Central auditory deficits also may arise from the aging process itself, leading to poorer neural synchrony and time-locking, slower refractory periods, decreased central inhibition, atypical interhemispheric asymmetry, and interhemispheric transfer deficits) (Bellis, Nicol, & Kraus, 2000; Bellis & Wilber, 2001; Jerger, Moncrieff, Greenwald, Wambacq, & Seipel, 2000; Pichora-Fuller & Souza, 2003; Tremblay, Piskosz, & Souza, 2003; Willott, 1999; Woods & Clayworth, 1986). Approximately one in three older adults 65 years of age and older present with peripheral hearing loss (Ries, 1994) that, in itself, may lead to neuroplastic alterations in central auditory function and interact multiplicatively with age-related central auditory deficits (Kim, Morest, & Bohne, 1997; Morest, Kim, Potashner, & Bohne, 1998; Willott, 1996). In fact, beginning in the seventh decade (age 60 year and older), central auditory function (as measured by behavioral tests) declines more rapidly than pure-tone sensitivity or outer hair cell function (as measured by distortion product otoacoustic emissions [DPOAE]) (Gates, Feeney, & Mills, 2008), and age-related decline in temporal processing may begin in the fourth decade of life (Kumar, 2011). Even in the presence of normal hearing sensitivity, changes in interhemispheric processing of auditory stimuli may occur as early as the third decade of life for men and the sixth decade for women (Bellis & Wilber, 2001; Bellis et al., 2000).

Moreover, poor speech-in-noise perception has been shown to correlate with a reduction in neural synchrony in older adults (Anderson, Parbery-Clark, Yi, & Kraus, 2011). The foregoing suggests that older adults should be screened for CAPD and that auditory training should be included along with amplification to strengthen central auditory processing in older adults with speech-in-noise perception difficulties. The reader is referred to Chapters 8 and 18 of Volume 1 of the Handbook for discussion of prevalence, and CANS changes coincident to aging, respectively, and to Chapter 15 of this volume for considerations for intervention with older adults with peripheral and/or central auditory deficits.

Neuroplasticity

Recent research suggests that the central nervous system (CNS) is plastic, that is, capable of reorganization or remapping (both cortical and brainstem), by experience, for some time prior to stabilization of neural function, and that neural modification is reflected in behavioral change (Aoki & Siekevitz, 1988; de Boer & Thornton, 2008; Johnson, Nicol, Zecker, & Kraus, 2008; Knudsen, 1998; Nicol & Kraus, 2005; Russo et al. 2005; Snyder, Bonham, & Sinex, 2008; Song, Skoe, Wong, & Kraus, 2008). Although brain plasticity may be greatest and most obvious during development, accumulating data further suggest that the brain remains malleable throughout the life span and that significant neural reorganization can occur in response to injury or learning even in mature nervous systems (Edeline & Weinberger, 1991; Irvine, Rajan, & Robertson, 1992; Keuroghlian &

Knudsen, 2007; Kolb, 1995; Moore, 1993; Singer, 1995; see Feldman & Brecht, 2005 and Ohl & Scheich, 2005 for reviews). Plasticity may account for the maintenance of cognitive control across many decades despite the slow but sustained loss of neurons seen beginning in adolescence and continuing throughout the aging process (Kolb, 1995). In fact, system-wide neural plasticity, including experience-dependent plasticity (as reported for musicians and adolescent bilingual speakers), benefits the interdependent bottom-up (i.e., perceptual) and top-down (i.e., cognitive) processes that support listening and language processing (Krizman, Marian, Shook, Skoe, & Kraus, 2012). The reader is referred to Chapters 3 and 5 of Volume 1 of the Handbook for additional discussion of neuroplasticity.

Long-term potentiation, the long-lasting increase in synaptic transmission induced by intense and repeated synaptic activity (Brown, Chapman, Kairiss, & Keenan, 1988) may be the physiological mechanism underlying a variety of plastic processes in the nervous system (Pascual-Leone, Grafman, & Hallett, 1994; Schuman & Madison, 1994). Studies of long-term potentiation suggest significant opportunity to induce cognitive change through stimulation (Gustafsson & Wigstrom, 1988).

Neuroplasticity is induced through experience and stimulation and leads to reorganization (i.e., remapping) of the cortex and brainstem, improved synaptic efficiency, increased neural density, and associated cognitive and behavioral change (de Boer &Thornton, 2008; Elbert, Pantev, Wienbruch, Rockstroh, & Taub, 1995; Johnson et al., 2008; Knudsen, 1998; Merzenich, Schreiner, Jenkins, & Wang, 1993; Moore, 1993; Recanzone,

Schreiner, & Merzenich, 1993; Robertson & Irvine, 1989; Russo et al. 2005; Snyder et al., 2008; Song et al., 2008; Weinberger & Diamond, 1987; Willott, Aiken, & McFadden, 1993). Even relatively low-level processes (e.g., pitch discrimination) are subject to experience-related change (Carcagno & Plack, 2011). Activity-dependent plasticity is thought to underlie learning and memory as the brain changes in response to use and the needs and experiences of the individual (Elbert, Pantev, Wienbruch, Rockstroh, & Taub, 1995; Weinberger & Diamond, 1987). The cortical changes induced by stimulation (i.e., experience and practice) appear to be widespread and long-lasting (Merzenich & Jenkins, 1995) and include at least four different types of cortical reorganization: (1) map expansion, or the enlargement of a region dedicated to a given function; (2) compensatory allocation, or novel allocation of particular process to another brain region; (3) crossmodal reassignment involving regions of the brain accepting input from a new sensory modality; and (4) homologous area adaptation in which the same area of the opposite hemisphere assumes responsibility for processing input that, typically, would have been lateralized to the other hemisphere (Grafman & Litvan, 1999). In addition, activation of previously inactive neuronal tissue may occur secondary to stimulation, as may the development of more efficient synaptic connections within the brain (Kaas, 1995). Recent findings suggest that cortical reorganization may be far more extensive than originally thought, and may extend into areas quite distant from the region of insult or injury (Dancause et al., 2005).

A substantial body of literature demonstrates that systematic auditory stimulation or lack thereof affects the physiological function of the auditory system. For example, Hassmannova, Myslivecek, and Novakova (1981) observed decreased evoked potential latencies and greater ribonucleic acid (RNA) concentrations in the auditory cortex of rat pups following a two-week period of auditory stimulation. Knudsen (1988) reported changes in the spatial tuning underlying the localization function of the auditory neurons of barn owls following unilateral plugging and unplugging of the owls' ears. Following a frequency discrimination task, Recanzone et al. (1993) demonstrated increased cortical representation and improved frequency discrimination of the trained frequencies in owl monkeys. Edeline and Weinberger (1991) reported changes in the tuning of the auditory cortex neurons of guinea pigs following frequency discrimination training. Weinberger and Bakin (1998) demonstrated receptive field changes in the auditory cortex in animals performing various types of discrimination tasks. In his excellent review, Syka (2002) provided a variety of examples of auditory plasticity related to training in both damaged and healthy auditory systems.

Documenting a remarkable example of auditory system plasticity in the human brain, Allen, Cranford, and Pay (1996) reported normal central auditory processing in an adult with congenital absence of the left temporal lobe. In fact, a rapidly accumulating body of literature provides definitive evidence of the impact of auditory stimulation in effecting behavioral change in humans, as well as in animals (Alonso & Schochat, 2009; Beitel, Vollmer, Raggio, & Schreiner, 2011; Hayes, Warrier, Nicol, Zecker, & Kraus, 2003; Kraus, McGee, Carrell, King, Tremblay, & Nicol, 1995; Musiek, Baran, & Shinn, 2004; Russo, Nicol, Zecker, Hayes,

& Kraus, 2005; Tremblay, 2007; Tremblay & Kraus, 2002; Tremblay, Kraus, Carrell, & McGee, 1997; Tremblay et al., 1998; Tremblay, Kraus, McGee, Ponton, & Otis, 2001; Warrier, Johnson, Hayes, Nicol, & Kraus, 2004). Moreover, learning-induced cortical plasticity appears to be associated with both functional and anatomical/structural changes (Draganski et al., 2004; May et al., 2007). See Chapters 3, 7, and 11 for discussion of the efficacy of auditory training.

Draganski and colleagues (2004) reported structural changes (e.g., expansion in gray matter) detectable in adult humans after only three months of training (juggling). Training-related gray matter signal changes in MRI may be related to synaptic remodeling (Ilg et al., 2008). Keller and Just (2009) reported improved connectivity in corticocortical white matter tracts as measured by diffusion tensor imaging) suggesting myelination had increased following 100 hours of intensive remedial reading instruction in 10-year-old poor readers. These connectivity changes correlated with improved phonological decoding skills. Physiologic changes as measured by the mismatch negativity response (MMN) was seen following one 45-minute speech (CV syllable) training session with adults and function (i.e., improved CV syllable identification) was seen as early as four days following training (Tremblay et al. 1998). Speech discrimination training resulted in significant improvements in adults' behavioral discrimination and changes in the duration and magnitude of cortical evoked potentials (e.g., the mismatch negativity response, or MMN) (Kraus et al., 1995). Tremblay and Kraus (2002) reported that auditory training induced changes in cortical P1–P2 amplitude and improved phoneme (i.e. voice-onset time)

perception in normal hearing adults. Further, the changes in the neurophysiologic representation of these stimuli preceded the behavioral improvement in discrimination of the phoneme contrasts, providing insight into the time-course of CANS plasticity secondary to stimulation and training. Demonstrating auditory system plasticity in children, Tallal et al. (1996) reported that progressive, adaptive, and intensive auditory training improves temporal processing and certain language skills. Musiek and Schochat (1998) and Musiek (1999) reported improvement in auditory processing and academic and communication performance of children diagnosed with CAPD following informal auditory training. Following auditory training, children diagnosed with learning disabilities and/or attention deficit hyperactivity disorder showed improved auditory closure and sound blending skills, as well as changes in cortical potentials in quiet and in noise (Hayes et al., 2003).

Russo et al. (2005) observed improvement in auditory brainstem potentials triggered by abbreviated speech stimuli after consistent use of a commercial auditory training program. These brainstem responses, which were measured over a 40 msec time period, yielded enhanced amplitude to a 40 msec /da/ stimulus for both positive and negative peaks over this time period. Although all children exhibited identical click ABRs, 3- to 4-year-old children displayed delayed and less synchronous onset and sustained neural response activity when ABR was elicited by speech compared with 5- to 12-year-olds (Johnson, Nicol, Zecker, & Kraus, 2008). Adult listeners trained for 10 hours on a pitch discrimination task showed significant improvement in pitch discrimination, as well as a more robust frequency-following response to the sound enveloped compared with a control group (Carcagno & Plack, 2011). Demonstrating the potential of FM systems to drive neuroplasticity, Hornickel, Zecker, Bradlow, and Kraus (2012) reported reduced variability (i.e., improved neural [subcortical] response consistency as evidenced by a larger correlation between first and second halves of the speech-evoked auditory brainstem response [cABR] recordings to the formant transitions of speech syllables) in children with dyslexia, with no changes seen in a matched control group. These findings provide evidence of plasticity at the brainstem level.

Implications of Neuroplasticity for Rehabilitation

The foregoing studies have demonstrated that the CNS is not immutable: The brain has the capacity to remap or reorganize itself to best meet auditory processing demands (Moore, 1993; Recanzone et al., 1993; Robertson & Irvine, 1989; Willott, Aitken, & McFadden, 1993). Stimulation and training induce plasticity. We sculpt the brain the way we sculpt muscle. Activation of previously inactive neuronal tissue and/or improved neural synchrony, as well as the development of more efficient synaptic connections within the brain may occur secondary to stimulation (Edelman & Gally, 2001; Schnupp, Nelken, & King, 2011). These neurophysiologic modifications are reflected in behavioral change (i.e., learning). The inherent plasticity of the CNS has provided a foundation for renewed interest in various treatment and management approaches, including auditory training (see Chapters 3, 7, 8, and 9). Plasticity enables the CNS to accommodate and

offers speech-language pathologists and audiologists the opportunity to improve central auditory processing (Chermak & Musiek, 1992, 1997). The array of neuroplastic changes underlying different cortical reorganization strategies (as discussed above) bodes well for successful outcomes when intervention is undertaken comprehensively and broadly, engaging and exploiting the multimodal, crossmodal, and supramodal neural interfaces that support auditory performance. Stimulation enables plasticity and may extend the brain's so-called sensitive or critical periods for learning particular behaviors, thereby maximizing the potential for successful rehabilitative efforts (Hassmannova et al., 1981). In fact, experience promotes neuroplasticity (Hayes, Warrier, Nicol, & Kraus, 2003; Hyde et al., 2009; Kraus & Banai, 2007; Moreno et al., 2009; Skoe & Kraus, 2012; Threlkeld, Hill, Rosen, & Fitch, 2009) and continued practice results in overlearning that leads to automaticity wherein auditory skills can be accomplished with less metacognitive control (i.e., reduced self-allocation of attention or memory resources), thereby releasing internal resources for deployment to other tasks (Chermak & Musiek, 1997; Merzenich & Jenkins, 1995; Piquado, Cousins, Wingfield, & Miller, 2010). Moreover, the cortex remains plastic through adulthood (see Feldman & Brecht, 2005 and Ohl & Scheich, 2005 for reviews). Even mature sensory systems retain the potential for extensive plasticity triggered by changes in prevailing stimulation and/or by learning driven by behavioral demands (Pienkowski & Eggermont, 2011, 2012)

Because neural changes are dependent on activity and stimulation, neural plasticity affords opportunity for functional change only insofar as intervention is initiated in a timely manner (Aoki & Siekevitz, 1988; Bolshakov & Siegelbaum, 1995; Hassmannova et al., 1981). Intervention efforts should be aggressive and implemented as early as possible following either confirmed diagnosis or the time the individual, particularly the child, is identified as at risk for CAPD (Chermak & Musiek, 1992, 1997). However, because the absolute time course of the critical or sensitive periods prior to which time neural function begins to stabilize has not yet been established and may extend into adulthood (Keuroghlian & Knudson, 2007; Merzenich et al., 1984), intervention efforts should never be viewed as too late. Presumably, children and adults with CAPD present cortical plasticity and capability to learn. Therefore, with training and practice, these individuals should be able to resolve auditory events and information to a degree that is more compatible with the demands inherent to spoken language processing.

Change in neural substrate is facilitated by presenting stimulation in an organized manner that progressively challenges the client with the proper gradation of difficulty level and by integrating that stimulation into everyday activities (Rumbaugh & Washburn, 1996). Furthermore, active participation in the training on the part of the patient, along with inclusion of immediate feedback, salient reinforcement, and activities that work at or near the patient's skill threshold maximize neuroplasticity (Ahissar et al., 1992; Beninger & Miller, 1998; Blake, Strata, Churchland, & Merzenich, 2002; Danzl, Etter, Andreatta, & Kitzman, 2012; Holroyd, Larson, & Cohen, 2004). Because the remapping of the brain underlying improvements in auditory function probably requires some as yet unknown period of time that most likely varies widely among

individuals and as a function of task demands, clinicians must demonstrate patience and counsel the client similarly, giving the intervention program ample opportunity to activate the neural processes of plasticity that will lead to change (Chermak & Musiek, 1997). Intensive training seems to accelerate the remapping and relearning process (Merzenich et al., 1996; Tallal et al., 1996). Our inability to quantify the requisite time period for remapping complicates clinical decisions to maintain or modify a particular therapeutic course based on progress to date. Neurophysiologic markers of cortical reorganization may in fact precede behavioral markers of learning; therefore, electrophysiologic techniques may serve an important role in monitoring treatment and making clinical decisions (Tremblay et al., 1998). Although we (and others) have recommended 5 to 7 half-hour to one-hour sessions weekly for at least 4 to 6 weeks, neurophysiological and functional changes may occur more quickly, perhaps within a single training session (Atienza, Cantero, & Dominguez-Marin, 2002; Gottselig, Brandeis, Hofer-Tinguely, Borberly, & Achermann, 2004). The present uncertainty surrounding the time required to induce and to stabilize cortical reorganization and learning underscores the importance of appropriately selected outcome measures, as discussed below.

CANS plasticity compels us to provide direct treatment (i.e., auditory training) to improve central auditory processes and skills (see Chapters 3, 7, 9, and 11). However, the array of neuroplastic changes that may occur (e.g., compensatory allocation, cross-modal assignment) augments and broadens the potential for successful efforts undertaken to strengthen related systems through central resources training. Because the auditory system is extensive and overlaps other systems, we find tremendous opportunities for intervention focused on both bottom-up (i.e., auditory training and signal enhancement) and top-down (e.g., central resources and compensatory training) by a multidisciplinary team. As Hugdahl and Helland elaborate in Chapter 6 of Volume 1 of the Handbook, central auditory processing can be viewed as

> . . . the interaction of bottom-up, sensory, and top-down, cognitive factors that shape and modulate how a simple speech sound, like a CV-syllable, is processed in natural surroundings, as when people are talking to each other, which requires decoding of the phonology, but also correct attention and focus, and selective cognitive filtering of the signal to be processed. (p. 177)

They note:

> Without the ability to use higher cognitive processes and functions to inhibit or enhance lower level acoustic input, much of the flexibility and adjustability seen in human language communication would be lost. . . . Central auditory processing deficits are deficits where one or several of the components of the interaction is not functioning, causing failure of either low level perceptual processing or higher level cognitive modulation of the signal, or both. (p. 178)

Therefore, comprehensive intervention for CAPD should be designed to build listening skills and strategies, instill compensatory strategies to minimize functional listening deficits, and promote efficient allocation of perceptual and higher order (central) resources (e.g., language, memory, attention) to the task of spoken language processing (Chermak & Musiek, 2007). As discussed in Chapter 10, central resources training engages supramodal systems that interface with the CANS and can, through those interactions, increase treatment effectiveness by reducing the functional impact of CAPD and enhancing listening, communication, social and learning outcomes. (The reader is referred to Chapters 1, 3, and 5 of Volume 1 of this Handbook for additional discussion of neuroplasticity.)

Auditory Deprivation

As stimulation can induce change, so too can auditory deprivation induce cortical reorganization. In a plastic CNS, lack of effective practice can stabilize deficits and reinforce defective brain function (Evans, Webster, & Cullen, 1983). The observations of altered cortical tonotopicity secondary to partial cochlear hearing loss in guinea pigs (Robertson & Irvine, 1989) and differences in Heschl's gyrus subsequent to auditory deprivation in hearing impaired infants, including increased gray matter and decreased white matter and the absence of the typical left larger than right asymmetry (Smith et al., 2011), underscores this possibility.

In contrast, studies of children with histories of chronic otitis media confirm the resilience of the auditory system in rebounding from at least mild degrees of auditory deprivation. Following myringotomy and intubation, masking level differences of children with histories of chronic otitis media returned to normal suggesting recovery of binaural function (Hall, Grose, & Pillsbury, 1995). Similarly, Schwaber, Garraghty, and Kaas (1993) found extensive reorganization of adult macaque monkeys' auditory cortex following induced cochlear hearing loss. The deprived region of the auditory cortex became responsive to frequencies of an adjacent auditory region to ensure the viability of the neural tissue. Findings of cortical changes in adult monkeys suggests that auditory training may be successful regardless of the subject's age or duration of auditory deprivation, including deprivation caused by an auditory processing deficit (Seki & Eggermont, 2002; and Thai-Van, Veuillet, Norena, Guiraud, & Collet, 2010 for a review).

Brain Organization, Nonmodularity of the Central Nervous System, and Comorbidity

The neural activity of the brain is temporally coupled across the cortex, modalities, and hemispheres; therefore, dysfunction, especially deficient timing, can impose limitations that spread or ripple across brain regions and modalities (Hayes et al., 2003; Merzenich et al., 1993). These cascading effects may reduce the degree of neural synchronization and connectivity among brain regions, leading to the frequently observed range of comorbid conditions (e.g., CAPD and attention deficit disorder, language impairment, learning disability).

Recent studies demonstrate a great deal of interaction among even those areas that were considered previously to be sensory specific. The auditory system is extensive and overlaps with the neural substrate and networks of other sensory, language, cognitive, executive, and motor control systems (Bayazit, Oniz, Hahn, Gunturkun, & Ozgoren, 2009; Petacchi, Kaernbach, Ratnam, & Bower,

2011; Poldrack et al., 2001; Poremba et al., 2003; Wong et al., 2009; Salvi et al., 2002). Considerable evidence points to the multimodal convergence or interaction of sensory neurons responsive to stimulation of different sensory modalities, as well as the modulation of activity evoked by one modality on that evoked by another (Kayser & Logothetis, 2007). Many nuclei across the brainstem (e.g., dorsal cochlear nucleus, inferior colliculus, medial geniculate body) are sites of integration of acoustic and multimodal sensory inputs (Shore, 2005). Polysensory processing areas have been shown to exist within the cortex (e.g., superior temporal sulcus, prefrontal areas) (Meredith, Allman, Keniston, & Clemo, 2009). Most domain-specific functions (including language) typically activate multiple areas across widespread regions of the brain and most neural regions support multiple functions (Musiek, Bellis, & Chermak, 2005). The assumption of spatially segregated cortical areas subserving attention, memory, and individual sensory systems has been replaced by the recognition that widespread cortical networks span across cortical areas (Gaffan, 2005; Merzenich et al., 1993; Thiebaut de Schotten et al., 2005). A given brain region may be recruited for many different functions (Lopez-Aranda et al., 2009.) Auditory tasks (e.g., listening in noise) activate auditory and nonauditory areas of the brain, including areas involved in attention, executive control, working memory, language processing, and motor planning (Salvi et al., 2002). Moreover, there is growing evidence of the involvement of cognitive processes in basic perceptual events. For example, working memory has been shown to be integral to numerous auditory processes, including localization, temporal resolution, pattern recognition, speech identification and recognition in noise, and dichotic listening (Akeroyd, 2008; Jancke & Shah, 2002; Marler, Champlin, & Gillam, 2002; Martin, Jerger, & Mehta, 2007; Martinkauppi, Rama, Aronen, Korvenoja, & Carolson, 2002; Salvi et al., 2002; Wong et al., 2009; Zattore, 2001; Zatorre, Belin, & Benhune, 2002). Focusing attention to a given acoustic feature not only increases neural activity level, it also enhances neuronal selectivity to that feature in the particular part of the auditory cortex specialized in processing it (Kauramaki, Jaaskelainen, & Sams, 2007). Conversely, deficient auditory processing may affect neural organization and plasticity of multiple brain systems responsible for efficient auditory and auditory-language processing (e.g., executive control, attention, working memory) (Ciccia, Meulenbroek, & Turkstra, 2009). Consistent with a network model, emphasizing the distributed nature of information processing within the nervous system, perceptual responses to sensory stimuli are mediated across a large number of brain regions involving multiple serial, parallel, and dispersed neural networks (AAA, 2010; ASHA, 2005a; Masterton, 1992; Price, Thierry, & Griffiths, 2005; Ungerleider, 1995).

That CAPD co-occurs with other disorders is expected given the complexity, as well as the geographic proximity of *auditory areas* to polymodal association areas (Musiek et al., 2005). Dysfunction in or insult to (primarily) auditory regions is likely to spread beyond the artificial boundary of the so-called auditory-*specific* area (Musiek et al., 2005). Although some brain regions have been characterized as *auditory specific*, neurons in these areas respond primarily, though not exclusively, to auditory stimuli (Cacace & McFarland, 2005; Musiek et al., 2005).

An accumulating body of literature demonstrates the absence of complete modality specificity. Indeed, the neurophysiologic substrate of auditory processing includes nonprimary auditory areas of the CNS (e.g., thalamus) that are multimodal in nature (Kraus, McGee, Littman, Nicol, & King, 1994; Poremba et al., 2003). Diffusion tensor imaging has documented direct white matter connections between the auditory and visual cortices, in addition to subcortical, temporal and parietal connections (Beer, Plank, & Greenlee, 2011).

Visual Input (e.g., lip movements) can alter neurophysiologic representation of acoustic events (in response to both speech and nonspeech) in the primary auditory cortex (Besle, Bertrand, & Giard, 2009; Kislyuk, Mottonen, & Sams, 2008; Pekkola et al., 2005). Sams et al. (1991) demonstrated that neuronal activity in even the primary auditory cortex is modified by visual input. Similarly, Calvert et al. (1997) demonstrated that areas formerly thought to be sensitive only to auditory stimuli are activated during solely visual tasks. Using functional magnetic resonance imaging, Wright, Pelphrey, Allison, McKeowin, and McCarthy (2003) characterized the superior temporal sulcus as a polysensory area, observing that the response to bimodal stimuli in this area was greater than that to either modality alone. Poremba et al. (2003) observed that bimodal stimulation enhances neuronal response from areas of overlap. Behavioral responses to multimodal inputs presented in close spatial and temporal proximity are faster and more accurate than responses to unimodal stimuli (Stein & Meredith, 1993). Booth et al. (2002) observed b*oth* modality-specific and polysensory activations during judgments of semantic relatedness of words presented in the visual and auditory modalities. In fact, auditory neurons in the cerebrum exhibit interconnectedness with a variety of neurons in other nonauditory areas of the brain. In reviewing this topic, Streit-feld (1980) emphasized the interconnec-tions between specific brain regions and other areas with totally different func-tions. For example, she noted that the auditory cortex in primates has direct and indirect connections to the limbic system, cingulate gyrus, hippocampus, and frontal lobe. Bamiou, Musiek, and Luxon (2003) reported the presence of considerable auditory activity in the insula—a structure not usually consid-ered an auditory region. Additional areas of the brain not generally considered as auditory regions that have been identi-fied as auditory responsive include the amygdala, striatum, and frontal lobe, among others (e.g., Poremba et al., 2003; Salvi et al., 2002). Similarly, the corpus callosum provides interhemispheric con-nections subserving sensory, cognitive, and language functions, with auditory functions supported particularly in the posterior region of the corpus callosum Although most fibers of the corpus cal-losum are homolateral, connecting the two hemispheres at the same loci, some fibers are heterolateral connecting the two hemispheres at different loci (i.e., auditory regions with auditory and pos-sibly nonauditory regions). Therefore, the corpus callosum is responsible for interconnections among brain regions with different functions, further under-scoring the complex interconnectedness of the brain. Moreover, dysfunction in the corpus callosum has been demonstrated to lead to central auditory deficits and may, indeed, be one of the most com-mon regions of the brain that contributes

to central auditory dysfunction in both children and older adults (e.g., Bellis et al., 2000, 2001, 2011; Musiek & Gol-legly, 1988).

Taken together, a considerable cor-pus of research questions the ecologi-cal validity of modality-exclusive brain regions and demonstrates clearly that polysensory regions are located within so-called modality-specific regions, rais-ing serious questions regarding the like-lihood a disorder will affect one small, possibly modular area, leaving a poly-sensory area a micron away unaffected. It seems clear that *complete* modality specificity is neurophysiologically unten-able and that the organization of the brain underlies comorbidity (AAA, 2010; ASHA, 2005a; Bellis, 2002a; 2003; Musiek et al., 2005).

Implications of Brain Organization for CAPD Intervention

Individuals are referred for central audi-tory processing evaluation because of lis-tening problems that typically are impact-ing communication, learning, language processing, attention, and related areas. The nonmodularity and nonexclusively segregated organization of the brain underlies the heterogenous nature of CAPD and the comorbidity frequently observed between CAPD and commu-nication, language, learning, attention, and social deficits (Musiek et al., 2005). Individuals often present central auditory dysfunction comorbidly with other valid diagnoses such as dyslexia, specific lan-guage impairment, attention deficit, and learning disability (e.g., Cunningham,

Nicol, Zecker, Bradlow, & Kraus, 2001; Gomez & Condon, 1999; Iliadou, Bamiou, Kaprinis, Kandylis, & Kaprinis, 2009; Kraus et al., 1996; Moncrieff & Musiek, 2002; Pillsbury, Grose, Coleman, Conners, & Hall, 1995; Purdy, Kelly, & Davies, 2002; Riccio, Hynd, Cohen, Hall, & Molt, 1994; Sharma, Purdy, & Kelly, 2009; Sharma, Purdy, Newall, Wheldall, Beaman, & Dillon, 2006; Tillery, Katz, & Keller, 2000; Wible, Nicol, & Kraus, 2002, 2005; Warrier et al., 2004; Wright et al., 1997). Although links between inefficient auditory processing and language or learning problems have been documented both behaviorally and electrophysiologically (e.g., Banasich, Thomas, Choudhury, & Leppanen, 2002; Bellis & Ferre, 1999; Billiet & Bellis, 2011; Boscariol et al., 2011; Goswami et al., 2002; Kraus et al, 1996; Moncrieff & Musiek, 2002; Richardson, Thomson, Scott, & Goswami, 2004; Sharma et al., 2006; Wible, Nicol, & Kraus, 2005; Wright, Bowen, & Zecker, 2000), CAPD should not be viewed as a direct cause of all or even most cases of academic failure, learning disability, reading disability, or related disabilities. Nonetheless, as is true of many disorders, CAPD certainly can exacerbate academic challenge (e.g., listening in noisy classroom environments) even when direct causation is unlikely. In cases of comorbidity, the CAPD must be diagnosed fully and accurately and an intervention program must be developed and implemented by a team of professionals to address all significant functional deficits.

Based on the neurophysiologic foundations elaborated above, the framework underlying the conceptualization, diagnosis, assessment, and intervention for CAPD incorporates multidisciplinary and multimodal perspectives (AAA, 2010; ASHA, 2005a, 2005b; Bellis, 2002a; Bellis, 2003; Bellis & Ferre, 1999; Chermak & Musiek, 1997, 2007; Musiek et al., 2005). The complexity and interactive organization of the brain, comprising interfacing sensory, cognitive, and linguistic networks, underlies comorbidity of disorders and often exacerbates the functional impact of CAPD, resulting in associated difficulties in related areas, including language, learning, and social function. At the same time, however, these same interactions offer opportunities for more far-reaching and effective intervention for CAPD (Chermak & Musiek, 1997, 2007). A comprehensive approach to intervention capitalizes on the complex organization of the brain and its neuroplasticity. Cognitive, metacognitive, and language resources (i.e., central resources) can be engaged to buttress central auditory processing and complement direct auditory skills training, thereby minimizing the functional consequences of CAPD (Chermak & Musiek, 1997, 2007).

Auditory and Cognitive Neuroscience Foundations and Training Principles

A comprehensive approach to CAPD intervention is based on the accumulated auditory and cognitive neuroscience literature that demonstrates: (1) the plasticity of the auditory system, (2) the role of experience in reorganizing the cortex (and brainstem) and shaping auditory behavior, (3) that stimulation induces cognitive and behavioral change, and (4) that stimulation enables plasticity and may extend the time course of sensitive or critical periods, thereby maximizing the potential for successful rehabilitative efforts (Aoki & Siekevitz, 1988; Gustafsson & Wigstrom, 1988; Hassmannova, Myslivecek, & Novakova, 1981; Kolb, 1995; Schulte, Knief, Seither, Preisler, & Pantev, 2002; Skoe & Kraus, 2012). These findings translate into three principles that guide intervention (Merzenich & Jenkins, 1995). First, training should be *intensive* to exploit plasticity and cortical reorganization. The brain is malleable; however, change requires considerable practice as well as significant challenge by working near the patient's skill threshold (Blake et al., 2002; Hayes et al., 2003; Musiek et al., 2004; Musiek, Chermak, & Weihing, 2007; Russo et al., 2005; Tallal et al., 1996). Second, training should be *extensive* to maximize generalization, effectiveness, and reduce functional deficits. Training should incorporate various stimuli (nonverbal and verbal) and stimulus parameters, in multiple contexts, involving tasks that deploy cognitive, metacognitive and language resources (Chermak & Musiek, 1997, 2002, 2007). Such training exploits the extensive, shared and overlapping auditory, cognitive, metacognitive, and language systems, emphasizes interactions between bottom-up and top-down processing, as well as supramodal, cross-modal and polymodal interfaces, may extend the area of cortical reorganization, and serves to complement and supplement auditory training, and reduces functional deficits. Third, active participation and salient reinforcement and feedback must be incorporated into the training process to augment attention, engage motivation and maximize learning (Ahissar et al., 1992; Holroyd et al., 2004). This third principle also is derived from learning theory (Swanson & Cooney, 1991).

Integrating Learning Theory

In designing intervention programs, clinicians should integrate the third neuroscience-based training principle (i.e., active participation and salient reinforcement) with other longstanding tenets of learning theory (Swanson & Cooney, 1991). Following the principles of neuroscience as well as learning theory leads the clinician to recognize the importance of both the quality and the quantity (or intensiveness) of intervention. Learning theory emphasizes the efficiency of distributing practice over time rather than compressing the same amount of practice into a short period of time (Spence & Norris, 1950; Starch, 1912). Moreover, both the neuroscience-based training principles and the tenets of learning theory direct clinicians to sequence tasks to provide opportunities for correct performance and positive reinforcement (Ausubel & Robinson, 1969; Clifford, 1978; Hegde, 1993). Learning theory emphasizes the importance of engagement strategies to build trust and rapport, the use of feedback to reinforce and motivate learning, and self-monitoring to ensure integration of skills into real life situations. To achieve the latter, skills and strategies should be overlearned to the level of mastery and automaticity to increase retention.

Treatment Effectiveness, Efficacy, and Evidence-Based Practice

The efficacy and effectiveness of efforts to improve central auditory processing and strategy learning ultimately depend on the plasticity of the CNS, adherence to neuroscience-based training principles, and early and aggressive intervention. Efficacy refers to the extent to which a specific treatment has been shown to be beneficial under ideal (experimentally controlled) conditions (Office of Technology Assessment, 1978; Robey & Schulz, 1998). In contrast, effectiveness refers to the extent to which a specific treatment has been shown to be beneficial under typical (real-life) conditions (Office of Technology Assessment, 1978; Robey & Schulz, 1998). Clearly, treatment effectiveness is the goal to be achieved with each, individual client.

Effective intervention is beneficial to the client, efficient, persists in time, and generalizes beyond the training parameters and settings (Chermak & Musiek, 1997). Effective behavioral treatments depend on motivated and assertive clients. Treatment variables, however, determine the ultimate success of intervention efforts, including the use of the best available clinical strategies/interventions, intensive practice using engaging tasks of graded difficulty, generous feedback, and opportunities to generalize (Chermak & Musiek, 1997, 2007). Determining which treatments are the "best available" requires reliance on evidence-based practice (EBP).

Related to efficacy and effectiveness is the considerable interest in EBP. As defined by Sackett, Straus, Richardson, Rosenberg, and Haynes (2000), EBP is the "the integration of best research evidence with clinical expertise and patient values" (p. 1). EBP encourages clinicians to adopt treatment recommendations on the basis of a client's needs and values in concert with the best available data regarding the most effective methods for use in one's clinical practice. A five-step process, EBP encourages clinicians to undertake a systematic review of the literature to identify high levels evidence that establish the scientific validity of clinic practices. The clinician begins the process by generating a focused question. Next, databases must be searched to find the best available evidence to answer the question. After collecting the evidence, the clinician must evaluate the evidence (e.g., is the evidence of high quality—derived from a double-blinded, prospective, randomized clinical trials or from a less rigorous observational study, case study, or retrospective study). The clinician must then integrate the evidence with the client's profile and needs, make recommendations for intervention, and finally evaluate the results and identify ways to improve the outcomes (Sackett et al. 2000). (See Chapter 2 and Cox, 2005 for in-depth discussion of evidence-based practice and treatment efficacy.)

Although studies with high levels of evidence (e.g., randomized controlled trials; meta-analysis of randomized controlled trials) are lacking for specific intervention programs for a variety of disorders, including CAPD (Abrams, McArdle, & Chisolm, 2005), a solid base of research documents improved psychophysical performance, neurophysiologic representation of acoustic stimuli, and listening and related function in children and adults following targeted auditory training (e.g., Bao, Chang, Woods, & Merzenich, 2004; deVillers-Sidani, Alzghoul, Zhou, Simpson, Lin, & Merzenich, 2010; Hayes et al., 2003; Jirsa, 1992; Kraus & Disterhoft, 1982; Kraus et al., 1995; Merzenich, Grajski, Jenkins, Recanzone, & Peterson, 1991; Merzenich et al., 1996; Millward, Hall, Ferguson, & Moore, 2011; Moncrieff & Wertz, 2008; Murphy & Schochat, 2011; Musiek, Baran, & Pinheiro, 1994; Musiek et al., 2004; Pan, Zhang, Cai,

Zhou, & Sun, 2011; Pinheiro, & Capellini, 2010; Russo et al., 2005; Schochat, Musiek, Alonso, & Ogata, 2010; Strait & Kraus, 2011; Tallal et al., 1996; Tremblay, 2007; Tremblay & Kraus, 2002; Tremblay et al., 1997, 1998, 2001; Warrier et al., 2004). (See Chapter 3 for review of efficacy studies.) It should be noted further that although randomized controlled trials and similar research designs, are entirely appropriate for medical studies (e.g., drug trials), they may not apply as well to studies involving communication disorders, including CAPD, due in large part to the highly heterogeneous nature of speech, language, hearing, and related disorders, and to the difficulty in designing such large scale studies in this area.

As Chermak and Musiek elaborate in Chapter 22, several caveats are in order regarding the evidence-based ratings. Group studies reflect average performance, which might not be directly applicable to a particular clinical case. Case studies and retrospective studies (which are classified as lower level evidence) often provide evidence appropriate for a particular individual's profile and intervention (Barlow & Hersen, 1984). Indeed, "practice-based" evidence (PBE), wherein a clinician reports on the particular intervention outcomes of an individual patient, although not intended to replace randomized clinical trials, can provide another source of information to improve clinical practice (Horn & Gassaway, 2007). Although some disagree as to the quantity of evidence supporting the efficacy of CAPD interventions (see Fey et al., 2011 and Bellis, Chermak, Weihing, & Musiek, 2012), it is important to be clear: Limited evidence does not indicate limited effectiveness and the limitations of the evidence does not

mean that the interventions offer no benefit. Although it is assumed that research designs assigned high levels of evidence (e.g., meta-analyses and randomized controlled trials) are less likely to be influenced by measurement error and unintended or uncontrolled variables, Dollaghan (2007) noted, "studies with highly ranked designs can yield invalid or unimportant evidence, just as studies with less highly ranked designs can provide crucial evidence" (p. 6). As Pimentel and Inglebret emphasize in Chapter 2, it is important to go beyond the assignment of an evidence level to appraise the quality of each study. Moreover, as they note, the field of CAPD benefits from the quality of its outcome measures, which are increasingly including electrophysiological measures that:

> . . . are less likely to be influenced by confounding variables and lead to a higher level of validity, "objectivity," and certainty that change or differences associated with a particular intervention are "real." Thus, outcome measures of an electrophysiological nature contribute to higher evidence quality. (p. 53)

Regardless of one's view regarding the quantity or the quality of the published evidence, most would likely agree that additional research is needed to demonstrate the effectiveness and efficacy of various CAPD treatment approaches, using both auditory and other behavioral and electrophysiological outcome measures with individuals specifically diagnosed with CAPD (as opposed to individuals "suspected of CAPD" or other diagnoses). Nonetheless, it is our view that sufficient evidence is available today to guide intervention for CAPD using information gained from audiologic diagnosis and multidisciplinary assessment across functional domains (AAA, 2010; Alonso, & Schochat, 2009; Delhommeau, Micheyl, & Jouvent, 2005; Foxton, Brown, Chambers, & Griffiths, 2004; Loo, Bamiou, Campbell, & Luxon, 2010; Moncrieff & Wertz (2008); Murphy & Schochat, 2011; Schochat, Musiek, Alonso, & Ogata, 2010; Pinheiro & Capellini, 2010). Nevertheless, additional carefully designed clinical studies, controlling threats to internal validity and incorporating appropriate outcome measures, are needed to firmly establish the efficacy of a number of treatments currently recommended for CAPD.

Outcome Measures

Various outcome measures can be used to demonstrate the effectiveness of therapy. Outcome measures are dependent variables that measure aspects of benefit provided by intervention. Measures can incorporate quantitative or qualitative data and include physical, physiological, and behavioral measures obtained through observations, interviews, self-report, or direct measurement. Post-therapy changes on central auditory tests, psychoacoustic measures, and electrophysiologic procedures can be used to document the effectiveness of CAPD intervention directed toward improving central auditory processes.

To demonstrate treatment outcomes in a more ecologically relevant context, one should measure changes in listening (comprehension) or spoken language processing. For example, speech recognition for time-compressed speech or speech recognition in interrupted noise provide ecologically appropriate outcome measures to supplement pitch or duration patterns, gap detection, or masking level differences used to assess changes in temporal processing. Similarly, one can measure auditory discrimination by measuring difference thresholds for intensity, frequency, or duration, or one might assess auditory discrimination in a more functional context of phonemic analysis or synthesis.

One must exercise caution, however, in selecting ecological (i.e., functional) outcome measures. Even though improvements in language processing, academics, and social areas may be seen in some cases following intervention for central auditory deficits, many other variables, some of which are far removed from the auditory domain, also contribute to learning and socialization (Musiek et al., 2005). Moreover, gains in nonauditory domains are as much dependent, if not more dependent, on many nonauditory factors, most of which are beyond the control of the clinician administering auditory training. As such, the effectiveness (and efficacy) of CAPD intervention should not be gauged primarily by academic outcomes or social skills (or other more expansive measures), but rather by improvements in auditory function that, then, may support improvements in those domains that are dependent on audition (Musiek et al., 2005).

Collaboration Promotes Treatment Effectiveness/Efficacy

The potential adverse impact of CAPD on language, academic performance, and employment underscores the importance of multidisciplinary collaboration among professionals and with families (Bellis, 2003; Bellis & Ferre, 1999; Chermak & Musiek, 1997). As emphasized by Rumbaugh and Washburn (1996), optimizing brain plasticity in support of change requires that stimulation be integrated into one's everyday activities and lifestyle. Collaboration among professionals, clients, and families facilitates this integration.

Collaboration involves mutual deliberation in which participants collectively establish or clarify goals and values for the purpose of problem solving (Chermak, 1993). Engaging clients, families, and other professionals in planning, decision making, and program implementation maximizes problem resolution and successful therapeutic outcomes (Coufal, Hixson, & Stick, 1990; Crais, 1991; Luterman, 1990). Collaboration does not begin, however, with intervention. As discussed in Volume 1 of this Handbook, the diagnosis of CAPD is made on the basis of performance deficits demonstrated on valid tests of central auditory processing; however, other measures, particularly, speech-language measures and psychoeducational measures, provide needed information about language ability and communicative function, and academic achievement, respectively, which contribute to the differential diagnosis of CAPD, and illuminate functional deficits requiring intervention (AAA, 2010; ASHA, 2005a, 2005b). Hence, both audiologists and speech-language pathologists (SLPs) should assume lead roles in implementing comprehensive intervention for CAPD (see Chapter 17 for the role of the SLP). Typically, the audiologist leads the effort to improve signal quality by enhancing the acoustic signal and improving the listening environment. In serving patients

with CAPD, SLPs focus on enhancing the scope and use of language and other central resources. Auditory training should be undertaken by both professionals, as described in Chapter 7. Other professionals, including psychologists and/or neuropsychologists, regular and special educators, and others also are integral to the overall intervention program.

Collaborative consultation should lead to improved diagnostic and treatment strategies, more practical goals for intervention, and increased probability of successfully implementing diagnostic and treatment strategies (Coufal et al., 1990; Crais, 1991). Given family involvement in developing goals and designing strategies, and their subsequent motivation to implement treatment activities in the home and other natural environments, collaboration should maximize the transfer of skills (i.e., generalization) from treatment to daily routines (Crais, 1991). Because collaboration promotes the client's self-efficacy by emphasizing an active, metacognitive approach to problem solving and encouraging self-regulation, it is a particularly valuable component of central resources training and the comprehensive intervention approach (Chermak & Musiek, 1997). The reader is referred to Chermak (1993) and Chermak and Musiek (1997) for in depth discussion of the especially important role of collaboration in building partnerships that are both consistent with cultural paradigms and appropriate to the treatment needs of the client when working with culturally diverse individuals and families. The reader is referred to other chapters in this volume, including Chapters 5, 13, 14, 17, 19, and 20 for additional perspectives on the role of collaboration for effective intervention.

Foundations of Comprehensive Intervention

All auditory tasks, from pure-tone detection to spoken language processing, are influenced by higher order, nonmodality-specific systems such as attention and memory, as well as motivation and decision processes, and the underlying multimodal, crossmodal, and supramodal neural interfaces supporting performance of complex behaviors (Chermak & Musiek, 1997; Musiek et al., 2005). Conversely, and as elaborated above, successful spoken language comprehension requires the listener to coordinate various knowledge bases and skills, including auditory vigilance, auditory discrimination, and temporal processing to discern and organize basic acoustic features; segmentation skills to parse the continuous sound stream into constituent phonetic units; language knowledge; general knowledge; and metacognitive knowledge and executive control (Abbs & Sussman, 1971; ASHA, 1996; Chermak & Musiek, 1992, 1997; Danks & End, 1987; Fant, 1967; Kintsch, 1977; Massaro, 1975a, b; Ronald & Roskelly, 1985; Samuels, 1987). Effective listeners employ various self-regulation strategies to guide extraction of information and synthesis of the spoken message (Chermak & Musiek, 1997). Throughout the process, they must reflect continually on the processes and products of their listening. Experience, expectation, and motivation influence both the allocation of resources and the particular meaning derived from the acoustic signal. Given the number and range of skills and knowledge bases demanding coordination in service of central auditory processing and spoken language understanding, comprehensive intervention programs for CAPD must integrate specific skills development, general problem-solving strategies, and self-regulation of strategy use (Chermak & Musiek, 1997).

Because listening takes place within the multiple contexts of the acoustic, phonetic, linguistic, and social domains, simultaneous and integrated orchestration of multiple knowledge bases and skills is required for spoken language comprehension (Chermak & Musiek, 1997). Moreover, the complex organization of the brain and the resulting interdependence of sensory, cognitive, and language networks necessitate a comprehensive intervention program that includes intensive training via *bottom-up*, auditory training, signal enhancement and environmental modifications, coupled with extensive *top-down* training focused on central resources knowledge, skills, and strategy training (AAA, 2010; ASHA, 2005a, 2005b; Bellis, 2002b, 2003; Chermak & Musiek, 1997).

Bottom-up (stimulus driven) approaches include specific auditory training techniques, assistive listening systems, and clear speech. Top-down (internal, concept-driven) approaches include language and metalanguage strategies, cognitive strategies, metacognitive strategies, classroom, instructional, and learning strategies, and workplace, recreational and home accommodations. Generally, bottom-up and top-down treatment approaches are complementary and should both be incorporated to maximize treatment effectiveness—improving auditory skills through bottom-up auditory training and compensating for residual deficits by building top-down central resources. Combined, these bottom-up and top-down approaches exploit the interactions supported by supramodal, multimodal, and crossmodal interfaces in addressing the range of functional deficits that characterize CAPD and the often occurring comorbid disorders. Together, these approaches offer tremendous potential to mitigate listening difficulties stemming from CAPD.

Customizing Intervention

Central auditory diagnostic data is pivotal to intervention planning; however, comprehensive intervention cannot be designed on the basis of central auditory test results alone. Understanding the processes underlying successful task performance helps to bridge the gap between data collection and intervention strategies and techniques (Chermak & Musiek, 1992). Information from multidisciplinary evaluations combined with central auditory test outcomes reveal the full range of functional deficits and areas of concern relevant to intervention program planning (Bellis, 2002b, 2003; Bellis & Ferre, 1999). In fact, the practical relevance of data to intervention programming varies considerably across tests. For example, although both masking level differences (MLDs) and tests involving auditory performance with competing messages both provide useful diagnostic insights regarding site or level of CANS dysfunction and compromised central auditory processes, the abstract nature of the MLD paradigm and the absence of an everyday listening analog renders MLDs less useful for counseling purposes. Both tests, however, provide valuable information regarding appropriate foci for auditory

training (i.e., reduced MLDs indicate binaural interaction training; depressed auditory performance with competing messages suggest binaural integration and binaural separation training) (Chermak, 1996; Musiek & Chermak, 1994; Musiek & Chermak, 1995).

The heterogeneity of CAPD and its occurrence across the life span, as well as the imperative to intervene efficiently as well as effectively, leads to several questions regarding the distinctiveness of intervention. First, can we truly customize intervention to the specific auditory profile? Second, can distinctive intervention strategies be formulated to manage CAPD within a constellation of comorbid language or cognitive deficits? Third, should management strategies differ as a function of the client's age?

Functional Deficit CAPD Profiles

With a firm understanding of CAPD gained from auditory and cognitive neuroscience, it now may be possible to develop functional deficit profiles that reflect patterns of central auditory deficits and functional cognitive, language, learning, and communication sequelae (Bellis, 2002a, 2002b, 2003; Bellis & Ferre, 1999). These deficit profiles, which should conform to well-established neuroscience tenets that demonstrate the presence of brain-behavior relationships across a wide variety of functional areas, can be used to guide development of comprehensive intervention programs that address the cluster of central auditory and functional symptoms. Consider, for example, the difference in emphases for individuals diagnosed with CAPD who present similar auditory performance decrements with competing signals, but dissimilar temporal processing abilities. Both individuals would probably benefit from auditory training focused on degraded signal processing (e.g., filtered speech recognition, speech recognition in noise, reverberation, and competing messages), signal enhancement strategies (e.g., FM technology and preferential seating), and linguistic strategies that emphasize use of context to resolve messages (i.e., closure skills). The individual experiencing temporal processing difficulties, however, might also benefit from auditory training focused on temporal discrimination (e.g., gap detection) and time-compressed speech recognition exercises, as well as activities directed toward the use of prosody to predict degraded messages and recommendations that partners speak more slowly, pause more often, and emphasize key words.

Notwithstanding the utility of such subprofiling methods, clinicians are cautioned that there can and should be no "cookie-cutter" approach to CAPD diagnosis or intervention. Indeed, the degree of individual heterogeneity in both bottom-up and top-down functions precludes any simple one-to-one correlation between fundamental auditory behaviors and listening, learning, and related skills across large groups. This finding was underscored by Jutras, Loubert, Dupuis, Marcoux, Dumont, and Baril (2007), who found that a subprofiling method involving only one diagnostic test of central auditory function successfully "classified" more children than did a multidimensional approach involving a test battery that assessed various central auditory regions and loci as well as several different auditory behaviors. This is discussed further in Chapter 8 of Volume 1 of the Handbook.

Effectiveness of Deficit-Specific Intervention

CAPD profiling is based on theoretical constructs and relates test findings to observed day-to-day behaviors; however, they have not yet been fully validated empirically (AAA, 2010; ASHA, 2005a; Bellis, 2002b). The effectiveness of deficit-specific auditory intervention should be gauged, primarily, by improvements seen on central auditory tests, as well as concomitant improvement in functional listening skills. Nonetheless, given the neurophysiologic interdependencies across sensory, cognitive, and language networks, improvements in academic and social arenas may be anticipated, especially when the comprehensive approach is fully implemented.

Customized Deficit-Specific Intervention

It should be emphasized that the use of function deficit profiling for purposes of devising deficit-specific and individualized intervention programs should not be construed to be a *cookie-cutter* approach to CAPD intervention. The unique confluence of bottom-up and top-down abilities present in a given individual, along with his or her functional difficulties and complaints, will necessarily dictate the components of the intervention program that will be most appropriate in any given situation. With this caveat in mind, however, the following example illustrates the application of CAPD profiling and customized intervention.

The likelihood of an interhemispheric transfer deficit is inferred from findings of a significant left-ear deficit on dichotic tests and poor performance on temporal patterning tests in the linguistic labeling report condition. This test data is consistent with the child's functional deficit profile, which includes difficulty listening in noisy environments, little or no benefit seen from bimodal summation (i.e., looking and listening), some bipedal and bimanual (motor coordination) difficulties, and reading and spelling difficulties despite normal language levels. The customized intervention program derived from multidisciplinary assessment focuses on: (1) dichotic listening training; (2) interhemispheric transfer exercises; (3) classroom modifications, including the use of an FM system; (4) acoustic enhancements; (5) central resource compensatory strategies, including active listening, attribution training, cognitive problem-solving; and (6) continued reading and spelling resource services. Post-therapy improvements are observed in left-ear performance on the central auditory test battery, ability to listen in noise, ability to handle concurrently presented multimodality cues, as well as some improvement in reading and spelling.

Accommodating Comorbidity in Customizing Intervention

To formulate distinctive intervention strategies, the relative contribution of the constellation of concomitant auditory, language, cognitive, and learning deficits must be determined. Accurate differential diagnosis must precede efforts to customize therapy; however, notwithstanding careful assessment using an efficient, comprehensive, and multidisciplinary test battery, the relative contributions of auditory, language, and cognitive processes to spoken language comprehension problems may remain uncertain (ASHA, 1996). For example, several explanations can be offered to account for the fairly typical case of a child who presents with difficulty understanding spoken language in the presence of competing noise. The child may lack control over language resources, which prevents him or her from using language knowledge to compensate for the degraded acoustic signal. Alternatively, the nature and severity of the child's CAPD may contravene his or her ability to separate signal from noise, despite full use of normal language knowledge (Chermak & Musiek, 1997). In addition, the child may exhibit an attention-based deficit that interferes with his or her ability to selectively attend to auditory stimuli in the presence of distractors, despite intact language and central auditory function (Chermak, 2007). Similarly, it is often difficult to determine the relative contribution of cognitive, linguistic, and central auditory processing deficits for the language comprehension problems experienced by an adult with cognitive/linguistic disorders (e.g., aphasia) (ASHA, 1996). In fact, it is likely that spoken language comprehension problems in aphasia result from some combination of processing deficits. Distinguish between two or more conditions presenting with similar symptoms or attributes and disentangling impairments due to comorbid conditions can be challenging. Determining whether there is an auditory component to a child's language impairment, learning disability, or attention deficit or whether one condition is responsible for the symptoms seen in another can be quite challenging; however, making this determination is exceedingly important to ensure appropriately targeted intervention and requires comprehensive, multidisciplinary assessment. With information gleaned from a robust central auditory test battery interpreted in the context of a multidisciplinary test battery, clinicians can begin to disentangle the relative contributions of sensory, cognitive, and language processing deficits to a spoken language comprehension deficit and implement intervention directed toward improving the individual's functional abilities in appropriate contexts. (The reader is referred to Volume 1 of this Handbook for discussion of diagnosis, differential diagnosis and multidisciplinary assessment.)

Life Span Considerations

Children with CAPD frequently present with comorbid cognitive, language, and learning deficits. Older adults frequently present with both peripheral and central auditory disorders, as well as a range of age-related decline in cognitive abilities (e.g., working memory and speed of processing) and language processes that compound spoken language understanding difficulties, especially when there is reverberation and the competing signal is speech (Hickson & Worrall, 2003; McCoy et al., 2005; Pichora-Fuller, 2003; Pichora-Fuller & Sousa, 2003). Individual differences are expected, given the normal variation in brain organization and age-related change across individuals coupled with the variable manifestations of central auditory pathologies (Phillips, 1995, 2002). Only comprehensive assessment can determine the ultimate relative role of these factors in explaining the spoken language difficulties experienced by the older adult (Chermak & Musiek, 1997).

Although many of the strategies and techniques described in this volume are likely to benefit the great majority of clients with CAPD across the life span, specific emphases will vary depending on the nature of the processing deficits

identified, the functional consequences of these deficits, the presence of comorbid conditions, and the client's age. For example, given the inherent neural plasticity of the developing CNS, intervention for children with CAPD should emphasize direct auditory training and acoustic signal enhancement. Given the frequent comorbid constellation of attention, language, and learning issues, however, central resources training also is recommended and should be integrated with the academic curriculum (Bellis, 2002b, 2003; Chermak & Musiek, 1997).

Intervention goals and approaches with older adults with CAPD must take into account neurophysiologic changes, comorbid conditions, and the lifestyle and attendant demands of the older adult. The diminished plasticity of the older nervous system implies that management strategies in adults and older adults might necessarily be directed more toward compensation (i.e., assistive listening system, central resources training) rather than recovery of function (ASHA, 1996), although spontaneous and/or stimulus-induced recovery of function following acute brain injury may suggest a role for direct treatment (i.e., auditory training) approaches as well (e.g., Bellis, 2008; Sweetow & Henderson-Sabes, 2006). Opportunities to infuse multidisciplinary treatment and management strategies to address comorbid conditions in older adults (e.g., aphasia) should not be overlooked (Chermak & Musiek, 1997).

Intervention Strategies Appropriate Across Profiles

Notwithstanding the value of customizing intervention to achieve effective and efficient outcomes of the greatest functional significance, a number of intervention principles and strategies should be applied across clinical deficit profiles. Common principles guiding intervention across clinical populations include an emphasis on collaboration, self-regulation, and an ecological- and strategy-based orientation (Chermak & Musiek, 1997). Intervention strategies common across profiles include implementation of active listening techniques (e.g., listening empathetically, deploying closure, inferencing, deducing, and predicting, and communication repair strategies), using clear speech to enhance acoustic cues, and coupling auditory training with central resources (compensatory strategies) training, and collaboration with other members of the professional team. In many cases, trial of assistive listening systems (e.g., FM, infrared systems) may be indicated, as well. In producing clear speech, speakers attempt to produce every word and phrase in a precise and clear fashion, without exaggerating. Speakers are directed to speak clearly (e.g., as if speaking to someone with hearing loss or from a different language background), to focus on a slower and louder rate of speech, and to enunciate, emphasize key words, and pause more frequently and for longer durations. Acoustically, clear speech results in increased power of the consonants relative to vowels, wider pitch range, expanded vowel spaces, and more varied intonation and more prominent stress markers (Bradlow, Kraus, & Hayes, 2003; Picheny, Durlach, & Braida, 1985, 1986, 1989).

Musical training looms as an attractive intervention possibility. Clearly, musically trained individuals perform better than nonmusicians on a host of auditory tasks (see Chapter 7) However, using music as auditory training for adults with CAPD who present no previous musical experience is an area for which there remains a paucity of information. Therefore, it is difficult to determine whether this therapy approach would be effective for adults with no prior musical experience.

Summary

A clearer understanding of the brain's complex organization and plasticity carries considerable implications for intervention. The accumulated literature in auditory and cognitive neuroscience elucidates the nature of CAPD and helps explain the frequent comorbid presentation with related attention, language, and learning deficits. The new understanding translates into training principles grounded in neuroscience and learning theory. The overlapping and widespread distribution of sensory, cognitive, and language networks undergird auditory training and central resource intervention methods and strategies that harness the brain's potential to *remodel* itself through learning. The emerging understanding also provides a framework to begin developing deficit subprofiles of CAPD around clusters of symptoms and associated neurophysiologic bases to implement effective intervention directed to those functional deficit clusters.

References

AAA (American Academy of Audiology). *Guidelines for the diagnosis, treatment, and management of children and adults with central auditory processing disorder.* Retrieved from http://www.audiology.org/

resources/documentlibrary/Documents/ CAPD%20Guidelines%208-2010.pdf

Abbs, J. H., & Sussman, H. M. (1971). Neurophysiological feature detectors and speech perception: A discussion of theoretical implications. *Journal of Speech and Hearing Research*, *14*, 23–36.

Abrams, H. B., McArdie, R., & Chisolm, T. H. (2005). From outcomes to evidence: Establishing best practices for audiologists. *Seminars in Hearing*, *26*, 157–169.

Ahissar, E., Vaadia, E., Ahissar, M., Bergman, H., Arieli, A., & Abeles, M. (1992). Dependence of cortical plasticity on correlated activity of single neurons and on behavioral context. *Science*, *257*, 1412–1415.

Akeroyd, M. (2008). Are individual differences in speech reception related to individual differences in cognitive ability? A survey of twenty experimental studies with normal and hearing impaired adults. *International Journal of Audiology*, *47*(Suppl.), S53–S71.

Allen, R. L., Cranford, J. L., & Pay, N. (1996). Central auditory processing in an adult with congenital absence of left temporal lobe. *Journal of the American Academy of Audiology*, *7*, 282–288.

Alonso, R., & Schochat, E. (2009). The efficacy of formal auditory training in children with central auditory processing disorder: Behavioral and electrophysiological evaluation. *Brazilian Journal of Otorhinolaryngology*, *75*, 726–732.

Anderson, S., Parbery-Clark, A., Yi, H. G., & Kraus, N. (2011). A neural basis of speech-in-noise perception in older adults. *Ear and Hearing*, *32*, 750–757.

Aoki, C., & Siekevitz, P. (1988). Plasticity in brain development. *Scientific American*, *259*, 56–64.

ASHA (American Speech-Language-Hearing Association). (1996). Task Force on Central Auditory Processing Consensus Development. Central auditory processing: Current status of research and implications for clinical practice. *American Journal of Audiology*, *5*, 41–54.

ASHA. (2005a). *(Central) auditory processing disorders*. Retrieved from http://www .asha.org/members/deskref-journals/desk ref/default

ASHA. (2005b). *(Central) auditory processing disorders—the role of the audiologist* [Position statement]. Retrieved from http://www.asha.org/members/deskref -journals/deskref/default

Atienza, M., Cantero, J. L., & Dominguez-Marin, E. (2002). The time course of neural changes in underlying auditory perceptual learning. *Learning and Memory*, *9*, 138–150.

Ausubel, D. P., & Robinson, F. C. (1969). *School learning*. New York, NY: Holt, Rinehart, and Winston.

Bamiou, D. E., Musiek, F. E., & Luxon, L. M. (2001). Aetiology and clinical presentation of auditory processing disorders—a review. *Archives of Disease in Childhood*, *85*, 361–365.

Bamiou, D. E., Musiek, F. E. & Luxon, L. M. (2003). The insula (island of Reil) and its role in auditory processing: Literature review. *Brain Research Reviews*, *42*, 143–154.

Banasich, A., Thomas, J., Choudhury, N., & Leppanen, P. (2002). The importance of rapid auditory processing abilities to early language development: Evidence from converging methodologies. *Developmental Psychobiology*, *40*, 278–292.

Bao, S., Chang, E. F., Woods, J., & Merzenich, M. M. (2004). Temporal plasticity in the primary auditory cortex induced by operant perceptual learning. *Nature Neuroscience*, *7*, 974–981.

Baran, J. A., & Musiek, F. E. (1991). Behavioral assessment of the central auditory nervous system. In W. F. Rintelmann (Ed.), *Hearing assessment* (pp. 549–602). Austin, TX: Pro-Ed.

Barlow, D., & Hersen, M. (1984). *Single case experimental designs: Strategies for studying behavior change*. Oxford, UK: Pergamon Press.

Bayazit, O., Oniz, A., Hahn, C., Gunturkun, O., & Ozgoren, M. (2009). Dichotic listening revisited: Trial-by-trial ERP analyses reveal intra- and inter-hemispheric differences. *Neuropsychologia, 47,* 536–545.

Beer, A., Plank, T., & Greenlee, M. (2011). Diffusion tensor imaging slows white matter tracts between human auditory and visual cortex. *Experimental Brain Research, 213,* 299–308.

Beitel, R., Vollmer, M., Raggio, M., & Schreiner, C. (2011). Behavioral training enhances cortical temporal processing in neonatally deafened juvenile cats. *Journal of Neurophysiology, 106,* 944–959.

Bellis, T. J. (2002a). Considerations in diagnosing auditory processing disorders in school-aged children. *American Speech-Language-Hearing Association Special Interest Division 9 (Hearing and Hearing Disorders in Children), 12,* 3–9.

Bellis, T. J. (2002b). Developing deficit-specific intervention plans for individuals with auditory processing disorders. *Seminars in Hearing, 23,* 287–295.

Bellis, T. J. (2002c). *When the brain can't hear: Unraveling the mystery of auditory processing disorder.* New York, NY: Atria Books.

Bellis, T. J. (2003). *Assessment and management of central auditory processing disorders in the educational setting: From science to practice* (2nd ed.). Clifton Park, NY: Thomson Learning.

Bellis, T. J. (2008). Treatment options for patients with (central) auditory processing disorders. In R. Roeser, M. Valente, & H. Hosford-Dunn (Eds.), *Audiology: Treatment* (2nd ed., pp. 271–292). New York, NY: Thieme.

Bellis, T. J., Billiet, C. R., & Ross, J. (2011). The utility of visual analogs of central auditory tests in the differential diagnosis of (central) auditory processing disorder and attention deficit hyperactivity disorder. *Journal of the American Academy of Audiology, 22,* 501–514.

Bellis, T. J., Chermak, G. D., Weihing, J., & Musiek, F. E. (2012). Efficacy of auditory interventions for central auditory processing disorder: A response to Fey et al.

(2011). *Language, Speech, and Hearing Services in Schools, 43,* 381–386.

Bellis, T. J., & Ferre, J. M. (1999). Multidimensional approach to the differential diagnosis of central auditory processing disorders in children. *Journal of the American Academy of Audiology, 10,* 319–328.

Bellis, T. J., Nicol, T., & Kraus, N. (2000). Aging affects hemispheric asymmetry in the neural representation of speech sounds. *Journal of Neuroscience, 20,* 791–797.

Bellis, T. J., & Wilber, L.A. (2001). Effects of aging and gender on interhemispheric function. *Journal of Speech, Language, and Hearing Research, 44,* 246–263.

Beninger, R. J., & Miller, R. (1998). Dopamine D1-like receptors and reward-related incentive learning. *Neuroscience and Biobehavior Review, 22,* 335–345.

Besle, J., Bertrand, O., & Giard, M. (2009). Electrophysiological (EEG, sEEG, MEG) evidence for multiple audiovisual interactions in the human auditory cortex. *Hearing Research, 258,* 143–151.

Billiet, C. R., & Bellis, T. J. (2011). The relationship between brainstem temporal processing and performance on tests of central auditory function in children with reading disorders. *Journal of Speech, Language, and Hearing Research, 54,* 228–242.

Blake, D. T., Strata, E., Churchland, A. K., & Merzenich, M. M. (2002). Neural correlates of instrumental learning in primary auditory cortex. *Proceedings of the National Academy of Sciences USA, 99,* 10114–10119.

Bolshakov, V. Y., & Siegelbaum, S. A. (1995). Regulation of hippocampal transmitter release during development and long-term potentiation. *Science, 269,* 1730–1733.

Booth, J. R., Burman, D. D., Meyer, J. R., Gitelman, D. R., Parrish, T. B., & Mesulam, M. M. (2002). Modality independence of word comprehension. *Human Brain Mapping, 16,* 251–261.

Boscariol, M., Guimarães, C.A., Hage, S.R., Garcia, V., Schmutzler, K., Cendes, F., & Guerreiro, M. (2011). Auditory processing disorder in patients with language-learning impairment and correlation with malformation of cortical development. *Brain Development, 33,* 824–831.

Bradlow, A. R., Kraus, N., & Hayes, E. (2003). Speaking clearly for children with learning disabilities: Sentence perception in noise. *Journal of Speech, Language, and Hearing Research, 46,* 80–97.

Brown, T. H., Chapman, P. F. E., Kairiss, W., & Keenan, C. L. (1988). Long-term synaptic potentiation. *Science, 242,* 724–728.

Cacace, A., & McFarland, D. (2005). The importance of modality specificity in diagnosing central auditory processing disorder (CAPD). *American Journal of Audiology, 14,* 124–127.

Calvert, G. A., Bullmore, E. T., Brammer, M. J., Campbell, R., Williams, S. C. R., McGuire, P., . . . David, A. S. (1997). Activation of auditory cortex during silent lipreading. *Science, 276,* 593–596.

Carcagno, S., & Plack, P. (2011). Subcortical plasticity following perceptual learning in a pitch discrimination task. *Journal Association Research Otolaryngology, 12,* 89–100.

Chermak, G. D. (1993). Dynamics of collaborative consultation with families. *American Journal of Audiology, 2,* 38–43.

Chermak, G. D. (1996). Central testing. In S. E. Gerber (Ed.), *Handbook of pediatric audiology* (pp. 206–253). Washington, DC: Gallaudet University Press.

Chermak, G. D. (2003). It takes a team to differentially diagnose APD. *Hearing Journal, 56,* 32.

Chermak, G. D., & Musiek, F. E. (1992). Managing central auditory processing disorders in children and youth. *American Journal of Audiology, 1,* 61–65.

Chermak, G. D. & Musiek, F. E. (1997). *Central auditory processing disorders: New perspectives.* San Diego, CA: Singular.

Chermak, G. D., & Musiek, F. E. (Eds.). (2007). *Handbook of (central) auditory processing disorder: Comprehensive intervention* (Vol. 2). San Diego, CA: Plural.

Chermak, G. D., & Musiek, F. E. (2011). Neurological substrate of central auditory

processing deficits in children. *Current Pediatric Reviews, 7,* 241–251.

Ciccia, A. H., Meulenbroek, P., & Turkstra, L. S. (2009). Adolescent brain and cognitive developments. Implications for clinical assessment in traumatic brain injury. *Topics in Language Disorders, 29,* 249–265.

Clifford, M. M. (1978). Have we underestimated the facilitative effects of failure? *Canadian Journal of Behavioral Science, 10,* 308–316.

Cooper, J. C. Jr., & Gates, G. A. (1991). Hearing in the elderly—the Framingham Cohort, 1983–1985: Part II. Prevalence of central auditory processing disorders. *Ear and Hearing, 12,* 304–311.

Coufal, K. L., Hixson, P. K., & Stick, S. L. (1990, November). *Collaborative consultation—an alternative treatment: Efficacy data and policy issues.* Paper presented at the annual Convention of the American Speech-Language-Hearing Association, Seattle, WA.

Cox, R. (2005). Evidence-based practice in provision of amplification. *Journal of the American Academy of Audiology, 16,* 419–438.

Crais, E. R. (1991). Moving from "parent involvement" to family-centered services. *American Journal of Speech-Language Pathology, 1,* 5–8.

Cunningham, J., Nicol, T., Zecker, S. G., Bradlow, A., & Kraus, N. (2001). Neurobiologic responses to speech in noise in children with learning problems: Deficits and strategies for improvement. *Clinical Neurophysiology, 112,* 758–767.

Dancause, N., Barbay, S., Frost, S. B., Plautz, E. J., Chen, D., Zoubina, E. V., . . . Nudo, R. J. (2005). Extensive cortical rewiring after brain injury. *Journal of Neuroscience, 25,* 10167–10179.

Danks, J. H., & End, L. J. (1987). Processing strategies for reading and listening. In R. Horowitz & S. J. Samuels (Eds.), *Comprehending oral and written language* (pp. 271–294). San Diego, CA: Academic Press.

Danzl, M., Etter, N., Andreatta, R., & Kitzman, P. (2012). Facilitating neurorehabilitation through principles of engagement. *Journal Allied Health, 41*, 35–41.

de Boer, J., & Thornton, A. R. D. (2008). Neural correlates of perceptual learning in the auditory brainstem: Efferent activity predicts and reflects improvement at a speech-in-noise discrimination task. *Journal of Neuroscience, 28*, 4929–4937.

deVillers-Sidani, E., Alzghoul, L., Zhou X., Simpson, K., Lin, R., & Merzenich, M. (2010). Recovery of functional and structural age-related changes in the rat primary auditory cortex with operant training. *Proceedings of the National Academy of Sciences USA, 107*, 13900–13905.

Dollaghan, C. A. (2007). *The handbook of evidence-based practice in communication disorders*. Baltimore, MD: Paul H. Brookes.

Domitz, D., & Schow, R. (2000). A new CAPD battery—multiple auditory processing assessment (MAPA): Factor analysis and comparisons with the SCAN. *American Journal of Audiology, 9*, 101–111.

Draganski, B., Gasert, C., Busch, V., Schuierer, G., Bogdahn, U., & May, A. (2004) Neuroplasticity: changes in grey matter induced by training. *Nature, 427*, 311–312.

Edeline, J. M., & Weinberger, N. M. (1991). Thalamic short-term plasticity in the auditory system: associative retuning of receptive fields in the ventral medial geniculate body. *Behavioral Neuroscience, 105*, 618–639.

Edelman, G. M, & Gally, J. (2011). Degeneracy and complexity in biological systems. *Proceedings of the National Academy of Sciences USA, 98*, 13763–13768.

Elbert, T., Pantev, C., Wienbruch, C., Rockstroh, B., & Taub, E. (1995). Increased cortical representation of the fingers of the left hand in string players. *Science, 270*, 305–306.

Evans, W. J., Webster, D. B., & Cullen, J. K. (1983). Auditory brainstem responses in neonatally sound deprived CBA/J mice. *Hearing Research, 10*, 269–277.

Fant, G. (1967). Auditory patterns of speech. In W. Wathen-Dunn (Ed.), *Models for the perception of speech and visual form* (pp. 111–125). Cambridge, MA: MIT Press.

Feldman, D. E., & Brecht, M. (2005). Map plasticity in somatosensory cortex. *Science, 310*, 810–815.

Fey, M. E., Richard, G. J., Geffner, D., Kamhi, A. G., Medwetsky, L., Paul, D., . . . Schooling , T. (2011). Auditory processing disorder and auditory/language interventions: An evidence-based systematic review. *Language, Speech, and Hearing Services in Schools, 42*, 246–264.

Gaffan, D. (2005). Widespread cortical networks underlie memory and attention. *Science, 309*, 2172–2173.

Gates, G., Feeney, M. P., & Mills, D. (2008). Cross-sectional age-changes of hearing in the elderly. *Ear and Hearing, 29*, 865–874.

Golding, M., Carter, N., Mitchell, P., & Hood, L. (2004). Prevalence of central auditory processing (CAP) abnormality in an older Australian population: The Blue Mountains Hearing Study. *Journal of the American Academy of Audiology, 15*, 633–642.

Gomez, R., & Condon, M. (1999). Central auditory processing ability in children with ADHD with and without learning disabilities. *Journal of Learning Disabilities, 32*, 150–158.

Goswami, U., Thomson, J., Richardson, U., Stainthorp, R., Hughes, D., Rosen, S., & Scott, S. K. (2002). Amplitude envelope onsets and developmental dyslexia: A new hypothesis. *Proceedings of the National Academy of Sciences, 99*, 10911–10916.

Gottselig, J. M., Brandeis, D., Hofer-Tinguely, G., Borberly, A. A., & Achermann, P. (2004). Human central auditory plasticity associated with tone sequence learning. *Learning and Memory, 11*, 151–171.

Grafman, J., & Litvan, I. (1999). Evidence for four forms of neuroplasticity. In J. Grafman & Y. Christen (Eds.) *Neuronal plasticity: Building a bridge from the laboratory to the clinic* (pp. 131–139). New York, NY: Springer-Verlag.

Gustafsson, B., & Wigstrom, H. (1988). Physiologic mechanisms underlying long-term potentiation. *Trends in Neuroscience, 11,* 156–162.

Hall, J. W., Grose, J. H., & Pillsbury, H. C. (1995). Long-term effects of chronic otitis media on binaural hearing in children. *Archives of Otolaryngology-Head and Neck Surgery, 121,* 847–852.

Hassamannova, J., Myslivecek, J., & Novakova, V. (1981). Effects of early auditory stimulation on cortical areas. In J. Syka & L. Aitkin (Eds.), *Neuronal mechanisms of hearing* (pp. 355–359). New York, NY: Plenum Press.

Hayes, E. A., Warrier, C. M., Nicol, T. G., Zecker, S. G., & Kraus, N. (2003). Neural plasticity following auditory training in children with learning problems. *Clinical Neurophysiology, 114,* 673–684.

Hegde, M. N. (1993). *Treatment procedures in communicative disorders.* Austin, TX: Pro-Ed.

Hickson, L., & Worrall, L. (2003). Beyond hearing aid fitting: Improving communication for older adults. *International Journal of Audiology, 42*(Suppl. 2), S84–S91.

Holroyd, C. B., Larsen, J. T., & Cohen, J. D. (2004). Context dependence of the event-related brain potential associated with reward and punishment. *Psychophysiology, 41,* 245–253.

Horn, S. D., & Gassaway, J. (2007). Practice-based evidence study design for comparative effectiveness research. *Medical Care, 45,* S50–S57.

Hornickel, J., Zecker, S., Bradlow, A., & Kraus, N. (2012). Assistive listening devices drive neuroplasticity in children with dyslexia. *Proceedings of the National Academy of Sciences USA, 109,*16731–16736.

Hyde, K., Lerch, J., Norton, A., Forgeard, M., Winner, E., Evans, A., & Schlaug, G. (2009). Musical training shapes structural brain development. *Journal of Neuroscience, 29,* 3019–3025.

Ilg, R., Wohlschlager, A. M., Gaser, C., Liebau, Y., Dauner, R., Woller, A., . . . Muhlau, M. (2008). Gray matter increase induced by practice correlates with task-specific activation: A combined functional and morphometric magnetic resonance imaging study. *Journal of Neuroscience, 28,* 4210–4215.

Iliadou, V., Bamiou, D-E., Kaprinis, S., Kandylis, D., & Kaprinis, G. (2009). Auditory processing disorders in children suspected of learning disabilities—a need for screening. *International Journal of Pediatric Otorhinolaryngology, 73,* 1029–1034.

Irvine, D. R. F., Rajan, R., & Robertson, D. (1992). Plasticity in auditory cortex of adult mammals with restricted cochlear lesions. In R. Naresh Singh (Ed.), *Nervous systems: Principles of design and function* (pp. 319–350). New Delhi, India: Wiley-Eastern.

Jancke, L., & Shah, N. (2002). Does dichotic listening probe temporal lobe function? *Neurology, 58,* 736–743.

Jerger, J., Moncrieff, D., Greenwald, R., Wambacq, I., & Seipel, A. (2000). Effect of age on interaural asymmetry of event-related potentials in a dichotic listening task. *Journal of the American Academy of Audiology, 11,* 383–389.

Jerger, J., Thibodeau, L., Martin, J., Mehta, J., Tillman, G., Greenwald, R., . . . Overson, G. (2002). Behavioral and electrophysiologic evidence of auditory processing disorder: A twin study. *Journal of the American Academy of Audiology, 13,* 438–460.

Jirsa, R. E. (1992). The clinical utility of the P3 AERP in children with auditory processing disorders. *Journal of Speech and Hearing Research, 35,* 903–912.

Johnson, K. L., Nicol, T., Zecker, S. G., & Kraus, N. (2008). Developmental plasticity in the human auditory brainstem. *Journal of Neuroscience, 28,* 4000–4007.

Kaas, J. H. (1995). Neurobiology. How cortex reorganizes. *Nature, 375,* 735–736.

Kauramaki, J., Jaaskelainen, I., & Sams, M. (2007). Selective attention increases both gain and feature selectivity of the human auditory cortex. *PLoS ONE, 9,* e909.

Kayser, C., & Logothetis, N.K. (2007). Do early sensory cortices integrate cross-modal information? *Brain Structure and Function, 212,* 121–132.

Keuroghlian, A. S., & Knudsen, E. I. (2007). Adaptive auditory plasticity in developing and adult animals. *Progress in Neurobiology, 82*, 109–121.

Kim, J., Morest, D. K., & Bohne, B. A. (1997). Degeneration of axons in the brain stem of the chinchilla after auditory overstimulation. *Hearing Research, 103*, 169–191.

Kintsch, W. (1977). On comprehending stories. In M. A. Just & P. A. Carpenter (Eds.), *Cognitive processes in comprehension* (pp. 33–62). Hillsdale, NJ: Lawrence Erlbaum.

Kislyuk, D., Mottonen, R., & Sams, M. (2008). Visual processing affects the neural basis of auditory discrimination. *Journal Cognitive Neuroscience, 20*, 2175–2184.

Knudsen, E. I. (1988). Experience shapes sound localization and auditory unit properties during development in the barn owl. In G. Edelman, W. Gall, & W. Kowan (Eds.), *Auditory function: Neurobiological basis of hearing* (pp. 137–152). New York, NY: John Wiley.

Knudsen, E. (1998). Capacity for plasticity in the adult owl auditory system expanded by juvenile experience. *Science, 279*, 1531–1533.

Kolb, B. (1995). *Brain plasticity and behavior*. Mahwah, NJ: Lawrence Erlbaum.

Kraus, N., & Banai, K. (2007). Auditory-processing malleability: Focus on language and music. *Current Directions in Psychological Science*, 16, 105–110.

Kraus, N., & Disterhoff, J. F. (1982). Response plasticity of single neurons in rabbit auditory association cortex during tone-signalled learning. *Brain Research, 246*, 205–215.

Kraus, N., McGee, T., Carrell, T., King, C., Tremblay, K., & Nicol, T. (1995). Central auditory system plasticity associated with speech discrimination training. *Journal of Cognitive Neuroscience*, 7, 25–32.

Kraus, N., McGee, T., Carrell, T., Zecker, S., Nicol, T., & Koch, D. (1996). Auditory neurophysiologic responses and discrimination deficits in children with learning problems. *Science, 273*, 971–973.

Kraus, N., McGee, T., Littman, T., Nicol, T., & King, C. (1994). Nonprimary auditory thalamic representation of acoustic change. *Journal of Neurophysiology, 72*, 1270–1277.

Krizman, J., Marian, V., Shook, A., Skoe, E., & Kraus, N. (2012). Subcortical encoding of sound is enhanced in bilinguals and relates to executive function advantages. *Proceedings of the National Academy of Sciences USA, 109*, 7877–7881.

Kumar, A.U. (2011). Temporal processing abilities across different age groups. *Journal of the American Academy of Audiology, 22*, 5–12.

Lopez-Aranda, M. F., Lopez-Tellez, J. F., Navarro-Lobato, I., Masmudi-Martin, M., Gutierrez, A., & Khan, Z. U. (2009). Role of layer 6 of v2 visual cortex in object-recognition. *Memory, 325*, 87–89.

Luterman, D. M. (1990). Audiological counseling and the diagnostic process. *American Speech-Language-Hearing Association, 32*, 35–37.

Marler, J. A., Champlin, C. A., & Gillam, R. B. (2002). Auditory memory for backward masking signals in children with language impairment. *Psychophysiology, 39*, 767–780.

Martin, J., Jerger, J., & Mehta, J. (2007). Divided-attention and directed–attention listening modes in children with dichotic deficits: An event-related potential study. *Journal of the American Academy of Audiology, 18*, 34–53.

Martinkauppi, S., Rama, P., Aronen, H. J., Korvenoja, A., & Carolson, S. (2002). Working memory of auditory localization. *Cerebral Cortex, 10*, 889–898.

Massaro, D. W. (1975a). Language and information processing. In D. W. Massaro (Ed.), *Understanding language: An information-processing analysis of speech perception, reading, and psycholinguistics* (pp. 3–28). New York, NY: Academic Press.

Massaro, D. W. (1975b). *Understanding language: An information-processing analysis of speech perception, reading, and psycholinguistics*. New York, NY: Academic Press.

Masterton, R. B. (1992). Role of the central auditory system in hearing: The new direction. *Trends in Neuroscience, 15,* 280–285.

May, A., Hajak, G., Gänssbauer, S., Steffens, T., Langguth, B., Kleinjung, T., & Eichhammer, P. (2007). Structural brain alterations following 5 days of intervention: Dynamic aspects of neuroplasticity. *Cerebral Cortex, 17,* 205–210.

McCoy, S. L., Tun, P. A., Cox, L. C., Colangelo, M., Stewart, R. A., & Wingfield, A. (2005). Hearing loss and perceptual effort: Downstream effects on older adults' memory for speech. *Journal of Experimental Psychology, 58,* 22–33.

Meredith, M. A., Allman, B. L., Keniston, L. P., & Clemo, H. R. (2009). Auditory influences on nonauditory cortices. *Hearing Research, 258,* 64–71.

Merzenich, M. M., Grajski, K., Jenkins, W., Recanzone, G., & Peterson, B. (1991). Functional cortical plasticity: Cortical network origins of representations changes. *Cold Spring Harbor Symposium on Quantum Biology, 55,* 873–887

Merzenich, M., & Jenkins, W. (1995). Cortical plasticity, learning and learning dysfunction. In B. Julesz & I. Kovacs (Eds.), *Maturational windows and adult cortical plasticity: sfi studies in the sciences of complexity* (Vol. XXIII, pp. 247–272). Reading, PA: Addison-Wesley.

Merzenich, M., Jenkins, W. M., Johnston, P., Schreiner, C., Miller, S. L., & Tallal, P. (1996). Temporal processing deficits of language-learning impaired children ameliorated by training. *Science, 271,* 77–80.

Merzenich, M., Schreiner, C., Jenkins, W., & Wang, X. (1993). Neural mechanisms underlying temporal integration, segmentation, and input sequence representations: Some implications for the origin of learning disabilities. *Annals of the New York Academy of Sciences, 682,* 1–22.

Merzenich, M., Nelson, R. J., Stryker, M. P., Cynader, M. S., Schoppmann, A., & Zook, J. M. (1984). Somatosensory cortical map changes following digit amputation in adult monkeys. *Journal of Comparative Neurology, 224,* 591–605.

Millward, K., Hall R., Ferguson, M., & Moore, D. (2011). Training speech-in-noise perception in mainstream school children. *International Journal of Pediatric Otorhinolaryngology, 75,* 1408–1417.

Moncrieff, D., Jerger, J., Wambacq, I., Greenwald, R., & Black, J. (2004). ERP evidence of a dichotic left-ear deficit in some dyslexic children. *Journal of the American Academy of Audiology, 15,* 518–534.

Moncrieff, D., & Musiek, F. (2002). Interaural asymmetries revealed by dichotic listening tests in normal and dyslexic children. *Journal of the American Academy of Audiology, 13,* 428–437.

Moncrieff, D., & Wertz, D. (2008). Auditory rehabilitation for interaural asymmetry: Preliminary evidence of improved dichotic listening performance following intensive training. *International Journal of Audiology, 47,* 484–497.

Moore, D. R. (1993). Plasticity of binaural hearing and some possible mechanisms following late-onset deprivation. *Journal of the American Academy of Audiology, 4,* 227–283.

Moreno, S., Marques, C., Santos, A., Santos, M., Castro, S. L., & Beeson, M. (2009). Musical training influences linguistic abilities in 8-year-old children: More evidence for brain plasticity. *Cerebral Cortex, 19,* 712–723.

Morest, D. K., Kim, J., Potashner, S. J., & Bohne, B. A. (1998). Long-term degeneration in the cochlear nerve and cochlear nucleus of the adult chinchilla following acoustic overstimulation. *Microscopy Research and Technique, 41,* 205–216.

Murphy, C., & Schochat, E. (2011).Effect of nonlinguistic auditory training on phonological and reading skills. *Folia Phoniatrica Logopaedica, 63,* 147–153.

Musiek, F. E., Baran, J. A., & Pinheiro, M. L. (1994). *Neuroaudiology case studies.* San Diego, CA: Singular.

Musiek, F. E., Baran, J. A., & Shinn, J. (2004). Assessment and Remediation of an auditory processing disorder associated with head trauma. *Journal of the American Academy of Audiology, 15*, 117–132.

Musiek, F. E., Bellis, T. J., & Chermak, G. D. (2005). Nonmodularity of the CANS: Implications for (central) auditory processing disorder: A critique of Cacace and McFarland's "The importance of modality specificity in diagnosing central auditory processing disorder (CAPD)." *American Journal of Audiology, 14*, 128–138.

Musiek, F. E., & Chermak, G. D. (1994). Three commonly asked questions about central auditory processing disorders: Assessment. *American Journal of Audiology, 3*, 23–27.

Musiek, F. E., & Chermak, G. D. (1995). Three commonly asked questions about central auditory processing disorders: Management. *American Journal of Audiology, 4*, 15–18.

Musiek, F. E., Chermak, G. D., & Weihing, J. (2007). Auditory training. In G. D. Chermak & F. E. Musiek (Eds.), *Handbook of (central) auditory processing disorder: Vol. 2. Comprehensive intervention* (pp. 77–106). San Diego, CA: Plural.

Musiek, F. E., & Gollegly, K. (1988). Maturational considerations in the neuroauditory evaluation of children. In F. Bess (Ed.), *Hearing impairment in children* (pp. 231–252). Parkton, MD: York Press.

Musiek, F. E., Gollegly, K., Lamb, L., & Lamb, P. (1990). Selected issues in screening for central auditory processing of dysfunction. *Seminars in Hearing, 11*, 372–384.

Musiek, F. E., Lenz, S., & Gollegly, K. M. (1991). Neuroaudiologic correlates to anatomical changes of the brain. *American Journal of Audiology, 1*, 19–24.

Musiek, F. E., Pinheiro, M. L., & Wilson, D. (1980). Auditory pattern perception in split-brain patients. *Archives of Otolaryngology, 106*, 610–612.

Musiek, F. E., & Schochat, E. (1998). Auditory training and central auditory processing disorders. *Seminars in Hearing, 19*, 357–365.

Nicol, T., & Kraus, N. (2005). How can the neural encoding and perception of speech be improved? In M. Merzenich & S. Syka (Eds.), *Plasticity and signal representation in the auditory system* (pp. 259–270). New York, NY: Kluwer Plenum.

Office of Technology Assessment. (1978). Assessing the efficacy and safety of medical technologies. *OTA-H-75.* Washington, DC: U.S. Government Printing Office.

Ohl, F. W., & Scheich, H. (2005). Learning-induced plasticity in animal and human auditory cortex. *Current Opinions in Neurobiology, 15*, 470–477.

Palfery, T. D., & Duff, D. (2007). Central auditory processing disorders: Review and case study. *Axon, 28*, 20–23.

Pan, Y., Zhang, J., Cai, R., Zhou, X., & Sun, X. (2011). Developmentally degraded directional selectivity of the auditory cortex can be restored by auditory discrimination training. *Behavioral Brain Research, 225*, 596–602.

Pascual-Leone, A., Grafman, J., & Hallett, M. (1994). Modulation of cortical motor output maps during development of implicit and explicit knowledge. *Science, 263*, 1287–1292.

Pekkola, J., Ojanen, V., Autti, T., Jaaskelainen, I., Mottonen, R., Tarkiainen, A., & Sams, M. (2005). Primary auditory cortex activation by visual speech: An fMRI study at 3T. *NeuroReport, 16*, 125–128.

Petacchi, A., Kaernbach, C., Ratnam, R., & Bower, J. M. (2011). Increased activation of the human cerebellum during pitch discrimination: a positron emission tomography (PET) study. *Hearing Research, 282*, 35–48.

Phillips, D. P. (1995). Central auditory processing: A view from auditory neuroscience. *American Journal of Otology, 16*, 338–352.

Phillips, D. P. (2002). Central auditory system and central auditory processing disorders: Some conceptual issues. *Seminars in Hearing, 23*, 251–261.

Pichney, M. A., Durlach, N. I., & Braida, L. D. (1985). Speaking clearly for the hard of hearing. I: Intelligibility differences between clear and conversational speech. *Journal of Speech and Hearing Research, 28,* 96–103.

Pichney, M. A., Durlach, N. I., & Braida, L. D. (1986). Speaking clearly for the hard of hearing. II: Acoustic characteristics of clear and conversational speech. *Journal of Speech and Hearing Research, 29,* 434–446.

Picheny, M. A., Durlach, N. I., & Braida, L. D. (1989). Speaking clearly for the hard of hearing: III. An attempt to determine the contribution of speaking rates to differences in intelligibility between clear and conversational speech. *Journal of Speech and Hearing Research, 32,* 600–603.

Pichora-Fuller, M. K. (2003). Cognitive aging and auditory information processing. *International Journal of Audiology, 42,* 26–32.

Pichora-Fuller, M., & Souza, P. (2003). Effects of aging on auditory processing of speech. *International Journal of Audiology, 42,* 2S11–2S16.

Pienkowski, M., & Eggermont, J. J. (2011). Cortical tonotopic map plasticity and behavior. *Neuroscience and Biobehavioral Reviews, 35*(10), 2117–2128.

Pienkowski, M., & Eggermont, J. (2012). Reversible long-term changes in auditory processing in mature auditory cortex in the absence of hearing loss induced by passive, moderate-level sound exposure. *Ear and Hearing, 33,* 305–314

Pillsbury, H. C., Grose, J. H., Coleman, W. L., Conners, C. K., & Hall, J. W. (1995). Binaural function in children with attention-deficit hyperactivity disorder. *Archives of Otolaryngology-Head and Neck Surgery, 121,* 1345–1350.

Pinheiro, F., & Capellini, S. (2010). Auditory training in students with learning disabilities. *Pro Fono, 22,* 49–54.

Piquado, T., Cousins, K., Wingfield, A., & Miller, P. (2010). Effects of degraded sensory input on memory for speech: Behavioral data and a test of biologically constrained computational models. *Brain Research, 1365,* 48–65.

Poldrack, R., Temple, E., Protopapas, A., Nagarajan, S., Tallal, P., Mezenich, M., & Gabrieli, J. (2001). Relations between neural bases of dynamic auditory processing and phonological processing: Evidence from fMRI. *Journal of Cognitive Neuroscience, 13*(5), 687–697.

Poremba, A., Saunders, R. C., Crane, A. M., Cook, M., Sokoloff, L., & Mishkin, M. (2003). Functional mapping of the primate auditory system. *Science, 299,* 568–571.

Price, C., Thierry, G., & Griffiths, T. (2005). Speech-specific auditory processing: Where is it? *Trends in Cognitive Science, 9,* 271–276.

Purdy, S., Kelly, A., & Davies, M. (2002). Auditory brainstem response, middle latency response, and late cortical evoked potentials in children with learning disabilities. *Journal of the American Academy of Audiology, 13,* 367–382.

Recanzone, G. H., Schreiner, C. E., & Merzenich, M. M. (1993). Plasticity in the frequency representation of primary auditory cortex following discrimination training in adult owl monkeys. *Journal of Neuroscience, 13,* 87–103.

Riccio, C. A., Hynd, G. W., Cohen, M. J., Hall, J., & Molt, L. (1994). Comorbidity of central auditory processing disorder and attention-deficit hyperactivity disorder. *Journal of the American Academy of Child and Adolescent Psychiatry, 33,* 849–857.

Richardson, U., Thomson, J., Scott, S., & Goswami, U. (2004). Auditory processing skills and phonological representation in dyslexic children. *Dyslexia, 10,* 215–233.

Ries, P. W. (1994). *Prevalence and characteristics of persons with hearing trouble: United States.* National Center for Health Statistics, *Vital Statistics, 24,* 188.

Robertson, D., & Irvine, D. R. F. (1989). Plasticity of frequency organization in auditory cortex of guinea pigs with partial unilateral deafness. *Journal of Comparative Neurology, 282,* 456–471.

Robey, R., & Schulz, M. (1998). A model for conducting clinical-outcome research: An adaptation of the standard protocol for use in aphasiology. *Aphasiology, 12,* 787–810.

Ronald, K., & Roskelly, H. (1985, March). *Listening as an act of composing*. Paper presented at the Annual Meeting of the Conference on College Composition and Communication, Minneapolis, MN.

Rumbaugh, D. M., & Washburn, D. A. (1996). Attention and memory in relation to learning: A comparative adaptation perspective. In G. R. Lyon & N. A. Krasnegor (Eds.), *Attention, memory, and executive function* (pp. 199–220). Baltimore, MD: Paul H. Brookes.

Russo, N., Nicol, T., Zecker, S., Hayes, E., & Kraus, N. (2005). Auditory training improves neural timing in the human brainstem. *Behavioural Brain Research, 156,* 95–103.

Sackett, D., Straus, S., Richardson, W. S., Rosenberg, W., & Haynes, B. (2000). *Evidence-based medicine: how to practice and teach EBM*. London, UK: Churchill Livingstone.

Salvi, R. J., Lockwood, A. H., Frisina, R. D., Coad, M. L., Wack, D. S., & Frisina, D. R. (2002). PET imaging of the normal human auditory system: Responses to speech in quiet and in background noise. *Hearing Research, 170,* 96–106.

Sams, M., Aulanko, R., Hamalainen, M., Hari, R., Lounasmaa, O. V., Lu, S. T., & Simola, J. (1991). Seeing speech: Visual information from lip movements modifies activity in the human auditory cortex. *Neuroscience Letters, 127,* 141–145.

Samuels, S. J. (1987). Factors that influence listening and reading comprehension. In R. Horowitz & S.J. Samuels (Eds.), *Comprehending oral and written language* (pp. 295–325). San Diego, CA: Academic Press.

Schnupp, J., Nelken, I., & King, A. (2011). *Auditory neuroscience: Making sense of sound*. Cambridge, MA: MIT Press.

Schochat, E., Musiek, F. E., Alonso, R., & Ogata, J. (2010). Effect of auditory training on the middle latency response in children with (central) auditory processing disorder. *Brazilian Journal of Medical and Biological Research, 43,* 777–785.

Schow, R. L., & Chermak, G. D. (1999). Implications from factor analysis for central auditory processing disorders. *American Journal of Audiology 8,* 137–142.

Schow, R. L., Seikel, J. A., Chermak, G. D., & Berent, M. (2000). Central auditory processes and test measures: ASHA 1996 revisited. *American Journal of Audiology, 9,* 63–68.

Schulte, M., Knief, A., Seither-Preisler, A., & Pantev, C. (2002). Different modes of pitch perception and learning-induced neuronal plasticity of the human auditory cortex. *Neural Plasticity, 9,* 161–175.

Schuman, E. M., & Madison, D. V. (1994). Locally distributed synaptic potentiation in the hippocampus. *Science, 263,* 532–536.

Schwaber, M. K., Garraghty, P. E., & Kaas, J. H. (1993). Neuroplasticity of the adult primate auditory cortex following cochlear hearing loss. *American Journal of Otology, 14,* 252–258.

Seki, S., & Eggermont, J. (2002). Changes in cat primary auditory cortex after minor-to-moderate pure-tone induced hearing loss. *Hearing Research, 173,* 172–186.

Sharma, M., Purdy, S., & Kelly, A. (2009). Comorbidity of auditory processing, language, and reading disorders. *Journal of Speech, Language, and Hearing Research, 52,* 706–722.

Sharma, M., Purdy, S., Newall, P., Wheldall, K., Beaman, R., & Dillon, H. (2006). Electrophysiological and behavioral evidence of auditory processing deficits in children with reading disorder. *Clinical Neurophysiology, 117,* 1130–1144.

Shore, S. (2005). Multisensory integration in the dorsal cochlear nucleus: Unit responses to acoustic and trigeminal ganglion stimulation. *European Journal of Neuroscience, 21,* 3334–3348.

Singer, W. (1995). Development and plasticity of cortical processing architectures. *Science, 270,* 758–764.

Skoe, E., & Kraus, N. (2012). A little goes a long way: how the adult brain is shaped by musical training in childhood. *Journal of Neuroscience, 32*, 11507–11510.

Smith, K. M., Mecoli, M. D., Altaye, M., Komlos, M., Maitra, R., Eaton, K. P., . . . Holland, S. K. (2011). Morphometric differences in the Heschl's gyrus of hearing impaired and normal hearing infants. *Cerebral Cortex, 21*, 991–998.

Snyder, R. L., Bonham, B. H., & Sinex. D. G. (2008). Acute changes in frequency responses of inferior colliculus central nucleus (ICC) neurons following progressively enlarged restricted spiral ganglion lesions. *Hearing Research, 246*, 59–78.

Song, J. H., Skoe, E., Wong, P. C., & Kraus, N. (2008). Plasticity in the adult human auditory brainstem following short-term linguistic training. *Journal of Cognitive Neuroscience, 20*(10), 1892–1902.

Spence, K. W., & Norris, E. B. (1950). Eyelid conditioning as a function of the intertrial interval. *Journal of Experimental Psychology, 40*, 716–720.

Stach, B. A., Spretnjak, M. L., & Jerger, J. (1990). The prevalence of central presbycusis in a clinical population. *Journal of the American Academy of Audiology, 1*(2), 109–115.

Starch, D. (1912). Periods of work in learning. *Journal of Educational Psychology, 3*, 209–213.

Stein, B. E., & Meredith, M. A. (1993). *The merging of the senses*. Cambridge, MA: MIT Press.

Strait, D., & Kraus, N. (2011). Can you hear me now? Musical training shapes functional brain networks for selective auditory attention and hearing speech in noise. *Frontiers in Psychology, 2*, 113.

Streitfeld, B. (1980). The fiber connections of the temporal lobe with emphasis on Rhesus monkey. *International Journal of Neuroscience, 11*, 51–71.

Swanson, H. L., & Cooney, J. B. (1991). Learning disabilities and memory. In B. Y. L. Wong (Ed.), *Learning about learning disabilities* (pp. 104–127). San Diego, CA: Academic Press.

Sweetow, R. W., & Henderson-Sabes, J. H. (2006). The need for and development of an adaptive listening and communication (LACE™) Program. *Journal of the American Academy of Audiology, 17*, 538–558.

Syka, J. (2002). Plastic changes in the central auditory system after hearing loss, restoration of function and during learning, *Physiology Review, 82*, 601–636

Tallal, P., Miller, S., Bedi, G., Byma, G., Wang, X., Nagarajan, . . . Merzenich, M. M. (1996). Language comprehension in language-learning impaired children improved with acoustically modified speech. *Science, 271*, 81–84.

Thai-Van, H., Veuillet, E., Norena, A., Guiraud, J., & Collet, L. (2010)Plasticity of tonotopic maps inhumans: influence of hearing loss, hearing aids and cochlear implants. *Acta Otolaryngolica,130 (3)*, 333–337.

Thiebaut de Schotten, M., Urbanski, M., Duffau, H., Volle, E., Levy, R., Dubois, B., & Bartolomeo, P. (2005). Direct evidence for a parietal frontal pathway subserving spatial awareness in humans. *Science, 309*, 2226–2228.

Threlkeld, S. W., Hill, C. A., Rosen, G. D., & Fitch, R. H. (2009). Early acoustic discrimination experience ameliorates auditory processing deficits in male rats with cortical developmental disruption. *International Journal of Developmental Neuroscience, 27*, 321–328.

Tillery, K. L., Katz, J., & Keller, W. D. (2000). Effects of methylphenidate (Ritalin) on auditory performance in children with attention and auditory processing disorders. *Journal of Speech, Language, and Hearing Research, 43*, 893–901.

Tremblay, K. (2007). Training-related changes in the brain: Evidence from human auditory evoked potentials. *Seminars in Hearing, 28*, 120–132.

Tremblay, K., & Kraus, N. (2002). Auditory training induces asymmetrical changes in cortical neural activity. *Journal of Speech, Language, and Hearing Research, 45*, 564–572.

Tremblay, K., Kraus, N., Carrell, T., & McGee, T. (1997). Central auditory system plasticity: Generalization to novel stimulation following listening training. *Journal of the Acoustical Society of America, 102,* 3762–3773.

Tremblay, K., Kraus, N., & McGee, T. (1998). The time course of auditory perceptual learning: Neurophysiological changes during speech-sound training. *NeuroReport, 9,* 3557–3560.

Tremblay, K., Kraus, N., McGee, T., Ponton, C., & Otis, B. (2001). Central auditory plasticity: Changes in the N1-P2 complex after speech-sound training. *Ear and Hearing, 22*(2), 79–90.

Tremblay, K., Piskosz, M., & Sousa, P. (2003). Effects of age and age-related hearing loss on the neural representation of speech cues. *Clinical Neurophysiology, 114,* 1332–1343.

Ungerleider, L. G. (1995). Functional brain imaging studies of cortical mechanisms for memory. *Science, 270,* 769–775.

Warrier, C. M., Johnson, K. L., Hayes, E. A., Nicol, T., & Kraus, N. (2004). Learning impaired children exhibit timing deficits and training-related improvements in auditory cortical responses to speech in noise. *Experimental Brain Research, 157,* 431–441.

Weinberger, N., & Bakin, J. (1998) Learning induced physiological memory in the adult primary auditory cortex: Receptive field plasticity, model and mechanisms. *Audiology and Neuro-otology, 3,* 145–167.

Weinberger, N. M., & Diamond, D. M. (1987). Physiological plasticity in auditory cortex: Rapid induction by learning. *Progress in Neurobiology, 29,* 1–55.

Wible, B., Nicol, T., & Kraus, N. (2002). Abnormal neural encoding of repeated speech stimuli in noise in children with learning problems. *Clinical Neurophysiology, 113,* 485–494.

Wible, B., Nicol, T., & Kraus, N. (2005). Correlation between brainstem and cortical auditory processes in normal and language-impaired children. *Brain, 128,* 417–423.

Willott, J. F. (1996). Physiological plasticity in the auditory system and its possible relevance to hearing aid use, deprivation effects, and acclimatization. *Ear and Hearing, 17*(Suppl.), 66S–77S.

Willott, J. F. (1999). *Neurogerontology: Aging and the nervous system.* New York, NY: Springer.

Willott, J. F., Aitken, L. M., & McFadden, S. L. (1993). Plasticity of auditory cortex associated with sensorineural hearing loss in adult mice. *Journal of Comparative Neurology, 329,* 402–411.

Wong, C., Jin, J., Gunasekera, G., Abel, R., Lee, E., & Dhar, S. (2009). Aging and cortical mechanisms of speech perception in noise. *Neuropsychologia, 47,* 693–703.

Woods, D. L., & Clayworth, C. C. (1986). Age-related changes in human middle latency auditory evoked potentials. *Electroencephalography and Clinical Neurophysiology, 65,* 297–303.

Wright, B., Bowen, R., & Zecker, S. (2000). Nonlinguistic perceptual deficits associated with reading and language disorders. *Current Opinion in Neurobiology, 10,* 482–486.

Wright, B. A., Lombardino, L. J., King, W. N., Puranik, C. S., Leonard, C. M., & Merzenich, M. M. (1997). Deficits in auditory temporal and spectral resolution in language-impaired children. *Nature, 387,* 176–178.

Wright, T. M., Pelphrey, K. A., Allison, T., McKeown, M. J., & McCarthy, G. (2003). Polysensory interactions along lateral temporal regions evoked by audiovisual speech. *Cerebral Cortex, 13,* 1034–1043.

Zatorre, R. J. (2001). Neural specialization for tonal processing. *Annals of the New York Academy of Sciences, 930,* 193–210.

Zatorre, R. J., Belin, B., & Benhune, V. B. (2002). Structure and function of auditory cortex: music and speech. *Trends in Cognitive Sciences, 6,* 37–46.

CHAPTER 2

EVIDENCE-BASED PRACTICE AND TREATMENT EFFICACY

JANE T. PIMENTEL and ELLA INGLEBRET

Clinical decision making for audiologists and speech-language pathologists has been oriented historically toward providing the best quality service possible to meet the individual needs of specific clients. To ensure optimal service delivery, clinicians have built their professional expertise through both formal and informal education, as well as through experience. Educational programs in communication disorders equip clinicians with strong foundational knowledge in their respective fields (i.e., audiology, speech-language pathology), with exposure to a variety of clients to begin building their experiential base, and with theoretical and scientific background regarding expertise in a given topic area such as central auditory processing disorder (CAPD). Professionals traditionally take this foundation, pair it with continuing education opportunities, and build their clinical proficiency through formal and informal interactions and observations of clients' performance to influence future clinical decision making (Cox, 2005). Although very important, this approach alone no longer suffices. Rather, each clinician is responsible for determining the best course of action for a client based on this traditional approach *in combination with the current, best external scientific evidence along with client/family values* (American Speech-Language-Hearing Association [ASHA], 2005c; Robey, 2011).

Today's work environment has placed additional demands on professionals in both educational and medical settings to provide empirical evidence that the approaches used in service delivery result in the intended outcomes. To address the demands for increased accountability set forth by legal mandates, such as the Individuals with Disabilities Education Act (IDEA), and those of third-party payers, evidence-based practice (EBP) has become the cornerstone for decision making regarding client care. ASHA (2004c) especially highlights the need to apply principles of EBP to complex diagnostic categories like CAPD where heterogeneous clinical profiles and frequent comorbidity (e.g., attention deficit hyperactivity disorder, language impairment, learning disability) render differential diagnosis crucial to effective and efficient intervention.

The purpose of this chapter is to provide the background and principles of EBP in relation to CAPD. Examples illustrate how clinicians can utilize EBP in their clinical work. This chapter also elucidates the differences between treatment outcomes, treatment efficacy, treatment effectiveness, and cost/benefit or public policy research so the clinician can better determine the level of evidence available for a specific treatment approach. The reader is referred to other chapters in this Handbook for comprehensive reviews of the evidence in specific topic areas regarding CAPD. Finally, the importance of the clinician evaluating the treatment approach based on best evidence is emphasized.

Principles of Evidence-Based Practice

The most widely cited definition of evidence-based medicine (of which EBP has its origins) is that by Sackett, Richardson, and Rosenberg (1997): "Evidence based medicine is the conscientious, explicit and judicious use of current best evidence in making decisions about the care of individual patients" (p. 2). This definition implies a tripartite focus. First, the practitioner's clinical judgment comes into play with "conscientious, explicit and judicious" selection and use of particular practices. Second, "best evidence" suggests that practice is supported by high-quality, scientific research and, third, the "individual" patient's needs are considered. The American Speech-Language-Hearing Association (ASHA) has reframed these three components into a triad of clinical expertise, current best evidence, and client/family values. ASHA's position is that all three components converge for the best clinical decision making (ASHA, 2005c). Robey (2011) and Straus, Glasziou, Richardson, and Haynes (2010) proposed that the model be extended to include a fourth component that focuses on identification of each client's clinical characteristics and service delivery environment. For the purposes of the current discussion, this fourth component is addressed as part of the client/family values leg of the triad. Each of the three components delineated by ASHA are now further described.

Consideration of client/family values, perspectives, and needs forms one leg of the EBP triad. The ultimate goal of service delivery is "improving the lives of individuals with communication disorders in terms of sense-of-wellness and functional health through high-quality services that they consider important and valuable" (ASHA, 2004c, p. 7). This is best accomplished when the clinician carefully considers the disorder as it is framed by the background of the client and his or her family. The International Classification of Functioning, Disability, and Health (ICF) (World Health Organization, 2001), which has been integrated into ASHA's Scope of Practice for Audiology (2004a) and Speech-Language Pathology (2007), provides a useful framework to ensure that the client's situation is examined comprehensively and is inclusive of strengths, disorder characteristics, and service delivery options. Using the first domain of the ICF, the clinician examines body functions and structures (e.g., central auditory processing in a formal testing situation), as well as gathers information regarding the client's activity and participation in daily life (e.g., responding to verbal directions given by a parent at home or teacher in the classroom, understanding spoken language in noise). The second domain of the ICF involves examination of contextual factors, including those of either an environmental or personal nature. Environmental variables might include acoustic characteristics of a classroom space or availability of speech, language, and hearing services; whereas, personal factors include cultural and linguistic background, age, gender, and lifestyle. Underlying the ICF framework is the intent to identify both barriers and facilitators that can be addressed to achieve specific targeted outcomes in the client's specific circumstances.

Although all aspects of the ICF model are equally important to consider, personal factors related to cultural and linguistic diversity are highlighted here. Due to rapid shifts in demographics (U.S. Bureau of the Census, 2012), audiologists and speech-language pathologists are faced with greater cultural and linguistic diversity (CLD) in their clientele than ever before. ASHA (2011) advocates that professionals use approaches that respond to cultural diversity inclusive of "age, ability, ethnicity, experience, gender, gender identity, linguistic back-

ground, national origin, race, religion, sexual orientation, and socioeconomic status" (p. 1), as well as to linguistic variations associated with English language learners or dialectal variations. Consideration of these personal factors is very important in the context of CAPD, as it is possible to mistake characteristics associated with CLD for symptoms often associated with CAPD. For example, an English language learner may misunderstand messages or respond inconsistently to verbal directions, particularly when background noise is present, as a normal part of second language acquisition. These characteristics are also common to CAPD (ASHA, 2005a). As another example, individuals from some cultural backgrounds may pause for an extended period before responding to a communication partner's statement or question (Covarrubias, 2007; Wallace, Inglebret, & Friedlander, 1997), another behavior often observed in individuals with CAPD due to inherent temporal processing deficits (ASHA, 2005a). Consequently, IDEA's mandate to identify disorders using multiple measures in multiple contexts becomes particularly important for accurate diagnosis of CAPD for members of CLD populations.

Cultural and linguistic diversity carries additional implications for intervention. Inherent in the diverse values, beliefs, and norms associated with cultural background are variations in attitudes and preferences regarding particular treatment practices. Therefore, it is of paramount importance to actively involve each client and appropriate family members in determining which evidence-based practices will be included in the therapy plan. The client and family should continually have an active voice in evaluating the ongoing course of treatment to ensure that a "sense-of-wellness and functional health" (ASHA, 2004c, p. 7) for the individual with CAPD is consistently facilitated. To this end, it may also be appropriate to access a cultural informant who can assist with identifying culturally relevant materials and techniques that can be meaningfully integrated into functional situations (ASHA, 2004e; Davis & Banks, 2012). As an additional consideration, the clinician will need to determine the appropriate language(s) for intervention with English language learners.

Expertise of the clinical service provider forms the second leg of ASHA's EBP triad. Clinical expertise is dependent on the type of experience a clinician has with a certain clinical population, such as individuals with CAPD. Multiple variables factor into a clinician's experience, including years of experience, number of cases treated, and knowledge and skills from advanced training and self-study. For beginning clinicians, as well as those more experienced, it is imperative to have a theoretical model on which to base a treatment approach. For example, in the area of CAPD, a clinician may be interested in using a cognitive approach to assist a child in developing problem solving skills and to monitor and self-regulate message comprehension (Keith, 1999). This approach may be supported by a "top-down" theory that builds on the assumption that a child's language abilities and general knowledge can buttress a disordered auditory system. The approach based on this theory is considered metalinguistic or metacognitive in orientation (Chermak & Musiek, 1997). It is the responsibility of the clinician to understand the theory, including its possible shortcomings, and determine if it supports a particular approach for treatment and make decisions accord-

ingly. For example, the above treatment approach may be applicable to clients evidencing CAPD regardless of the hypothesized etiology for the disorder, a breakdown at the perceptual level for speech (i.e., speech-specific hypothesis) or a more general auditory impairment (i.e., general auditory hypothesis; Friel-Patti, 1999).

Independent of the treatment approach chosen, the prudent clinician also takes data to generate evidence pertaining to specific interventions. Professional education programs provide clinicians with data collection skills that are a valuable resource in clinical practice. A typical starting point is to collect data prior to initiation of an intervention, which serves as a baseline measure of targeted behavior. Data pertaining to the target behavior then continue to be collected regularly throughout intervention, culminating in collection of postintervention data. This practice-based evidence takes the clinician beyond minimal data collection to document increases in target behavior in a manner allowing the clinician to determine if the increase was due to the intervention itself or to other outside variables, such as maturation(Lemoncello & Fanning, 2011). One means to accomplish this is through collection of multiple baseline data (Bain & Dollaghan, 1991). Rather than collecting data that only pertains to the target behavior, the clinician also collects data for one or more behaviors in need of remediation but not targeted in intervention. These latter data then serve as control data. If similar increases are observed for both the target and control behaviors, then the evidence suggests that gains were not due specifically to the intervention. However, if the target data show more gains than the control data, the clinician can be more confident in saying that evidence exists indicating the gains were due to the intervention for that client.

The manner in which multiple baseline data is gathered can take on several forms; the above example represents one of a variety of single-subject research designs that are available to the clinical service provider (Byiers, Reichle, & Symons, 2012; Hayes, Barlow, & Nelson-Gray, 1999; Richards, Taylor, Ramasamy, & Richards, 1999). Practitioners may interject elements of systematic control into data collection by examining behaviors under intervention across settings, time periods, and individual subjects. Treatment may also be periodically withdrawn so that comparisons can be made between behaviors during intervention and nonintervention periods. When possible, a second observer, who is unfamiliar with the client, should review the behavioral records via audio- or videotape to establish interrater reliability and, thus, limit potential bias (Dollaghan, 2007). It should be noted that all of these approaches involve collection and analysis of descriptive data for only one client. Since the calculation of parametric statistics is inappropriate, the results do not allow for generalization of the findings to other clients. Thus, it will be necessary for the clinician to apply the principles of single-subject design to each client served.

Representing a particular strength, single-subject research designs provide a powerful tool for practitioners interested in examining functional outcomes associated with the ICF model (World Health Organization, 2001). For example, data can be gathered to examine outcomes of intervention involving socially important behaviors at home or in the community (e.g., participation in daily life activities). Data to document meaningful treatment outcomes also may include measures of generalization to activities critical to the client's success, such as academic performance in the classroom (Horner et al., 2005). By adopting multiple baseline data collection or other single-subject designs, clinicians compile their own evidence, enriching their experience, and hence, the *clinical expertise* leg of the evidence-based triad. This method of systematic data collection provides a means of documenting *treatment outcomes* to support practice-based evidence for a particular client, but does not determine if a treatment is efficacious.

When Is Treatment Efficacious?

A lack of agreed upon terminology in and across professions regarding efficacious treatment has resulted in some confusion and possible misinterpretation of evidence supporting treatments. Wertz and Katz (2004) wisely advised some "rules to live by" in regard to more precise definitions and uniform methods to conduct research and to evaluate the scientific literature. The terms most confusing are these: treatment outcome, treatment efficacy, and treatment effectiveness. First and foremost, these terms are not interchangeable as they are not synonyms. Second, the definitions provided by Robey and Schultz (1998), largely based on those proposed by the Office of Technology Assessment (OTA; 1978), provide consistency and mutual exclusivity of terms. In general, an *outcome* refers to any measurable change between two points in time; this can be positive or negative. For example, to measure an environmental modification outcome one might select a sample of school-aged children, or a single client, diagnosed with CAPD, document their classroom performance before treatment (i.e., pretreatment) with an outcome measure (e.g., listening behavior rating scale), apply the treatment (i.e., environmental modifications), and reevaluate performance posttreatment with the same outcome measure. If listening behavior improved in the classroom for the group, then a positive outcome has occurred. This outcome, however, does not document efficacy or effectiveness. This outcome indicates only that treatment is "active"; that is, something happened when the treatment was applied that resulted in the children's performance improving on the measurement. Based on the design of this sample study, improvement cannot be attributed exclusively to the treatment because there are no controls. If a similar study were conducted with methodological rigor and ideal conditions and the same positive outcomes were documented, then those findings would support the treatment as efficacious.

Demonstration of treatment *efficacy* requires that multiple conditions be met. The treatment protocol being tested must be clearly specified to allow for replication (i.e., treatment fidelity is demonstrated). Likewise, the population being examined must be clearly defined and the study subjects must represent that population; this allows for generalization of the findings to the population. Lastly, the conditions under which the study occurs are optimal (OTA, 1978). These ideal conditions include "ideal treatment candidates, ideally trained therapists, ideal dosage (intensity and duration of treatment), and ideal outcome measures" (Wertz & Katz, 2004, p. 231). As the treatment literature is reviewed in the area of

CAPD, it quickly becomes apparent that a limited number of studies meet these ideal criteria. Thus, treatment efficacy studies conducted with this rigor are necessary to inform the profession regarding whether a treatment can work under conditions more akin to a laboratory setting. It is important to stress that, given the ideal conditions required, efficacy studies do not indicate if a treatment does work under routine conditions, such as those confronted by clinicians across practice settings (Robey& Schultz, 1998). Nonetheless, if a treatment does not work under these "ideal" conditions, then it is doubtful that the treatment would work under "less ideal," real-world conditions. Therefore, the establishment of efficacy for our treatments is a critical phase of research in order to build our evidence. See Chapters 3 and 11 for reviews of auditory training efficacy studies.

Treatment *effectiveness* indicates that a treatment works under typical conditions (e.g., typical caseload, typical duration and intensity of treatment protocol) (Wertz & Katz, 2004). Studies of treatment effectiveness must occur after efficacy has been demonstrated for a given treatment. If a study demonstrates positive outcomes following a treatment applied in typical conditions but that same treatment is not yet established as efficacious, then the study can only say the treatment is active but cannot say the treatment is effective. Of course, this information is still valuable and serves to provide preliminary data for future studies.

Cost-benefit and public policy research is another aspect of EBP that is used when referring to treatment outcomes (Mullan, 2007). The term "treatment efficiency" is the terminology Wertz and Irwin use to denote research around the cost/benefit of a particular treatment (2001). They define efficiency as, "acting or producing effectively with a minimum of waste, expense, or unnecessary effort, essentially, exhibiting a high ratio of output to input" (p. 236). Cost-benefit studies regarding a particular treatment ideally occur after efficacy and effectiveness have been established. For example, issues of treatment "dosage" (intensity and/or duration) might be investigated to determine how much treatment is required to achieve the desired outcome.

Treatment, then, is efficacious when high quality studies, with adequate control, have documented positive outcomes. Recall, an "outcome" simply denotes any measurable change between two points in time but does not, by itself, imply controls, conditions or purpose of the measurement. It should be clear that the terms efficacy, effectiveness, and cost-benefit should not be used casually when referring to the treatment literature in CAPD. Understanding the appropriate use of the outcome terminology allows more accurate interpretation of the literature and professional communication. Similarly, when using an EBP framework, the term 'intervention' refers to the processes of prevention, screening, assessment, and/or treatment protocols targeting a disorder, in this case, CAPD (Robey, 2011).

Selection and Interpretation of the Literature

Perhaps the most considered leg of ASHA's EBP triad is the use of external scientific evidence, that is, the research literature available regarding the intervention for a particular clinical population. This literature search should go beyond traditional speech and hearing journals (e.g., *American Journal of Audiology*) to relevant journals in related areas (e.g., *Journal of Neuroscience*). Searching for the most pertinent literature and interpreting its relevance for a given case can present a daunting task to a clinician, especially one with a large caseload. Developing an appropriate clinical question and having a method for determining the quality of the literature will make this task more efficient and clinically applicable. Figure 2–1 illustrates the steps involved in such a search. Each of these steps is discussed in the following sections.

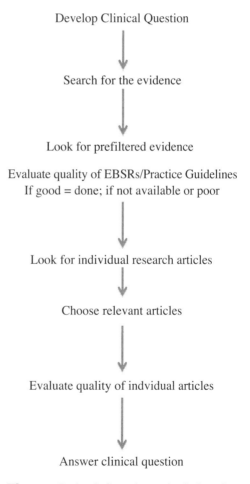

Develop Clinical Question

↓

Search for the evidence

↓

Look for prefiltered evidence

↓

Evaluate quality of EBSRs/Practice Guidelines
If good = done; if not available or poor

↓

Look for individual research articles

↓

Choose relevant articles

↓

Evaluate quality of indvidual articles

↓

Answer clinical question

Figure 2–1. A flowchart depicting the steps involved with finding and evaluating literature for evidence-based practice.

Guiding the Scientific Literature Quest

In order to seek the evidence specifically related to a given client and intervention, it is first necessary to frame an answerable clinical question to guide the search. According to ASHA (2005d), PICO is one accepted approach to developing a question. PICO stands for "population, intervention, comparison, and outcome." A relevant example follows: the population is children with CAPD; the intervention of interest is auditory training; the comparison approach is auditory integration training; and the intended outcome would be improved central auditory processing skills as measured through behavioral tests and electrophysiological procedures. Therefore, the clinical question might read: "Does auditory training result in better central auditory processing skills as compared with auditory integration training for children with CAPD?"

The next step is to operationalize terminology included in the question. Mullen (2010) pointed out that precise definitions used to refer to disorder types, such as CAPD, are necessary to determine which research literature is pertinent to a specific clinical question. In addition, intervention approaches included in the question will need to be described, again to ensure alignment between the research literature examined and the intervention of interest. In the example question, this would include distinguishing "auditory training" from "auditory integration training." At this point clinicians can access clinical practice documents and guidelines for CAPD developed by ASHA (2005a, 2005b) and more recently by the American Academy of Audiology (2010a) to locate information about the definition of CAPD and auditory training. Clinicians can also access position statements on auditory integration training (AIT) from ASHA (2004) and AAA (2010b) to clarify distinctions between auditory training and AIT.

It is recognized that the question developed largely depends on the level of functioning targeted with a client and that, indeed, often a combination of treatment approaches may be utilized and multiple levels of functioning may be targeted and outcomes measured concurrently. This would simply result in guiding separate literature searches with different clinical questions. In the example above, the clinical question guides the clinician in finding the literature regarding outcomes when the auditory impairment itself is targeted. Certainly it would also be appropriate to search literature regarding interventions targeting the functional activities of the child (e.g., use of FM systems to increase academic performance in the classroom) and the environment itself (e.g., acoustic considerations in the classroom). These considerations are consistent with the International Classification of Functioning, Disability, and Health framework (ICF; WHO, 2001).

Searching For The Evidence

Clinicians are being pressed to critically evaluate the scientific literature to determine both the quality of the experimental design (Mullan, 2007; Robey & Schultz, 1998) and the cumulative level of evidence (Cox, 2005; Reilly, Douglas & Oates, 2004) available to support their assessment and treatment decisions. The first challenge for the clinician in all service delivery settings is to access this literature in an efficient and meaningful manner to determine best practices. Understandably, clinicians may be concerned regarding additional burdens placed on an already stressed caseload. Barriers to clinicians include limited time to search for the evidence, limited search skills and limited access to the experimental evidence (Choi, 2005; Reilly, Douglas & Oates, 2004; Worrall & Bennett, 2001; Zipoli & Kennedy, 2005). Despite these challenges, the astute clinician knows that by equipping oneself with knowledge regarding the most valid and reliable assessment tools and the treatments most likely to work will ultimately aid all involved through better intervention efforts.

Finding the Relevant Literature

A number of search engines and databases are available to search from any Internet connection. Google Scholar (http://scholar.google.com/), for example, provides easy access to multiple types of scholarly publications; however, critical content may be omitted and searches reveal inconsistent results (Jacso, 2005). Internet search engines such as Google and Bing access about one billion documents. Although that sounds like a huge amount, consider that the part of the web that Internet search engines do not access has nearly 550 billion documents—this is termed the "Invisible Web" (Devine & Effer-Sider, 2004; Pimentel & Munson, 2004). Two of the reasons Internet search engines cannot get to the Invisible Web is: (a) login authorization is required or (b) the information is in databases.

Two public domain databases most pertinent to speech-language pathology and audiology are PubMed and ERIC. PubMed is provided free of charge from the National Library of Medicine. It provides access to bibliographic information in the field of medicine, nursing, dentistry, veterinary medicine, the health care system and the preclinical sciences. Bibliographic citations and author abstracts are drawn from more than 4,800 peer-reviewed biomedical journals published in the United States and abroad. PubMed (http://www.nlm.nih.gov) contains links for a few, free full-text journal articles. ERIC (http://www.eric.ed.gov) is provided free from the Education Resources Information Center, which is sponsored by the U.S. Department of Education. This database includes journal and non-journal education literature of more than 1.1 million citations going back to 1966. Both PubMed and ERIC databases are relevant to the area of CAPD as pertinent literature is housed both in the medically oriented research and the educational research. Although helpful, all databases have limitations. To help counteract these limitations, clinicians should scan the references of relevant articles and bibliographies of current texts, such as this one, to provide key leads for their literature search.

Professional organizations, which require login authorization, also provide a quick means to search available literature in their sponsored journals; often providing links to other professional resources as well. The American Speech-Language-Hearing Association's (http://www.asha.org/default.htm) entire website is searchable for documents that can guide the clinician in utilizing best practices. For example, two relevant and recent documents are the position statement (ASHA, 2005b) and accompanying technical report on CAPD (ASHA, 2005a). The position statement clearly defines CAPD, the primary role of the audiologist as the diagnostician, and the interdisciplinary nature of intervention utilizing the skills of the speech-language pathologist. The technical report provides a valuable resource for the clinician regarding appropriate terminology to use in a search for evidence. It also provides a theoretical framework for the disorder and guides the clinician in selecting assessment and treatment approaches. Reports such as these serve to inform and update the clinician regarding best practices. From these types of documents, then, the clinician can better develop a clinical question. In addition, clinicians can capitalize on valuable resources in the EBP section of the ASHA website (http://www.asha.org/members/ebp/) including ASHA-sponsored evidence-based systematic reviews (EBSRs; e.g., Fey et al., 2011), evidence maps and a compendium of links to other prefiltered evidence and practice guidelines. For example, ASHA's National Center of Evidence-Based Practice in Communication Disorders (N-CEP) staff search 28 electronic databases (e.g., Cochrane Library, HighWire Press, Neuroscience Abstracts) to compile best evidence made available in the compendium. Furthermore, the creation of evidence maps provides a "one-stop shop" for the clinician specific to populations and disorders. Unfortunately, there is not currently a map for CAPD but ASHA continues to add to this resource.In regard to EBSRs, the reader may wish to read Bellis, Chermak, Weihing, and Musiek (2012) who highlighted shortcomings of systematic searches that fail to take into consideration a number of aspects elaborated below. Similarly, The American Academy of Audiology (AAA) provides members with search capability on their Internet site. Documents and positions of the association can be accessed, including Guidelines for the Diagnosis, Treatment, and Management of Children and Adults with CAPD (AAA, 2010a). This document provides a comprehensive review of the research literature and analysis of levels of evidence based on types of research design. In addition, the PubMed database can be easily accessed from the AAA site to search for relevant articles indexed from the *Journal of the American Academy of Audiology (JAAA)*.

Another benefit of belonging to professional organizations is the ability to easily access the full-text of the most prestigious journals in the field. ASHA provides online access dating back to 1990 for the *Journal of Speech-Language-Hearing Research (JSLHR), American Journal of Audiology (AJA), American Journal of Speech-Language Pathology (AJSLP)*, and *Language, Speech, and Hearing Services in the Schools (LSHSS)*. Given the interdisciplinary nature of CAPD, searching all of these journals for pertinent literature is appropriate. Specific to audiologists, The AAA offers a similar benefit, again back to 1990, to access the full text of its journal (*JAAA*).

Another useful database supported and maintained by our Australian colleagues is SpeechBite (http://www.speechbite.com). This is a free access, searchable database for scientific articles based on selecting variables such as population, intervention, age, service delivery setting, and experimental design. Users may select as many or as few variables to search as desired. For instance, when searching for "auditory processing" treatment articles,greater success was achieved placing the quoted terms in the key word box than indicating search variables.

Developing and adding to a list of key words to use in database searching facilitates an efficient search. The clinical question and the clinician's expertise about CAPD direct key word selection. Key words in the area of CAPD may include: central auditory processing, central auditory nervous system, aural rehabilitation, auditory processing, auditory evoked potentials, auditory perceptual disorders, auditory training, acoustic signal enhancement, metacognitive, cognitive, and language strategies. As literature searches become routine to support best practices, key word lists should be kept, expanded, and drawn upon for future searches. It is also important to note what key words did not aid a search for a particular database (Garrard, 2011). In addition, noting the database search dates (e.g., 2006–2010) will allow for a more narrow, repeated search in the future as more literature becomes available in the speech/hearing and neuroscience fields.

Regardless of the database searched and the key words used, it is important to employ search strategies to aid efficiency. These strategies include the appropriate use of Boolean operators and knowing the database terminology. Boolean operators allow the searcher to combine words or phrases in specific ways by the appropriate use of the words AND, OR, and NOT. "AND" should be used to narrow your search as AND requires that all words be present in the retrieved articles (e.g., metacognitive AND metalinguistic). Alternatively, OR is used to broaden a search because it allows any of the words to be present in the article; this is especially helpful in the case of synonyms (e.g., central auditory processing disorder OR auditory processing disorder). The use of the term NOT allows the searcher to exclude terms; that is, NOT requires that the chosen word is not present in any of the retrieved articles (e.g., NOT auditory integration). It is

suggested that NOT be used cautiously as it can eliminate relevant articles from the search.

Phrase searching and truncation are two other useful strategies to enlist. Phrase searching keeps words together as a phrase via the use of quotation marks around the phrase (e.g., "best practices"). If a phrase is used without quotations, most databases will assume the Boolean "and" between words; thus, an article may be retrieved that has all the words in your phrase but not necessarily together. For example, if *auditory processing* without quotes is used, all articles that include the word *auditory* or the word *processing* will be revealed. Truncation allows a search for words beginning with specific characters. Many databases use an asterisk (*) to truncate. For example, practic* retrieves practice, practices, practicing, etc. (Pimentel & Munson, 2004). Truncating can be helpful to speed up your search; however, it is not advisable to truncate short words as too many possibilities exist and your search will become unwieldy. For example, hear* retrieves hear, hearing, heart, hearse, heard, and so on.

As mentioned previously, each database has its specific terminology. The terms for PubMed may well differ from the terms used to search ERIC. The appropriate keywords for a given database can be determined via a key word search. Also, try searching the thesaurus or the MeSH headings index (PubMed) for better words or phrases, or use a different combination of words. Lastly, correct spelling does matter as databases do not spell check; thus, you could end up with no results due to a misspelled word! Quite a bit of literature is available on CAPD regarding description and assessment; however, the same is not true of the treatment literature. Because of this, the search key terms and phrases often need to be expanded beyond the original clinical question to find the relevant literature.

As the search is underway, the databases will provide article abstracts to review. Abstracts provide windows to screen the article and determine if it is relevant to your clinical question. Searching the Internet, the databases, and the professional organizations, results in a number of abstracts regarding possibly relevant literature. It is important to take the time to read the abstracts prior to accessing the full text, as titles can be misleading. For example, a search of PubMed revealed an article entitled "The clinical management of perceptual skills disorders in a primary care practice" (Rosner & Rosner, 1986). When examining the abstract it was clear that this article pertained to visual and not auditory perception.

Once the selection of relevant articles has been made, they need to be accessed. Some relevant papers and journal articles are available full text via the Internet search. As mentioned previously, this is the case with ASHA and AAA journals accessed from the organizations' websites. PubMed and ERIC occasionally provide free access to full text for their references. Otherwise, clinicians can: (a) request articles through their employer, as many hospitals and school districts maintain library services, (b) utilize area community colleges and universities, as many institutes of higher education are open to the public for on-site use, and (c) purchase full-text articles through online resources such as http://www.ingentaconnect.com/

As was previously discussed, the EBP triad includes not only the scientific literature but also clinician expertise and client/family values. In searching for the evidence, it is wise to consult professional writings by experts in the field typically in the form of textbooks and clinical tutorials in periodicals (e.g., *Seminars in Hearing* [2002]) that focused on management of CAPD. This body of professional literature is extremely helpful in building the clinician's expertise, in pointing out relevant research literature and in providing references. However, a caution is in order in that non-peer-reviewed texts should not be used as the sole basis for clinical decision making (ASHA, 2004d), and clinical tutorials, while helpful in learning how to do the job of providing services better (Cox, 2005), do not evaluate a treatment approach for efficacy or effectiveness.

Evaluating the Evidence

Not all literature is created equal: The quality of the research design, data collection tools and procedures, outcome measures and their analyses are variable. Therefore, once the clinician has accessed the relevant literature, judgments must be made regarding the value of the literature (ASHA, 2005c). Professional literature, in most cases, is trustworthy based on the peer-review process and codes of ethics that guides our professions. Nonetheless, even quality literature deserves various rankings of worthiness, which is dependent on a number of factors.

ASHA has recognized the need for a common EBP framework to guide speech-language pathologists and audiologists in evaluating research evidence. In 2005, ASHA's Advisory Committee on Evidence-Based Practice (ACEBP) was formed and began partnering with the

National Center for Evidence-Based Practice in Communication Disorders (N-CEP) to examine existing EBP frameworks (Mullen, 2007). They found a multitude of research design hierarchies available to use in assigning a level of quality. However, problems in adopting existing frameworks were identified. First, a preponderance of existing systems focused on hierarchies of research design without quality indicators to use in discriminating high from low quality studies conducted using the same research designs. As Dollaghan (2007) noted, "studies with highly ranked designs can yield invalid or unimportant evidence just as studies with less highly ranked designs can provide crucial evidence" (p. 6). Secondly, the EBP frameworks grew out of a medical model focused on large group epidemiologic and treatment studies whose findings reflect "average" behavior that may not be applicable in the treatment of specific individuals (AAA, 2010a). In fact, in many EBP frameworks, single-subject designs are not considered to be a source of evidence. In the fields of speech-language pathology and audiology, single-subject design is considered an important source of evidence as it provides in-depth investigation of individual behavior, particularly for low prevalence communication disorders (AAA, 2010a; Mullen, 2007). Based on limited applicability of existing frameworks to our professions, ASHA developed its own levels of evidence (LOE) system (Mullen, 2007). The ASHA LOE system is implemented using four steps: (1) evaluate the quality of individual studies related to the clinical question, (2) identify the research stage associated with individual studies, (3) assess the quality of each study in relation to the research stage represented, and (4) synthesize the findings pertaining to a specific clinical question. Each of these steps is described in more detail.

Step 1: Evaluating Quality of Individual Studies

ASHA's LOE system (2007) focuses on eight explicit indicators to use when evaluating the quality of available evidence addressing a specific clinical question. These indicators include: (1) research design, (2) blinding, (3) sampling, (4) subjects, (5) outcomes, (6) significance, (7) precision, and (8) intention to treat (for clinical trials only). Each study is examined to determine the extent to which the indicators are represented. A description of each indicator follows.

Research Design

Evaluation of research evidence begins with identification of the research design used in a particular study. The intent underlying the evaluation of research design is to increase certainty that the research evidence accurately represents the targeted phenomena and that it is "objective" (Dollaghan, 2007). ASHA's LOE system (Mullen, 2007) involves five levels of research design that are listed in order of ranking, from highest to lowest: (1) controlled trial, (2) cohort study, (3) single-subject design OR case control study, (4) cross-sectional study OR case series, and (5) case study. Clinicians may find it helpful to refer to the EBP glossary developed by ASHA (ASHA, 2012) where definitions of specific research design terminology and other related concepts are provided. The order of the above listing is based on the assumption that the first research design, controlled trial, is the least likely to be influenced by measurement error and unintended or uncontrolled variables, whereas evidence derived from research designs of lesser ranking, such as a case study without controls, has the greatest potential for being influenced by confounding variables. Currently, the majority (but not all) of the literature in CAPD would receive a ranking of 2, 3, 4, or 5 (AAA, 2010a). However, as previously stated, it is important to go beyond a ranking of research design to account for multiple factors indicative of the quality of a study.

Blinding

As the literature is reviewed for quality of evidence, investigator subjectivity and possible bias should be considered. Ideally, subjectivity is avoided by conducting blind studies in which all involved with the study, including the assessors and the subjects themselves, are unaware of information that could bias the results (ASHA, 2004d; Dollaghan, 2007). Understandably, it is difficult if not impossible to conduct behavioral studies with complete blinding, but steps can be taken to minimize the tendency toward bias and studies should be evaluated regarding their rigor in controlling this variable. As clinicians read research articles, they should note who measured the treatment effects as it should be someone without knowledge of treatment assignments. Studies in which assessors are blinded receive a higher ranking than studies where no blinding is reported.

Sampling

The quality of research is largely dictated by the control demonstrated in its implementation. Experimental control refers to the ability to attribute the effects of an intervention to the intervention itself and

not to other factors. The best method to obtain control is via random assignment of subjects to treatment and no treatment groups. In ASHA's LOE system (Mullen, 2007), studies that use random sampling are ranked higher than studies using convenience or opportunistic samples. Adequacy in describing the sampling procedure also is considered.

Subjects

Detailed description of research subjects allows the practitioner to determine if the subject characteristics align with the group(s) identified in the clinical question. Criteria for inclusion and/or exclusion of subjects are generally provided. When comparisons are made between groups, enough information should be provided to ensure that relevant characteristics are comparable across groups at the outset of the study. Studies that adequately describe subjects and for which groups are judged to be comparable at baseline are ranked higher than studies that do not supply this information or include insufficient subject descriptions (Mullen, 2007). When a disorder type, such as CAPD, is a key characteristic of a target group, the subject selection criteria would be expected to involve accepted diagnostic methods and criteria specific to CAPD, as identified in clinical practice guidelines (AAA, 2010a; ASHA, 2005a; 2005b).

Outcome Measures

Outcome measures used in a study should validly and reliably represent the performance of target behaviors identified in the clinical question (Mullen, 2007). In general, standardized tests can provide a means to ensure a high level of measurement validity at the outset of a study; however, these tools are not intended for administration multiple times over a short period of time and often do not reflect small changes in behavior that might be targeted in a study (Dollaghan, 2007). Criterion-referenced measures provide a means to examine specific target behaviors and are often used in treatment outcomes research; however, fidelity of implementation is a concern when using criterion-referenced measures (Kaderavek & Justice, 2010). To reduce measurement error, studies should be designed to include procedures, such as training of the implementers, establishing interexaminer reliability, and collecting behavioral data at multiple points over time (Dollaghan, 2007).

It should also be considered that with technological advances, CAPD research has increasingly made use of electrophysiological procedures to accompany behavioral measures of central auditory processing. Neurobiological evidence of "structural reorganization and functional improvement of auditory skills, as well as neurophysiological representation of acoustic stimuli following auditory training" (Bellis, Chermak, Weihing, & Musiek, 2012, p. 384) have been reported (see, for example, Tremblay & Kraus, 2002 and Schochat, Musiek, Alonso, & Ogata, 2010). Furthermore, Chermak and Musiek (2011) suggested that common patterns found in central auditory nervous system (CANS) lesion studies for adults or children with CAPD "approximate a 'gold standard' for CAPD in children with no identifiable lesion" (p. 247). Results of electrophysiological measures are less likely to be influenced by confounding variables and lead to a higher level of validity, "objectivity" and certainty that change or differences associated with a particular intervention are "real." Thus, outcome measures of an electrophysiological nature contribute to higher evidence quality. See Chapters 3 and 7 in this volume and Chapters 7, 11, and 17 in Volume 1 of the Handbook.

Significance

The practitioner is ultimately concerned with the clinical significance of research results. Bain and Dollaghan (1991) have operationalized the concept of clinical significance to include three aspects of observed change: (a) it results from clinical services and not from extraneous variables, (b) it is real, reliable, and not random, and (c) it is important and not trivial. As was pointed out previously, researchers use experimental control to reduce the effects of extraneous variables, so the focus of this section will be on the second two components of clinical significance: determining whether research findings represent real phenomena, versus random occurrences, and measuring the importance of the results to clinical practice.

To measure whether or not observed change is real, scientific research papers have traditionally reported results of data analysis in relation to their statistical significance (Goldstein, 2005). Measures of statistical significance allow the researcher to determine whether or not the original null hypothesis can be rejected and, thus, rule out the possibility that the results were due to chance. Statistical procedures used vary depending on whether or not basic criteria regarding the target population(s) are met. When it can be assumed that a normal distribution exists, interval or ratio data is involved, and the sample size is large, parametric statistics can be calculated.

When these assumptions cannot be met, nonparametric statistics are often calculated (Shiavetti, Metz, & Orlikoff, 2011). Meline (2005) points out, however, that the relevance of either statistical analysis to actual clinical practice can be limited, as statistical significance is largely influenced by sample size. Statistically significant differences between groups also may be found when the observed behavior for both groups falls within a normal range. Limitations in applicability of statistical significance to clinical practice have led the fields of audiology and speech-language pathology, as well as other health and education related fields, to look for other means to systematically identify patterns in data pertaining to service delivery outcomes (Meline & Wang, 2004). As a result, measures of practical significance are now more commonly reported in research articles.

Kazdin (1999) differentiated between statistical significance and, what he termed, clinical significance defined as "the practical or applied value or importance of the effect of the intervention, that is, whether the intervention makes any real (e.g., genuine, palpable, practical, noticeable) difference in everyday life to the clients or to others with whom the client interacts" (p. 332). Noting the relevance of a study's findings to the particular client or patient group and clinical situation is important. The closer the subjects studied are to the characteristics of those being served, the more relevant the evidence. In addition, Bothe and Richardson (2011) identified the need to consider *personal significance*, which is different from clinical significance in the perspective represented.

Clinical significance reflects the clinician's perspective, whereas personal significance represents the client's perspective on the extent of improvement in his or her activities and participation in daily life contexts. Measurement of personal significance is based on use of tools developed to focus on each individual client's condition and situation (Franic & Bothe, 2008). In fact, a movement to include patient reported outcomes (PROs) is gaining momentum as an important means of documenting meaningful change in addition to the more traditional reporting by the clinician of the patient's progress (U.S. Food and Drug Administration, 2009, p. 2). For children with CAPD, this includes both the child's and parent's impressions of change based on intervention. In addition to relevance reflected through clinical and personal significance, the practical implications of applying the research findings to clinical practice need to be addressed.

Precision

Practical significance reflects the importance or meaningfulness of research findings to clinical outcomes (Meline & Paradiso, 2003; Meline & Schmitt, 1997). Effect sizes are the calculated measures used to determine the extent of practical significance or precision for particular results. An effect size represents the magnitude of difference or correlation between data sets independent of the sample size (Cohen, 1988). Various metrics are used to calculate effect sizes depending on the research design used (Meline & Wang, 2004). Practitioners should expect effect sizes to be reported in research articles and should also look for interpretation of the effect sizes (Bothe & Richardson, 2011; Goldstein, 2005). For example, based on Lipsey and Wilson's (1993) meta-analyses of 302 studies of psychological, educational, and behavioral treatments, general guidelines exist for interpreting effect size (ES) for one type of metric, Cohen's d (i.e., ES greater than or equal to 0.67 is meaningful, ES equal to 0.50 may be meaningful, ES less than or equal to 0.30 is not meaningful). However, Cohen cautions that degree of magnitude of effect sizes are discipline specific (Cohen, 1988). Since the fields of audiology and speech-language pathology have only recently begun including calculation of effect sizes as a part of research reporting, discipline-specific interpretation standards have not yet been developed (Goldstein, 2005).

Effect size calculations are increasingly being seen in research utilizing single-subject designs (Byiers et al., 2012). According to Byiers and colleagues, the most common ES metric used for single-subject designs is the percentage of nonoverlapping data (PND). Basically, PND calculates the percent of intervention phase B data above the highest baseline data point in phase A; that is, the number of data points that fall above (or below) baseline is tallied and divided by the total number of intervention data points (Byiers et al., 2012).

Practitioners also should expect to find the confidence intervals for the effect sizes reported in research articles (ASHA, 2004d; Bothe & Richardson, 2011). Confidence intervals represent a range of values in both positive and negative directions within which the true effect size is likely to occur (Guyatt, Rennie, Meade, & Cook, 2008; Straus et al., 2010). Focusing on a range of possible values allows the researcher to examine precision of the effect size and possible measurement error (Meline & Schmitt, 1997). A commonly used confidence interval is 95%. This means that in 95 out of 100 instances the true effect size will fall within the specified range of values. Examination of confidence intervals aids the practitioner in determining the strength of the difference between outcomes for treatment types or for treatment versus control groups. For example, when the confidence interval surrounding the calculated effect size is small, it is considered a more precise representation of the true effect size so that a stronger argument can be made for applicability of the clinical practice to a broader population.

Calculation of effect sizes and confidence intervals is dependent on agreement as to what constitutes normal versus pathological behavior. While some argue that damage to the brain in adults may not be identical to CANS dysfunction seen in developmental disorders involving the CANS in children, the sensitivity and specificity of a number of behavioral tests and electrophysiological measures of the CANS have been documented in patients with confirmed lesions of the CANS and an "accumulating body of research supports the presence of deficit patterns in central auditory test battery performance in children that mirror those of lesion studies in populations with circumscribed disorders of the CANS" (AAA, 2010, p. 15). Audiologists have a sensitive and specific battery of behavioral tests and electrophysiological procedures capable of detecting central auditory dysfunction across populations, notwithstanding variability due to plasticity, age, etiology, and other factors (AAA, 2010).

Intention to Treat

An analysis of intention to treat is conducted only for controlled trials (ASHA, 2012; Mullen, 2007). This analysis involves examination of the extent to which all subjects are retained in their originally assigned groups. In controlled trials, participants may drop out, miss treatment sessions, or receive treatments other than that originally intended. Retention of data for all participants in their initially enrolled groups retains randomization and, thus, stronger research quality. In contrast, when data for some subjects are excluded, the study loses its original randomization resulting in a lower ranking.

Single-Subject Experimental Designs

The importance of single-subject experimental designs (SSEDs) in the evaluation of the evidence supporting our interventions in audiology and speech-language pathology should not be overlooked. In fact, as our field looks less at the research design and more at the quality of scientific rigor, SSEDs can be evaluated as critically as group studies. Byiers et al. (2012) presented a means of doing just this specific to EBP. In their tutorial, Byiers and colleagues presented criteria by the What Works Clearing House (WWCH) to assist researchers and clinicians in identifying interventions studied using an SSED as evidence-based (Kratochwill et al., 2010). Each of four criteria has descriptions to judge as meeting standards, not meeting standards, or meeting with reservations. These four criteria are: (1) independent variable(s), (2) dependent variable(s), (3) length of phases, and (4) replication of effect. According to the WWCH criteria, determining if a SSED qualifies as evidence-based involves three steps. First, it must have an adequate experimental design that meets the standards for the four criteria indicated. Second, there must be adequate visual analysis,

including a baseline with established stability, as evidenced by no improvement trend with a minimum of three data points in the preintervention phase and data inspection in other phases (e.g., treatment, withdrawal) for level, trend, and variability. Third, the treatment effect must be replicated either within or across subjects. More specifically, the WWCH panel recommends an intervention have a minimum of five supporting SSED studies by different researchers in different locations with a total minimum of 20 subjects to provide sufficient evidence. These are rigorous and well-defined criteria for evidence clinicians can believe in when it comes to SSEDs.

Byiers et al. (2012) also discussed the use of "pre-experimental" SSEDs—the AB design, which is particularly useful in generating clinical or practice-based evidence. This baseline (A) followed by intervention (B) design does not allow for experimental control, but does offer insight as to whether a treatment is active, and also provides preliminary objective data for the clinician and researcher (Kazdin, 2010).

Step 2: Identify the Research Stage Associated With Individual Studies

A variety of research designs are utilized in a progression of stages to answer different types of research questions. Mullen (2007) described a four-stage model, that is, I: exploratory, II: efficacy, III: effectiveness, and IV: policy, adapted from the work of Robey (2004). Stage I studies are largely exploratory in nature where researchers are seeking to determine if a treatment is active; that is, if there is any therapeutic effect and, if there is, the magnitude of the effect (Robey, 2004; Mullen, 2007). Stage I studies also can provide clinical insights leading to valuable hypotheses for research to move into Stage II and beyond (Cox, 2005). Stage I studies also build on previous findings by further establishing treatment protocols as well as reliability and validity of measurements, by finalizing operational definitions, and confirming the therapeutic effect and the amount of therapy required (optimal intensity and duration). Case studies, single-subject designs, and small sample size studies are appropriate for Stage I in this four-phase model. When these research parameters are well defined and the treatment protocols are well established, then Stage II research is conducted.

Stage II research involves the randomized clinical trial. Only at Stage II are the terms "trial" and "efficacy" used appropriately (Mullen, 2007; Robey, 2004). A clinical trial is characterized by large sample sizes and, through the control of variables, answers treatment efficacy questions. Robey and Schultz (1998) referred to treatment efficacy as defined by the Office of Technology Assessment (OTA, 1978) as "the probability of benefit to individuals in a defined population from a medical technology applied for a given medical problem under ideal conditions of use" (p. 16). The ideal condition implies control and is not meant to be mistaken for what clinicians can accomplish in their everyday, real-world settings. Nonetheless, it can be argued that if efficacy cannot be demonstrated for a treatment in ideal conditions (e.g., well-established and followed treatment protocols, reliable and valid measures, adequate treatment time, high quality treatment materials), then this same treatment cannot be expected to work in less than ideal conditions.

Stages III and IV studies seek to expand the therapeutic effect found in ideal conditions to day to day clinical practice (Mullen, 2007; Robey, 2004). The goal of Stage III studies is to document treatment effectiveness. Treatment effectiveness is defined by the Office of Technology Assessment (1978) as "the probability of benefit to individuals in a defined population from a medical technology applied for a given medical problem under average conditions of use" (p. 16). As indicated earlier, when using this model, efficacy must first be established prior to conducting effectiveness research. Finally, Stage IV studies seek to validate the treatments via cost/benefit analyses and expand the questions asked to those affecting regulations and policy (Mullen, 2007; Robey, 2004). The methodological rigor appropriate for these different phases will, to a large extent, dictate the level of evidence supported by a given study.

Step 3: Assess the Quality of Each Study in Relation to its Research Stage

After determining where a study falls on the continuum of stages (i.e., I, exploratory; II, efficacy; III, effectiveness; and IV, policy), quality indicators are applied. Ratings for each of the eight indicators (i.e., research design, blinding, sampling, subjects, outcomes, significance, precision, intention to treat) will vary depending on the associated research stage. For example, case studies in an exploratory stage would not be expected to involve the randomized control of a clinical trial, a very costly and time intensive process.

According to scoring methods developed for ASHA (Mullen, 2007), exploratory studies receive a maximum score of 7 as intention to treat would not be applied. A rating of 7 reflects "high quality," ratings of 5 or 6 reflect "good quality," and a rating of 4 or lower reflects "low" quality. Thus, quality of evidence is rated regardless of the stage of research. Other systems for rating the quality of studies using specific research designs are available. See for example, Robey (2011) and Dollaghan (2007).

Step 4: Synthesize Findings

The larger the corpus of studies supporting a specific intervention approach, the greater the strength of the evidence for that approach. As a search is completed, it is the cumulative evidence regarding the clinical question that bears weight. A formal example of a synthesis of research findings is a meta-analysis or a systematic review conducted on a given topic for a population. Lemoncello and Fanning (2011) referred to this as "prefiltered evidence." This level of information is emerging in the CAPD literature. For example, Sweetow and Palmer completed a systematic review of the evidence supporting auditory training in adults (2005) and Strong, Torgerson, Torgerson, and Hulme (2011) completed a meta-analysis regarding the effectiveness of Fast ForWord for language intervention. Fey et al. (2011) conducted a systematic review of research published between 1978 and 2008 examining auditory/language interventions for school-age children reported to have auditory processing disorders. Just as the evaluation of the quality of individual studies is warranted, evaluation of the quality of systematic reviews is recommended. Dol-laghan (2007) has developed a system for critically appraising a meta-analysis or systematic review of research evidence. Her system focuses on examining the transparency and explicitness of the procedures used. Examples of questions asked include: "Were clear and adequate criteria used to include and exclude studies from the analysis?" and "Were individual studies rated independently?" (p. 109). In addition, Baylor and Yorkston (2007) recommended evaluating the literature search in regard to where the authors looked and how they conducted the review. They also suggested evaluating the evidence based on what time span was covered in the review and when the review was published. Indeed, one limitation of a systematic review is that it may lag behind current trends. For example, the time elapsed between conducting a systematic review and its publication may be several years. Rapid changes in technology that increasingly allow for more "objective" neurophysiological measures of auditory processing may not be taken into account in systematic reviews of older literature. Lastly, the individual studies included in the review should be assessed for quality, and the conclusions the authors offer also need to be evaluated especially as related to an individual case. A careful and critical evaluation of Fey et al.'s systematic review is evident as represented by letters to the editor expressing differing views on terminology used and overall findings and conclusions (Bellis et al., 2011; Fey, Kamhi, & Richard, 2011).

It is also possible that a practitioner will develop a clinical question for which a review is not available. In this case, the individual studies found regarding a clinical question require examination to determine if there is a converging body of evidence coming together regarding a specific treatment. For example, in the CAPD literature, positive outcomes are being reported in the use of auditory training in adults and children as measured by psychophysical performance and neurophysiological responses to acoustic stimuli since 2008 (e.g., Alonso & Schochat, 2009; Millward, Hall, Ferguson, & Moore, 2011; Murphy & Schochat, 2011; Pantev & Herholz, 2011; Schochat et al., 2010; Strait & Kraus, 2011). Clearly, there is an emerging convergence of evidence in this area from more than one research lab; this begins to demonstrate independent confirmation.

What About "Expert" Opinion?

Conducting a search will often yield expert reports and links to other resources, such as monographs, rather than high quality peer-reviewed documents. These resources are helpful given the paucity of research evidence to support many of our treatment practices. When utilizing these resources, the clinician must determine how expert in the field of CAPD the "expert" is in order to pass judgment on the worthiness (i.e., validity) of the information. The individual clinician's acquired foundational knowledge is relevant here as both students and clinicians can utilize information from respected authorities on CAPD from texts, from exposure via continuing education, and from relying on respected colleagues in their fields for insight. Examples of "expert opinions" of high quality are two noteworthy reports. The expert opinions expressed in the so-called *Bruton* report from fourteen senior scientists and clinicians regarding the appropriate diagnosis of auditory processing disorders in school-aged children was published in

the *Journal of the American Academy of Audiology*, the peer-reviewed journal of the American Academy of Audiology, confirming the quality the "expertness" of the opinions expressed in this report. The second, more recent, example is the Clinical Practice Guidelines regarding intervention for children and adults with CAPD published by the American Academy of Audiology (AAA, 2010a). As clinicians become more familiar with the literature in CAPD, so too will the names of the respected authorities writing in the area.

Additional resources are available to aid the clinician in evaluating the literature, especially in regard to research articles. For example, Law et al. (1998) developed protocols to aid in the critical review of both quantitative and qualitative research articles. The protocols present a series of questions addressing the study's purpose, rationale, design, subjects, outcome measures, intervention, results, and conclusion to guide the clinician in the evaluation. These protocols, and accompanying guidelines, are available online at http://www.fhs.mcmaster.ca/rehab/ebp/. After examining the level of quality for indicators represented in a particular study, the stage of research where the study fits is identified (i.e., Stage I, II, III, or IV). Based on the stage of research represented, the study is given a quality rating as "high," "good," or "low" (see Mullen, 2007).

After evaluation of research evidence is completed, the clinician returns to the client/patient and family to present the evidence regarding treatment options to ensure the best practice for that particular client or patient. In this way, individuals with CAPD and their families are active participants in selecting from best practices in choosing the optimal course of action (ASHA, 2004c). Returning to the EBP triad, the client and family values, as well as clinician expertise, are considered along with the scientific evidence available to make the best treatment decision.

The clinician finally applies the evidence to his or her assessment and/or treatment plan. Importantly, it is the clinician's duty to evaluate the outcomes achieved in clinical work in light of the research evidence in the literature. This is considered the evaluation phase or follow-up component of evidence based practice (Cox, 2005). In evaluating the EBP approach, especially in the area of intervention, the clinician can apply a number of methodologies—from single-subject design to addressing social validation by gaining input from the clients themselves or significant others regarding the results of the treatment efforts (Schlosser & Raghavendra, 2004). Degree of success of the assessment/treatment plan is then reviewed and interpreted in order to either: (1) stay the course and apply the findings to future cases, or (2) make modifications to the assessment or treatment plan to achieve greater success. Either way, clinicians learn about the clinical applicability of the evidence and build their knowledge base for future application.

Summary

This chapter has presented information to take the clinician from a traditional approach regarding intervention to the more current approach of incorporating the available literature and client/patient and family values along with clinical expertise in practicing evidence-based,

clinical decision making. Clinicians can build expertise through critical evaluation of the literature followed up by changes in their practice based on the evidence. This follow-up includes documenting change through data collection methods (i.e., practice-based evidence) to determine if the external scientific evidence supporting a given assessment and/or treatment is realized in the service delivery setting. In this way, the clinician makes sound judgments regarding the value of the evidence for an individual client.

EBP requires a profession to become more deliberate and systematic in provision of the best assessment and treatment practices both in research and in clinical work. No doubt, applying the methodology of EBP will take some effort. This will be effort well expended on behalf of all clients with CAPD as clinicians become better informed, better equipped, and better at serving their clientele.

References

AAA (American Academy of Audiology). (2010a). *Guidelines for the diagnosis, treatment, and management of children and adults with central auditory processing disorder.* Retrieved from http://www.audiology.org/resources/document library/Documents/CAPD%20Guidelines%208-2010.pdf

AAA. (2010b). *Position statement: Auditory integration training (AIT).* Retrieved from http://www.audiology.org/resources/documentlibrary/Documents/AIT_Position%20Statement.pdf

Alonso, R., & Schochat, E. (2009). The efficacy of formal auditory training with (central) auditory processing disorder: Behavioural and electrophysiological evaluation. *Bra-*

zilian Journal of Otorhinolaryngology, 75, 726–732.

ASHA. (2004a). *Auditory integration training* [Position statement]. Retrieved from http://www.asha.org/docs/html/PS2004-00218.html

ASHA. (2004b). *Scope of practice in audiology*. Rockville, MD: Author.

ASHA. (2004c). *Report of the joint coordinating committee on evidence-based practice*. Rockville, MD: Author.

ASHA. (2004d). *Evidence-based practice in communication disorders: An introduction* [Technical report]. Retrieved from http://www.ash.org/members/deskref-journals/deskref/default

ASHA. (2004e). Knowledge and skills needed by speech-language pathologist and audiologists to provide culturally and linguistically appropriate services. *ASHA Supplement, 24*, 152–158.

ASHA (American Speech-Language-Hearing Association). (2005a). *(Central) auditory processing disorders*. Retrieved from http://www.asha.org/members/deskref-journals/deskref/default

ASHA. (2005b). *(Central) auditory processing disorders—the role of the audiologist* [Position statement]. Retrieved from http://www.asha.org/members/deskref-journals/deskref/default

ASHA. (2005c). *Evidence-based practice in communication disorders* [Position Statement]. Retrieved from http://www.asha.org/members /deskref-journals/deskref/default

ASHA. (2005d, October 28). *Introduction to evidence-based practice*. Retrieved from http://www.asha.org/members/ebp/

ASHA. (2007). *Scope of practice in speech-language pathology*. Rockville, MD: Author.

ASHA. (2011). *Cultural competence in professional service delivery* [Position statement]. Retrieved from http://www.asha.org/policy

ASHA. (2012). *Evidence-based practice glossary*. Retrieved from http://www.asha.org/members/ebp/Glossary.htm

Bain, B. A., & Dollaghan, C. A. (1991). The notion of clinically significant change. *Language, Speech, and Hearing Services in Schools, 22*, 264–270.

Baylor, C. R., & Yorkston, K. M. (2007).Using systematic reviews and practice guidelines: A how-to guide for clinicians. *Perspectives: Neurophysiology and Neurogenic Speech and Language Disorders, 17*, 6–10.

Bellis, T. J., Chermak, G. D., Weihing, J., & Musiek, F. E. (2012). Efficacy of auditory interventions for central auditory processing disorder: A response to Fey et al. (2011). *Language, Speech, and Hearing Services in Schools, 43*, 381–386.

Bothe, A. K., & Richardson, J. D. (2011). Statistical, practical, clinical, and personal significance: Definitions and applications in speech-language pathology. *American Journal of Speech-Language Pathology, 20*, 233–242.

Byiers, B. J., Reichle, J., & Symons, F. J. (2012). Single-subject experimental design for evidence-based practice. *American Journal of Speech-Language Pathology, 21*, 397–414.

Chambless, D. L., & Hollon, S. D. (1998). Defining empirically supported therapies. *Journal of Consulting and Clinical Psychology, 66*, 7–18.

Chermak, G. D., Hall, J. W., & Musiek, F. E. (1999). Differential diagnosis and management of central auditory processing disorder and attention deficit hyperactivity disorder. *Journal of the American Academy of Audiology, 10*, 289–303.

Chermak, G. D., & Musiek, F. E. (1997). *Central auditory processing disorders: New perspectives*. San Diego, CA: Singular.

Chermak, G. D., & Musiek, F. E. (2011). Neurological substrate of central auditory processing deficits in children. *Current Pediatric Reviews, 7*, 241–251.

Choi, D. M. (2005). *Evidence-based practice in speech-language pathology: Dysphagia treatment approaches*. (Unpublished master's research project). Washington State University, Spokane, WA.

Cohen, J. (1988). *Statistical power analysis for the behavioral sciences* (2nd ed.). Hillsdale, NJ: Erlbaum.

Covarrubias, P. (2007). (Un)biased in Western theory: Generative silence in American Indian communication. *Communication Monographs, 74,* 265–271.

Cox, R. M. (2005). Evidence-based practice in provision of amplification. *Journal of the American Academy of Audiology, 16,* 419–438.

Davis, P. N., & Banks, T. (2012). Intervention for multicultural and international clients with communication disorders. In D. E. Battle (Ed.), *Communication disorders in multicultural and international populations* (p. 279–295). St. Louis, MO: Elsevier.

Devine, J., & Egger-Sider (2004). Beyond Google: The invisible web in the academic library. *Journal of Academic Librarianship, 30,* 265–269.

Dollaghan, C. A. (2007). *The handbook of evidence-based practice in communication disorders.* Baltimore, MD: Paul H. Brookes.

Fey, M. E., Kamhi, A. C., & Richard, G. J. (2012). Auditory training for children with auditory processing disorder and language impairment: A response to Bellis, Chermak, Weihing, and Musiek. *Language, Speech, and Hearing Services in Schools, 43,* 387–392.

Fey, M. E., Richard, G. J., Geffner, D., Kamhi, A. G., Medwetsky, L., Paul, D., . . . R Schooling , T. (2011). Auditory processing disorder and auditory/language interventions: An evidence-based systematic review. *Language, Speech, and Hearing Services in the Schools, 42,* 246–264.

Franic, D. M., & Bothe, A. K. (2008). Psychometric evaluation of condition-specific instruments used to assess health-related quality of life, attitudes, and related constructs in stuttering. *American Journal of Speech-Language Pathology, 17,* 60–80.

Friel-Patti, S. (1999).Clinical decision-making in the assessment and intervention of central auditory processing disorders. *Language, Speech, and Hearing Services in Schools, 30,* 345–352.

Garrard, J. (2011). *Health sciences literature made easy: The matrix method* (3rd ed.). Sudbury, MA: Jones and Bartlett Learning.

Goldstein, B. A. (2005). From the editor. *Language, Speech, and Hearing Services in Schools, 36,* 91.

Gunnarson, A. D., & Finitzo, T. (1991). Conductive hearing loss during infancy: Effects on later auditory brain stem electrophysiology. *Journal of Speech and Hearing Research, 34,* 1207–1215.

Guyatt, G., Rennie, D., Meade, M., & Cook, D. (2008). *Users' guide to the medical literature: A manual for evidence-based clinical practice* (2nd ed.). Chicago, IL: American Medical Association.

Hayes, S. C., Barlow, D. H., & Nelson-Gray, R. O. (1999). *The scientist practitioner: Research and accountability in the age of managed care.* Boston, MA: Allyn & Bacon.

Horner, R. H., Carr, E. G., Halle, J., McGee, G., Odom, S., & Wolery, M. (2005). The use of single-subject research to identify evidence-based practice in special education. *Exceptional Children, 71,* 165–179.

Jacso, P. (2005). Google scholar: The pros and the cons. *Online Information Review, 29,* 208–214.

Jerger, J., & Musiek, F. (2000).Report of the consensus conference on the diagnosis of auditory processing disorders in school-aged children. *Journal of the American Academy of Audiology, 11,* 467–474.

Kadaravek, J. N., & Justice, L. M. (2010). Fidelity: An essential component of evidence-based practice in speech-language pathology. *American Journal of Speech-Language Pathology, 19,* 369–379.

Kazdin, A. E. (1999). The meanings and measurement of clinical significance. *Journal of Consulting and Clinical Psychology, 67,* 332–339.

Kazdin, A. E. (2010). *Single-case research designs: methods for clinical and applied settings.* (2nd ed.). New York, NY: Oxford University Press.

Keith, R. W. (1999). Clinical issues in central auditory processing disorders. *Language,*

Speech, and Hearing Services in Schools, 30, 339–344.

Kratochwill, T. R., Hitchock, J., Horner, R. H., Levin, J. R., Odom, S. L., Rindskipf, D. M., & Shadish, W. R. (2010). *Single case design technical documentation*. Retrieved from http://ies.ed.gov/ncee/wwc/pdf/wwc.scd.pdf

Law, M., Stewart, D., Pollock, N., Letts, L., Bosch, J., & Westmorland, M. (1998). *Critical review form—quantitative studies*. Retrieved from http://www.fhs.mcmaster.ca/rehab/ebp

Lemoncello, R., & Fanning, J. (2011, November). *Practice-based evidence: Strategies for generation your own evidence*. Short course presented at the Annual Convention of the American Speech-Language-Hearing Association, San Diego, CA.

Lipsey, M. W., & Wilson, D. B. (1993). The efficacy of psychological, educational, and behavioral treatment: Confirmation from meta-analysis. *American Psychologist, 48*, 1181–1209.

Meline, T. (2005, November). *Statistics for evidence-based practice (EBP): Statistics and their relevance for evidence-based speech-language pathology*. Seminar presented at the Annual Convention of the American Speech-Language-Hearing Association, San Diego, CA.

Meline, T., & Schmitt, J. F. (1997). Case studies for evaluating significance in group designs. *American Journal of Speech-Language Pathology, 6*, 33–41.

Meline, T., & Paradiso, T. (2003). Evidence-based practice in schools: Evaluating research and reducing barriers. *Language, Speech, and Hearing Services in the Schools, 34*, 273–283.

Meline, T., & Wang, B. (2004). Effect-size reporting practices in AJSLP and other AHSA journals, 1999–2003. *American Journal of Speech-Language Pathology, 13*, 202–207.

Millward, K. E., Hall, R. L., Ferguson, M. A., & Moore, D. R. (2011). Training speech-in-noise perception in mainstream school children. *International Journal of Pediatric Otorhinolaryngology, 75*, 1408–1417.

Mullen, R. (2007, March 6). The state of the evidence: ASHA develops levels of evidence for communication sciences and disorders. *ASHA Leader.*

Mullen, R. (2010, October 12). Clarifying our terminology: Moving the discipline forward by defining terms and sharing data. *ASHA Leader.*

Murphy, C. F., & Schochat, E. (2011). Effect of nonlinguistic auditory training on phonological and reading skills. *Folia PhoniatricaLogopedics, 63*, 147–153.

Musiek, F. E., Kurdziel-Schwan, S., Kibbe, K. S., Gollegly, K. M., Baran, J. A., & Rintelmann, W. F. (1989). The dichotic rhyme task: Results in split-brain patients. *Ear and Hearing, 10*, 33–39.

Office of Technology Assessment. (1978, September). *Assessing the efficacy and safety of medical technologies*. OTA-H-75. Washington, DC: U.S. Government Printing Office.

Pantev, C., & Herholz, S. C. (2011). Plasticity of the human auditory cortex related to musical training. *Neuroscience and Biobehavioral Reviews, 35*, 2140–2154.

Pimentel, J., & Munson, D. (2004). *Searching for evidence: Supporting best practices*. Annual Washington State Speech and Hearing Convention. Spokane, WA.

Reilly, Douglas J., & Oates, J. (2004). *Evidence based practice in speech pathology*. Philadelphia, PA: Whurr.

Richards, S. B., Taylor, R. L., Ramasamy, R., & Richards, R. Y. (1999). *Single-subject Research: Applications in educational and clinical settings*. San Diego, CA: Singular.

Robey, R. (2004). A five-phase model for clinical outcome research. *Journal of Communication Disorders, 37*, 401–411.

Robey, R. (2011). Treatment effectiveness and evidence-based practice. In L. LaPointe (Ed.), *Aphasia and related neurogenic language disorders* (4th ed., pp. 197–210). New York, NY: Thieme.

Robey, R., & Schultz, M. (1998). A model for conducting clinical/outcome research: An adaptation of the standard protocol for use is aphasiology. *Aphasiology, 12*, 787–810.

Rosner, J., & Rosner, J. (1986). The clinical management of perceptual skills disorders in a primary care practice. *Journal of the American Optometry Association, 57,* 56–59.

Russo, N. M., Nicol, T. G., Zecker, S. G., Hayes, E. A., & Kraus, N. (2005). Auditory training improves neural timing in the human brainstem. *Behavioral Brain Research, 156,* 95–103.

Sackett, D. L., Richardson, W. S., & Rosenberg, W. M. C. (1997). *Evidence based medicine.* London, UK: Churchill Livingstone.

Schiavetti, N., Metz, D. E., & Orlikoff, R. F. (2011).*Evaluating research in communicative disorders* (6th ed.). Upper Saddle River, NJ: Pearson.

Schlosser, R. W., & Raghavendra, P. (2004). Evidence-based practice in augmentative and alternative communication. *Augmentative and Alternative Communication, 20,* 1–21.

Schochat, E., Musiek, F. E., Alonso, R., & Ogata, J. (2010). Effect of auditory training on the middle latency response in children with (central) auditory processing disorder. *Brazilian Journal of Medical and Biological Research, 43,* 777–785.

Seminars in Hearing. (2002). Management of auditory processing disorders. *Seminars in Hearing, 23.* New York, NY: Thieme.

Strait, D. L., & Kraus, N. (2011). Can you hear me now? Musical training shapes functional brain networks for selective auditory attention and hearing speech in noise. *Frontiers in Psychology, 2,* 113.

Strauss, S. E., Glasziou, P., Richardson, W. S., & Haynes, R. B. (2010). *Evidence-based medicine: How to practice and teach it* (4th ed.). London, UK: Churchill Livingstone.

Strong, G. K., & Torgerson, C. J., Torgerson, D., & Hulme, C. (2011). A systematic meta-analytic review of evidence for the effectiveness of the 'Fast ForWord' language intervention program. *Journal of Child Psychology and Psychiatry, 52,* 224–235.

Sweetow, R., & Palmer, C. V. (2005). Efficacy of individual auditory training in adults: A systematic review of the evidence. *Journal of the American Academy of Audiology, 16,* 494–504.

Tremblay, K., & Kraus, N. (2002). Auditory training induces asymmetrical changes in cortical neural activity. *Journal of Speech, Language, and Hearing Research, 45,* 564–572.

U.S. Bureau of the Census. (2012). *The 2012 statistical abstract.* Retrieved from http://www.census.gov/compendia/statab/cats/population.html

U.S. Food and Drug Administration. (2009, December). *Guidance for industry-patient-reported outcome measures: Use in medical product development to support labeling claims.* Retrieved from http://www.fda.gov/downloads/Drugs/GuidanceComplianceRegulatoryInformation/Guidances/UCM071975.pdf

Wallace, G., Inglebret, E., & Friedlander, R. (1997). American Indians: Culture, communication, and clinical considerations. In G. L. Wallace (Ed.), *Multicultural neurogenics: A resource for speech-language pathologists* (pp. 193–225). Tucson, AZ: Communication Skill Builders (A Division of the Psychological Corporation).

Wertz, R. T., & Irwin, W. H. (2001). Darley and the efficacy of language rehabilitation in aphasia. *Aphasiology, 15,* 231–247.

Wertz, R. T., & Katz, R. C. (2004).Outcomes of computer-provided treatment for aphasia. *Aphasiology, 18,* 229–244.

World Health Organization. (2001). *ICF: International classification of functioning, disability, and health.* Geneva, Switzerland: Author.

Worrall, L. E., & Bennett, S. (2001). Evidence-based practice: Barriers and facilitators for speech language pathologists. *Journal of Medical Speech-Language Pathology, 9,* xi–xvi.

Zipoli, R. P., & Kennedy, M. (2005). Evidence-based practice among speech-language pathologist: Attitudes, utilization, and barriers. *American Journal of Speech-Language Pathology, 14,* 208–220.

CHAPTER 3

THE EFFICACY OF AUDITORY TRAINING IN CHILDREN AND ADULTS WITH CENTRAL AUDITORY PROCESSING DEFICITS

JEFFREY WEIHING, GAIL D. CHERMAK, FRANK E. MUSIEK, and TERI JAMES BELLIS

Overview

As discussed in Chapter 7, the efficacy of auditory training is examined across a wide range of auditory training paradigms and populations. These studies highlight how the plastic human central auditory system is able to take advantage of frequent and demanding auditory listening tasks to improve the central processing of auditory stimuli. These studies include many different types of research subjects, from individuals who had a developmental issue concerns (e.g., learning disability) to subjects with normal peripheral and central auditory function. There, therefore, is an emphasis on examining auditory training efficacy in a very broad sense, using studies across which samples were very heterogeneous.

Although these studies are extremely important in demonstrating the ability of the human auditory system to adapt to complex auditory demands and to change with stimulation, they do not directly address the question of the efficacy of auditory training, specifically in cases of central auditory processing disorder (CAPD). Studies that look at training-based remediation in individuals with CAPD are important for a variety of reasons. Foremost among these is that such studies speak specifically to whether these paradigms benefit the very individuals toward which these therapies are targeted—those with auditory disorders. Auditory training is focused toward individuals with CAPD, and only though an examination of the effectiveness of these therapies in patients with the disorder do we achieve an understanding of the utility of training.

To this end, this chapter provides a more detailed discussion of those research studies that have examined auditory training in individuals with CAPD. For each study considered in this chapter, some discussion is given to how CAPD is diagnosed. Best practice recommendations are to diagnose CAPD using a test battery of measures that are sensitive and specific to CAPD (AAA, 2010; Musiek et al., 2011). Failure of two tests (at least two standard deviations below the norm) along with an intra- and intertest patterns of performance that are consistent with underlying CANS dysfunction is necessary for the diagnosis of the disorder. It is also important to demonstrate that difficulties on central auditory tests can be attributed to auditory-specific issues, and not to a more global, supramodal issue such as attention, memory, cognition, or to a speech-language related issue (AAA, 2010; ASHA, 2005). Unfortunately, not all of the studies reviewed in this chapter meet these criteria precisely, as there has been much variation, historically, in the manner in which CAPD has been diagnosed. However, all the studies reviewed examine the application of auditory training techniques to individuals with confirmed difficulties on at least one or more diagnostic measures of central auditory function.

It will become clear in this chapter that examination of auditory training efficacy in patients specifically diagnosed and who meet current guidelines for CAPD is an emerging line of research. This population has not been examined in as much as detail as the normal hearing population nor individuals with developmental disorders, including dyslexia and other auditory-based, language-learning disorders. The initial studies reviewed here, however, provide an important, preliminary look into how well auditory training benefits those with CAPD. These studies and our focus here is on the efficacy of a range of auditory training paradigms for individuals presenting various central auditory processing deficits.

The Nature of Auditory Training as a Treatment for CAPD

Some discussion of best practice recommendations for auditory training in cases of CAPD is considered here. The most recently published guidelines for diagnosis of and intervention for CAPD highlight the important role that auditory training plays in treatment of the disorder (AAA, 2010). These guidelines recognize that interventions for CAPD can benefit the central auditory nervous system (CANS) in both a bottom-up, or stimulus driven, and top-down, or cognitively driven, manner. Although the group of studies highlight that auditory training mainly targets the first of these networks, an argument can be made that training recruits both bottom-up and top-down resources. The work of Recanzone described in Chapter 7 demonstrates that structural, bottom-up changes to the CANS can be expected following repeated exposure to a demanding training task. Additionally, the work of Moore and colleagues, also described in Chapter 7, has shown that cognitive, top-down modifications also can occur as the patient better understands tasks demands and adopts improved strategies for completing the task successfully. Thus, in implementing auditory training as a treatment for patients with CAPD, one would expect to recruit both bottom-up and top-down processes.

The AAA guidelines also identify characteristics of effective auditory training for patients with CAPD. These include, but are not limited to,

> . . . varying stimuli and tasks; presenting stimuli at comfortable listening levels (or slightly louder and slower . . .); presenting tasks systematically and graduated in difficulty to be challenging and motivating but not so difficult as to be overwhelming . . . ; targeting a moderate degree of accuracy with generous feedback and reinforcement; requiring at least a moderate degree of accuracy or performance of poorer ear comparable to that of the better ear before proceeding to a more demanding task; providing intensive practice . . . distributed in regard to length of training sessions, number of training sessions, time intervals between sessions and period of time over which training is conducted. (AAA, 2010, p. 25)

Importantly, these guidelines recognize that benefits obtained will be dictated by individual-specific and task-specific variables, such that no single auditory training approach will be equally effective in all individuals with CAPD. Therefore, training needs to be individualized to the patient's deficit and needs.

Training Studies for Patients With CAPD

What follows is a consideration of published research that meets specific inclusion criteria (i.e., the application of auditory training techniques to individuals with confirmed difficulties on at least one or more diagnostic measures of central auditory function) that has examined auditory training in individuals with CAPD. The following types of training were examined in these studies: dichotic auditory training, temporal processing training, binaural interaction training, and training batteries that incorporate a range of auditory processing tasks. Following a review of these studies, we consider the effect size for each of the studies and provide a preliminary meta-analysis that provides a quantitative approach to summarizing these findings. The reader is referred to Chapter 10 for discussion of many of the types of training included in the studies reviewed below.

Dichotic Auditory Training

Dichotic auditory training is administered to patients with CAPD who typically have been diagnosed with an asymmetric dichotic processing deficit. (See Chapter 9 for a discussion of dichotic interaural intensity difference [DIID] training.) Several studies have reported the efficacy of dichotic training in individuals with dichotic deficits confirmed via CAPD tests.

Moncrieff and Wertz (2008) administered a dichotic listening therapy (Auditory Rehabilitation for Interaural Asymmetry [ARIA]) to children with dichotic deficits in two experiments. The children's dichotic deficits were either unilateral left ear weakness or bilateral deficits. In both experiments, dichotic stimuli were administered through two speakers in the sound field and difficulty was adaptively modified by gradually increasing the level of the acoustic signal coming from the right speaker. The initial interaural intensity difference was 30 dB HL;

as patients improved, this difference was decreased over time by 1 to 5 dB to maintain performance between 70% and 100%. Eight children ranging in age between 7 and 13 years participated in experiment 1. The children trained for 30 minutes per session, three times a week, for four weeks.

Results revealed that left ear performance for dichotic digits was significantly greater following training, with an average improvement of approximately 15%. In experiment 2, a larger sample of children was recruited (n = 13) of children aged 6.5 through 11 years. In addition to a larger sample, some children in experiment 2 trained over a longer duration (ranging from 12 to 24 sessions), and they were administered additional nondichotic listening comprehension outcome measures. Significant left and right ear improvements were noted posttraining for both dichotic digits and competing words, with an approximately 20% improvement in performance for the left ear. Improvements in the right ear were much smaller in magnitude; however, pretraining performance for the right ear generally was also much higher than the left ear score, which allowed for a smaller margin of improvement. A significant correlation was observed between improvements in left ear performance on both dichotic measures and the listening comprehension measures (i.e., Brigance Comprehensive Inventory of Basic Skills Revised).

Musiek, Weihing, and Lau (2008) administered a DIID-like therapy to 14 children with dichotic issues for 10 weeks. Although typically the paradigm attempts to improve weaker ear performance by manipulating interaural level differences, this particular study utilized interaural timing differences instead. The authors referred to this variant as the DIID II. By having the stimulus in the weaker ear arrive slightly later than the stimulus in the better ear, a dichotic advantage is created for the weaker ear. As the patient improves, the lag between the ears is decreased to make the task more challenging.

The authors found a significant improvement in pre- versus posttraining dichotic listening performance that was, on average, 30%. Benefits of DIID training also translated into reduction of symptoms, as determined by parent or teacher report. Respondents were given a questionnaire that asked about the child's improvements in ability to follow directions, communication ability, academic performance, attention, and ability to hear in noise. Scores ranged from 0 = no improvement, to 5 = problem is no longer apparent. Overall, the group demonstrated average or greater than average improvement, with scores on these items showing means of 3 or greater.

Temporal Processing Training and Auditory Discrimination Training

Temporal processing refers to a range of auditory processing tasks, all of which incorporate some aspect of processing acoustic stimuli over time. Of all the central auditory processes, this is perhaps the broadest, and includes deficits in areas such as frequency, intensity, and duration discrimination; temporal sequencing; backward and forward masking; and others. The specific training tasks that target temporal processing ability are generally quite varied given the many types of temporal processes. Many temporal processing exercises are included in some computer-based auditory training packages, as discussed below.

McArthur, Ellis, Atikinson, and Coltheart (2008) recruited children with specific reading disability or specific language impairment who also showed below normal performance on auditory temporal processing measures. As such, although a comprehensive central auditory test battery was not administered, the poor performance on tests of temporal processing indicated the likelihood of CAPD in this sample. A total of 28 children ranging in age from 6 through 15 years of age participated in the study. Subjects were trained on one of the following auditory discrimination tasks: frequency discrimination, vowel discrimination, consonant-vowel discrimination, or backward masking. Training was adaptive in difficulty, and was administered for 30 minutes a day, 4 days a week, for 6 weeks. Psychoacoustic tasks similar to the training paradigms were administered before training was initiated and then again after the last training session. Approximately 90% of the sample showed psychoacoustic performance that was within normal limits following the end of training. These improvements did not appear to be related to a more global change in how participants approached the tasks as evidenced by the finding that participants did not show similar improvements on visual discrimination or sustained attention tasks. Control subjects who were not trained also showed a degree of improvement on outcome measures on retest; however, the magnitude of improvement was smaller than that seen for the trained group. The control group generally had better temporal

processing skills than the trained group when measured at pretesting and, therefore, did not have as much potential for gains as the experimental group.

Sharma, Purdy, and Kelly (2012) recruited 55 children who were diagnosed with CAPD per AAA guidelines (AAA, 2010). Participants ranged in age from 7 through 13 years, with a mean age of 9.7 years. All subjects had normal peripheral hearing sensitivity. Children were randomly enrolled in one of the following interventions: auditory discrimination training, auditory discrimination training and FM system, language therapy, or language therapy and FM system. Training consisted of 12 hours of intervention comprised of exercises performed both in the clinic and at home. Training was divided into one-hour clinical sessions a week and 15 minutes of exercises at home, five days a week, for five weeks. Home exercises for the auditory training group included use of Earobics (http://www.earobics.com, Houghton Mifflin Harcourt) specifically the phonological training components of the software. For the language therapy group, home exercises included reading aloud with an emphasis on correct stress and intonation, and appreciating differences in meaning that result from the use of different stress and timing patterns. Results showed that all interventions yielded some degree of effectiveness. Both the auditory discrimination training and the language therapy yielded improvements in temporal processing posttraining. Additional benefits were seen in language and reading outcomes. Although these results might suggest equal effectiveness of auditory training and language therapy, it should be noted that it is generally expected that training that specifically targets an affected auditory process(es) will yield the most benefit to the patient (AAA, 2010). Since children were randomly assigned to training paradigms that did not necessarily target their specific deficient auditory process(es), lesser gains might have accrued to the participants, with little difference seen relative to the particular treatment administered.

Krishnamurti, Forrester, Rutledge, and Holmes (2013) examined Fast ForWord (FFW training), which targets temporal processing and auditory discrimination skills in a speech-language context. They reported on two pediatric cases, both of whom presented normal peripheral hearing sensitivity and ranged in age from 7 to 8 years. Both children showed difficulties on the researchers' central auditory test battery that included one highly sensitive and specific nonverbal measure of disorders of the CANS (Musiek et al., 2011) (i.e., Frequency Patterns [Musiek, 1994]), as well as several language-based measures that some argue assess central auditory aspects as well (i.e., SCAN-C [Keith, 2000], Phonemic Synthesis [Katz & Medol, 1972], and TAPS-R [Martin & Brownell, 2005]). (Musiek et al., 2011). The children also were administered the Test of Nonverbal Intelligence (TONI) (Brown, Sherbenou, & Johnsen, 1997), Clinical Evaluation of Language Fundamentals (CELF) (Semel, Wiig, & Secord, 2003), and the speech auditory brainstem response (seABR) (Wong, Skoe, Russo, Dees, & Kraus, 2007). The children engaged in training over an 8 to 12-week period, 5 days a week, for 50-minute sessions.

For the first participant, improvement was seen on the FFW tasks, which was expected given the intensity of the training. Improved performance also was seen on the SCAN, Frequency Patterns, Phonemic Synthesis, and the CELF. Benefits seemed to generalize beyond the central auditory and language measures, as evidenced by gains in cognition measured via the TONI. Improvements also were observed electrophysiologically on the seABR, which presented as an increase in amplitude of the V-A response, post-training. The second child showed similar improvements following training on the verbal and nonverbal central auditory test measures and the seABR (i.e., shorter latencies); however, benefits did not generalize to the TONI or the CELF.

Binaural Interaction

Cameron and Dillon (2011) have defined the term "spatial processing disorder" (SPD) as a type of CAPD that originates from a deficit in the binaural system. They state that SPD arises from an inability of the CANS to make use of the spatial location of sounds to suppress competing acoustic information. Spatial processing is most similar to the binaural interaction auditory process described by AAA (2010). (See Chapter 8 for discussion of SPD and Chapter 16 of Volume I of the Handbook for discussion of binaural interaction.) Children with SPD do not show the expected improvement in speech recognition ability when the location of a noise source is separated from the location of the speech signal. As treatment for SPD, Cameron and Dillon (2011) introduced the LiSN and Learn auditory training software program. This program trains users to utilize spatial processing skills to achieve better listening performance, particularly in the presence of noise. The authors recruited nine children ranging in age from 6 through 11 years. The children participated in the LiSN and Learn program 15 to 20 minutes a day, five times a week, for approximately three months. Results documented that the children were better able to utilize spatial separation cues following training.

Battery Approach to Training

Several studies have examined the use of a battery of treatment approaches for individuals diagnosed with CAPD and others who might not have been diagnosed as CAPD but who presented deficits on specific auditory processing tests. Characterizing the training battery approach is the inclusion of multiple types of auditory training exercises, spanning a range of auditory processes, and in some cases, the addition of top-down instruction and compensatory modifications. Although the training battery approach used in some of the studies described below did not necessarily target training to processes that were shown to be deficient, the training battery approach has some inherent ecological validity as individuals with CAPD typically present deficits in more than one auditory process. Moreover, multiple auditory processes underlie listening and its deficits (e.g., listening difficulty in noise might be due to binaural separation issues, spatial processing issues, temporal processing issues) and a training battery may be beneficial when the affected auditory process cannot be precisely identified, as would occur if the central auditory deficits were revealed primarily from electrophysiological measures and not behavioral tests of central auditory processing.

Musiek and Schochat (1998) reported a case study in which a 15-year-old with CAPD received benefit from a task battery approach to auditory training. Diag-

nosis of CAPD was accomplished using four tests: Dichotic Digits (Musiek, 1983), Compressed Speech (Wilson, 1993), Frequency Patterns (Musiek & Pinheiro, 1987), and Duration Patterns (Musiek, Baran, & Pinheiro, 1990). Pretraining, the youngster scored below normal limits on all measures, except the duration patterns. The formal auditory training protocol consisted of one-hour sessions, three times a week, for six weeks. Additional informal exercises also were provided to work on at home for 15 to 30 minutes, two to three times a week. Formal training tasks focused on the following auditory processes: auditory discrimination (i.e., intensity discrimination, frequency discrimination, CV discrimination), dichotic processing (i.e., DIID training), and monaural low redundancy (i.e., speech in noise training). Difficulty level of the formal tasks was adaptive to maintain performance at 70% correct. Informal training tasks included reading aloud with good intonation and rhythm (which is a top-down approach that targets discrimination and temporal processing), and identifying target lyrics in songs (which also targets temporal [sequencing] processing).

Following the termination of training, the participant showed improved central auditory processing, particularly for the compressed speech task and dichotic processing, which was within normal limits following training. The participant's mother completed a hearing processing questionnaire that was designed to assess degree of improvement from the training. Several areas of improvement were rated from 0, no improvement, to 5, no longer has a problem in this area. Following directions, communication ability, academic ability, attention span, speech recognition in noise ability, and alertness were all indicated as areas in which the participant showed considerable (score of 3) to marked improvement (score of 4). The wide range of areas in which improvements were noted following training may speak to the breadth of the auditory training paradigm used in this case and/or to the primacy of CAPD in contributing to the patient's symptoms.

Putter-Katz, Adi-Bensaid, Feldman, and Hildesheimer (2008) administered a combination of dichotic listening and speech in noise auditory training coupled with use of an FM system, as well as some top down interventions (e.g., modification of learning strategies, cognitive and metacognitive approaches, and classroom and home modifications) to 20 children, ranging in age from 7 to 14 years, with a mean age of 9 years. Ten control subjects who ranged in age from 6 to 11 years, with a mean age of 8 years, received neither training nor interventions. Both groups were diagnosed with CAPD based on performance below one standard deviation in at least one ear on one or more of the central auditory tests used in the study—dichotic (binaural separation) listening, monaural low redundancy, temporal processing (i.e., gap detection ability), and binaural interaction. All children with CAPD presented listening difficulties, as reported by parents, teachers, and/or clinical professionals working with the child. Eleven children were diagnosed with a monaural low-redundancy deficits only (i.e., "noise group"), and nine children were diagnosed with a combination of monaural low-redundancy and dichotic processing issues (i.e., "noise + dichotic group"). The same training was administered to both groups for 45 minutes, once a week, for 4 months, and training was the same for both trained groups. Outcome measures included the central auditory tests administered prior to training. Results revealed that central auditory test scores improved for participants in both the "noise" and "noise+dichotic" groups following the four-month interval. Similar improvements were not seen for the control group.

Alonso and Schochat (2009) recruited 29 children with CAPD ranging in age from 8 to 16 years to examine the efficacy of auditory training. Two measures of monaural low redundancy and two measures of dichotic processing were administered in the diagnostic central auditory test battery. Diagnosis of CAPD was made based on the child failing at least two central auditory tests. These central auditory tests and the auditory P300 served as outcome measures. Training consisted of eight 50-minute sessions, once per week for eight weeks. Training was similar to that employed by Musiek and Schochat (1998) (described above). The difficulty of tasks was modified each week to maintain performance at approximately 70%. Following training, significant improvements were observed on most of the outcome measures, including the P300 latency and all four central auditory measures. Nearly 73% of the participants presented normal auditory processing ability following training.

Schochat, Musiek, Alonso, and Ogata (2010) recruited 30 children with CAPD and 22 without, ranging in age from 8 to 14 years. Children were diagnosed with CAPD using the criteria set forth by ASHA (2005) and AAA (2010). All participants had normal peripheral hearing. The children with CAPD were enrolled in training: 50-minute sessions, once weekly, for eight weeks. Training included a combination of frequency discrimination, intensity discrimination, duration discrimination, gap detection, dichotic interaural intensity difference, localization, and speech perception training. Informal exercises comprised of word-recognition tasks also were given to subjects to be completed at home for 15 minutes daily.

Posttraining measures included speech recognition in quiet and in noise, verbal and nonverbal dichotic listening and the auditory middle-latency response (MLR). Results confirmed that the children displayed significant improvement on central auditory measures following training. Additionally, the children receiving training showed an increase in MLR amplitude measured over the left hemisphere that was not seen in the control group.

Several case studies with neurological patients also have examined the efficacy of auditory training using a battery of auditory exercises and interventions. Musiek and Baran (2004) reported on a young adult patient who experienced a hemorrhage in the pons that was a result of an arteriovenous malformation. The patient was first evaluated audiologically three months after this event, at which point she had reported she had significant listening difficulties particularly when in the presence of background noise. An audiogram performed at this time revealed relatively normal hearing in the left ear and a sensorineural loss that ranged to severe in the high frequencies in the right ear. Two monaural low-redundancy tests were administered: Performance was 0% in the right ear and ranged between 50% and 75% in the left ear. She was enrolled in an informal rehabilitation protocol, which included the following recommendations: Wear an earplug in the right ear to prevent distortion, use an assistive listening device, and engage in auditory training that consisted of auditory discrimination of numbers, consonants, vowels, words, and sentences. These tasks were performed over the phone (to simulate a monaural low-redundancy, filtered speech context) with a friend reading her the stimuli. Each session began with the better ear first, and then proceeded to the poorer performing right ear. The patient did this for approximately 15 to 20 minutes daily for approximately six months. Her central auditory function was reassessed twice during that time. Subjectively, she reported significant improvements in listening, although some situations were still problematic for her, such as listening in noise. Her right ear performance on one of the monaural low-redundancy tests improved from 0% to approximately 50%. Interestingly, the high-frequency sensorineural hearing loss also improved from severe to mild/moderate, though it is likely this improvement was seen because a portion of her hearing loss was related to central changes that may have been coincident with the hemorrhage in her pons. Auditory training would not be expected to improve peripheral hearing loss.

In another case, Musiek, Charette, Morse, and Baran (2004) reported on a 21-year-old patient with a subarachnoid bleed that affected the inferior colliculi bilaterally. Initially, the patient was centrally deaf and unresponsive to sounds, despite showing normal otoacoustic emissions and auditory brainstem response through wave III. Steady improvements were seen in his hearing over the course of 12 weeks, and by 10 months his hearing sensitivity was equivalent to a moderately severe hearing loss. He noted significant difficulties hearing in noise despite his gains in hearing sensitivity. Intensity discrimination was assessed at 5 and 11 weeks post-episode. The difference limen to intensity was elevated at the two sessions, but was slightly improved at 11 weeks for the right ear and for binaural administration. Central auditory issues also were confirmed by abnormal middle latency responses and event related potentials.

An auditory rehabilitation program was initiated one month after the patient left the hospital. Therapy sessions were administered formally, once a week for approximately an hour, for 14 weeks. Training was adaptive to maintain difficulty at a moderate level. Informal exercises also were given for home use, which included auditory directives, discrimination tasks, and music listening. Initially, the formal training consisted of having the patient answer questions about himself, administration of discrimination tasks, and speechreading. Approximately midway through the program, focus of the therapy switched to identification and discrimination of voices and environmental sounds, speech recognition in noise, identification of nonword speech sounds, and reading aloud. The patient made obvious progress in auditory discrimination ability throughout these stages of therapy. In the final stages of the program, an emphasis was placed on significantly increasing the difficulty of therapy as the patient was making noticeable gains. Discrimination tasks utilized sounds that were more similar, and sentence level material was introduced. An assistive listening device also was introduced around this time. Despite the gains seen by this patient during this training, Musiek et al. acknowledged that it was difficult to separate out gains made from therapy versus spontaneous recovery, although they cited research showing that training facilitates recovery in neurological cases.

Musiek, Baran, and Shinn (2004) also reported an auditory training case in which hearing difficulties were noted following a mild head trauma. The 41-year-old patient noted that it was difficult to attend for long periods of time, particularly when auditory information was being presented, and she reported difficulty when presented with multistep directions. She also felt she had more difficulty hearing from the left ear than the right ear, despite normal and symmetrical hearing sensitivity bilaterally. A central auditory evaluation that included the dichotic digits, competing sentences, frequency patterns, duration patterns, and compressed speech revealed performance consistent with CAPD. Specifically, she showed a bilateral dichotic deficit that was poorer in the left ear, a left ear deficit on compressed speech, and below normal performance on the duration patterns. She enrolled in an auditory training program that included training in advocating for clear speech, reading aloud, dichotic interaural intensity difference training, auditory memory enhancement training, auditory speech discrimination training, temporal sequence training, and instruction on metacognitive strategies. Post-training, the patient showed significant gains in central auditory processing: performance on the dichotic digits and right ear scores on the compressed speech and competing sentences were now within normal limits. Significant improvements also were seen in the left ear on compressed speech and competing sentences, though performance only bordered normal limits.

Effect Size of Results From CAPD Training Studies

As a means to demonstrate the relative strength of the training effects for individuals with CAPD reviewed in this chapter, we report the Cohen's d or η^2 effect size we derived from statistics reported in these studies. Details on which statistic reported in each study was used for computations of Cohen's d, along with other important study specific information, are included in Table 3–1. Only studies that included data in aggregate (i.e., not individual case studies) were included in this analysis. Two studies (McArthur et al., 2008; Putter-Katz et al., 2008) that could have contributed an effect size are not included in Table 3–1 because appropriate statistics or mean values could not be reliably derived from the original papers.

In general, each study had several statistics that could have been used to compute effect size; however, we elected to present one effect size per study sample. In our attempt to describe these effects at their most robust, we derived the effect size from the statistic reported in the original paper related to the outcome measure and ear that demonstrated the greatest auditory benefit in the study. In some cases, more than one effect size was computed but each statistic reflected different participants (e.g., the study employed multiple treatment groups). Cohen's d was calculated based on methods described by Cohen (1988), Rosenthal (1991), and Rosenthal and Rosnow (1991); η^2 was reported by Cameron and Dillon (2011).

Cohen (1988) provides the following classification for interpretation of effect sizes: .2 is a small effect, .5 is a medium effect, and .8 or more is a large effect. The η^2 statistic is best understood as percent variance associated with the main effect or interaction and is interpreted by multiplying the statistic value by 100. Most of the studies included in Table 3–1 show a large effect size. The largest effect sizes generally were seen for studies that

included dichotic training therapy in isolation (i.e., Moncrieff & Wertz, 2008; Musiek et al., 2008). A very strong effect size was seen for the LiSN and Learn (i.e., binaural interaction/spatial processing) training (Cameron & Dillon, 2011), which indicated that 87% of variance was associated with the main effect of training. Undoubtedly, some of the strengths of these two training approaches as used in the studies cited is that they directly trained on tasks that were targeting deficits shown to be below normative values on the central auditory processing tests, and these same tests served as outcome measures. This approach is justified as the goal of auditory training is to remediate the deficient auditory processing. Thus, identifying the affected auditory processes, training them, and then re-evaluating those auditory processes would seem the most direct way to evaluate training. As emphasized by Bellis, Weihing, Chermak, and Musiek (2012), although auditory training may indirectly benefit related skills (e.g., language, reading), especially when auditory training is combined with interventions that target central resources and environmental modifications, auditory training is designed to improve auditory deficits that have been identified by valid tests of auditory function in a targeted, deficit-specific manner. Therefore, the efficacy of auditory training must be measured most directly using auditory tasks similar to those used in training.

Studies that measured auditory outcomes that were not specifically trained tended to have smaller effect sizes (i.e., Sharma et al., 2012). Additionally, battery approaches to auditory training tended to have smaller effect sizes than more targeted therapies (i.e., Alonso & Schochat, 2009; Schochat et al., 2010).

Table 3–1. Effect Size Values Reflecting Training Effects for Selected Studies Reported In the Present Chapter

Study	Type of Process Trained	Outcome Measure	Effect Size: Cohen's d or η^2	Statistic Type Used to Compute d or η^2	N	Notes
Moncrieff and Wertz (2008)	Dichotic Processing	Dichotic Test	d: 1.02	Pre-Post Mean Difference	8	Outcome is left ear improvement on dichotic digits
Moncrieff and Wertz (2008)	Dichotic Processing	Dichotic Test	d: 2.11	Pre-Post Mean Difference	13	Outcome is left ear improvement on dichotic digits
Musiek et al. (2008)	Dichotic Processing	Dichotic Test	d: 2.33	Pre-Post Mean Difference	14	Mean values used reflect dichotic digits improvement. They were not reported in paper but were obtained from the study's authors
Sharma et al. (2012)	Temporal Processing	Frequency Patterns	d: 1.23	Pre-Post Mean Difference	12	Outcome reflects right ear performance
Cameron and Dillon (2011)	Binaural Interaction	LiSN	η^2: 0.873	F	10	Effect size reported in original paper
Alonso and Schochat (2009)	Battery Approach	SSI - CCM	d: 1.29	Pre-Post Mean Difference	29	Other outcome measures showed similar effect sizes
Schochat et al. (2010)	Battery Approach	Nonverbal Dichotic	d: 1.12	Pre-Post Mean Difference	30	Other outcome measures showed similar effect sizes

Despite these trends, all of the studies reviewed produced large effect sizes, although they did not approach the magnitude of effects seen in dichotic and binaural interaction therapies. It is possible that potential benefits are reduced in the training battery approaches used in the studies reviewed due to the distribution of training across multiple tasks. This may lead to less intensive training on actual deficits and poorer outcomes. Additionally, not utilizing outcome measures that assess the affected auditory process may yield smaller effect sizes than had more relevant outcome measures been utilized.

Conclusions

A review of all auditory training studies that met the authors' inclusion criteria was presented in this chapter. These studies examined the effectiveness of specific, targeted training as well as training batteries as interventions for individuals diagnosed with CAPD or individuals who demonstrated difficulties on central auditory processing measures. Most of these studies confirm that auditory training can successfully remediate the auditory skills of individuals with CAPD and/or central auditory processing deficits. As this a new area of inquiry, as demonstrated by the limited number of studies that met our stringent inclusion criteria, there is a need for training studies of individuals diagnosed with CAPD based on best practice guidelines that direct training in a targeted fashion those processes that are shown to be deficient using valid and sensitive measures, as recommended by AAA (2010). There is also need for additional stud-

ies that employ proper controls, including patients with CAPD who undergo a "sham" intervention (e.g., patients with CAPD exposed to a visual analog of the auditory training). Carefully designed research can help to further establish the robustness of auditory training in cases of CAPD. The available research in this area strongly suggests that auditory training is a viable approach to addressing the auditory difficulties encountered by individuals with CAPD. This conclusion, based on the effect sizes reported here certainly comports with the authors' collective clinical experience.

References

AAA (American Academy of Audiology). (2010). *Clinical practice guidelines—diagnosis, treatment, and management of children and adults with central auditory processing disorder.* Retrieved from http://www.audiology.org/resources/document library/Documents/CAPD%20Guidelines%208-2010.pdf

Alonso, R., & Schochat, E. (2009). The efficacy of formal auditory training in children with (central) auditory processing disorder: Behavioral and electrophysiological evaluation. *Brazilian Journal of Otorhinolaryngology, 75,* 726–732.

ASHA (American Speech-Language-Hearing Association). (2005). *(Central) auditory processing disorders* [Technical report]. Retrieved from http://www.asha.org/policy

Bellis, T., Chermak, G., Weihing, J., & Musiek, F. (2012). Efficacy of auditory interventions for central auditory processing disorder: A response to Fey et al (2011). *Language, Speech, and Hearing Services in School, 43,* 381–386.

Brown, R., Sherbenou, S., & Johnsen, S. (1997). *Test of Nonverbal Intelligence* (3rd ed.). Austin, TX: Pro-Ed.

Cameron, S., & Dillon, H. (2011). Development and evaluation of the LiSN & learn auditory training software for deficit-specific remediation of binaural processing deficits in children: Preliminary findings. *Journal of the American Academy of Audiology, 22*, 678–696.

Cohen, J. (1988). *Statistical power analysis for the behavioral sciences* (2nd ed.). Hillsdale, NJ: Lawrence Earlbaum Associates.

Katz, J., & Medol, E. (1972). The use of phonemic synthesis in speech therapy. *Menorah Medical Journal, 3*, 10–13.

Keith, R. (2000). *SCAN-C Test for Auditory Processing Disorders in Children-Revised*. San Antonio, TX: Psychological Corporation.

Krishnamurti, S., Forrester, J., Rutledge, C., & Holmes, G. (2013). A case study of the changes in the speech-evoked auditory brainstem response associated with auditory training in children with auditory processing disorders. *International Journal of Pediatric Otorhinolaryngology, 77*, 594–604.

Martin, N., & Brownell, R. (2005). *Test of Auditory Processing Skills* (3rd ed.). Novato, CA: Academic Therapy.

McArthur, G., Ellis, D., Atikinson, C., & Coltheart, M. (2008). Auditory processing deficits in children with reading and language impairments: Can they (and should they) be treated? *Cognition, 107*, 946–977.

Moncrieff, D., & Wertz, D. (2008). Auditory rehabilitation for interaural asymmetry: Preliminary evidence of improved dichotic listening performance following intensive training. *International Journal of Audiology, 47*, 84–97.

Musiek, F. (1983). Assessment of central auditory dysfunction: The Dichotic Digit Test Revisited. *Ear and Hearing, 4*, 79–83.

Musiek, F. (1994). Frequency (pitch) and duration pattern tests. *Journal of the American Academy of Audiology, 5*, 265–286.

Musiek, F., & Baran, J. (2004). Audiological correlates to a rupture of a pontine anteriovenous malformation. *Journal of the American Academy of Audiology, 15*, 161–171.

Musiek, F., Baran, J., & Pinheiro, M. (1990). Duration pattern recognition in normal subjects and patients with cerebral and cochlear lesions. *Audiology, 29*, 304–313.

Musiek, F., Baran, J., & Shinn, J. (2004). Assessment and remediation of an auditory processing disorder associated with head trauma. *Journal of the American Academy of Audiology, 15*, 117–132.

Musiek, F., & Pinheiro, M. (1987). Frequency patterns in cochlear, brainstem, and cerebral lesions. *Audiology, 26*, 79–88.

Musiek, F., & Schochat, E. (1998). Auditory training and central auditory processing disorders—a case study. *Seminars in Hearing, 19*, 357–366.

Musiek, F., Charette, L., Morse, D., & Baran, J. (2004). Central deafness associated with a midbrain lesion. *Journal of the American Academy of Audiology, 15*, 133–151.

Musiek, F., Chermak, G., Weihing, J., Zappulla, M., & Nagle, S. (2011). Diagnostic accuracy of established central auditory processing test batteries in patients with documented brain lesions. *Journal of the American Academy of Audiology, 22*, 342–358.

Musiek, F., Weihing, J., & Lau, C. (2008). Dichotic interaural intensity difference (DIID) training—a review of existing research and future directions. *Journal of the Academy of Rehabilitative Audiology, 41*, 51–65.

Putter-Katz, H., Adi-Bensaid, L., Feldman, I., & Hildesheimer, M. (2008). Effects of speech in noise and dichotic listening intervention programs on central auditory processing disorders. *Journal of Basic Clinical Physiology and Pharmacology, 19*, 301–316.

Rosenthal, R. (1991). *Meta-analytic procedures for social research*. Newbury Park, CA: Sage.

Rosenthal, R., & Rosnow, R. (1991). *Essentials of behavioral research: Methods and data analysis*. New York, NY: McGraw-Hill.

Schochat, E., Musiek, F., Alonso, R., & Ogata J. (2010). Effect of auditory training on the middle latency response in children with (central) auditory processing disorder. *Brazilian Journal of Medical and Biologi-*

cal Research, 43, 777–785. Oakland CA: Fast Forword. Scientific Learning,

Semel, E., Wiig, E. H., & Secord, W. A. *(2003). Clinical Evaluation of Language Fundamentals, fourth edition* (CELF-4). Toronto, Canada: Psychological Corporation/Harcourt Assessment.

Sharma, M., Purdy, S., & Kelly, A. (2012). A randomized control trial of interventions in school-aged children with auditory processing disorders. *International Journal of Audiology, 51,* 506–518.

Wilson, R. (1993). Development and use of auditory compact discs in auditory evaluation. *Journal of Rehabilitation Research and Development, 30,* 342–351.

Wong, P., Skoe, E., Russo, T., Dees, N., & Kraus, N. (2007). Musical experience shapes human brainstem encoding of linguistic pitch patterns. *Nature Neuroscience, 10,* 420–422.

CHAPTER 4

ACOUSTIC FOUNDATIONS OF SIGNAL ENHANCEMENT AND ROOM ACOUSTICS

JACEK SMURZYNSKI

Introduction

Architectural design is an essential element for providing good acoustical characteristics in spaces where speech communication occurs. For example, excessive background noise may interfere with speech communication and present an acoustical barrier to learning, thus making learning more difficult, less sustained, and more fatiguing. Appropriate acoustical characteristics of a classroom provides an environment for more effective and less stressful teaching, especially of young children and students with communication disabilities, including those with central auditory processing disorder (CAPD). Since adult-like ability to recognize speech in noisy or reverberant backgrounds is not

reached until the age of approximately 14 to 15 years, adequate acoustic cues delivered to the immature auditory and linguistic system are essential, especially in children with CAPD. Several studies have reported that the majority of classrooms do not meet recommended criteria of appropriate listening environment; therefore, it is important to follow proper recommendations when new classrooms are designed or to conduct appropriate modifications of existing classrooms (e.g., American National Standards Institute [ANSI], 2010).

The purpose of this chapter is to summarize several topics that should be taken into account to improve the quality of education by decreasing or eliminating acoustical barriers for teachers and students, including those with communication disabilities. The chapter begins with a description of the propagation of sounds in free field. However, in most listening conditions, including classrooms, major departures from the free-field condition occur. Therefore, several topics related to more common sound-field conditions, particularly with reference to maximizing the acoustic characteristics of classrooms, as well as the basics of sound measurement and elements of sound reinforcement systems are discussed to provide the foundation for many bottom-up (stimulus driven) and top-down (concept driven) interventions for CAPD. See Section 2 for elaboration of these interventions.

Sound Wave Phenomena

Air molecules while being in constant random motion create static air pressure that is proportional to the density of the molecules. Under particular conditions, changes in existing air pressure may be perceived as sounds. Those pressure variations may be local or spread out, minuscule or massive, slow or fast. The task of the auditory system is to detect and to process them in such a way that a meaningful message may be sent to the brain.

Sound originates from the vibration of an object. When the object moves outward away from its resting position, the molecules next to it are jammed into the adjacent molecules and create an area of increased density (condensation), that is, an area of pressure higher than the static one. Through multiple collisions, extra energy given to the molecules is transferred to other molecules and the region of condensation moves away from the vibrating object. When the object moves back toward its original position,

an area of a partial vacuum (rarefaction) is created before molecules fill the space vacated by the vibrating object. Now the density of air molecules has decreased locally. Thus, the movement of an object to and fro around its resting position creates a disturbance or a local variation of air pressure and that disturbance initiates a wave that may travel through a medium, for example, air. The object represents a source that delivers energy to the medium and a wave carries this energy away from the source. It is important to recognize the fact that even though the air through which the wave travels may experience some local oscillations as the wave passes, the air particles do not travel with the wave. A sound wave in air is an example of a longitudinal wave: The displacement of the medium (air particles) occurs along an axis that is aligned with the direction of sound propagation.

The disturbance that initiates the wave may have a variety of shapes, from a short pulse to a long-lasting oscillation. An impulsive wave may be generated by a single short stimulation of a vibrating object. Common examples of impulsive sounds are those produced from plucked or struck musical instruments (e.g., the guitar, the piano, and most percussion instruments). It is important to point out that a wave that travels on a guitar string when it is plucked is a transverse wave; the particles of the string move perpendicular to the direction in which the wave travels (along the string). However, the energy of a vibrating string creates a longitudinal wave propagated in the air and traveling away from the instrument. An impulsive wave may be also created by an abrupt change of air pressure (e.g., a hand clap, an explosion). Oscillatory waves have a pattern that is repeated over and over. A sine wave, the simplest type of sound, is created when displacement of a vibrating object to and fro around its resting position over time can be described mathematically by a sine function. A vibrating tuning fork produces a sine wave, also called a simple tone or a "pure tone." Musical instruments generate oscillatory waves that are complex but can be represented by a sum of sine waves by doing Fourier analysis.

Three parameters must be specified to describe an oscillatory wave: amplitude, wavelength, and the period (or the frequency that is the reciprocal of the period). The amplitude of the wave represents the greatest amount by which the instantaneous pressure is changing above and below the existing static air pressure. The distance between each successive condensation (or rarefaction) is the wavelength of sound, symbolized by the Greek letter λ. The time interval that separates the arrival of the two condensations at any fixed location is called the period of the wave (often written as T). The wave's period (in seconds) or its frequency and the wavelength(in meters) are related as follows:

$$\lambda = cT \text{ or } \lambda = c/f \qquad \text{(Eq. 4–1)}$$

where c is the speed of sound (in meters per second) and f is the frequency (in Hz) or the number of times per second the waveform repeats itself. The speed of sound in dry air at 20 degrees Celsius is approximately 343 meters per second; however, it varies as a function of the temperature, density, and humidity of air (Cramer, 1993).

The simplest three-dimensional source of sound waves may be described by a uniformly pulsating sphere whose radius alternately expands and contracts accord-

ing to a sine function. If the size of such a sphere is much smaller than the wavelength of sound it emits (λ), it can be represented by a "monopole" or a "point source." This source radiates sound equally well in all directions under a free-field condition. The point source model is a good approximation for the sound field created by a boxed loudspeaker at low frequencies. The concept of a free field assumes that the space has no boundaries and the medium (air) is homogeneous and motionless; thus, there are no reflections. Under free-field conditions, the sound intensity is described by the inverse square law, which states that the intensity varies inversely with the square of the distance from the source. Therefore, sound intensity I (in W/m^2) measured at distance r (in m) from the source producing the power P (in W) is described as:

$$I = P/(4\pi r^2) \qquad \text{(Eq. 4–2)}$$

Thus, if distance is doubled, sound intensity decreases by a factor of 4. When expressed in decibels, level decreases by 6 dB for each doubling of the distance from the source to the point of measurement.

During the process of wave generation, some of the energy delivered by a source is dissipated in the form of heat and therefore some degree of damping must be anticipated. With resistance added to the system, the amplitude of oscillation will not have a constant value but rather will decay over time. The amount of resistance is associated with how rapidly damping occurs. The greater the amount of resistance in the system, the more the oscillation is damped. As resistance is increased, a condition known as critical damping will be reached when the system no longer oscillates but simply relaxes to the equilibrium position. Thus, damping provides a force that acts to stop objects vibrating. The effect of damping may be used beneficially to control acoustical properties of a room, as discussed later in this chapter.

Sound Reflection, Absorption, Diffusion, and Transmission

Major departures from the inverse square law occur in most listening conditions (including in the classroom) whenever there is an obstacle in the sound path. These obstacles may alter the sound wave in a number of ways, including reflection, absorption, diffusion, and transmission. These alterations occur any time there is a change in the physical properties of the medium through which a wave travels (e.g., when a wave propagating in air strikes a brick wall). Then, part of the acoustic energy carried by the wave is reflected from the barrier, part is absorbed by it, and part is transmitted through into the space beyond it. Also, a sound/surface interaction may create a scatter of the wave in many directions (i.e., diffusion).

The characteristic impedance, Z, represents the opposition of a medium to the passage of sound waves; a medium with high impedance obstructs the movement of acoustic energy more than a medium with low impedance. Impedance is proportional to both the density of the medium (ρ; mass per unit volume) and the speed of sound propagation (c) or $Z = \rho c$. How much energy is reflected or transmitted depends on the impedance of the medium in which the wave is ini-

tially traveling, Z_1 (e.g., air), the impedance of the material in which the wave travels when it crosses the boundary, Z_2, and on the size of the boundary in relation to the wavelength of the sound. Reflection is quantified by the reflection coefficient, R (i.e., the ratio of pressure amplitude in reflected and incident wave) and it depends on the acoustic impedances of the two media, Z_1 and Z_2. If the wave is normally incident to the boundary between the two media, the pressure reflection coefficient is expressed by:

$$R = (Z_2 - Z_1) / (Z_2 + Z_1). \qquad \text{(Eq. 4–3)}$$

The ratio of intensities in reflected and incident waves is called intensity reflection coefficient, R_{int}. It shows what fraction of the energy reaching the boundary is reflected from it:

$$R_{int} = |R|^2 = |(Z_2 - Z_1) / (Z_2 + Z_1)|^2. \qquad \text{(Eq. 4–4)}$$

Absorption coefficient, α, is defined as:

$$\alpha = 1 - R_{int} \qquad \text{(Eq. 4–5)}$$

and it represents energy of the incident wave minus that of the reflected sound. For example, if $\alpha = 0.9$, 90% of acoustic energy is transported into the second medium and 10% is reflected from the boundary. It needs to be kept in mind that some energy absorbed by a barrier may be transmitted into the space beyond it, that is, sound may penetrate the barrier. This is an important aspect of room acoustics because a part of acoustic energy created by a source in a room will be transmitted outside through walls or ceiling, between spaces within a building, through ventilation systems and other structures of a building.

Acoustic isolation is a measure of the decrease in sound level (attenuation) when sound passes from one room to another. It depends on the sound reduction through building elements, on their size, on sound leakage around their periphery, and on the frequency of the sound.

Transmission loss (TL) describes the amount of sound pressure level reduction that a partition imparts to the transmitted acoustic wave. Typically, TL decreases with a decrease of frequency and it increases with an increase in the mass of a partition. Attenuation properties of partitions are described quantitatively by a single number rating called sound transmission class (STC). The STC value is determined in an acoustical testing laboratory by measuring the transmission loss of partitions in 1/3-octave bands (e.g., ANSI, 2010). A higher STC rating provides more sound attenuation through a partition. Similarly, noise isolation class (NIC) is a single-number rating of the noise isolation between two enclosed spaces that are connected acoustically by one or more paths. The procedure used for calculating NIC is the same as that used for calculating STC except that noise reduction between the two spaces in 1/3-octave bands is used instead of transmission loss.

Reflection and diffraction provide the possibility of hearing sound around barriers. Diffraction involves a change in direction of a wave as it passes through a small opening or around a barrier in its path. The effects of diffraction are more pronounced for low rather than for high frequencies; in other words, the effects increase with decreasing the frequency. When the wavelength of a wave (see Equation 4–1) is smaller than the obstacle no noticeable diffraction occurs; small objects present no barrier to sound waves that have a wavelength longer than the object's size. Larger objects create shadows for sound with wavelengths shorter than the object's size; longer wavelengths bend (diffract) in behind the object. This principle is also important for binaural hearing; the interaural level difference is considered as one of several cues available for sound source localization. Low-frequency sounds have a wavelength that is long compared with the size of the head. Therefore, the sound bends around the head and, due to diffraction, no shadow is cast by the head. At high frequencies, the wavelength is short compared with the size of the head, little diffraction occurs, and a shadow is cast by the head creating an interaural level difference that is a useful cue for pure tones with frequencies above 2 kHz.

Another aspect of diffraction is exhibited when waves spread out past small openings. A small (relative to the wavelength) gap between acoustic spaces causes the sound waves to be re-radiated; the small opening is a source of a sound wave itself. Larger gaps between barriers are no obstacle to the waves; lower frequencies bend around the edges of the gap and higher frequencies are shadowed.

Standing Waves

When two waves pass though a medium simultaneously, the resulting acoustic pressure is the sum of the acoustic pressure of each individual wave at that particular location and at that moment. An interesting wave interference pattern, called a standing wave, is produced by two sine waves of equal amplitude and frequency traveling in opposite directions.

Standing waves are characterized by the absence of propagation and by alternating nodal and antinodal regions, where the pressure is zero and maximum, respectively.

When a wave is incident on a boundary, an acoustic field is created with wave interference resulting from an interaction between the incident and reflected waves. In the case of total reflection, that is, for $R = R_{int} = 1$, the amplitude of reflected pressure is the same as that of the incident pressure. A standing wave may be created if a sound is perfectly reflected back and forth between two parallel surfaces located at a distance L from each other. In such a simple one-dimensional room model, resonance frequencies at which standing waves occur (f_n) are given by:

$$f_n = nc/2L \qquad \text{(Eq. 4–6)}$$

where n is an integer ($n = 1, 2, 3, \ldots$) and c is the speed of sound in the air. In other words, a standing wave exists when a frequency is such that the distance L is equal to an integer multiple of one-half of a wavelength λ, or:

$$L = n\lambda/2. \qquad \text{(Eq. 4–7)}$$

For example, if the room has a length of L = 10 m, then the longest wavelength of the standing wave (for $n = 1$) is 20 m. Therefore, assuming that $c = 343$ m/s, the lowest resonance frequency is approximately 17 Hz (c/λ; 343/20). Consecutive resonance frequencies are 34, 51, 68 Hz, and so forth.

The pressure is always at a maximum at the wall when the room is driven at any of its resonance frequencies. When the sound source is located at an anti-node for a given resonance frequency, the maximum pressure is twice the source amplitude because the incident and reflected waves are in phase at the wall. With the source located at a node, the room response drops to zero; the amplitude of the pressure wave as a function of position in the room will be zero regardless of the pressure amplitude at a source.

A standing wave pattern will only occur when the room is driven at a resonance frequency. At any other frequency, the wave radiated from the source reflects from the walls, but it does not combine to create a standing wave. Thus, there are no antinodes and nodes, and the pressure may reach zero at a wall. Typically, an incident wave is not completely but rather partially reflected, that is, $R < 1$. Standing waves may be still formed by an interaction of incident and partially reflected waves; however, the maximum pressure will be smaller than twice the source amplitude and will be greater than zero at a node.

In a three-dimensional enclosed space, a complicated pattern of three-dimensional standing waves, or room modes, exists. There are three basic types of room modes. Axial modes take place between two opposing parallel surfaces as described above for a one-dimensional model. Axial modes are a function of the linear dimensions of a room. Tangential modes occur between four surfaces and oblique modes between all six surfaces of the room. Therefore, tangential and oblique modes are a function of two or all three of the dimensions of the room, respectively.

Modes are described by mode numbers *n1, n2, n3*, which are integers (0, 1, 2, etc.). For a rectangular room of dimensions L (length), W (width), and H (height), the frequencies of the room modes are given by the equation:

$$f_{n1n2n3} = c/2\,[(n1/L)^2 + (n2/W)^2 + (n3/H)^2]^{1/2}. \qquad \text{(Eq. 4–8)}$$

If two mode numbers are zero, then Equation 4–8 represents axial modes (e.g., $f_{1,0,0}$). When one of three mode numbers is zero, the equation provides values of frequencies of tangential modes. If all three numbers are different from zero, oblique modes may be described. The combination of these three mode types forms a set of possible standing wave frequencies in a room. Rooms designated for clinical activities involving patients with communication disorders should have highly absorptive materials placed appropriately to limit or to eliminate the possibility of creating multiple reflections, especially between parallel surfaces—for example, between the ceiling and the floor (see subsequent sections of this chapter).

A distribution of room modes is important because it directly affects the frequency response of a room when stimulated by a sound source, especially at low frequencies, because of the relatively low modal density in small rooms. It is desirable to space room modes as evenly as possible to avoid the situation of multiple modal frequencies falling within a small bandwidth or bandwidths with absence of modes. If a room is a perfect cube, there will be a large resonance at a low frequency corresponding to the lowest axial mode that is the same for all three dimensions ($f_{1,0,0}$, $f_{0,1,0}$, and $f_{0,0,1}$). Therefore, it is better to design a room where all three dimensions are different. Equation 4–8 also shows that if any of

the dimensions are integer multiples of each other, then some of the frequencies of the room modes will be the same. Therefore, it is better to choose noncommensurate (i.e., not harmonically related) ratios for the room dimensions to obtain the modes that are spread out as much as possible.

Many methods and optimum room ratios have been suggested over the last 65 years to minimize the absence or boosting of certain frequencies in the room response. Often the most favorable dimensions are given in terms of the ratios to the smallest room dimension. Bolt (1946) provided a chart to determine good room ratios under the assumption that evenly spaced modal frequencies would create fewer problems with peaks and dips in the modal response. He suggested the ratio of 1:1.26:1.59, but also noted that there was a broad area over which the average modal spacing criterion would be acceptable. Louden (1971) used the standard deviation of the intermode spacing and recommended a room ratio of 1:1.4:1.9.

In general, the number of resonances within a given frequency bandwidth increases with frequency. The top panel of Figure 4–1 displays frequencies of modes up to 275 Hz for a rectangular room with a height of 3.5 m and the ratio of dimensions of 1:1.26:1.59, as suggested by Bolt. Modal frequencies are relatively equally spaced with no coincident modes as indicated by the same mode strength for all components depicted. However, some of the frequencies are very close to each other (e.g., a tangential mode and an axial mode around 63 Hz).

Bonello (1981) developed criteria for assessing the modal behavior in a room based on perceptual terms. The number

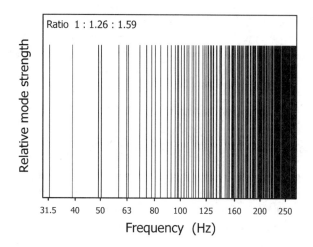

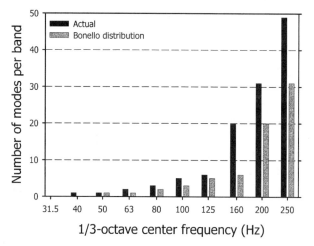

Figure 4–1. *Top:* Distribution of room modes for a rectangular room with a height of 3.5 m and the ratio of dimensions as indicated. Relative mode strength is shown in arbitrary units. There are no coincident modes as indicated by the same mode strength of all components. *Bottom:* Distribution of modes in 1/3-octave bands for the room with modal frequencies depicted in the top (*black bars*) and for Bonello's criteria (*gray bars*). See text for more information.

of modes is counted in 1/3-octave bands, which represent an approximation of critical bands (Moore, 2003). If the number of modes per band increases monotonically, then it is assumed that the room will be perceived as having a smooth frequency response. In addition, modes with coincidental frequencies are not expected to create perceptually noticeable response peaks in a band when there are at least three additional noncoincident resonances to balance the two that are coincident. The bottom panel of Figure 4–1 represents the distribution of modes per 1/3-octave bands for the room with modal frequencies depicted in the top panel. It is assumed that if the bar calculated according to Bonello's criteria (gray) in any 1/3-octave exceeds the actual bar (black) in the same 1/3-octave, the room is "nonideal." If this is the case, an alternate ratio of room dimensions should be considered, or if altering the room dimensions may not feasible, adaptation of the room acoustics should be planned. The frequency range below approximately 200 Hz is acoustically the most challenging because of the spatially and frequency-wise distribution of room modes. Computer programs are available that provide the calculations of the resonant modes of a given room and suggestions for optimum sound source (e.g., a loudspeaker) and listener placements.

Reverberation

Below approximately 200 Hz the acoustics of different locations in the room are dominated by a particular distribution of discrete room resonances. For frequencies above 200 Hz, these modes become tightly packed in frequency (see Figure 4–1), the room behaves more uniformly, and is better described by its reverberation properties. When a sound source, such as a loudspeaker or a talker, is located inside a room, the waves from the source travel in diverging directions. Part of a sound that arrives directly to the listener's ears is called direct sound. The rest strikes surrounding boundaries. At each encounter with the boundaries of the room, the waves are partly absorbed (representing the loss of energy) and partly reflected. Reflected waves, after a single or multiple reflections, reach the

listener's ears with a delay of some milliseconds after the direct sound. Thus, the direct sound is followed by the reverberant sound arriving at the ears with a variety of delays and intensities. In a room with a sound source emitting a constant acoustic power, the reverberant sound builds up to a constant level. The equilibrium level occurs when the total loss of energy related to sound absorption by the boundaries of the room equals the rate at which the energy is being injected into the enclosure by the source. To predict reverberation characteristics of a room with given acoustic properties, one needs to know the total sound absorption, which depends on the areas and absorptive properties of the materials covering room boundaries.

The room absorption (also known as absorptivity or room constant), A, is described by the sum of absorption coefficients, α, weighted by their areal contribution to the room:

$$A = \alpha_1 S_1 + \alpha_2 S_2 + \alpha_3 S_3 + \ldots \quad \text{(Eq. 4–9)}$$

where α_n is an absorption coefficient of a material covering a boundary surface segment with the area of S_n. Note that A has a unit of square meters. It is called metric sabin (named after W. C. Sabine) and it is equivalent to one square meter having an absorption coefficient α of 1, as would be the case for an open window (no energy reflected back to the room). It is important to point out that α depends on frequency and it is usually measured at 125, 250, 500, 1000, 2000, and 4000 Hz. Also, the sum expressed in Equation 4–9 includes dissipation of energy in the medium within the room and absorptions due to objects (including people) placed in a room. Statistical approach assumes that except close to the source or to the absorbing surfaces, the energy distribution in the room is uniform and has random local directions of flow. In such conditions, the intensity of the reverberant sound created by the source producing the power P is given by:

$$I = 4P/A. \qquad \text{(Eq. 4–10)}$$

Note that all the information on the room is expressed by the room absorption A. Let us assume that in a busy classroom with the initial value of $A = 40$ sabins, all internal sources (e.g., air conditioning and conversation) generate a sound level of 60 dB. After installing wall and ceiling acoustic treatments, A increased to 400 sabins. Then, the reverberant sound level would be reduced by 10 dB, from 60 to 50 dB.

Most rooms have a mixture of reverberant and direct sound. At a point that is close to the sound source, more energy comes directly from the source than from the reverberant field. Then, the directivity factor of the source needs to be taken into account. That aspect of energy propagation may be related to the source per se or to a location of a source relative to room boundaries. As described above, a monopole radiates sound equally well in all directions under a free-field condition. However, if the monopole is placed on a floor that is a perfectly reflecting surface ($\alpha = 0$), then it radiates only into the upper half of the space. Therefore, the intensity at a distance r from it would be twice that given by Equation 4–2; the extra power would come from the floor reflection. Similarly, if the source is located in a three-surface corner of a room (e.g., where two walls and the ceiling meet), then the intensity would be eight times higher than that of a free-field condition.

Most sound sources—for example, the human mouth—do not radiate energy equally well in all directions, that is, they are not omnidirectional. They are characterized by their directionality. The directivity factor, Q, is defined as the ratio of the intensity of a source in some specified direction (usually along the acoustic axis of the source) to the intensity at the same point in space due to an omnidirectional point source with the same acoustic power. Thus, Q indicates how much more effectively a directional source concentrates its available acoustic power into a preferred direction. Typically, the value of Q increases with an increase of frequency and therefore it must be expressed as a function of f or $Q(f)$. For a source that is different from a monopole (then $Q = 1$), Equation 4–2 should be modified:

$$I = Q(f)\, P/(4\pi r^2). \qquad \text{(Eq. 4–11)}$$

The total intensity obtained by combining the direct and reverberant sound is given by:

$$I = Q(f)\, P/(4\pi r^2) + 4P/A. \qquad \text{(Eq. 4–12)}$$

Converting the above equation into a logarithmic scale would allow calculating contributions of the direct and reverberant sound in terms of sound intensity level:

$$L = L_p + 10\log[Q(f)/(4\pi r^2) + 4/A] \qquad \text{(Eq. 4–13)}$$

where L_p is the power level from the source referenced to one picowatt or 10^{-12} watts.

At any point in a room, a listener receives both direct sound, which follows the inverse square law (or the 6-dB rule), and reverberant sound, the level of which is independent of distance from the source. Equation 4–13 is presented graphically in Figure 4–2 assuming that a sound source is a talker with a directivity factor $Q = 3.5$ placed in a small room ($9 \times 6 \times 2.75$ m) with the room constant $A = 50$ sabins. When the listener (e.g., a child in a classroom) is close to the source, the level of the direct sound exceeds that of the reverberant sound. When the listener is far from the source, the reverberant sound dominates. The so-called critical distance, D, is defined as the distance from a sound source at which direct sound and reverberant sound are at the same level. For the example depicted in Figure 4–2, $D = 1.9$ m. At distances less than approximately one-third of the critical distance, the direct sound level is at least 10 dB stronger than the reverberant sound (open circle in Figure 4–2) and the contribution of reverberation can generally be ignored. The sound level depends on the directionality of the source and, therefore, may vary with a change in the position of a listener or of a microphone measuring sound pressure distribution across different locations. At distances greater than approximately three times

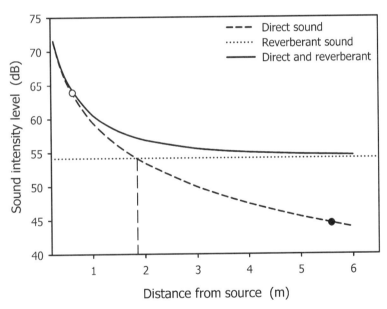

Figure 4–2. Sound intensity level in a room, with parameters described in the text, as a function of a distance from a source. The dashed line corresponds to direct sound, dotted line to reverberant sound, and solid line to total sound energy. The dashed vertical line corresponds to the critical distance from the source at which the levels of direct and reverberant sounds are equal. The open circle corresponds to one-third of the critical distance, where the direct sound level is at least 10 dB stronger than the reverberant sound. The filled circle corresponds to three times the critical distance, where the direct sound is at least 10 dB weaker than the reverberant sound.

the critical distance, the direct sound is at least 10 dB weaker than the reverberant sound(filled circle in Figure 4–2) and the contribution of the direct signal is negligible.

Reverberation Time

Equations 4–12 and 4–13 represent an equilibrium situation of a uniformly diffuse acoustic field reached when a sound source emits a constant acoustic power and the reverberant sound builds up to a constant level. When the sound source is turned off, the reverberant sound level begins to decrease because the waves emitted by the source have repeated collisions with the room boundaries losing energy with each collision as determined by the absorption coefficients. The energy will gradually decay until all sound energy gets absorbed by the boundaries. The time taken for the energy density to decrease to one-millionth of its initial value, that is, for the sound level to drop by 60 dB, is defined as the reverberation time, T_r. Sabine (1927) developed an equation for calculating the reverberation time, which remains a fundamental parameter in studies of room acoustics:

$$T_r = (0.161V)/A \qquad \text{(Eq. 4–14)}$$

where V is the cubic volume of a room in cubic meters.

Following the pioneering work of Sabine, reverberation time was measured by exciting a room into a steady state by a noise signal and recording graphically the decay curves (sound pressure level plotted against time) after the sound source was turned off. The shortcoming of that procedure was a substantial test/retest variability of decay curves, especially in the initial portion of the curves, due to the randomness of the amplitudes and phases of the normal room modes at the moment when the excitation signal was turned off. To minimize the effect of the fluctuations in decay curves, multiple measurements were performed and the results were averaged to determine the reverberation time. Schroeder (1965) proposed a new method based on applying tone bursts to excite the enclosure and then calculating the backward integration of room response. In that method, the last energy is integrated first and the initial arrival is integrated last, similar to the integration of a backward-played tape recording of the decaying signal. The data obtained from a single measurement result in a decay curve that theoretically equates to the ensemble average of infinitely many decay curves measured using interrupted noise. The work of Schroeder started a new area of research and practical applications based on the impulse response of a room.

Early and Late Reflections

The impulse response describes the propagation of a brief pressure impulse that is generated at some point inside a room and recorded by a microphone placed in another location. An example of the impulse response of a room is presented in Figure 4–3. The direct sound arrives first at the point of the microphone with a short latency, t_0, relative to the time of the initial pulse generation. The second impulse is smaller than the direct sound and it corresponds to the first reflection from the surface closest

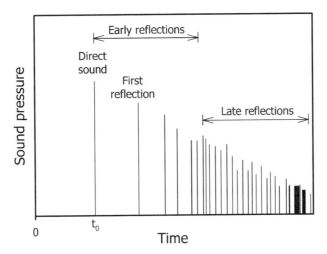

Figure 4–3. An example of the impulse response of a room. A brief pressure impulse is generated at time equals zero. Direct sound arrives first at the point of the measurement, followed by single and multiple early reflections, and a series of late reflections coming closer and closer in time.

to the microphone. Then, other pulses corresponding to single reflections from the walls, the ceiling, and the floor are recorded followed by a series of multiple reflections coming closer and closer in time. The reflected sounds become smaller and smaller because they have more encounters with the boundaries and thus are increasingly absorbed by the surface. Sounds that strike multiple surfaces represent the reverberant energy that persists for some extended period of time (expressed quantitatively by the reverberation time).

The impulse response can be used to evaluate acoustic properties of an existing room and to suggest modifications that can be made to improve communication in the room. In addition, the analysis of a predicted impulse response is useful during the process of designing a room. Many computer programs have the capability of creating models of acoustical properties of a room by simulating propagation of signals generated by virtual sound sources placed in various locations within the room of a particular shape, dimensions, and materials used to cover the boundaries (e.g., Siebein, 2004).

When analyzing the impulse room response, it is important to distinguish between early and late components (see Figure 4–3). Hass (1972) described the beneficial effect of sound reflections arriving at a listener's ears within short time periods after the direct sound. Two brief sounds are heard as a single sound if the interval between them is short. The limit is about 5 ms for clicks but may be 40 ms for complex signals such as speech. The lagging sound is suppressed. If two successive sounds are heard as fused, the location of the total sound is determined largely by the location of the first sound; a listener makes his or her localization judgments instantly based on the earliest arriving waves in the onset of a sound. This phenomenon is called the precedence effect (or Haas effect) because the earliest arriving sound wave, the direct sound with accurate localization information, is given precedence over the reverberation that conveys inaccurate information.

The precedence effect influences speech perception in rooms designed for the purpose of speech communication, such as small meeting rooms, classrooms, and auditoria. Early reflections (occurring within a 50 to 80-ms time window after the direct sound) can be integrated with the direct sound. They are considered a useful portion of the energy because they generally increase the audibility of a speech source without degrading intelligibility (e.g., Bradley, Sato, & Picard, 2003). A study of Nábělek and Robinette (1978) performed for normal and hearing-impaired listeners indicated that reflections arriving shortly after the direct sound may enhance word identification in both groups of subjects if the direct sound level was not sufficient. Later reflections (greater than 50–80 ms) are perceived as a prolongation of the sound and "smear out" the temporal information. For speech signals, those later reflections cause a decrease in intelligibility. Therefore, in a room where speech communication is the deciding factor for evaluating its acoustical quality, reverberation is often considered in negative terms, together with background noise that can originate from outside or inside a room. Some of the most common sources of noise include air and road traffic, heating, ventilating and air conditioning systems, human activity in adjacent rooms, and internal human activity (including speech). The effect of

noise can be considered negligible if its level is at least 10 dB below that of the late reverberation. Similarly, the effect of late reverberation is insignificant if its level is at least 10 dB below that of the noise. See Chapter 2 of Volume 1 of this Handbook for discussion of psychoacoustic considerations and implications.

The effects of background noise and reverberation should not be viewed as two room properties occurring separately but rather as combining in a synergistic manner. Thus, a combination of noise and reverberation may potentially induce a more significant decrease of speech recognition than the sum of those two effects being treated separately (Smaldino, Crandell, Kreisman, John, & Kreisman, 2008). It has been suggested that this synergistic effect results from reverberation filling in temporal gaps in background noise. Therefore, the temporal structure of noise becomes steadier and the noise acts as a more effective masker. Consequently, it has been suggested that in order to provide adequate classroom acoustics necessary for creating a desirable learning environment, especially for children with communicative disorders, both a reduced reverberation time and high signal-to-noise (S/N) ratios are needed (ANSI, 2010).

Several approaches to quantify acoustical qualities related to speech intelligibility in rooms have been reported (Smaldino et al., 2008). For example, Lochner and Burger (1961) introduced the useful-to-detrimental energy ratios as a measure of different contributions of early versus late reflections to speech intelligibility. These measures relate the useful portion of energy in a signal (e.g., in speech), consisting of the direct sound and early reflections, to the detrimental energy, which consists of reverberant energy and background noise. Bradley (1986) evaluated different acoustical measures as predictors of speech intelligibility in rooms of varied size and acoustical conditions. He showed high predictive accuracy of the U_{80} parameter, that is, a useful-to-detrimental energy ratio calculated with the value of 80 msselected as the dividing point between the early energy that is useful and contributes to the loudness of the direct sound and the detrimental energy. Similarly, there are other early/late ratio measures, U_{35}, U_{50}, U_{90}, when the value of 35, 50, or 95 ms is defined as the dividing point between the early and late energy, respectively. These latter parameters are related to the effective S/N ratio; the effective signal is a combination of the direct signal and early reverberation, whereas the effective noise is a combination of actual noise (from external and internal sources) and late reverberation. It is generally agreed that if the listener is to have access to all the useful information in the speech signal, the effective S/N needs to be at least 15 dB across a broad frequency region (e.g., Boothroyd, 2004). One possibility for reaching this requirement would be to minimize T_r.

Maximizing Room Acoustics

The recent ANSI standard (ANSI, 2010) specifies maximum reverberation times in unoccupied, furnished learning spaces measured in octave bands with center frequencies of 500, 1000, and 2000 Hz. The recommended value of T_r is 0.6 seconds or lower in small to medium class-

rooms (with enclosed volume ≤10,000 ft^3 or ≤283 m^3) and 0.7 seconds or lower in large classrooms (with enclosed volume >10,000 ft^3 and ≤20,000 ft^3). The presence of 20 to 25 students in a room is expected to lower T_r by approximately 0.05 seconds. A position statement of the American Speech-Language-Hearing Association (ASHA, 2005) recommended acoustical criteria that are essentially identical to the ANSI standard.The ANSI and ASHA recommendations suggest a need for minimizing reverberation times. Very short values of T_r may be obtained by increasing absorption of room surfaces. However, that solution is likely to lead to reduced early reflection energy and therefore to reduced speech intelligibility (see above). Bradley et al. (2003) reported data on speech intelligibility tests in simulated sound fields for normal-hearing and hearing-impaired listeners. The results showed that increased early reflection energy (arriving within the first 50 ms after the direct sound) had the same effect in increasing speech intelligibility scores as increased direct sound level; therefore, adding early reflections increases the effective S/N. Moreover, both groups of subjects benefitted similarly from added early reflections. The results also confirmed that listeners with hearing-impairment required approximately 5 dB higher S/N values to have similar intelligibility scores as normal-hearing listeners (Bradley et al., 2003). Furthermore, it needs to be realized that several populations of children—for example, children with learning disabilities, dyslexia, or (central) auditory processing deficit—may experience difficulty recognizing speech in noise despite their normal hearing sensitivity (Smaldino et al., 2008). Those children require a much more favorable S/N in order to access the classroom instruction; a +15 S/N value has been recommended.

The directionality of the humanvoice may also influence the amount of the direct energy available to a listener. For example, when the talker's head is turned away from the listener, the listener will experience reduced direct speech sound, especially for the high frequencies, which are critical for speech recognition. By modifying the spectrum of the direct speech sound, Bradley et al. (2003) simulated changes in the talker's head angle relative to the listener. When early reflections were added, there was only a small reduction in intelligibility scores for the situation of the talker's head turned 180 degrees (i.e., facing away from the listener) compared with the zero-degree position (i.e., the talker situated straight ahead). Those results clearly indicated that in many situations, where the direct sound is reduced due to the talker who is not facing the listener, speech understanding is possible only because of the benefits of early reflections.

Analyses of impulse response measurements in typical rooms used for speech communication included in the study of Bradley et al. (2003) indicated that the effect of early reflections in rooms is equivalent to an increase in the direct speech level of up to 9 dB. Moreover, the benefit of the early reflection energy tended to increase with an increase of a distance between a source (talker) and a receiver (listener). That finding emphasizes that a correct design that enhances early reflections provides the greatest increase in intelligibility where it is most needed, that is, the farthest from the source.

In recent years, many computer programs have been developed to assist architects, acousticians, and engineers in designing new rooms and modifyingexisting rooms (e.g., Bradley, et al., 2003; Siebein, 2004). Software resources may be used to construct computer models for evaluating and maximizing room acoustics at different stages of such projects. As described above, the major goal in the acoustical design of rooms for speech communication should be to maximize the energy of the direct sound and early reflections.

Computer models allow evaluation of different options for placement of sound-reflecting surfaces to enhance the signal. Optimal locationof acoustic reflectors on a ceiling depends on teaching strategy and may be different for a typical lecture-type classroom than for a room designated for small group instruction with general movement throughout the classroom by the teacher. Different options for spatial distribution of absorbing materials also may be tested using computer models to ensure that there is no excessive later arriving reflection energy and to optimize frequency characteristics of the reverberation time.

Clearly, model studies are helpful in evaluating the geometry of a room in terms of a distribution of room modes that should be spaced as evenly at low frequencies as possible. Strong specular (mirrorlike) reflections should be limited in small rooms where standing waves modes are well separated at low frequencies. One method of reducing specular reflections involves placing diffusing surfaces (Kleiner, 2012). A diffusing surface, for example a roughened or a textured one, creates random scattering of incident waves. Such an option is relatively easy to implement; however, the response of a diffusing surface is difficult to predict due to random characteristics of the reflections. Specially designed diffusers provide a uniform diffraction pattern over a specified frequency range, defined as the operating bandwidth.

Very often the term "damping" rather than "absorption" is used to describe properties of absorbers that are designed to maximize the conversion of acoustic energy to heat and thus result in minimizing late reflections and detrimental resonances. In physics, damping describes an effect that tends to reduce the amplitude of oscillations. It seems more appropriate, therefore, to relate damping to the characteristics of a sound source and absorption to a decrease of acoustic energy that has been generated by the source and decays, while propagating in a room, due to the characteristics of the boundaries. During the process of designing acoustical properties of a room, placement of absorbing materials should be carefully arranged to enhance speech communication in the room.

Presence of students in a classroom or in an auditorium, as well as of the audience in a performance space represents "natural absorbers" together with sound-absorptive surfaces, such as furniture, walls, ceilings, and floors. In many cases "added absorbers" are used to achieve the desired acoustic properties of a room. There are two general categories of sound absorbers. Nonresonant absorbers, also known as porous absorbers, made of materials such as mineral wool, fiberboard, or plastic foams dissipate acoustic energy by friction that air molecules encounter while moving through pores. When such absorbers are applied directly to a reflecting surface (e.g., to a hard wall of a room), their effectiveness depends on the thicknessof the matter. For a sound wave that is incident on a rigid wall, the maximum parti-cle velocity occurs at $\lambda/4$. If the thickness of the absorber is less than one quarter of the wavelength, the absorption effect is small. Therefore, even relatively thick porous sheets placed on a solid wall are effective primarily for high frequencies with short wavelengths (see Equation 4–1).

The second type of absorbers, the resonant absorbers, is designed using the resonance properties of air columns, membranes, and plates. For example, panel absorbers are often used when low-frequency absorption is required. Thin wood panels are mounted away from the wall, creating an air cavity. Incident sound at a particular frequency causes the panel to vibrate. Due to inherent resistance of the panel to rapid flexing and to the resistance of the enclosed air to compression, some of the sound energy is converted into heat by the internal damping. Panel absorbers are most effective at their resonant frequency (typically around 100 Hz), which depends upon density of the surface material and the width of the enclosed space. Filling the cavity with a porous material results not only in broadening the frequency range over which some absorption occurs, but also in decreasing the peak value of the absorption coefficient (i.e., the "tuning" characteristics of the absorber becomes shallow).

Cavity absorbers (a type of resonant absorber), also known as resonators or Helmholtz resonators, represent alarge cavity with a port on its front to couple the enclosed volume of the airspace to the air in the room. These absorbers give a high absorption coefficient in a narrow frequency band around the resonant frequency, which is defined by the cross-sectional area and the length of the port and by the volume of air trapped in the cavity. At resonant and neighboring frequencies, the air moves in and out of the cavity, causing the acoustic energy to be converted into heat. Cavity absorbers are often used in noise control applications when energy of noise generated by machines occurs in a narrow range of frequencies. An absorber "tuned" to a targeted frequency provideshigh absorption efficiency.

All three of the mechanisms described above may be combined in slot and perforated panel absorbers. The panel itself may be plywood, hardboard, or metal and, therefore, it may act as a membrane absorber. The panel is spaced away from one of the walls and may have perforations, holes, or slots that create multiple cavity resonators. Absorption properties are improved by placement of porous materials between the wall and the panel. The frequency characteristic of the absorption coefficient depends on the width and depth of slots, pattern of perforations (hole size and spacing), the thickness of the panel and its distance from the wall, and the thickness and the placement of the porous material. There are various commercially available products that may provide required absorption properties and those are often used to reduce low-frequency reverberation time without affecting it in the high-frequency range.

Annex C to the ANSI standard (ANSI, 2010) titled "Design Guidelines for Controlling Reverberation in Classrooms and Other Learning Spaces" and a chapter by Smaldino et al. (2008) describe useful procedures towards achieving appropriate acoustical characteristics in learning spaces. The initial step involves selecting sound-absorbing materials to be installed and determining their surface areas, thus allowing calculating the total sound absorption (A) needed to apply the room acoustics Equations 4–9 and 4–14. In a classroom with a height smaller than 3 m (10 ft) and with no fixed teacher-students configuration, it is recommended to place all sound-absorbing material on the ceiling (ANSI, 2010). For ceiling heights greater than 3 m, some sound-absorbing material should be also placed on the walls. Carpeting alone in a classroom, even though it helps to reduce the level of noise in the room, does not provide enough absorption, especially at low frequencies. In rooms with greater teacher-to-student distances (e.g., in high schools), it is useful to place sound-reflecting surfaces to assure adequate S/N ratio of speech in the back of the room. If the teacher-student configuration is fixed, that is, one area (typically in the front) can be designated as the "teaching-lecturing" area, beneficial reflections are provided by sound-reflecting surfaces placed above the teacher, also extending over the students' section on the ceiling and/or sidewalls. Such an arrangement adds useful early reflections to reinforce the direct sound of the teacher's voice and increases acoustic energy reaching students in the classroom. It is important to assure, especially in small classrooms, that sound waves traveling across the room are scattered to avoid a possibility of creating continued multiple reflections between two opposite parallel surfaces. Typically, acoustic modifications include placing absorbing materials on the ceiling and additionally carpeting the floor, thus limiting or eliminating the possibility of creating continued multiple reflections between the ceiling and the floor. However, extending the placement of absorbing materials, at least partially, on one of the parallel walls can reduce potential strong excitation of room modes (see Equations 4–6 and 4–8).

Measuring Sound

The pascal (or N/m²) is a unit of the amplitude of the pressure fluctuations created by sound propagation. Due to the wide dynamic range of the human auditory system the decibel (dB) scale, which is a logarithmic measure, is more useful for measuring sound affecting human listeners. A signal with a root-mean-square (RMS) pressure, p, has a sound pressure level, L (in dB SPL), of:

$$L = 20\log(p/p_0) \qquad \text{(Eq. 4–15)}$$

where p_0 is the reference value of 20 µPa. The RMS value of a time-varying signal is defined as the numerical value of a constant that would have the same average power as the signal. For a sine wave, the RMS value is 0.707 times the amplitude of the sine.

Sound pressure levels are measured by a sound level meter (SLM) that consists of a pressure-sensitive microphone, amplifier, weighting filter, temporal averaging circuit, and a display providing the result in dB SPL re: 20 µPa. Typically, condenser microphones are used in SLMs because of high precision and stability. The electrical signal produced by the microphone is relatively small and needs to be amplified before being further processed.

The weighting filters are designed to simulate the equal loudness contours by attenuating low- and high-frequency signals. There are three internationally standardized characteristics termed A, B, and C weightings (IEC, 2002); however, the B-weighting filter is not widely used. The A-weighting filter resembles the response of the human auditory system to sine signals of low to intermediate levels (e.g., Moore, 2003). It attenuates low frequencies substantially, for example, by 19 dB at 100 Hz relative to 1 kHz. The A-weighted measures are most often used in evaluating sound annoyance. The C-weighting filter approximates equal loudness contour at high SPLs. Its response is almost flat with a small attenuation for frequencies below 200 Hz (e.g., 2 dB at 40 Hz) and above 1250 Hz (e.g., 3 dB at 8 kHz).

Most sounds that need to be measured fluctuate in level over time. Different settings of the temporal averaging circuit of an SLM allow a selection of response characteristics most appropriate to obtain an RMS value of a signal depending on its rate of fluctuation. A time constant of 125 ms (a "fast" setting) enables one to measure and follow signals fluctuating slowly. A time constant of one second (a "slow" option) gives a response that averages out fast fluctuations. For measurements of very short (impulse) signals, SLMs have impulse characteristics with a time constant of 35 ms, which is short enough to enable detection of a transient sound. In addition, some SLMs include a circuit for measuring the peak and the maximum RMS values of the sound level, regardless of its duration and fluctuations. Modern SLMs have digital displays that depict results and information of settings (e.g., A-weighting, fast versus slow averaging time constant).

Annoyance of noise depends not only on its level, but also on its duration. For constant sound levels, the measurement is straightforward. If the signal varies over time, the level must be sampled repeatedly over a specified time period. Most commonly, level-fluctuating sounds are described in terms of an average level that has the same acoustical energy as the summation of all the time-varying events. This energy-equivalent sound descriptor is called the equivalent continuous sound level, L_{eq}. The most common averaging period is hourly. For example, a one-hour-average A-weighted sound level is a single-value measure corresponding to the time-mean-square A-weighted sound pressure averaged over a one-hour period.

Noise Sources in a Classroom

In addition to specifying maximum reverberation times, the ANSI standard (ANSI, 2010) provides criteria for background noise in classrooms. The one-hour-average A-weighted steady background noise in a classroom shall not exceed 35 dB. For large spaces with volumes >20,000 ft^3, the limit is 40 dBA SPL. These limits apply to the noisiest continuous one-hour period during times when learning activities take place and while exterior and interior noise sources are operating simultaneously.

According to Siebein (2004), poorly designed heating, ventilation, and air conditioning (HVAC) systems are the primary sources of noise in classrooms. Siebein provided recommendations for designing air handling units to achieve background noise criteria of ANSI. Noise from students within the classroom, in adjoining rooms, and in outdoor areas adds significant amounts of energy to the unwanted background (Smaldino et al., 2008). Absorbers placed in a classroom reduce noise from students' activities within the room, in addition to optimizing reverberation. Installing carpet on the floor may decrease impact sounds propagating within multistory school buildings. Walls, windows, and doors with high transmission loss also lower the noise level of exterior sources. This is especially important if a site for a school is located near a major road, airport, railway line, or industrial noise source. One needs to keep in mind that acoustic isolation of a classroom is limited by the weakest element in the entire acoustic system. For example, a gap between a window frame and a wall can negate high transmission loss of the wall.

In some situations, a sufficient S/N ratio cannot be achieved by modifying room acoustics or by lowering the influence of noise sources. In such cases, amplification provided by personal FM or sound-field technology systems should be considered. These systems consist of a wireless microphone used by a teacher, an amplifier, and loudspeakers carefully located in the classroom to increase the level of speech signals (see Chapter 12).

High-Fidelity Transducers

High-fidelity or *hi-fi* reproduction is defined as the reproduction of sounds that is as close as possible to the original. A hi-fi system contains several different devices and any device within that system may distort signals in various ways or add some amount of noise. The performance of the entire system is determined by the performance of its weakest element. A set of measurements is performed to assess the sound quality of each element.

One specification that is commonly evaluated is frequency response. A sine wave of constant amplitude and varying frequency is used as an input signal to the device and the output signal is expected not to vary as a function of frequency. Typically, there are some irregularities in the response and the frequency range that is reproduced is limited. For example, the frequency response of a loudspeaker may be stated as 60 to 18,000 Hz ± 3 dB, meaning that the sound level would not vary over more than a 6-dB range for any frequency from 60 Hz to 18 kHz. From a perceptual standpoint, it is not necessary to extend the response of a hi-fi device below 30 Hz, as there is little audible energy in musical signals below that frequency, except for synthesized sounds and some organ sounds of a very low pitch. Due to the frequency limits of hearing, generally stated to lie between 20 Hz and 20 kHz for normal young human ears, it is also assumed that in the absence of distortions, energy in the range above 16 kHz would not make a significant contribution to the perceived sound quality. Thus, a frequency response extending from 30 Hz to 16 kHz is perfectly sufficient for hi-fi reproduction (Moore, 2003).

Significant irregularities in the frequency response may affect the timbre of the reproduced sound. A series of studies reported by Green (1988) on a so-called profile analysis suggested that listeners cannot detect changes in spectral shape when the level in a given frequency region is changed by less than 2 dB relative to the level in other frequency bands. A response that is flat within ±1 dB, therefore, would not be perceptually different from a completely flat one. A frequency response specified as 30 to 16,000 Hz ±1 dB would be ideal in term of perceptual relevance.

In general, all elements of a hi-fi system exhibit some degree of nonlinearity or, in other words, they generate distortion (i.e., the presence of some frequency components in the output signal that are not present in the input signal).

One method of evaluating the degree of nonlinearity is to measure harmonic distortions. A pure tone of a particular frequency is used as an input signal. Due to nonlinearities, the output signal would contain a fundamental component with the same frequency as that of the input signal and a series of harmonics, that is, components with frequencies corresponding to integer multiplications of the fundamental frequency. The total amplitude of the second and higher order harmonics, expressed as a percentage of the amplitude of the fundamental, is called the total harmonic distortion (THD). The audibility of harmonic distortion depends on the spectrum of the input signal and on the distribution of energy among harmonics. If the second and third harmonics dominate, THD of 2 to 3% will not be noticed if the signal is a piece of music; however, if the distortion produces significant energy at high-order harmonics, TDH above approximately 0.1% may be audible (Moore, 2003).

Another method of measuring distortion is to apply simultaneously two pure tones (primary tones) with frequencies f_1 and f_2 at the input and to measure combination products in the output signal with frequencies such as $f_1 - f_2$, $2f_1 - f_2$, or $f_1 + f_2$ (intermodulation distortions). The total amplitude of the intermodulation signals is expressed as a percentage of the amplitudes of the primary tones. The audibility of intermodulation distortion may be difficult to predict; however, in general a value smaller than 0.5% is not expected to be detected (Moore, 2003).

Some amount of undesired noise, in the form of a low-frequency hum due to the frequency of the alternating current (AC) power supply and/or in the form of a high-frequency hiss, may be expected to be added to the signal by many devices. The S/N ratio, expressed in decibels, is specified as the ratio of the output power for a relatively high-level signal to the output power due to hum and noise alone. A ratio greater than 70 dB is adequate for listening to music at moderate sound levels (Moore, 2003).

A basic sound reinforcement (i.e., amplification) system consists of an input device (e.g., a microphone, a CD or an MP3 player), an amplifier, and an output device (one loudspeaker or a set of loudspeakers). The primary goal of the sound system in a room designed for speech communication is to deliver clear, intelligible speech to each listener. The performance of modern hi-fi amplifiers and CD players is likely to be more than adequate for limits required by the ear (Moore, 2003). The sound quality of the entire system, therefore, typically is determined by the performance of the microphone and loudspeakers. The microphone, which is an electroacoustic transducer converting the waveform of sound pressure to an electrical signal, is the first link in the audio system. The ideal microphone should generate the output (electrical) signal having the same waveform as the input (acoustical) signal. Thus, a poor quality microphone may result in preventing the rest of the system from functioning to its full potential.

The sensitivity of a microphone is defined as the level of its electrical output for a sound of a particular level at its input. For weak sounds, a microphone of high sensitivity is desirable. The directional characteristic of a microphone is defined as the variation of its output when it is oriented at different angles relative to the direction of the sound source. An omnidirectional microphone is equally sensitive to sound coming from all directions and its characteristics will show on a polar graph as a smooth circle. Since all microphones have a finite size, they become directional at sufficiently high frequencies, for example, over frequencies of a few kHz. A unidirectional microphone is most sensitive to sound coming from a particular direction. A cardioid microphone, with a heart-shaped polar pattern, is the most common type of unidirectional microphones (Kleiner, 2012). The cardioid microphone is most sensitive to sound coming from the front of the microphone and least sensitive to sound from the rear; therefore, it may be directed toward the desired sound source and away from the undesired source. In addition, a cardioid microphone picks up less ambient noise than an omnidirectional microphone. Directional characteristics may vary as a function of frequency, but high-quality microphones maintain their directivity pattern over a wide frequency range.

Active microphones, including some types of condenser microphones, need to be supplied with electrical power to operate, usually through the output cables. Since the power signal uses a very high frequency or it is a direct current (DC) source, it does not interfere with the microphone output (audio) signal. The most common design, *phantom power*, provides a simple solution of canceling both the power supply signal and its noise (Kleiner, 2012).

Two microphone transducer types, that is, condenser (or capacitive) and electrodynamic, are the most widely used microphone systems (Kleiner, 2012). The transducer of a condenser microphone is a plate capacitor in which the distance between the plates varies due to sound pressure. A passive condenser microphone that uses an electrically conductive diaphragm and a back plate to form the transducer has to be supplied with a polarization voltage to generate a static charge between the plates. Fast variations in capacitance created by sound pressure lead to voltage variations corresponding to the input (acoustical) signal. Most recently designed condenser microphones use an electret, that is, an electrostatically charged material, typically a plastic film to permanently charge the microphone transducer, so that no polarization voltage is necessary. The film, for example made from polymers, can be used both as a diaphragm, after metallization, and as a layer on the back plate. Together with a preamplifier, the electret microphone can be made very small and it can be manufactured at a relatively low cost. The condenser microphones designed using recent technologies have fairly flat frequency response and low directivity. The major advantage of condenser microphones over the other types is their low distortion. However, due to their low output level, condenser microphones always require a microphone preamplifier.In a dynamic microphone, a coil of wire is mounted on a diaphragm surrounded by a magnetic field. When the diaphragm is moved by a change of air pressure (sound), the resulting fluctuations in the magnetic field create the electric signal corresponding to the sound picked up by a microphone. Since the magnetic field can be relatively strong, the microphone can have fairly high sensitivity. Dynamic microphones are self-powered, economical, but still provide excellent sound quality. Therefore, they are the most widely used in general sound reinforcement systems. In an environment like a boardroom, audi-

torium, or a courthouse, when the highest sound quality is desired, a condenser microphone rather than a dynamic microphone might be preferred.

Microphones used for speech communication include several designs: hand-held, user-worn (clip-on, lavalier styles worn on a lanyard around the neck, or head-worn types), and free-standing mounted or surface mounted. For optimum operation of a microphone, it should be placed much closer from a talker than the critical distance (D) to get an acceptable ratio of direct-to-reverberant sound. In general, an omnidirectional microphone should be placed no farther from the talker than 30% of D, and a unidirectional microphone should be positioned closer than 50% of D. In the example depicted in Figure 4–2, those values would be approximately 55 cm and 90 cm, respectively.

Any type of microphone (except phantom-powered condensers) may be used as part of a wireless system, which needs to include a radio transmitter and a radio receiver to replace the microphone cable with a radio link. The transmitter uses the audio signal from the microphone to vary frequency of a radio signal based on frequency modulation (FM) and broadcasts the microphone signal to the receiver. See Chapter 12 for discussion of FM technology.

Loudspeakers are transducers that convert electrical energy of a signal delivered by an amplifier into an acoustic pressure signal. Retaining the waveform of the signal as close as possible is the goal of designing a high-quality loudspeaker. The loudspeaker's diaphragm driven by a force of an electromechanical transducer moves the surrounding air particles. The term "loudspeaker" is widely used to describe both the loudspeaker driver (motor) and its box. The acoustic design of the loudspeaker box modifies sounds radiated by the driver. In a horn loudspeaker, the diaphragm radiates through a horn placed in front; thus, it is possible to dramatically change the acoustical properties of the output signals. Horn loudspeakers are typically used in outdoor and indoor arenas, theatres, and cinemas. Loudspeaker drivers use electrodynamic, piezoelectric, and electrostatic transduction principles (Kleiner, 2012). An electrodynamic driver uses the force generated by electric current in a coil of metal wire attached to a diaphragm and placed in the magnetic field provided by a permanent magnet. The frequency response of a loudspeaker is typically measured in an anechoic chamber where there are no reflections from walls, ceiling, or floor. A loudspeaker's efficiency is expressed in dB/W by measuring the sound pressure level at a distance of one meter from the loudspeaker for an input of one watt. The electrodynamic loudspeakers are the most widely used due to a simple and inexpensive design, sufficient acoustic power output, and good frequency response. However, their efficiencies typically do not exceed 5% and amplifiers are needed to produce a particular sound level. Loudspeakers often generate significant amounts of harmonic and intermodulation distortion, with a common THD value of approximately 1 to 2%; therefore, a loudspeaker is most likely to be the weakest element of a hi-fi system (Moore, 2003).

It is desirable to reproduce the full range of audio frequencies (from 30 to 16,000 Hz) uniformly for the playback frequency band of the speaker system, but it is difficult for one loudspeaker unit to reproduce such a wide range of frequencies. Even a high fidelity loudspeaker driver may provide a uniform frequency response limited to a frequency range of three octaves. Therefore, it is common practice to subdivide the frequency range and use different loudspeaker drivers for high, middle, and low frequency ranges. These designs are called two- or three-way systems, depending on how many drivers are used in a single loudspeaker box to cover the desired frequency range. Electrical low- and high-pass filters, called crossover filters, divide the frequencies of a signal to reach the designated loudspeaker driver. Using more than one driver also helps to partially solve the problems related to the directional characteristics of a loudspeaker (see earlier discussion on the directivity factor Q for sound sources.) The frequency response of a loudspeaker is typically measured with a microphone placed directly in front of the loudspeaker. If the microphone is placed at some angle to the loudspeaker but at the same distance from it, the measured sound pressure level may decrease due to directional characteristics. In conventional loudspeakers, the beam of energy radiated by a loudspeaker grows narrower as the frequency increases. By using multiple drivers, each of which produces a reasonable wide beam over the range of frequencies it reproduces, directional characteristics that are more independent of frequency than that of a single-transducer speaker are created (Moore, 2003).

Room acoustics also influence the perceived sound quality reproduced by a loudspeaker because: (1) reflections are always present, (2) high frequencies are usually absorbed more than low frequencies, and (3) at low frequencies room resonances may be excited by acoustic energy radiated by the loudspeaker. Peaks and dips of the frequency response measured in an anechoic chamber may be combined with peaks and dips produced by room acoustics to produce a substantially irregular response of the loudspeaker in a particular room. To minimize this effect, the frequency response recorded in the anechoic chamber should be as smooth as possible. If loudspeakers are part of a sound system in a room, their parameters and location should be carefully designed to provide the most even distribution of sound throughout the space and to minimize acoustic feedback that arises when the sound from the loudspeakers recirculates and is picked up by a microphone. The ANSI (2010) standard underscores the need of achieving the acoustical design of classrooms first, while treating the audio distribution system as an additional element of a complex room design. Such a system should assist persons with low-amplitude voice levels or those with certain hearing conditions. Installed classroom audio distribution systems should have uniform coverage within ±2.5 dB for octave-band sound pressure levels with midband frequencies of 0.5, 1, 2, and 4 kHz.

Summary

Sound waves carry acoustic energy generated by a source (e.g., loudspeaker, musical instruments, or a speaker) away from that source. In a free-field condition (i.e., in a space with no boundaries), the sound intensity decreases inversely with the square of the distance from the source. Major departures from the inverse square law occur in most listening conditions (including the classroom) due to obstacles in the sound path resulting in reflection, absorption, diffusion, and altered transmission of sound waves. Interference of waves reflected within a three-dimensional enclosed space may create a complicated pattern of standing waves. Computer programs are available to optimize room geometry and the placement of sound sources (e.g., loudspeakers) and listeners to maximize the uniformdistribution of acoustic energy within the room. Some of the sound generated by a source located inside a room arrives directly at the listener's ears. Other waves reflected by the boundaries of the room reach the listener's ears with a delay subsequent to the direct sound. The listener is able to integrate early reflections (occurring within 50 ms) with the direct sound) and increase speech intelligibility. Excessive reverberation (i.e., extended persistence of sound in a room due to multiple reflections) may reduce intelligibility; therefore, a room design that enhances early reflections and controls reverberation (but not necessarily decreasing it too much) benefits room acoustics. It is important to recognize that acoustic conditions of a room that are tolerable for normally hearing adults in informal conversation can be difficult for children in learning situations. Even though adequate classroom acoustics is an important prerequisite for learning for all children, it is especially a critical factor for individuals with deficits of hearing, language, attention, or processing. A carefully designed amplification system may be helpful to deliver clear speech signals to each listener within the room.

References

American National Standards Institute. (2010). *Acoustical performance criteria, design requirements, and guidelines for schools. Part 1: Permanent schools.* ANSI S12.60. New York, NY: Author.

American Speech-Language-Hearing Association. (2005). *Acoustics in educational settings: Position statement.* Retrieved from http://www.asha.org/policy/PS2005-00028.htm

Bolt, R. H. (1946). Note on normal frequency statistics for rectangular rooms. *Journal of the Acoustical Society of America, 18,* 130–133.

Bonello, O. J. (1981). New criterion for the distribution of normal room modes. *Journal of the Audio Engineering Society, 29,* 597–605.

Boothroyd, A. (2004). Room acoustics and speech perception. *Seminars in Hearing, 25,* 155–166.

Bradley, J. S. (1986). Predictors of speech intelligibility in rooms. *Journal of the Acoustical Society of America, 80,* 837–845.

Bradley, J. S., Sato, H., & Picard, M. (2003). On the importance of early reflections for speech in rooms. *Journal of the Acoustical Society of America, 113,* 3233–3244.

Cramer, O. (1993). The variation of the specific heat ratio and the speed of sound in air with temperature, pressure, humidity and CO_2 concentration. *Journal of the Acoustical Society of America, 93,* 2510–2516.

Green, D. M. (1988). *Profile analysis.* Oxford, UK: Oxford University Press.

Haas, H. (1972). The influence of a single echo on the audibility of speech. *Journal of the Audio Engineering Society 20,* 146–159.

International Electrotechnical Commission. (2002). *Electroacoustics—sound level meters. Part 1: Specifications.* IEC 61672-1. Geneva, Switzerland: Author.

Kleiner, M. (2012). *Acoustics and audio technology.* Fort Lauderdale, FL: J. Ross.

Lochner, J. P. A., & Burger, J. F. (1961). The intelligibility of speech under reverberant conditions. *Acustica, 11,* 195-200.

Louden, M. M. (1971). Dimension ratios of rectangular rooms with good distribution of eigentones. *Acustica, 24,* 101–104.

Moore, B. C. J. (2003). *Psychology of Hearing.* San Diego, CA: Academic Press.

Nábělek, A. K., & Robinette, L. (1978). Influence of the precedence effect on word identification by normally hearing and hearing-impaired subjects. *Journal of the Acoustical Society of America, 63,* 187–194.

Sabine, W. C. (1927). *Collected papers on acoustics.* Cambridge, MA: Harvard University Press.

Schroeder, M. R. (1965). New method of measuring reverberation time. *Journal of the Acoustical Society of America, 37,* 409–412.

Siebein, G. W. (2004) Understanding classroom acoustic solutions. *Seminars in Hearing, 25,* 141–154.

Smaldino, J. J., Crandell, C. C., Kreisman, B. M., John, A. B., & Kreisman, N. V. (2008). Room acoustics for listeners with normal hearing and hearing impairment. In M. Valente, H. Hosford-Dunn, & R. J. Roeser (Eds.), *Audiology treatment* (pp. 418–451). New York, NY: Thieme Medical.

CHAPTER 5

SCHOOL POLICIES, PROCESSES, AND SERVICES FOR CHILDREN WITH CENTRAL AUDITORY PROCESSING DISORDER

GEORGINA T. F. LYNCH and CYNTHIA M. RICHBURG

Introduction

Before services for children with central auditory processing disorders (CAPD) can be fully presented and described, the reader must be conversant on three specific topics: (1) terminology used within the educational environment, (2) historical developments of special education law within the United States, and (3) how CAPD fits into the realm of special education. Therefore, when discuss school-based audiology and speech-language pathology service provision as it relates to CAPD across the United States, there are several terms and concepts that need to be described for a reader unfamiliar with the educational system to make sense of them all. For example, in education, enforcement of federal legisla-

tion concerning students with special needs is provided by the United States Office for Civil Rights (OCR) within the United States Department of Education (ED). The OCR enforces 504 services (described below) and certain sections of the Americans with Disabilities Act (ADA). The Office of Special Education and Rehabilitative Services (OSERS; a part of the U.S. ED) enforces IDEA (also described below) and the services provided under it.

Each state has its own Department of Education (DE). Under the DE within each state, there are local education agencies (LEAs), which are synonymous with the term "school district." An LEA/school district is a state-level governmental agency that supervises the educational services to the community within its public primary and secondary schools.

Some school districts directly employ their audiologists and speech-language pathologists (SLPs), while other school districts contract with their audiologists and SLPs. Audiology and speech-language pathology are referred to in legislative documents as related services (along with counseling and psychological services, physical and occupational therapy services, nursing and nutrition services), but they can also be the primary special education service that is provided to students. The legislative documents (described more fully below) are typically referred to as Public Law (PL). Therefore, the reader will note references to "PL 94-142" or "PL 93-112," but many of those public laws also have names attached to them (e.g., "The Educational for All Handicapped Children Act," "Section 504 of the Rehabilitation Act").

Because there are many states in which school districts are small, some states have resorted to forming educational cooperative agencies, or "co-ops." Therefore, in some cases, audiology and speech-language pathology services are provided in a state under this cooperative system to individual districts. Different states use different terms for cooperatives. Thus, the reader needs to be aware that Education Service Cooperatives (ESCs), Board of Cooperative Education Services (BOCES), Intermediate Units (IUs), Area Education Agencies (AEAs), and Regional Educational Service Agencies (RESAs) all refer to cooperative agencies within a state's educational system.

LEAs, or cooperatives in some cases, are charged with the responsibility of providing Individualized Education Programs (IEPs) and 504 Plans for school-age children and Individual Family Service Plans (IFSPs) for children ages birth to 3 years. An IEP defines individualized instruction and learning objectives for a child who has been labeled with a "disability," as specifically defined by federal regulations. An IEP is tailored to a student's individual needs and is intended to help that child reach educational goals. It is also intended to help educators understand the student's disability and how that disability affects the learning process.

An IFSP, on the other hand, is a plan for special services that are provided for children, ages 0 to 3 years, who have been identified, or who are at risk, for developmental delays. An IFSP identifies supports and services that will augment the identified child's development. Due to the young child's age, family members are strongly encouraged to be active with these services. Prior to the child's third birthday, a transition component is included within the IFSP to ensure continuity of services when transitioning individualized services to an IEP.

Finally, a "504" or "504 Plan" refers to Section 504 of the Rehabilitation Act (1973). This is the plan that fully describes the modifications and accommodations a school-age child might need in order to have the opportunity to perform at the same level as her peers. In the case of CAPD, this may simply mean a classroom amplification system or a test environment free of background noise.

There are components of current federal grant funding of special education programs that allow LEAs the option of utilizing portions of the funding, depending upon the intervention model used within their educational system. An example of this kind of caveat within the law is specifically cited in the Individuals with Disabilities Education Improvement Act (IDEIA; 2004) federal grant regarding the allocation of funds used to implement a Response to Intervention (RTI) model (IDEA § 300.309 (b) (613) (f); U.S. Department of Education, 2006). The National Center on Response to Intervention describes RTI as integrating "assessment and intervention within a multilevel prevention system to maximize student achievement and to reduce behavioral problems" (NCRTI, 2010, p. 2). The development of RTI over the last 10 years or so has dramatically changed the way in which public school systems identify students in need of special education services, as well as the way in which classroom instruction is delivered. The effects RTI has had on the services provided for students diagnosed with CAPD are explained later in this chapter.

These terms and concepts, along with their liberally used acronyms, make it difficult for the unfamiliar reader to fully comprehend all of the underlying forces surrounding the educational environment. Further descriptions of these and other terms will be presented throughout the chapter. For more information about terms related to audiology and speech-language pathology services in the educational setting, see works by Johnson and Seaton (2012), Richburg and Smiley (2012), and Dodge (1999).

Federal Mandates and Special Education Services

When a student's LEA is charged with identifying or remediating a CAPD, depending on how CAPD is recognized within that specific state and that specific LEA, an IEP or a 504 Plan may be implemented. But where did these terms and concepts come from? Are these plans used with all school students, or just those requiring special education services? Therefore, in addition to reviewing new terminology and concepts, a brief history about the development and evolution of special education law should help the reader understand how students access special education services and benefit from special education instruction.

Students who are identified with disabilities have civil rights, and ensuring those rights is an educator's key responsibility when developing an IEP for a student. The Education for All Handicapped Children Act of 1975, passed as PL 94-142, included seminal federal laws governing the provision of special education services to all individuals, ages 3 to 21 years. The 1980s, and specifically Public Law 99-457 (Education of the Handicapped Act Amendments of 1986), amended PL 94-142 laws by including and expanding services for children ages birth to 3 years. The Early Intervention (EI) movement, which allows service providers to identify children earlier, has benefited from this inclusion of services for preschool-age children and their families.

After multiple amendments to 1970s and 1980s federal legislation, the Individuals with Disabilities Education Act was enacted in 1990 and is known as "IDEA," or PL 101-476. Any agency receiving federal funds under IDEA must adhere to the requirements as outlined in great detail on the U.S. Department of Education's website (http://www.ed.gov/policy/speced/ guide/idea/idea2004.html). IDEA dictates that special education and related services should be designed to meet the unique learning needs of eligible children with disabilities, preschool through age 21.

IDEA was reauthorized in 2004 as the Individuals with Disabilities Education Improvement Act (IDEIA) and was most recently amended in 2006 to include supplemental requirements to govern and regulate the provision of special education services. The reader should be aware that individual states can take a great deal of time implementing and developing administrative codes that regulate the provision of special education services. Each state interprets the federal regulations, then the states develop administrative codes to align with the IDEIA codes. The process of developing state administrative codes and passing them through the state legislature can take years. The reader is encouraged to review the most recently amended version of IDEIA for current regulations, as these regulations will continue to change.

The acronyms IDEIA and IDEA are frequently interchanged when referenced in other readings, and many professionals refer to the 2004 and 2006 versions of the act simply as "IDEA." These differences in terminology can make comprehending the legislation, and appreciating the subtle contributions of each amendment, difficult. Yet, in order to fully understand how any student accesses and benefits from special education services, foundational knowledge in the area of disabilities and education policy is necessary. The policies and procedures used to evaluate, identify, and secure subsequent intervention services for students with disabilities are complex, as can be seen in the IDEIA. These policies and procedures must be taken into consideration within the context of each LEA and how the LEA interprets and implements such matters. As clinicians (specifically audiologists and SLPs) advocate for students with CAPD in the school setting, it is helpful to have a thorough understanding of the IDEIA and current federal guidelines that exist regarding the provision of special education services. Although these rules apply to all federally funded educational agencies and are amended as the law is revised, we cannot stress enough that a great variance from state to state, and from LEA to LEA, exists with respect to interpretation of these federal regulations.

For a more complete history and description of federal special education law, it is recommended that the reader see the studies by Johnson and Seaton (2012) and Richburg and Smiley (2012). In addition, to supplement these readings, the U.S. Department of Education and one's own state department of education are important and appropriate resources for acquiring a better understanding of current special education legislation.

Central Auditory Processing Disorder in the Realm of Special Education

Where We Have Been

First and foremost, the reader should be aware that IDEIA does not have a disability category for CAPD. Therefore, over the past decade, students with a diagnosis of CAPD have been at a disadvantage in terms of accessing special education services. This fact was primarily due to the nature of how federal laws guided educators through the decision-making process for children receiving special education services. That is, the influence of the term "adverse educational impact" (which was added to the 1997 reauthorization of IDEA) played a key role in the decision-making process and dictated that a student must have a disability that *interfered* with some aspect of learning. In addition, decisions were made using the "discrepancy model" under the specific learning disability (SLD) category. (Special education law requires the assignment of students to funding categories under strict eligibility guidelines, and the most frequently used funding category for CAPD has been the SLD category.) The discrepancy model required that there exist a difference (or discrepancy) between a student's IQ and academic performance. Therefore, a student with a CAPD diagnosis may not have been seen as having "enough" of a disability, or there may have been no discrepancy between the student's IQ and academic performance. Because of this lack of discrepancy, a student with a CAPD diagnosis might not have even been able to access special education services in the past. This example shows how federal regulations historically tied the hands of educators by providing a "wait to fail" model for identification instead of a preventative model of intervention.

In the earlier years of special education resource allocation, the amount of funding per student was linked to the disability category under which the child was identified, as outlined by IDEA. Under this funding model, more severe disabilities (such as the category of "multihandicapped") garnished more resources. This was because resource allocation operated under the notion that the student with multiple disabilities had "more need" than a child with a communication disorder, for example. This kind of thinking has shifted and resources are

no longer allocated in this manner. Now LEAs identify students eligible for special education services under IDEIA and report these numbers to the state. LEAs are then allocated full time equivalent (FTE) dollars per special education student, and all FTE dollars are equivalent to one another. That is, regardless of disability, the FTE is the same. Therefore, over the course of time, school districts could potentially save special education dollars if a student's need is identified earlier and intervention approaches are provided sooner using accurate and sound, evidence-based practices.

In addition to the problems encountered by educators during the decision-making process established by federal regulations, another problem arose from the variation in interpretation of the regulations, which was mentioned previously. When state education and LEA officials do not interpret the laws in the same manner, the variation that exists for implementing protocols and identifying students needing assistance is great. In the case of CAPD, this variation has led to some states (and LEAs) acknowledging CAPD as a disability, while others do not. For example, the DE for Arkansas (as well as many states) does not acknowledge CAPD as a stand-alone disability category; however, the state of Colorado's DE does acknowledge CAPD as a disability category and has very detailed guidelines for diagnosing and treating it (Colorado Department of Education, 2008). If a state or LEA does not define CAPD as a disability category, parents, students, and educators have fewer options when it comes to remediating the problems in the schools, especially if the student is not exhibiting an adverse effect on language or learning.

Where We Are Going

Fortunately, as IDEA has been amended and has evolved in its terminology and requirements, the focus on SLD as it pertains to a CAPD diagnosis and the provision of appropriate services is now being looked at differently in many states. The kindergarten through third-grade emphasis for intervention delivery now allows educators more flexibility in terms of early intervention; thus, the "wait to fail" approach is no longer acceptable in many LEAs. The advent of RTI has brought about positive change in the way some LEAs identify students needing special education services, as well as the way in which classroom instruction is delivered. (Services directly targeting academic deficiencies that coincide with risk factors for CAPD would be recommended during the early stages of development, but no label should be placed on the child at that time. Due to the difficulty level required of behavioral central auditory tests to identify dysfunction in the central auditory nervous system, formal assessment for CAPD is not possible until the child is about 7 years of age. Therefore, a diagnosis and label of CAPD typically is not reliable for a younger child, but early academic support for a child exhibiting behaviors suggestive of CAPD is a true benefit of the RTI model of education.) See Chapter 11 of Volume 1 of this Handbook for an overview of the central auditory test battery and limitations in testing young children.

What Bridges We Still Must Cross

Although we have alluded more than once to the fact that great variation from state to state exists with respect to interpretation of IDEIA regulations, we would be remiss if we did not relate this variation to the larger picture: the lack of the development of consistent evidence-based practices that could be considered *the standard* of service delivery for CAPD in the educational system. The changes in terminology and the changes to the SLD criteria mentioned previously also contribute to the variation in professional opinion for how best to serve students with this diagnosis and what kinds of services can be made available. All too often, LEAs will utilize the SLD category for determining eligibility and then offer services that do not "best fit" the student's needs. Evidence-based services for other communication disorders have been in place for a significant number of years, with consensus among professionals for what constitutes appropriate educational service delivery models. Examples of these disorders include autism, deaf or hard of hearing, and learning disability. National committees and councils focusing on these disabilities have established guidelines for the use of evidence-based practices in the educational setting (American Psychological Association, 2012; National Association of School Psychologists, 2007; National Autism Center, 2010; National Joint Committee on Learning Disabilities, 2006; National Research Council, 2001). A review of special education litigation (Jacobs, 2010; Weatherly, 2006) cites court cases in which evidence-based educational practices for these diagnoses were used to support rulings in terms of appropriate services. The professional organizations citing the use of evidence-based educational practices mentioned in those cases were the National Association of School Psychologists (NASP), the American Speech-Language-Hearing Association (ASHA), the National Autism Center (NAC), the National Reading Panel (NRP), and the National Research Council.

So, why is having a "gold standard" for identification and service delivery of CAPD in the educational system so important? The simple answer to this is "litigation." The development of evidence-based practices (or gold standards) specifically established for the educational system has proven to be helpful in resolving disputes between parents and schools. These disputes are frequently over what constitutes appropriate services and what does not. Therefore, attorneys and school systems need evidence-based practice to support their cases and address those services. In addition, evidence-based practice provides guidance to those professionals who serve students posing specific challenges for teachers. To date, guidelines containing evidence-based practice for CAPD specific to the educational setting do not exist; however, a large body of research supporting positive outcomes for children with CAPD does exist. The reader is encouraged to review ASHA's *Technical Report on Central Auditory Processing Disorders ([C]APD)* developed in 2005 and the American Academy of Audiology's *Guidelines for the Diagnosis, Treatment, and Management of Children and Adults with Central Auditory Processing Disorder* (AAA, 2010). The authors of these documents thoroughly review the literature and provide guidance in the areas of diagnosis and treatment of CAPD.

Because children with CAPD demonstrate deficits that can be masked, or that may appear to be the result of another underlying (comorbid) disability, it is imperative that service providers

practicing in the schools follow current research regarding intervention practices that support positive long-term outcomes specific to this disability and its diagnosis. Interventions should be implemented within the framework of service delivery established by the service providers' respective LEAs. In doing so, service providers (i.e., the multidisciplinary team of professionals who work with these students, including audiologists and SLPs) are encouraged to utilize the policies and procedures identified through federal guidelines when creating a model of service delivery that offers the most benefit to the student (i.e., creates the most optimal scenario for the student to make academic gains).

Response to Intervention (RTI) and CAPD

Although not fully understood by all educators, RTI, a comprehensive system of academic intervention, is being used by at least 17 out of 50 states, based on the 2009/2010 reporting year cited by the Department of Education Data Accountability Center (DAC, 2010). RTI is based on a system of universal screenings and successive tiers of intervention. These tiers of intervention are sometimes referred to as "primary," "secondary," and "tertiary" levels of intervention. The addition of this option of a tiered intervention system within the IDEIA to determine eligibility for services turns the discrepancy model of years past on its head and requires educators and specialists to consider services at the earliest stage possible. As students are monitored for progress under an RTI system, the students performing below grade-level expectation are "targeted" for additional academic support. All students in an educational system operating under the RTI model receive instruction under "Tier I," which is the general education curriculum. The student with a diagnosis of CAPD would typically receive support services right away under Tier II, or the secondary level of intervention, if that child is not progressing in the general education curriculum at grade-level expectation. This additional academic support is typically provided for an initial period of six to eight weeks. During this period, data are collected by the teacher or support personnel working with the student. At the end of the first period of intervention, progress is reviewed. If there is little or no positive response to this initial intervention, a team of educators and specialists may seek solutions for how best to meet the student's needs. Instructional approaches may then be modified, based on the student's performance. This problem-solving approach could result in a referral for a special education evaluation, but most importantly, it would ensure that additional academic support is continued while the evaluation process is under way. The struggling student would not have to wait for the special education evaluation to be completed in order to receive additional help. This component of IDEIA allows for greater flexibility in the prevention of lifelong learning disabilities and potentially prevents a disproportionate number of high-risk populations being identified as disabled. In theory, this model also emphasizes the use of evidence-based practices and prevents poor academic instruction as a potential variable, or cause, of a student's academic challenges.

The use of RTI requires LEAs to identify students in need of intervention, not as a special education-specific model, but rather as a broader school district-based system of intervention for every student. Under an RTI system, every student has access to additional support regardless of diagnosis. Those students not succeeding, who are performing within the secondary tier relative to their grade-level, are given additional support to move forward through the curriculum. Schools have begun to form RTI "teams" that may include reading specialists, SLPs, and additional paraprofessionals to work one-on-one with students, counselors, and school psychologists. This team approach is another hallmark component of a schoolwide intervention model. In addition, all RTI educational interventions must follow evidence-based, or scientifically validated, practices.

Some proponents of RTI would claim that the addition of RTI takes the initial intent of IDEA and further expands the "access for all" concept within the general education curriculum to a level that has not yet been seen. The most recent amendment to the IDEIA in 2006 allows LEAs to allocate federal funds to "early intervening services" if the LEA is utilizing an RTI model with particular emphasis being placed on identifying students in need of Title I and special education services in kindergarten through third grade. Because RTI is an optional model that may be used to replace the outdated SLD discrepancy model, and because it takes years to establish a true RTI model within a school system, many LEAs across the nation are still in the very early stages of developing this form of service delivery. A review of the code outlined in IDEA §300.309 (a) (2) (i) 2006 and §300.311 (a) (7) 2006, and a review of the components of RTI as described by the National Center on Response to

Intervention (NCRTI, 2010), is helpful in fully understanding the intent of the law with this additional amendment.

The NCRTI (2010) document describes how LEAs may implement the RTI service delivery model. The use of an RTI model is discretionary on the part of the LEA and only mandated when it has been found that disproportionality in the special education population exists. This disproportionality compliance provision is what drove some of the states identified in the Department of Education Data Accountability Center (2010) report to implement this model. The federal government required the use of early intervention services as a result of negative findings on prior compliance reviews. Suffice it to say that the procedures for the establishment of appropriate services for a child with CAPD must be taken into consideration based on the type of educational intervention system in which the child participates. Based on what we know about current research for effective CAPD intervention, the student with a CAPD diagnosis stands to gain

better services under an RTI framework because of the focus on response to prior interventions and close monitoring of progress early on.

Under the RTI model, universal screenings are performed multiple times per year for all students in an educational system, resulting in the identification of most students progressing at grade-level expectation (approximately 80% of the population), some students being at risk for potential learning delay/disability (approximately 15% of the population), and the remaining students performing significantly below their peers (approximately 5% of the population). The second and third tiers are closely monitored for progress, utilizing evidence-based interventions to "treat" academic deficits. A conceptual framework for understanding this model is presented in Figure 5–1.

Fortunately, many educators are beginning to see the benefits of implementing this RTI kind of comprehensive educational intervention system based on a decrease in the number of students disproportionately identified as disabled,

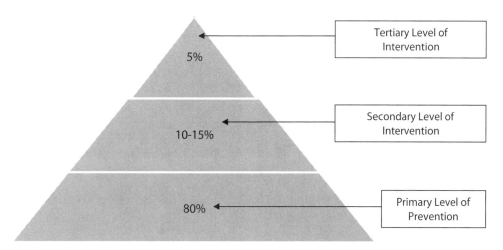

Figure 5–1. Multilevel system of prevention using a response to intervention model. Adapted from the National Center on Response to Intervention (NCRTI, 2012).

specifically English language learners, African American students, and Native American students. Other benefits of utilizing this model include an increase in reading scores and a decrease in behavioral issues (Vaughn, 2011).

Discrepancy Model Versus Response to Intervention Model for Students With CAPD

If an LEA is not operating under a similar model as outlined above, then the LEA must be utilizing a discrepancy model described previously as a model based upon a discrepancy between academic performance and a student's academic potential or intellectual quotient (IQ). That is, the child must demonstrate an IQ score that significantly deviates from performance on other academic measures (as outlined in established discrepancy tables published by each state) in order to receive any intervention services. Because there are validity issues associated with measuring IQ, and because a student typically does not begin to show this kind of discrepancy until the age of 8 or 9 years, this discrepancy model of eligibility determination prevents a student with difficulties processing auditory information from accessing special education services that could benefit the student in the form of early intervention. Historically, the student with deficits in auditory or listening behaviors would not have been supported with specially designed instruction until well into the third or fourth grade despite having persistent problems and a widening gap in skills when compared with her same-grade peers. By contrast, if a child diagnosed with CAPD (or about whom

concerns have been raised regarding the child's auditory and/or listening skills) is monitored for progress under an RTI system, indicators of at-risk performance, or significant deficits, can be identified earlier and deficits can be successively targeted to allow the student more access to instructional support (thus improving classroom performance).

Free Appropriate Public Education (FAPE) and CAPD

Before appropriate educational services can be identified and discussed as they relate to a diagnosis of CAPD, the way in which students are identified for special education services under "free and appropriate public education," or FAPE, must be considered. Regardless of whether or not an LEA is utilizing an RTI model, the obligation of the LEA is to provide the student a *free appropriate public education*, a definition that has been disputed in almost every court of law in this country, including the U.S. Supreme Court. The hallmark case example of the dispute over FAPE is the *Board of Education of Hendrick Hudson Central School District v. Rowley*, 458 US 176, 200 (1982). In that case, "free and appropriate" was interpreted as being an obligation of the school district to provide services that offered "some educational benefit" to the student. This concept of "some educational benefit" was frequently referred to in later court cases as the "Cadillac versus Chevrolet" argument, whereby under the law, a student receiving special education services was entitled to a "serviceable Chevrolet, not a Cadillac." Although this concept has been stated and referenced multiple times in subsequent special education litigation, it has since been established clearly in other Supreme Court cases that the Rowley decision does not mean that LEAs can provide the bare minimum of services, as some less supportive LEAs may contend. Rather, the team of educators and specialists contributing to the IEP process must be sure to propose *reasonable* services that would allow the student to demonstrate progress toward the special education goals identified within the IEP. With this term "reasonable" in mind, it is essential that service providers advocating for services for children with CAPD understand what the student is entitled to under the law and also understand that these services will vary greatly. As is often the case, services proposed in a clinical setting vary from those proposed by an IEP team, and this is primarily due to the concepts of "reasonable" and FAPE. Service providers advocating for intervention services must be aware of how a student's deficits impact overall performance and progress academically, as well as socially within the realm of communication.

With respect to FAPE, the reader must keep in mind that the interpretation of what constitutes FAPE for a given student and the allocation of funds toward services are often the basis of litigation initiated on the part of the parents. A "disconnect" between school districts and families in terms of identifying shared goals often spurs litigation that may take months, if not years, to resolve. Meanwhile, the student continues to receive instruction under a stalled IEP in which nothing can change (i.e., no goals can be updated and no progress can be addressed). For a student diagnosed with CAPD, this could add to increased frustration levels, continued poor academic performance, and a higher chance of dropping out of school.

Evaluating CAPD From a Special Education Perspective

FAPE is an important concept to understand because it serves as the central framework upon which an IEP is developed. The special education evaluation must address essential components to ensure that a student is correctly identified as being eligible for services under IDEIA. In order to progress to the step of developing the IEP and ensuring that FAPE is being delivered, a disability must be identified and eligibility must be established. To help sort through this process, the evaluation team must consider what is known as the "three prong test." Any student being evaluated for special education services due to a suspected disability must meet all three prongs of this assessment, as outlined in IDEIA§ 300.306 (U.S. Department of Education, 2006). The questions presented below summarize the considerations that must be made with respect to determining eligibility for special education services. These considerations are made as a culminating step in the decision-making process once all data are gathered and reviewed by the evaluation team:

a. *Does the student possess a disability?*

b. *Do the data gathered indicate an "adverse educational impact"?*

c. *Is there a need for specially designed instruction?*

If an evaluation of the data results in an answer of "yes" to all three questions, an IEP would be developed addressing "specially designed instruction" (SDI). However, a combination of "yes" and "no" answers from the reviewed data would lead the evaluation team to recommend the development of a 504 Plan of accommodations, which would include physical and educational accommodations rather than SDI. The term "specially designed instruction" implies that the teaching approach for a student needing an IEP differs from the instruction used within the general education curriculum. Thus, a student receiving special education services may demonstrate proficiency of the specially designed curriculum in a very different manner than students following the general education curriculum. In contrast to that, a 504 Plan would ensure that a student has appropriate accommodations to access the general education curriculum, not specially designed curriculum. Examples of accommodations may include extra time to complete assignments, taking tests in a quiet environment, or the use of special equipment and/or technology.

Getting back to the idea of the three prong test and determining special education eligibility, even if the answer to the first question (Does the student have a disability?) is "yes," a disability in and of itself does not constitute the need for special education services based on the disability alone. For example, a child with cerebral palsy may be extremely physically disabled, but the child may be able to access all components of the general education curriculum with appropriate accommodations in place. This student may possess a disability that results in an adverse educational impact, but for whom SDI is not warranted; this student is merely in need of physical accommodations. Therefore, this student may utilize the same eighth-grade textbook, access the same science curriculum, and follow the same grade-level common

core standards as nondisabled peers; however, this student may need assistive technology and adaptive equipment to access that curriculum. The student in this example would not meet special education eligibility under the IDEIA definition for an IEP, but would meet eligibility for accommodations and related services under Section 504. Over time, for some students, the 504 Plan would become unnecessary and the goal would be to gradually withdraw accommodations so that the students would be more reliant on their own auditory systems; however, for others, the 504 Plan may be carried forward to support the student through post-secondary education.

It is essential to know that the student with CAPD may benefit from either of these options (504 Plan or IEP), as long as the services provided as part of one plan or the other aligns with what is considered evidence-based practice. Furthermore, any established plan, either 504 or IEP, should be drafted in a way that will benefit the student as it relates to that child's individual deficits and needs resulting from the CAPD. Additionally, the child's strengths must be taken into consideration in order to capitalize on the child's ability to benefit from the instruction and/or accommodations set forth in the established plan.

Important Distinctions Between the 504 Plan and IEP With Respect to CAPD

To summarize the concepts presented earlier, when a team has identified the primary need of a student as one of "access," the consideration of a 504 Plan of accommodations needs to be discussed rather than an IEP. These kinds of accommodations are not considered to be SDI. Neither the curriculum nor the teaching approaches have to be changed. The IEP, however, does utilize specially designed instruction, and a student receiving services under an IEP uses the special curriculum rather than the general curriculum alone. These two concepts appear to be laid out clearly and should be easy enough to grasp; however, But as the reader will learn, the decision to implement a 504 Plan versus an IEP can be challenging.

Ideally, educators will identify areas of need early on in the general education academic program of a student. Once a student has been identified as needing special education, the educational team develops an IEP, and that student transitions from the IEP to a 504 Plan as progress is made (usually seen as the student develops and matures). As a general rule, when accommodations are determined to be the primary means for targeting specific deficits associated with CAPD, a 504 Plan of accommodations is chosen. However, accommodations are still an integral part of an IEP and should be included along with identified goals, if SDI is also needed. This means, if a student with a CAPD only needs accommodations, then that student will get a 504 Plan. If a student with CAPD needs accommodations *and* SDI, then the student gets an IEP.

We can think of the distinction in services for CAPD in alignment with the types of interventions that are typically recommended. These recommendations can be identified within the guidelines of the 504 Plan and/or IEP based on the type of service delivery associated with them. Recommendations for CAPD are often provided under the following categories: direct skills remediation, compensatory strategies, and environmental considerations (ASHA, 2005*).* These intervention approaches support the use of "top-down" and "bottom-up" intervention strategies. These intervention strategies use "systems theory" to support a collaborative and ecologic- or context-based model of intervention that emphasizes central resources training, in addition to environmental interventions (Chermak, 2007). The educational setting requires this model of intervention in order to fully meet the needs of students with CAPD. Following this model, an individual's intervention needs can be met, and resources can then be allocated. Some types of intervention are clearly considered SDI because the type of instruction taking place differs substantially from the general education curriculum. Other types of intervention may merely provide access to the general education curriculum and are more appropriate as an accommodation. Table 5–1 provides a framework for aligning forms of intervention for CAPD with an IEP or within a 504 Plan.

It is important for teams to dialogue about all of the options available to the student in order to ensure success. It is equally important for the teams to determine which professionals will develop the goals, monitor the progress, and oversee the SDI for given areas (should the team choose to develop an IEP). When considering the various professionals' scopes of practice and expertise, some areas, skills, and knowledge may overlap. It is likely that, as outlined above, the educational audiologist or the SLP will take a lead role in the instruction of specific skills.

Table 5–1. Types of Services and Options for Service Delivery

Description of Intervention	SDI	504 Plan	Type of Intervention
Redirection of competing signals		X (*)	(EM)
Use of visual aids		X (*)	(EM)
Preferential seating		X (*)	(EM)
Use of an FM system		X (*)	(EM)
Schema induction	X		(CS)
Discourse cohesion devices	X		(CS)
Context-derived vocabulary building	X		(CS)
Phonological awareness	X		(CS)
Semantic network expansion	X		(CS)
Assertiveness training	X		(CS)
Self-instruction training	X		(CS)
Procedures targeting: intensity, frequency, and duration discrimination	X		(DSR)
Phoneme discrimination & phoneme to grapheme discrimination	X		(DSR)
Temporal gap discrimination	X		(DSR)
Temporal order discrimination	X		(DSR)
Pattern recognition	X		(DSR)
Localization/lateralization training	X		(DSR)
Recognition of auditory information when presented with background noise	X		(DSR)
Peer note-takers		X (*)	(CS)
Previewing questions/visual organizers		X (*)	(CS)
Use of "pen script" audio-recording device for lectures		X (*)	(EM)

Types of Intervention: Environmental Modification (*EM*); Compensatory Strategies (*CS*); Direct Skills Remediation (*DSR*). An asterisk (*) denotes that the intervention can be identified as an accommodation on a 504 Plan or allowable as an accommodation on an IEP if there is an additional need for specific specially designed instruction.

Collaboration Essentials for CAPD

Until now, we have been mentioning "educational teams" and "multidisciplinary" approaches to evaluating and remediating CAPD. However, we have not specifically addressed these professionals and approaches as they relate to the educational environment.

Formulation of the appropriate team members and the collating of all essential evaluation data help to ensure that a suitable plan of service is developed for students with CAPD. In order to meet this requirement, a team of professionals knowledgeable about the disability and trained in the diagnosis and intervention of hearing disorders and/or language impairments should be established (AAA, 2010; Sharma, Purdy, & Kelly, 2009; Witton, 2010). This team of professionals will assist with the interdisciplinary or multidisciplinary approach needed for accurate assessment and remediation of CAPD. Typically, but not always, the evaluation process is initiated by the school psychologist who facilitates the special education evaluation and whose primary role is to ensure all components of the evaluation and eligibility determination have been followed legally in alignment with the IDEIA.

Two of the members of the multidisciplinary team who are uniquely qualified to identify and provide services for school children with CAPD are the audiologist and the SLP. As mentioned previously, these two professionals need to be singled out as important players in managing CAPD in the educational setting. Although the audiologist and the SLP may look at central auditory processing from different angles and perspectives, they are fully capable of working together to fully evaluate a student with CAPD, determine what, if any, additional testing needs to be included subsequent to the audiological diagnosis, and arrive at a sound management plan that incorporates school policies and procedures (AAA, 2010; ASHA, 2005).

An audiologist employed in a school setting may be called an "educational audiologist" or a "school-based audiologist." This audiologist plays many different roles under the umbrella terms of "diagnostician," "technology expert," "manager," and "remediator." This professional may be hired by the LEA as a full-time employee or on a contractual basis. Educational audiologists are the professionals with specialized knowledge about school-age children and hearing, classroom acoustics, and hearing assistance technology (HAT) options. For a thorough description of the roles an educational audiologist is expected to carry out, it is recommended that the reader access the Educational Audiology Association's *Recommended Professional Practices for Educational Audiology* (EAA, 2009) and the American Speech-Language-Hearing Association's *Guidelines for Audiology Service Provision in and for Schools* (ASHA, 2002). Due to the plethora of differences among school systems and within school administrations, it is impossible to list *all* of the roles and responsibilities of an educational audiologist. However, a few of the roles that would be expected of an educational audiologist working with a student diagnosed with a CAPD would include:

- performing classroom observations and evaluating auditory behaviors
- evaluating speech perception capabilities, in noise and in quiet

- evaluating the need for and selection of HATs, both personal and classroom
- counseling parents, teachers, administrators, and other team members about the CAPD and HAT
- troubleshooting the HAT on a routine basis and instructing the student and/or classroom teacher to perform daily listening checks
- staying abreast of current ideology and research about CAPD and HAT
- providing in-service trainings to staff/administrators regarding CAPD and HAT
- possessing a working knowledge of special education law and state policies relating to CAPD
- establishing communication between the school setting and outside clinics or personal audiologists.

School-based SLPs also possess valuable knowledge and skills for working with children diagnosed with a CAPD. Like the school-based audiologist, this school-based SLP must be knowledgeable in many of the areas outlined above. However, the school-based SLP approaches a CAPD from a slightly different perspective and will be focusing on the language comprehension and phonological aspects of the child's development, specifically as those relate to academic progress in the classroom. Testing techniques will be different, and intervention and remediation will vary from any intervention and remediation techniques provided by the school-based audiologist. A few of the roles that would be expected of a school-based SLP working with a student diagnosed with a CAPD, aside from testing and diagnosing the disorder, would include:

- performing classroom observations and evaluating auditory behaviors

- evaluating speech perception capabilities, in noise and in quiet
- reviewing performance on school-based measures of, and enhancing, development of early emerging literacy skills (rhyming, phonological awareness games/activities, story retelling)
- considering overall language development across the areas of vocabulary, morphology, semantics, and pragmatics and how deficits here may be impacted by the auditory processing disorder
- linking IEP goals to the common core standards of the curriculum
- building vocabulary and story grammar structure to assist the student in improving the ability to apply auditory information to the verbal retelling of a story
- teaching students how to identify and expand knowledge of key vocabulary linked to content areas; teaching multiple meaning words and formulation of inference working with teachers on ensuring the use of compensatory strategies in the classroom environment.

No matter what, all audiologists and SLPs practicing in the schools must remain vigilant to keep their roles within the scope of practice spelled out by ASHA (2004, 2007) and adhere to its code of ethics (ASHA, 2010). The *Working Group on Auditory Processing Disorders* (ASHA, 2005) warns of the pitfalls of assessing and treating CAPD without proper training or familiarity with topics such as neurophysiology, neuropsychology, and auditory neuroscience (p. 5). Not every school-based audiologist or SLP arrives on the job with the knowledge and skills to work with cases of CAPD; however, if an audiologist or SLP plans to stay employed in an educational setting, he or she also needs to plan to obtain the professional development (continuing education) necessary for developing familiarity and proficiency with CAPD. (See Chapters 12, 13, and 17 for discussion of HAT, classroom collaboration, and the SLP's role in assessment and treatment, respectively.)

Other professionals are involved in the collaboration process needed for an interdisciplinary or multidisciplinary approach to CAPD. Aside from the school psychologist, audiologist, and SLP mentioned previously, other professionals needed for their areas of expertise include educators, learning disabilities specialists, parents/caregivers, and in some cases, school nurses or the child's pediatrician. All of these professionals will allow for a broad, detailed overview of the student's strengths and weaknesses in the educational setting. A clear picture of the student's problem areas will not be available without input from all or most of these professionals.In addition, because not all professionals needed for a multidisciplinary approach to CAPD will be based in the educational environment, we would be remiss if we did not say something about the collaboration process between private service providers and educational service providers. In order to obtain a successful outcome for a student with CAPD, collaboration between private providers and public education providers must establish a mutually agreed-upon program and at the same time align with FAPE, evidence-based practices, goals of the parents, and other academic common core standards. This is no easy task, as one can imagine. However, if all of the professionals involved with a specific case are truly working in the student's best interest, collaborative efforts can be effective.

Equipment, Facilities, and Materials Needed for Proper Evaluation of CAPD

Any school-based audiologist's or SLP's ability to carry out the roles and responsibilities of his or her job includes having access to the appropriate equipment, facilities, and materials. In the ideal world, school-based audiologists and SLPs would have access to any and all equipment, facilities, and materials they need to fulfill their service delivery, but reality dictates that this is not always the case. The *Guidelines for Audiology Service Provision in and for Schools* (ASHA, 2002) lists much of the equipment needed to practice educational audiology. Equipment that may not be accessible to every educational audiologist (due to funding issues or resource allocation) includes two-channel audiometers or electroacoustical or electrophysiological equipment, such as otoacoustic emissions or auditory brainstem response. Therefore, not all school-based audiologists will be able to perform central auditory processing evaluations appropriately (i.e., as recommended by ASHA [2005] and AAA [2010]). In such cases, referral out of the school setting to a local clinical audiologist trained to perform central auditory processing evaluations is necessary.

Likewise, appropriate facilities may be hard to find in an educational setting. The term "facilities" typically refers to classrooms, offices, band halls, or broom closets found within schools. However, anyone who is familiar with schools knows that there is nothing typical or regular about these facilities. In the practice of audiology, an acoustically appropriate test area is needed. Some school-based audiologists may have access to sound-treated test booths, but most do not. Central auditory processing evaluations cannot provide accurate, reliable, and valid results if performed in poor acoustic environments. Therapies should be deliveredin environmentally a controlled (i.e., low-noise and low reverberation) environments.

The materials needed for screening and evaluating central auditory processing are addressed in the previously mentioned documents, *Working Group on Auditory Processing Disorders* (ASHA, 2005) and *Guidelines for the Diagnosis, Treatment, and Management of Children and Adults with Central Auditory Processing Disorder* (AAA, 2010). Chapters 10 and 11 in Volume 1 of this text fully address the screening and diagnostic measures used for evaluating central auditory processing abilities; therefore, we refer the reader to those chapters for a description of the screeners and tests recommended for a central auditory processing evaluation.

Suffice it to say that in some cases, school-based audiologists and SLPs may only use screening tools, and then refer students who perform poorly on those screeners to clinical audiologists or private service providers in the community. School-based audiologists and SLPs have a choice of many different screening tools (several not specific to central auditory processing and some intended for one group of professionals more than the other). These include:

- Children's Auditory Performance Scale (CHAPs; Smoski, Brunt, & Tannahill, 1998)
- Screening Instrument for Targeting Educational Risk (SIFTER; Anderson, 1989)
- Test of Auditory Perceptual Skills-Revised (TAPS-R; Gardner, 1997)

- Children's Home Inventory for Listening Difficulties, parent and student versions (CHILD; Anderson & Smaldino, 2000)
- Listening Inventory for Education, student version (LIFE; Anderson & Smaldino, 1999)
- Differential Screening Test of Processing (Richard & Ferre, 2006)
- Auditory Processing Domains Questionnaire (APDQ; O'Hare, 2006)
- Fisher's Auditory Problems Checklist (Fisher, 1976)
- Buffalo Model Questionnaire (BMQ; Katz, 2004,2006)
- SCAN-3:A (Keith, 2009)
- SCAN-3:C (Keith, 2009)

It needs to be reiterated here that these screening measures should only be used in appropriate listening environments, meaning in an area with few auditory distractions. Knowing that this type of environment is difficult to find in many school settings may help audiologists and SLPs with their decision to refer these students out. See Chapter 10 of Volume 1 of the Handbook for discussion of screening for CAPD.

Time Line Requirements Related to the Development and Implementation of an IEP for CAPD

An unfortunate drawback to accessing services in the public school system is the length of time it may take to identify a need for SDI and provide the necessary services. Time lines established under IDEIA are intended to assist LEAs with managing special education evaluation referrals, which may be large in number. A timeline also assists schools in: (1) ensuring that a thorough evaluation is completed by a multidisciplinary team, (2) allowing ample time for the team to review all of the evaluation results, and (3) developing an appropriate plan for intervention. When used to its maximum allowable timeframe, the process of evaluation and subsequent IEP development (i.e., from the first day of the referral) can take as long as 60 school days. An additional 30 calendar days is allowed to initiate a special education placement. IDEIA specifies that an evaluation should not take longer than 60 calendar days to complete; however, states vary on their use of this guideline, which may also be influenced by the number of special education referrals at a given time.

The example described here demonstrates how a time line can grow with respect to the amount of time needed for each step, from identification of a disability to development of an IEP. Each state adopts its own specific timeline for a special education evaluation. Professionals advocating for children with CAPD should consult the code of regulations for their respective states to ensure knowledge of the applicable timeline. To parents and professionals outside of the educational system, these timelines may appear to be counterproductive for obtaining services that capitalize on early intervention. The "school days" component of the evaluation timeline can add a significant delay in accessing services. For example, if a referral to special education is obtained the first or second week of school (most often beginning in September), the team could take 25 school days to review the relevant records containing referral information and then decide whether or not to accept the referral for further evalu-

ation. The team could use an additional 35 school days to administer all testing before meeting as a group to review the results. The team then has an additional 30 *calendar* days within which to decide to initiate the IEP. Based on this example and interpretation of the federal guidelines, if a team uses the maximum allowable time line, services might not begin until late December or early January, if vacations and holiday breaks are factored in. Therefore, it is quite possible that one-third to one-half of an academic year could be lost to accessing services while the evaluation process is under way. Under an RTI system, however, the child could be accessing some "Tier I" or "Tier II" interventions that would include some assistance as the evaluation process takes place. In a school district where an RTI system does not exist, the child would most likely be falling further and further behind academically.

Monitoring Progress on the IEP and Reevaluation

Monitoring progress toward goals identified on the IEP is a requirement under IDEIA and must be formally reviewed annually. That is, the IEP team is required to reconvene at least once a year to determine the appropriateness of identified goals and whether or not the student is making academic gains and progress toward those goals. In some cases, the IEP team may meet more than once a year, especially when a lack of progress is being made. At any time, any member of the IEP team (including the parent) may choose to initiate a request for an IEP meeting to discuss concerns. In those circumstances, the IEP team should come together to determine if other possible teaching methods should be used, and reconsider the goals included in the IEP. (The IEP team should take into consideration all team members' recommendations to support academic progress.)

In addition to the review, a reevaluation of the IEP is required at least every three years or whenever there is a question related to continued eligibility for services. A reevaluation is a separate requirement of the special education process, and it has specific provisions outlined within the requirements of IDEIA. Although a thorough evaluation should always be conducted, it is important to know that "re-administration" of standardized tests as part of the three-year re-evaluation is not required in order for a student to be determined eligible for continued special education services. This leniency within the regulations was put in place to support IEP teams working with students for whom administering repeated tests (i.e., IQ tests or other measures in which scores rarely change) would not be helpful in determining eligibility. Prior to the inclusion of this change in process, despite an IEP team's thorough knowledge about the child's needs without standardized testing (such as in the case of intellectual disability, in which IQ plays a role), teams had historically been required to keep administering unnecessary tests and reporting results to parents. Teams now have the flexibility to review all existing educational data, including, but not limited to, state assessments, progress toward goals on the IEP, private provider evaluation reports, parent report, and prior special education evaluation reports. Based on a review of existing relevant data, a team can choose which standardized tests may

be warranted to establish continued eligibility for services.

With this provision in mind, when it comes to reevaluation of the student with a CAPD diagnosis, under the guidance of the educational audiologist, the team may choose to continue prior services without new testing. However, one must consider the possible implications of choosing not to test, due to lack of resources or some other factor. Current testing related to performance on measures of central auditory processing should be considered when identifying intervention goals. Past performance on auditory measures may be very different from current auditory behavior after interventions have been in place. Thus, it is quite possible that something may be missed, or a given intervention approach could be applied incorrectly due to the lack of current testing and substantiation of the CAPD diagnosis. Flexibility is helpful when it comes to special education process; however, it is advisable that teams proceed with caution when it comes to reevaluation of a student with a CAPD diagnosis. Consultation with the educational audiologist, or a private clinical audiologist working with the student, would be necessary to ensure quality services.

Concluding Statements

Children often present with a myriad of issues or deficits; therefore, comprehensive and multidisciplinary evaluation is essential to determine eligibility for educational services and the appropriate mix of such services and supports. Comorbid diagnoses must be identified, and the evaluation team must take into consideration all of the student's needs, and consider other eligibility categories to ensure the child receives the services needed to succeed academically. The child with a CAPD who has no co-occurring condition should be eligible for, and gain access to, services regardless of the educational system under which the LEA operates. It is possible to establish eligibility for services under the category of "Other Health Impairment" (OHI) with a documented diagnosis of CAPD. However, if the child with a CAPD is deemed not eligible under the discrepancy model, teams should strongly be encouraged to develop a 504 Plan. The law requires the evaluation team to consider evaluation reports from private providers in order to establish eligibility for services. If the evaluation team is determining eligibility under a discrepancy model, a documented diagnosis of CAPD by a private clinical audiologist, when taken into consideration with an entire evaluation, would allow the team to utilize the category of OHI. Determining eligibility under the guidelines of the RTI model does not require the documented diagnosis and allows educators and evaluation teams to provide intervention services based on the child's "response" to prior interventions. The latter model focuses on addressing the unique academic needs of the student based on academic performance relative to grade-level standards, as opposed to meeting more constraining eligibility requirements, such as the influence of the IQ score on academic performance.

Although much of this chapter examines challenges with respect to the lack of standards for service delivery to students with CAPD, the dearth of evidence-based research, the lack of equipment and proper testing environments, and the length of time required for the evaluation and implementation process for the IEP, we want to make sure the reader understands that the identification and remediation of CAPD in the school environment is appropriate and necessary for the children struggling in their educational placements. Despite ambiguities in federal legislation and educational policies, as professionals in the field of communication sciences and disorders, we must resolve to overcome these barriers and develop sound methodologies for working with students diagnosed with CAPD in schools. Having a comprehensive understanding of the distinction between what constitutes specially designed instruction versus what constitutes accommodations is instrumental for assisting service providers with understanding how best to advocate for the needs of their students. Furthermore, the promise of including all students in an educational system that embraces a tiered system of intervention offers progress and hope for students diagnosed with CAPD. That is, special education in this country is heading in a positive direction by providing services earlier under RTI. This new system should keep children with a diagnosis of CAPD from falling further behind academically, as is the possibility under the more traditional models of evaluation (e.g., discrepancy model) and intervention currently in place. It is our hope that knowing more about educational policies, processes, and services will allow readers to fully appreciate a side of CAPD that may not have been described or explained before. Furthermore, we hope that this information will provide readers with the knowledge to advocate appropriately within their own educational systems.

Additional Recommended Readings

Fitzgerald, J. L. & Watkins, M. W. (2006). Parents' rights in special education: The readability of procedural safeguards. *Exceptional Children, 72*, 497–510.

Jerger, J., & Musiek, F. (2000).Report of the consensus conference on the diagnosis of auditory processing disorders in school-aged children. *Journal of the American Academy of Audiology, 11*, 467–474.

Moore, D. R. (2011). The diagnosis and management of auditory processing disorder. *Language, Speech, and Hearing Services in Schools, 42*, 303–308.

Richard, G. J. (2007). Cognitive-communicative and language factors associated with (central) auditory processing disorder: A speech-language perspective. In F. E. Musiek & G. D. Chermak (Eds.), *Handbook of (central) auditory processing disorders: Auditory neuroscience and diagnosis* (Vol. 1, pp. 397–416). San Diego, CA: Plural.

Smoski, W. J., Brunt, M. A., & Tannahill, J. C. (1992) Listening characteristics of children with central auditory processing disorders. *Language, Speech, and Hearing Services in Schools, 23*, 145–152.

References

AAA (American Academy of Audiology). (2010). *Guidelines for the diagnosis, treatment and management of children and adults with central processing disorder.* Retrieved from http://www.audiology.org/resources/documentlibrary/Pages/CentralAuditoryProcessingDisorder

Anderson, K. E. (1989). *Screening instrument for targeting educational risk.* Danville, IL: Interstate.

Anderson, K., & Smaldino, J. (1999). Listening Inventories for Education: A classroom measurement tool. *Hearing Journal, 52,* 74.

Anderson, K., & Smaldino, J. (2000) Children's Home Inventory of Listening Difficulties (CHILD). *Educational Audiology Review, 17, 3.*

ASHA (American Speech-Language-Hearing Association). (2002). *Guidelines for audiology service provision in and for schools.* Rockville, MD: Author.

ASHA. (2004). *Scope of practice in audiology.* Retrieved from http://www.asha.org/policy/SP2004-00192.htm

ASHA. (2005). *(Central) auditory processing disorders* [Technical report]. Retrieved from http://www.asha.org/policy

ASHA. (2007). *Scope of practice in speech-language pathology.* Retrieved from http://www.asha.org/policy/SP2007-00283.htm

ASHA. (2010). *Code of ethics.* [Ethics]. Retrieved from http://www.asha.org/policy/doi:10.1044/policy.ET2010-00309

Board of Education of Hendrick Hudson Central School District v. Rowley, 458 US 176, 200 (1982).

Chermak, G. D. (2007). Differential diagnosis of (central) auditory processing disorder and attention deficit hyperactivity disorder. In F. E. Musiek & G. D. Chermak (Eds.), *Handbook of (central) auditory processing disorder: Auditory neuroscience and diagnosis* (Vol. 1, pp. 397–416). San Diego, CA: Plural.

Colorado Department of Education. (2008). *(Central) auditory processing deficits: A team approach to screening, assessment and intervention practices.* Retrieved from http://www.cde.state.co.us/cdesped/download/pdf/APDGuidelines.pdf

Department of Education Data Accountability Center. (2010). *Data notes. Part B: Maintenance of effort reduction and coordinated early intervening services, 2009–2010 reporting year.* Retrieved from http://www.ideadata.org/docs

Dodge, E. P. (1999). *Survival guide for school-based speech-language pathologists.* San Diego, CA: Singular.

EAA (Educational Audiology Association). (2009). *Recommended professional practices for educational audiology.* Retrieved from http://www.edaud.org/displaycommon.cfm?an=1&subarticlenbr=4

Education of the Handicapped Act Amendments of 1986, Public Law 99-457, 20. U.S.C. 1400 *et seq.: U.S. Statutes at Large, 100*, 1145–1177 (1986).

Fisher, L. I. (1976). *Fisher Auditory Problem Checklist.* Cedar Rapids, IA: Grant Wood Area Educational Agency.

Gardner, M. Y. (1997). *Test of Auditory Perceptual Skills-Revised.* Austin, TX: Pro-Ed.

Individuals with Disabilities Education Improvement Act of 2004, Pub.L. No. 108-446, 20 U.S.C. §1400 et seq. (2004).

Jacobs, M. (2010). *Proceedings of the 30th Annual Pacific Northwest Institute on Special Education and the Law: Special education litigation: 2010 (An overview of the hottest and newest special education cases).* Palm Beach Gardens, FL: LRP Publications.

Johnson, C. D., & Seaton, J. B. (2012). *Educational audiology handbook* (2nd ed.). Stamford, CT: Cengage Learning.

Katz, J. (2004). *The Buffalo model questionnaire. SSW Reports, 26*, 5–6.

Katz, J. (2006). *Buffalo model questionnaire: Follow up. SSW Reports, 28*, 1–3.

Keith, R. W. (2009). *SCAN-3 for adolescents and adults: Tests for auditory processing disorders.* San Antonio, TX: Pearson.

Keith, R.W. (2009). *SCAN-3 for children: Tests for auditory processing disorders.* San Antonio, TX: Pearson.

National Association of School Psychologists. (2007). *Identification of students with specific learning disabilities (Position statement).* Bethesda, MD: Author.

National Autism Center. (2011) *Evidence-based practice and autism in the schools: A guide to providing appropriate interventions to students with autism spectrum disorders.* Randolph, MA: Author.

National Center on Response to Intervention. (2010, March). *Essential components of RTI-A closer look at Response to Intervention.* Washington DC: U.S. Department of Education, Office of Special Programs, National Center on Response to Intervention. Retrieved from http://www.rti4success.org/pdf/essentialcomponents

National Institute of Child Health and Human Development. (2000). *Report of the National Reading Panel. Teaching children to read: An evidence-based assessment of the scientific research literature on reading and its implications for reading instruction* (NIH Publication No. 00-4769). Washington, DC: U.S. Government Printing Office.

National Joint Committee on Learning Disabilities. (2006). *Learning disabilities and young children: Identification and early intervention.* Retrieved from http://www.ldonlline.org/article/Learning_Disabilities_and_You

National Research Council. (2001). *Educating children with autism: Committee on educational interventions for children with autism.* Division of Behavioral and Social Sciences and Education. Washington, DC: Academy Press.

O'Hare, B. (2006). *The listening challenge: Auditory processing domains questionnaire.* Retrieved from http://www.neuroaudiology.com/APDQ.pdf

Rehabilitation Act of 1973, Section 504, 29, U.S.C. 794: *U.S. Statutes at Large, 87*, 335–394 (1973).

Richard, G. J., & Ferre, J. M. (2006). *Differential screening test for processing.* LinguiSystems.

Richburg, C. M., & Smiley, D. F. (2012). *School-based audiology.* San Diego, CA: Plural.

Sharma, M., Purdy, S. C., & Kelly, A. S, (2009). Comorbidity of auditory processing, language, and reading disorders. *Journal of Speech, Language, and Hearing Research, 52*, 706–722.

Smoski, W. J., Brunt, M. A., & Tannahill, J. C. (1998). *Children's Auditory Performance Scale.* Tampa, FL: Educational Audiology Association.

U.S. Department of Education. (2006). Assistance to States for the Education of Children with Disabilities and Preschool Grants for Children with Disabilities, 71 Fed.Reg. 156 (August 14, 2006) (to be codified at 34 C.F.R § 300). Retrieved from http://www.ed.gov/legislation/FedRegister/finrule/2006-3/081406a.html

Vaughn, S. (2011). *Response to intervention in reading for English language learners.* Washington, DC: RTI Action Network, National Center for Learning Disabilities.

Retrieved from http://www.rtinetwork.org/learn/diversity/englishlanguagelearners

Weatherly, J. J. (2006). *Proceedings from the annual Pacific Northwest Institute on special education and the law.* Seattle, WA: LRP.

Witton, C. (2010). Childhood auditory processing disorder as a developmental disorder: The case for a multi-professional approach to diagnosis and management. *International Journal of Audiology, 49,* 83–87.

CHAPTER 6

HISTORICAL FOUNDATION OF CENTRAL AUDITORY PROCESSING DISORDER

JAMES W. HALL III and ANURADHA R. BANTWAL

*History teaches everything
including the future.*
(Lamartine, 1848)

Why an Historical Perspective Is Important

Introduction

Interest in and clinical assessment of central auditory processing disorder (CAPD) can be traced back to the earliest years of the profession of audiology. Our understanding of normal and disordered auditory processing has expanded and deepened remarkably during the past 60 years. Even a cursory historical overview of the topic yields at least three important lessons.

Lesson 1

Audiologists will encounter patients with hearing problems that involve the brain and not only the ear. It is no exaggeration to state unequivocally that "we hear with our brain." Extensive clinical experience with cochlear implants clearly confirms the importance of the central auditory nervous system (CANS) in auditory processing. Serious cochlear dysfunction and total deafness does not preclude useful hearing and effective communication.

Lesson 2

Basic research in neuroscience is the surest way to advance and improve clinical audiology services. Many examples could be cited in support of this statement. Perhaps the most dramatic is the impact of discovery during the "Decade of the Brain" of neural plasticity. Appreciation of the principle of neural plasticity continues to have a major impact on many aspects of clinical practice and, specifically, on techniques and treatments for CAPD. To get a glimpse into future clinical practice in the area of CAPD one must follow the research.

Lesson 3

An historical study of CAPD leads to one simple, obvious, and yet very important conclusion. Our understanding of CAPD and today's clinical techniques and technologies for diagnosis and intervention are due almost entirely to the insight and efforts of a relatively small number of hearing scientists and clinical scholars. We are indebted to pioneering men and women from the fields of psychology, neuroscience, and audiology who asked challenging research questions and then proceeded to answer them.

For many years more than a few skeptics dismissed the reality of CAPD. Some skeptics argued strongly that CAPD did not exist. Others grudgingly acknowledged that dysfunction within the CANS was possible, but they claimed that nothing could be done for patients with resulting CAPD. We are now well beyond this debate and controversy. CAPD involving the central nervous system is real and can be effectively managed using evidence-based strategies and treatments.

The Early Period

Introduction

We begin with a brief review of the critical contribution of a talented collection of scientists and clinicians who laid the foundation for diagnosis and treatment of CAPD. The field of CAPD emerged to a large extent from the research interests of several professionals other than audiologists. These pioneers included neurosurgeons, otolaryngologists, and psychologists.

Contributions of Italian Otolarygologists

Beginning in the early 1950s, Bocca and colleagues developed a set of tests they referred to as "sensitized speech tests." These otolaryngologists realized that pure tone audiometry was insufficient for detecting central auditory lesions and that disorders of the CANS could only be diagnosed using hearing tests that made listening more difficult. Their sensitized speech test battery included the use of binaurally switched, time compressed, distorted, and interrupted speech to investigate auditory deficits in individuals with brain lesions. Bocca and colleagues conducted clinical investigations over a period of 20 years. Results of their studies generated considerable interest among audiologists from other parts of the world and inspired the development of additional tests of CAPD that were applied in various patient populations.

In the 1960s and 1970s, Italian otolaryngologists Antonelli and colleagues described research with sensitized speech tests (SST) administered to patients with a variety of brain lesions. At the Danavox Symposium at Odense Denmark in 1970, Antonelli presented papers based on findings from their research with SST. The subjects consisted of three patient populations: with presbycusis (Antonelli, 1970a), lesions of the brainstem and "diffusive" central nervous system diseases

(Antonelli, 1970b), and brain lesions (Antonelli, 1970c). These researchers were some of the first to extensively study the effects of changes in test parameters such as various compression ratios or interruption rates on central auditory performance.

Antonelli and colleagues (Antonelli, 1970a) observed that older individuals had significantly poorer performance on SST compared with young adults even after peripheral hearing loss was taken into account. The authors offered two explanations for these findings: "some related to functional depression of the central mechanisms involving the overall sensory input integration; some, irreversible, connected with anatomical CNS lesions, typical with old age" (Antonelli, 1970a, p. 76). Today, it is widely recognized that older individuals are at risk for CAPD.

Calearo and Antonelli (Antonelli, 1970c) used the SST to investigate 22 subjects with temporal lobe lesions and 24 subjects with epilepsy who had undergone right temporal lobectomy. A formal language test was administered to each subject to rule out aphasia. These researchers emphasized the importance of differential diagnosis of symptoms caused by brain lesions. Data reported on the relationship between the side of lesion and laterality of abnormal SST scores indicated that normal hearing individuals presented comparable performance in both ears for interrupted and distorted sentence stimuli, whereas subjects with temporal lobe lesions showed a deficit in the ear contralateral to the lesion. Also, the extent of abnormal performance in the contralateral ear was similar for lesions on the right versus left side. Calearo and Antonelli concluded: "Thus, as far as the function of the auditory cortical area is concerned,

we can state that there are no phenomena connected with cerebral dominance in the SST discrimination" (1963, cited in Antonelli, 1970c, p. 180).

The Italian otolaryngologists increased our understanding of the relationship between extent of lesion and severity of auditory dysfunction. They compared data for two groups of patients: One group had undergone temporal lobectomy with removal of the auditory association area and the second group underwent removal of both auditory association area and primary auditory cortex. Auditory performance was evaluated over a period of one year. The patient group whose primary auditory cortex was spared showed faster improvement and recovery of auditory skills. Antonelli and colleagues concluded that an additional lesion in the primary auditory area did not contribute to worsening of auditory performance, but it did prolong the recovery period. Their reports highlighted the importance of longitudinal studies in understanding the effects of brain lesions and the function of different auditory areas within the brain (Antonelli, 1970c; Antonelli & Calearo, 1968).

Antonelli and colleagues observed that when compared with lesions of the brainstem, lesions of the auditory cortex resulted in relatively mild deficits in performance for degraded or interrupted speech. Performance on time-compressed speech appeared to be "peculiarly dependent on the functional state of reticular formation at the pontine level" (Antonelli, 1970b, p. 139). These pioneering researchers further noted that cortical lesions did not cause hearing loss as measured on pure-tone audiometry, whereas in contrast, brainstem lesions could be accompanied by hearing loss, either unilateral or bilateral (Antonelli 1970b, 1970c).

Pioneering Psychologists

Helmer Myklebust

Helmer Myklebust was one of the first professionals to stress the importance of assessing central auditory system function in addition to peripheral hearing loss in children. He earned a master's degree in psychology of deafness from Gallaudet University, a second master's degree in clinical psychology from Temple University, and a PhD from Rutgers University in 1945. Myklebust began his career as a teacher at the Tennessee School for the Deaf. Later in the Psychological Laboratory at the Vineland Training School, he became interested in issues concerning auditory behavior, language, learning disability, and brain injury (Hammill, 2012).

For most of his illustrious career, Myklebust was a faculty member in the Department of Audiology at Northwestern University where he also served as Director at the Institute for Language Disorders in Children (Hammill, 2012). The depth of his knowledge in areas related to hearing loss and auditory processing is reflected in a classic article published in the *Journal of Speech and Hearing Disorders*, in which he discussed assessment and management of children with a history of Rh incompatibility (Myklebust, 1956). Despite the rather limited audiological test battery at that time, Myklebust's clinical observations of symptoms in a subgroup of children with a history of Rh incompatibility were remarkably detailed. Taken together they suggested clinical patterns consistent with what we know today as auditory neuropathy spectrum disorder and CAPD.

Myklebust's rather prophetic diagnostic descriptions warrant more than a passing mention. In his article centered on the issue of whether children with Rh incompatibility have peripheral or central damage, Myklebust observed that high frequency hearing loss detected in a number of these children did not completely account for their auditory problems. He concluded that the clinical profile in these children was one of brain injury rather than of deafness. Myklebust noted that aphasia, auditory agnosia, dyspraxia, and learning disability all affect auditory behavior and language development. He recommended that central auditory disorders must be considered in the evaluation of these children. He stated: "The Rh child, if studied appropriately, frequently gives evidence of having an inability to *listen* rather than an inability to *hear*. His auditory disorder includes inability to integrate, structure, and perceive" (Myklebust, 1956, p. 424). Myklebust was committed to diagnostic evaluation and also remediation of auditory and other communication disorders. He suggested that in terms of education, children with Rh incompatibility should be considered "from the point of view of the psychology of brain injury whether or not a superimposed loss of hearing is present" (Myklebust, 1956, p. 424). He reflected in his writings an in-depth understanding of the symptoms of peripheral versus higher order disorders of the auditory system, and the possibility of their coexistence in some cases.

In the years between 1951 and 1997, Myklebust published articles, book chapters, and books on deafness, the psychology of deafness, and learning disability. He admonished clinicians (audiologists) not to restrict themselves to assessing hearing problems in children only based on an audiogram. Myklebust stressed the importance of evaluating auditory processing. His commitment to this principle is evident in the book titled *Auditory Disorders in Children: A Manual for Differential Diagnosis* (Myklebust, 1954). Myklebust's thinking strongly influenced a young scholar at Northwestern University during the early 1950s who later went on to be a giant in the field of audiology and an expert in the area of CAPD. The young scholar was James Jerger.

Donald Broadbent

Donald Broadbent was another psychologist making an enormous early contribution to assessment of central auditory processing. A well-known scientist in his profession, Broadbent started his research at the Applied Psychology Research Unit in Cambridge. He developed the dichotic listening paradigm with digit stimuli and applied the paradigm to the investigation of memory and selective attention. Broadbent was intrigued with the effects of attention, perception, and memory on communication. This interest was fueled by his experiences while in the British Royal Air Force and later by his work with air traffic controllers who had to listen and attend to multiple simultaneously occurring auditory signals. Broadbent proposed his theory of selective attention based on experiments with dichotic signals and described his findings in detail in his 1958 book *Perception and Communication.*

Doreen Kimura

In the early 1960s, Doreen Kimura joined the doctoral program at the Montreal Neurological Institute under the guidance of Dr. Brenda Milner. Their research probed right and left temporal lobe functions. Woodburn Heron, Kimura's mentor for her master's thesis work in the late 1950s, suggested she use dichotic digits for her doctoral research because the dichotic listening task would be sufficiently challenging to define the functions of the left temporal lobe (Kimura, 2011). Using digits from 1 to 10 in a three-pair dichotic format similar to that applied previously by Broadbent, Kimura noticed that the scores in normal hearing adults were consistently higher for the right ear than for the left ear. She called this the *right-ear effect.* Kimura also noted that this right-left difference was not replicated when the same stimuli were presented monaurally (Kimura, 1961a, 1967).

In a series of articles describing studies with a number of speech and nonspeech dichotic stimuli, Kimura reported a consistent pattern of ear differences in adults as well as children (Kimura, 1961a, 1963, 1967). She observed higher left ear scores compared with right for musical stimuli, which she attributed to dominance of the right temporal lobe for this task. The schematic diagram featured in her 1967 article on functional asymmetries of the brain formed the conceptual basis for explaining the dominance of contralateral pathways and suppression of ipsilateral pathways in dichotic listening (Kimura, 1967, p. 174). Contemporary articles and books about dichotic listening continue to use some variant of this diagram, a modified version of which is depicted in Figure 6–1.

Kimura's research examining auditory functions of the temporal lobes was innovative and insightful. She systematically studied and reported findings in 71 patients with temporal lobe lesions

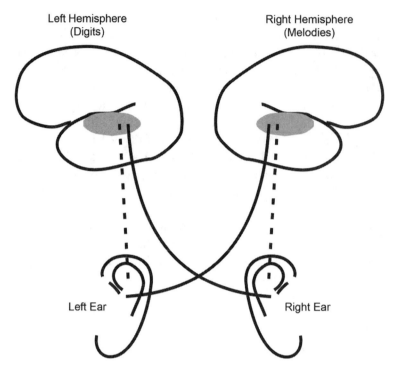

Figure 6–1. An adaptation of Kimura's diagram showing left temporal lobe dominance for digits and right temporal lobe dominance for melodies in a dichotic task.

(Kimura, 1961b), and she was one of the first to report the association between side of lesion and pattern of auditory deficits on dichotic tasks. Kimura's research on brain asymmetries and her theory of dichotic listening have endured the test of time. Although Broadbent developed the dichotic digit format, it was Kimura who applied the paradigm in clinical assessment much as we do today in the evaluation of CAPD. Dichotic tests with digits and other speech stimuli remain an essential part of the CAPD test battery. The right-ear effect discovered and explained by Kimura forms the basis for using the magnitude of ear difference as a diagnostic criterion for interpreting results from dichotic tests.

Early Audiologists

Introduction

Audiology is a young profession in comparison to otolaryngology and psychology. The immaturity of audiology in the 1950s and 1960s might explain why interested professionals from these other fields performed the early work in the area that we now refer to as CAPD. Before long, however, a small group of audiologists recognized the clinical value of test procedures for assessment of CANS function. These well-known leaders in our profession developed new tests for diagnosis of central auditory dysfunction and conducted necessary clinical studies to validate them. Among the audiologists who initially took great interest in understanding the mechanics of central auditory disorders were James Jerger, Jack Katz, Jack Willeford, and Robert Keith. These well-known audiologists are pictured in Figure 6–2.

James Jerger

Dr. James Jerger was a student of Raymond Carhart at Northwestern University. He then collaborated with Carhart on a variety of research projects. The majority of Jerger's numerous publications

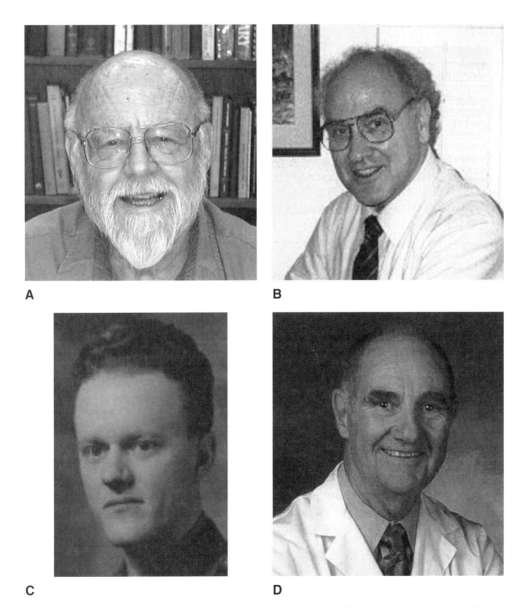

A　　　　　　　　　**B**

C　　　　　　　　　**D**

Figure 6–2. **A.** James Jerger, **B.** Jack Katz, **C.** Jack Willeford, and **D.** Robert Keith

and his landmark contributions to the field of CAPD were made during his 29-year tenure at the Baylor College of Medicine in Houston, Texas. Jerger is especially renowned for the diagnostic tests he developed, modified, or simplified to evaluate each part of the auditory system from the middle ear to the cortex.

In 1960, he wrote an article on audiological manifestations of lesions in the auditory nervous system (J. Jerger, 1960). Jerger proposed in this paper two concepts that are at the core of central auditory assessment that he referred to as the *subtlety* and *bottleneck* principles. He later stated in a book chapter:

> A tiny piece of wire inadvertently dropped into the labyrinth during surgery can cause severe or even total deafness in the ear; yet an entire temporal lobe can be removed and the effect on hearing is so slight that we must go to very great lengths indeed in our laboratory to show that patient's auditory system is not entirely normal. (J. Jerger, 1964, cited in Willeford, 1969, p. 1)

Jack Katz

Jack Katz completed his master's degree in audiology and speech pathology from Syracuse University and his PhD from University of Pittsburgh in 1961. He is probably best known for developing the Staggered Spondaic Word (SSW) test and for editing all six editions of *The Handbook of Clinical Audiology*. Katz first published his findings with the SSW test in 1962, soon after Kimura described clinical application of the dichotic listening paradigm (Katz, 1962). At the time, he held a position in the Department of Otolaryngology at the Tulane University School of Medicine in New Orleans. Katz explained in the article how the SSW test incorporated principles that enabled its use as a test of central auditory function. Over the next 50 years, Katz continued to study applications of the SSW test. Even today, it remains one of the most widely used commercially available central auditory tests.

Beginning of Formal Central Auditory Assessment

Research in the period before 1965 firmly established the need for specialized tests to assess the CANS. Researchers of the time faced several technical and professional hurdles. Tests needed to be designed so they could be administered with very basic equipment. In addition, clinical audiologists needed to be convinced that highly esteemed pure tone audiometry was grossly inadequate for assessing central auditory functioning, even though it had value in defining status of peripheral hearing function in individuals suspected of CAPD.

With reference to the pioneers of the early period, and especially to Dr. Doreen Kimura, James Jerger (2011) recently commented: "[M]any important breakthroughs were achieved by well-trained and clever people using what must be described by today's standards as exceedingly primitive equipment." Jerger went on to note that it was the sheer brilliance of these researchers coupled with their thorough understanding of neuroanatomy and neurophysiology that led them to take notice of what might be mistaken as aberrant results by the untrained eye.

The Second Phase

Introduction

The period from 1965 to 1990 witnessed prolific growth in assessment and intervention techniques for individuals with CAPD. Audiologists and speech-language pathologists played the major role in this effort. Research with patient populations who had confirmed lesions of the CANS validated assessment procedures. The earlier focus on individuals with brain lesions shifted slowly to include children and adults with no frank neurological or radiological evidence of brain lesions who nonetheless displayed symptoms of CAPD. Professionals began to recognize that children with learning disabilities were a population at risk for CAPD. While some researchers focused on the diagnostic aspect of CAPD, others additionally focused on developing training programs.

New Diagnostic Speech Audiometry Tests

In 1965, Charles Speaks and James Jerger developed synthetic sentences for the assessment of speech identification and soon after modified the test to include continuous discourse as a competing message (J. Jerger, Speaks, & Trammel, 1968). A few years later, Jerger reported various methods of using the Synthetic Sentence Identification (SSI) test for identifying retrocochlear pathology (J. Jerger, 1970). His clinical research showed that the most diagnostically useful approach was a comparison of performance for an ipsilateral competing message versus contralateral competing message (J. Jerger & Jerger, 1974; J. Jerger & Jerger, 1975a; J. Jerger & Jerger, 1975b).

Due to the language content (and working memory load), the SSI was appropriate only for adolescents and adults. When Susan and James Jerger developed the Pediatric Speech Intelligibility (PSI) Test for assessment of children between 3 to 8 years of age (S. Jerger & Jerger, 1984),

the same competing message format was applied effectively. It was common practice in the time to use, sometimes inappropriately in children, tests originally designed for adult populations. The PSI test was one of the first measures of central auditory function designed specifically for use with children. The Jergers reported extensive validation data for the PSI test from children with brain lesions who were suspected of having CAPD (S. Jerger, 1987; S. Jerger, Jerger, & Abrams, 1983; S. Jerger, Johnson, & Loiselle, 1988; S. Jerger & Zeller, 1989). Through their extensive follow up of the applications of the SSI and PSI tests, the Jergers contributed importantly to the understanding of the mechanisms underlying central auditory processing. Perhaps among their most important observations was that individuals with cortical lesions had difficulty with competing signals presented to the contralateral ear whereas those with brainstem lesions performed more poorly for ipsilateral competing signals.

Throughout the 1970s, Susan and James Jerger and colleagues at Baylor College of Medicine investigated the clinical application of objective auditory tests such as the acoustic reflex in identifying auditory nerve and lower brainstem dysfunction (S. Jerger & Jerger, 1977; S. Jerger, Jerger, & Hall, 1979). Also during this prolific period of research, the cross-check principle for diagnostic auditory assessment of children was recognized and implemented clinically (J. Jerger & Hayes, 1976).

Bottom-Up Versus Top-Down Thinking

Different viewpoints on the exact nature of CAPD began to emerge in parallel with progress in test development. Evolving opinions on the fundamental nature of CAPD, perhaps inevitably, contributed to controversies on intervention approaches. Some researchers agreed with Myklebust's theory that auditory problems in these children led to language disorders (Myklebust, 1954) whereas others strongly argued that language disorder was the cause of central auditory problems. The former was essentially a "bottom-up" view of auditory and language processing, whereas the latter constituted was a "top-down" perspective.

Contributions of Robert Keith

As early as the 1970s, Robert W. Keith pointed out that central auditory tests "present a confusing array of choices for the clinician. Some of the tests are designed for determining the anatomical site of lesion in the auditory system, while others assess auditory function as it relates to academic and behavioral functions, especially with regard to specific auditory problems in learning-disabled children" (Keith, 1977, p. vii). In part, to address the problem of inconsistency in assessment approaches, Keith spearheaded the organization of a symposium on central auditory dysfunction at the University of Cincinnati Medical Center. Invited distinguished speakers with experience in using central auditory tests presented papers covering a wide range of topics from traditional site-of-lesion tests, to test batteries, evaluation of children with learning disabilities, communicating results of auditory tests with other professionals, and team evaluation of children. Conference proceedings were compiled into a book edited by Keith (1977). This single-handed effort by Keith paved the way for broadening the scope of the audiologist's role in assess-

ment and intervention for CAPD. It was one of his many landmark contributions to the area of CAPD.

Keith further promoted the concept of compiling appropriate tests with adequate normative data from the same sample into a test battery. He developed the well-known SCAN: A Screening Test for Auditory Processing Disorders (Keith, 1986) for assessment of children aged 3 to 11 years. Keith later modified this test into a version suitable for adolescents and adults (SCAN-A [Keith, 1995]) and another version for children called the SCAN-C (Keith, 2000a). One of the strengths of the SCAN-C is the norms provided based on a large sample of typical children across the United States, with sample sizes from each region based on census data.

In addition, Keith published other tests for central auditory assessment, including the Auditory Fusion Test–Revised (McCroskey & Keith, 1996), the Random Gap Detection Test (Keith, 2000b), and the Time Compressed Sentences Test (Keith, 2002). He developed the Auditory Continuous Performance Test (Keith, 1994) for ruling out attention problems in children undergoing assessment for CAPD.

Over a span of nearly four decades, Robert Keith has contributed significantly and in many ways to the understanding of CAPD among audiologists, speech-language pathologists, and educators. His "case of the month" feature on the University of Cincinnati College of Medicine webpage, which is available for open Internet access, is an example of his continued efforts toward sharing knowledge and encouraging best practices in CAPD across the world.

Jack Willeford's Test Battery

Jack Willeford was one of the invited speakers at the Cincinnati symposium. He presented a paper on a three-test battery developed at the Colarado State University that became known as the "Willeford Test Battery." Willeford later expanded the battery to include six tests of central auditory processing. His stated aim was to "present a series of tests that were known to challenge the integrity of the CANS at several levels" (Willeford, 1977, p. 44). Willeford considered this a necessary feature of a test battery because auditory dysfunction could affect only one level or region of the CANS.

Willeford made a number of important points in his 1977 paper. For example, he cautioned professionals about the hazards of assessing children in uncontrolled settings such as a classroom or office where a child's responses could be highly affected by extraneous and nonauditory variables. He observed that audiologists were uniquely trained to assess the central auditory system, but few were involved in diagnosis or intervention of children with CAPD (at that time). He clarified that not all children with auditory processing deficits had language problems. Finally, Willeford opined that test results in children were best reported without comments on a site of lesion or dysfunction as it cannot usually be supported by neurophysiologic evidence. He stated: "We simply say that the child cannot do these types of auditory processing tasks" (Willeford, 1977, p. 72).

Richard Wilson and Speech Audiometry

Central auditory evaluation has become easier (and therefore more common) in clinical practice over the years due to the availability of a wide range of commercially available tests. Developing tools that are backed by strong norms, test-retest reliability, and validity data is a difficult task. Richard Wilson is among those audiologists who developed such tools, especially for adults suspected of CAPD. For most of his career, Wilson has held positions in audiology services and research facilities in Veterans Affairs (VA) Medical Centers in the USA. Among his most notable contributions is the development of a series of speech audiometry tests for central auditory assessment in adult patients. Available on compact discs, the tests have given audiologists in clinical practice easy access to well-researched test materials. In addition, his research collaborations with prominent audiologists from centers across the USA have led to a variety of publications on diagnosis and intervention for CAPD (e.g., Moncrieff & Wilson, 2009; Noffsinger, Martinez, & Wilson, 1994; Noffsinger, Wilson, & Musiek, 1994; Strouse & Wilson, 1999; Wilson, Moncrieff, Townsend, & Pillion, 2003).

Neuroaudiologist Frank Musiek

Frank Musiek has contributed importantly to establishing the connection of hearing to the brain and to promoting the unique role of audiologists in managing hearing disorders related to central auditory dysfunction. He coined the term "neuroaudiology" for this special area of the profession (J. Jerger, 2009). Working from the 1970s in close collaboration with neurologists, neurosurgeons, and otolaryngologists, Musiek honed his knowledge about the intricacies of the CANS and its evaluation. He has done much to increase understanding of the anatomic and physiologic bases of hearing, as demonstrated through extensive presentations and publications on the subject (e.g., Bamiou, Musiek, & Luxon,

2003; Musiek, 1986a; Musiek, 1986b; Musiek & Baran, 1986, 2006; Musiek, Weihing, & Oxholm, 2007).

Musiek has developed and validated several widely used clinical tests, such as the Dichotic Digits Test, Frequency Pattern Test and Duration Pattern Test, and the Gaps-In-Noise Test (Musiek, 1983a, 1983b; Musiek, Baran, & Pinheiro, 1990; Musiek, Gollegly, Kibbe, & Verkest-Lenz, 1991; Musiek & Pinheiro, 1985, 1987; Musiek et al., 2005; Musiek & Wilson, 1979). He also has played a crucial role in drafting important recommendations on CAPD, such as the ones made at the Bruton Conference in Dallas, Texas (J. Jerger & Musiek, 2000), the position statement of the American Speech-Language-Hearing Association (ASHA, 2005), and the recent clinical guidelines of the American Academy of Audiology (AAA, 2010). Through his work, Frank Musiek has demonstrated the essential role of audiologists in the diagnosis and intervention of CAPD.

Gail Chermak

Gail Chermak is another audiologist whose name has become synonymous with diagnosis and intervention for CAPD. For over 30 years, she has steadily researched and written about intervention for CAPD, particularly in children. In her 1992 article on management of CAPD (Chermak & Musiek, 1992), Chermak explained the rationale and techniques of intervention in a way that could be applied easily to routine clinical practice. Dr. Chermak is noted for her work on differentiating CAPD from attention deficit hyperactivity disorder (ADHD). Her research over the last nearly one and a half decades has proved that the two conditions are indeed clinically distinct, although they can coexist (e.g. Chermak, 2007, 2011; Chermak, Hall, & Musiek, 1999; Chermak, Somers, & Seikel, 1998; Chermak, Tucker, & Seikel, 2002). Her publications on using factor analysis to analyze the efficacy of test batteries (Schow & Chermak, 1999; Schow, Seikel, Chermak, & Berent, 2000) emphasize an often neglected area of work. She has traveled widely sharing her knowledge on CAPD with the audiology community around the world.

The Modern Era

Introduction

The modern era in the evolution of diagnosis and intervention for CAPD has highlighted the critical role that evoked responses serve in the diagnosis of CAPD. Diagnostic efforts in earlier periods were dominated by behavioral tests. Some of the pioneers of behavioral assessment techniques like James Jerger and Frank Musiek also advocated for including auditory evoked responses to further augment the central auditory diagnostic test battery. Actually, each of these researchers had first explored the clinical role of cortical auditory evoked responses years earlier. The emerging importance of auditory evoked responses is evidenced with the suggestion of J. Jerger and Musiek (2000) that behavioral and electrophysiological test measures should be combined in a minimal test battery for diagnosis of CAPD. Musiek also defined test performance for the auditory middle latency evoked response (AMLR) in patients with confirmed neurologic disorders (Musiek, Charette, Kelly, Lee,

& Musiek, 1999) and he described test combinations including various auditory evoked responses for assessing different levels of the CANS (e.g., Musiek & Chermak, 1994, 2009). See Chapter 17 in Volume 1 of the Handbook for discussion of electrophysiological measures in central auditory diagnostic test batteries.

Electrophysiological Evidence of CAPD From Nina Kraus

At this time, there is no *gold standard* test for diagnosis of CAPD. Evoked responses might in the future assume that role (AAA, 2010; J. Jerger & Musiek, 2000). Hughes Knowles Professor at the Northwestern University Nina Kraus has systematically studied evoked responses from various levels and regions of the CANS and also researched their application in assessing CAPD. In the 1980s, her publications featured the AMLR. Her research focus in the 1990s was the mismatch negativity (MMN) response, as well as the auditory late response (ALR) and the P300.

Most recently, Kraus has directed her attention to neural representation of speech processing in the brainstem as measured with the speech-evoked ABR, more recently known as complex ABR. The publications based on her research strongly reflect a commitment toward understanding the mechanisms underlying CAPD (e.g., Cunningham, Nicol, Zecker, Bradlow, & Kraus, 2001; Cunningham, Nicol, Zecker, & Kraus, 2000; Hornickel, Chandrasekaran, Zecker, & Kraus, 2011; Russo, Nicol, Zecker, Hayes, & Kraus, 2005; Warrier, Johnson, Hayes, Nicol, & Kraus, 2004). Not only has her research demonstrated that there is a difference between the speech-evoked

responses of typical individuals versus those with CAPD, as well as those with dyslexia, she has also confirmed that speech-evoked response measures can be applied as objective indicators of changes in neural and behavioral function. Kraus's research has established that the brainstem is directly involved in preservation and transmission of precise acoustic cues required for speech perception in quiet and noise. See Chapter 7 of Volume 1 of this Handbook for discussion of the research of Kraus's group.

Teri James Bellis

Teri James Bellis has shared her extensive clinical experience with CAPD in children through peer-reviewed journal articles, a popular audiology text book, and a "consumer" book written for patients with CAPD and their families. She has emphasized the importance of following up diagnosis with appropriate intervention by using test results to create an "auditory profile of strengths and weaknesses" and "deficit-specific intervention plans" (Bellis, 2002, 2003).

Innovative Tests From Australian Researchers

In recent years some of the most creative new tests of CAPD have been developed in Australia. Sharon Cameron, in collaboration with well-known fellow countryman Harvey Dillon, devised a test that assesses spatial listening under headphones. The Listening in Spatialized Noise Test (LiSN-S) examines the ability to use spatial separation to differentiate signal from noise (Cameron & Dillon, 2007; Cameron, Dillon, & Newall, 2006a,

2006b). There are adult and pediatric versions of the LiSN. Cameron's research has indicated that individuals with CAPD are often less able to take advantage of spatial auditory cues (Cameron & Dillon, 2008; Cameron, Dillon, & Newall, 2006a). Based upon her research, it is evident that traditional speech-in-noise tests administered under earphones do not tap into this very important aspect of everyday listening. Cameron and Dillon have also developed software for auditory training of spatial listening skills (see Chapter 8). Preliminary studies with children have yielded encouraging results (Cameron & Dillon, 2011).

Pioneers From the United Kingdom

Studies of the basic sciences underlying clinical phenomena are an important means of devising new strategies for intervention. Dr. Tim Griffiths used neuroimaging and psychoacoustics to study the brain processing that underlies auditory perception in normal individuals and those with CANS lesions (e.g. Griffiths, Bates et al., 1997; Griffiths, Dean, Woods, Rees, & Green, 2001; Griffiths, Rees, et al., 1997). Dr. Griffiths is Professor of Cognitive Neurology and the University of Newcastle upon Tyne in the United Kingdom. He has worked extensively investigating complex auditory processing in individuals with autism, dementia, and psychiatric disorders.

Dr. Doris-Eva Bamiou from the University College London Ear Institute also has contributed significantly to our understanding of CAPD. She has worked collaboratively with researchers around the world on publications related to basic

anatomy and physiology underlying central auditory processing (Bamiou, Musiek, & Luxon, 2003; Bamiou, Sisodiya, Musiek, & Luxon, 2007), as well as on central auditory assessment of children and adults (Bamiou, Musiek, & Luxon, 2001; Bamiou et al., 2006; Iliadou & Bamiou, 2012; Iliadou, Bamiou, Kaprinis, Kandylis, & Kaprinis, 2009; Iliadou et al., 2008).

International Collaborations

Research and clinical interest in CAPD has expanded in recent years to an international level. Collaboration among CAPD experts from around the world is now commonplace. The conference on Global Perspectives on Central Auditory Processing Disorder is an excellent example of the trend toward international collaboration. Organized by Frank Musiek, Doris Bamiou, and Program Chair Gail Chermak and held during the 2012 annual convention of the American Academy of Audiology in Boston, the conference included research presentations and panel discussions featuring many of the CAPD experts cited already. The titles of selected keynote addresses and featured sessions succinctly conveys some of the major themes of the global conference (e.g., The Mind's Ear: Structured Approaches to Normal and Abnormal Auditory Cognition; Defining CAPD and APD: Theoretical Constructs and Perspectives; Advances in Clinical Practice; Future Directions in Clinical Practice and Research). It is likely that the global conference is only the beginning of an international effort to better understand CAPD and how it can be best assessed and treated clinically.

Intervention for CAPD

Introduction

As already noted, professionals over the years have disagreed on the exact nature of CAPD and the best approaches for intervention. Indeed, some critics have even questioned the scientific basis and clinical effectiveness of intervention for CAPD, although the accumulating literature clearly demonstrates the utility of various treatments for CAPD (AAA, 2010; and Chapters 2 and 3). We conclude this overview of the historical foundations of CAPD with reference to advances in intervention technology, techniques, and strategies.

FM Technology

FM technology has a long-standing tradition in helping children and adults with CAPD. Classroom and personal FM systems to improve the signal-to-noise ratio (SNR) and listening environment are very appropriate for some individuals with CAPD. An enhanced SNR in the classroom benefits all children, and particularly those with special auditory or educational demands. Personal FM technology is remarkably effective in improving auditory performance in children with CAPD, as well as psychosocial status, academic performance, and perhaps auditory system efficiency and effectiveness (Hornickel, Zecker, Bradlow, & Kraus, 2012; Johnston, John, Kreisman, Hall, & Crandell, 2009).

Personal FM devices generally are not recommended for all individuals identified with CAPD. Individuals who show below normal performance on speech-in-noise tests and dichotic tests are likely to benefit from FM systems (AAA, 2010; ASHA, 2005; Bellis, 2003). In contrast, those with temporal processing deficits typically do not benefit from mere improvement of SNR. Chapter 12 includes a detailed review of signal enhancement technology.

Bottom-Up Auditory Training

Audiologists tend to gravitate toward bottom-up perception oriented approaches to intervention for CAPD. A bottom-up approach is based on the premise that difficulties in central auditory processing lead to impaired auditory perception, language, reading, and communication (Sloan, 1986). The focus of therapy is to improve speech perception through auditory training. Christine Sloan's book, *Treating Auditory Processing Difficulties in Children* was one of the first comprehensive guides to intervention for children with CAPD.

In the early 1990s, Katz devised the "Buffalo Model" for the assessment and remediation of CAPD (Katz, 1992; Katz & Smith, 1991). This model defined CAPD as "what we do with what we hear" (Katz, 2007). The classification of central auditory processing problems is based on an audiological test battery consisting of the SSW test, Phonemic Synthesis Test (Katz & Harmon, 1981), and a speech-in-noise test. Deficits are categorized into four subtypes: auditory-decoding deficit, auditory tolerance–memory fading deficit, auditory integration deficit, and auditory organization deficit. Management strategies are guided by the classification.

According to Katz, the rationale for this classification system is that functions evaluated with the test battery constitute skills that underlie both, basic central auditory processes (e.g., speech recognition in noise, dichotic listening), as well as higher level processes (e.g., short term/ working auditory memory, phoneme analysis and blending) (Katz, 2007).

Advances in neuroscience in the 1990s or the "Decade of the Brain" confirmed the principle of brain plasticity and its role in rehabilitation. This principle was applied in studies demonstrating the effectiveness of intensive computer-based training to address fundamental deficits of auditory processing (Tallal et al., 1996). However, well before the advent of software-based training programs, Alexander and Frost (1982) demonstrated in children with language delay that the ability to perceive fine phonemic contrasts could be improved through an intervention program incorporating decelerated synthesized speech. Slowing down of the speech apparently made critical formant cues easier to perceive. The program included systematically increasing the speed of the stimuli toward a normal rate.

There are now a variety of computer-based programs available that may have potential for remediation of individuals with CAPD using a "quasi" bottom-up approach, considered quasi because they are more appropriately considered auditory-language approaches (e.g., BrainTrain, 2010; Houghton Mifflin Harcourt Learning Technology, 2000; Scientific Learning Corporation, 1997). See Chapter 11 for an extensive review of computer-assisted training programs, and Chapters 7 and 9 for discussion of auditory training.

Combined Bottom-Up and Top-Down Approaches

Some well-known authorities on CAPD have combined top-down (i.e., language and cognitive oriented) and bottom-up (i.e., auditory perceptual) techniques in their training approaches. Dorothy Kelly (1995) developed strategies based on a combined approach that concentrated on auditory discrimination and auditory figure-ground (bottom-up focus), and auditory cohesion and auditory attention (top-down focus). Other auditory training approaches include a top-down focus on metacognition. Metacognitive strategies are useful in improving not only auditory processing skills, but also in minimizing the psychosocial problems associated with CAPD (Bellis, 2003; Chermak, 1998a; Chermak & Musiek, 1997; Ferre, 1998). Chermak and Musiek suggested several metacognitive and metalinguistic strategies for CAPD management (Chermak, 1998a, 1998b; Chermak & Musiek, 1997). See Chapter 1 for discussion of a comprehensive approach to intervention and Chapter 10 for elaboration of top-down, central resources training.

Multisensory Approach

The Auditory Discrimination in Depth (ADD) program of Patricia and Phyllis Lindamood is an example of an early auditory training approach that predated the advent of computer technology (Lindamood & Lindamood, 1971). The program was later renamed the Lindamood Phoneme Sequencing Program for Reading, Spelling, and Speech (LiPS). According to the Lindamoods, auditory processing consists of five processes: sensory input, perception, conceptualization, storage, and retrieval. The LiPS program is multisensory in nature. The technique utilizes auditory, visual, and oral-sensory/motor feedback to help patients better identify, classify, and label speech sounds.

Individualized Intervention

As experience in treating the auditory problems of individuals with CAPD has accumulated, there has been an increased realization that effective intervention programs are individualized, customized to the individual's deficits, needs, and lifestyle. No single strategy or approach suits all children and adults with CAPD. Katz and Wilde (1994) certainly appreciated this principle when they stated: "It is our belief that recommendations should be based on the individual's needs and the problem situations faced, rather than simply a generic approach" (p. 498).

Katz and colleagues edited a book in which most of the chapters were devoted to management strategies (Masters, Stecker, & Katz, 1998). They invited authors who were practicing different and individualized training techniques to contribute to the book (e.g., Chermak, 1998b; Cinotti, 1998; Ferre, 1998). Early and individualized training for central auditory processing deficits improves patient outcome. Intervention theory and clinical practice has evolved considerably during the past 60 years. There is now a general acceptance among members of the audiology and speech-language professional communities that the "one size fits all" approach is not effective in either assessment or intervention for CAPD. Deficit-specific intervention is most effective. The deficit-specific intervention approach uses a combination of management and treatment techniques and strategies to improve specific auditory skills. Together these strategies incorporate the strengths of the bottom-up and top-down intervention approaches. Teri Bellis (2003) and Jeanane Ferre (2002) have likened the combination of the three categories of intervention strategies (i.e., environmental modifications, remediation activities, and compensatory strategies) to the legs of a tripod.

Summary

Our understanding of central auditory processing and its disorders has increased considerably over the past 60 years. Debates and controversies about the nature of CAPD and intervention strategies are giving way to general agreement that the disorder can be identified, diagnosed, and remediated or adequately managed. Indeed, professional organizations like the American Academy of Audiology and the American Speech-Language-Hearing Association cite diagnosis of and intervention for CAPD as within the scope of practice of clinical audiology. The importance of a multidisciplinary approach for intervention of CAPD also is now well accepted by these professional organizations. To be sure, methods of diagnosis and intervention for CAPD are even today too often dependent to a large extent on preferences of individual clinicians rather than the needs of the patient. Nonetheless, we are optimistic about the steady progress toward patient-centered evaluation and intervention for CAPD.

References

AAA (American Academy of Audiology). (2010). *Clinical practice guidelines: Diagnosis, treatment and management of children and adults with central auditory processing disorder*. Retrieved from http://www.audiology.org/resources/documentlibrary/Documents/CAPD%20Guidelines%208-2010.pdf

Alexander, D. W., & Frost, B. P. (1982). Decelerated synthesized speech as a means of shaping speed of auditory processing of children with delayed language. *Perceptual and Motor Skills, 55*, 783–792.

Antonelli, A. (1970a). Sensitized speech tests in aged people. In C. Rojskaer (Ed.), *Speech audiometry* (pp. 66–79). Odense, Denmark: Second Danavox Symposium.

Antonelli, A. (1970b). Sensitized speech tests: Results in brainstem lesions and diffusive CNS diseases. In C. Rojskaer (Ed.), *Speech audiometry* (pp. 130–139). Odense, Denmark: Second Danavox Symposium.

Antonelli, A. (1970c). Sensitized speech tests: Results in lesions of the brain. In C. Rojskaer (Ed.), *Speech audiometry* (pp. 176–183). Odense, Denmark: Second Danavox Symposium.

Antonelli, A., & Calearo, C. (1968). Further investigations on cortical deafness. *Acta Oto-laryngologica, 66*, 97–100.

ASHA (American Speech-Language-Hearing Association). (2005). *(Central) auditory processing disorders* [Technical report]. Retrieved from http://www.asha.org/policy

Bamiou, D. E., Musiek, F. E., & Luxon, L. M. (2001). Aetiology and clinical presentation of auditory processing disorders: A review. *Archives of Disabilities in Childhood, 85*, 361–365. doi:10.1136/adc.85.5.361

Bamiou, D. E., Musiek, F. E., & Luxon, L. M. (2003). The insula (island of Reil) and its role in auditory processing: Literature review. *Brain Research Reviews, 42*, 143–154. doi:10.1016 /S0165-0173(03)00172-3

Bamiou, D. E., Musiek, F. E., Stow, I., Stevens, J., Cipolotti, L., Brown, M. M., . . . Luxon, L. M. (2006). Auditory temporal processing deficits in patients with insular stroke. *Neurology, 67*, 614–619. doi:10.1212/01.wnl.0000230197.40410.db

Bamiou, D. E., Sisodiya, S., Musiek, F. E., & Luxon, L. M. (2007). The role of the interhemispheric pathway in hearing. *Brain Research Reviews, 56*, 170–182. doi:10.1016/j.brainresrev.2007.07.003

Bellis, T. J. (2002). Developing deficit-specific intervention plans for individuals with central auditory processing disorders. *Seminars in Hearing, 23*, 287–295.

Bellis, T. J. (2003). *Assessment and management of central auditory processing disorders in the educational setting: From science to practice* (2nd ed.). New York, NY: Thomson and Delmar Learning.

BrainTrain. (2010). *SoundSmart*. Richmond, VA: Author. Retrieved from http://www.braintrain.com/soundsmart

Cameron, S., & Dillon, H. (2007). Development of the Listening in Spatialized Noise–Sentences Test (LISN-S). *Ear and Hearing, 28*, 196–211. doi:10.1097/AUD.0b013e318031267f

Cameron, S., & Dillon, H. (2008). The Listening in Spatialized Noise–Sentences Test (LISN-S): Comparison to the prototype LISN and results from children with either a suspected (central) auditory processing disorder or a confirmed language disorder. *Journal of the American Academy of Audiology, 19*, 377–391. doi:10.3766/jaaa.19.5.2

Cameron, S., & Dillon, H. (2011). Development and evaluation of the LiSN & learn auditory training software for deficit-specific remediation of binaural processing deficits in children: preliminary findings. *Journal of the American Academy of Audiology, 22*, 678–696. doi:610.3766/jaaa.3722.3710.3766

Cameron, S., Dillon, H., & Newall, P. (2006a). The Listening in Spatialized Noise Test: An auditory processing disorder study. *Journal of the American Academy of Audiology, 17*, 306–320. doi:10.3766/jaaa.17.5.2

Cameron, S., Dillon, H., & Newall, P. (2006b). The Listening in Spatialized Noise Test: Normative data for children. *International Journal of Audiology, 45,* 99–108. doi:10.1080/14992020500377931

Chermak, G. D. (1998a). Managing central auditory processing disorders: Metalinguistic and metacognitive approaches. *Seminars in Hearing, 19,* 379–392.

Chermak, G. D. (1998b). Metacognitive approaches to managing central auditory processing disorders. In M. G. Masters, N. A. Stecker, & J. Katz (Eds.), *Central auditory processing disorder: Mostly management* (pp. 49–62). Boston, MA: Allyn & Bacon.

Chermak, G. D. (2007). Differential diagnosis of (central) auditory processing disorder and attention deficit hyperactivity disorder. In F. E. Musiek & G. D. Chermak (Eds.), *Handbook of (central) auditory processing disorder: Auditory neuroscience and diagnosis* (Vol. I, pp. 365–394). San Diego, CA: Plural.

Chermak, G. D. (2011). Considerations for treatment and management of individuals with co-morbid CAPD and ADHD. *Hearing Journal, 64,* 6–8.

Chermak, G. D., Hall, J. W. III., & Musiek, F. E. (1999). Differential diagnosis and management of central auditory processing disorder and attention deficit hyperactivity disorder. *Journal of the American Academy of Audiology, 10,* 289–303.

Chermak, G.D., & Musiek, F.E. (1992). Managing central auditory processing disorders in children and youth. *American Journal of Audiology, 1,* 61–65.

Chermak, G. D., & Musiek, F. E. (1997). *Central auditory processing disorders: New perspectives.* San Diego, CA: Singular.

Chermak, G. D., Somers, E. K., & Seikel, J. A. (1998). Behavioral signs of central auditory processing disorder and attention deficit hyperactivity disorder. *Journal of the American Academy of Audiology, 9,* 78–84.

Chermak, G. D., Tucker, E., & Seikel, J. A. (2002). Behavioral characteristics of audi-tory processing disorder and attention-deficit hyperactivity disorder: Predominantly inattentive type. *Journal of the American Academy of Audiology, 13,* 332–338.

Cinotti, T. M. (1998). The Fast ForWord program: A clinician's perspective. In M. G. Masters, N. A. Stecker, & J. Katz (Eds.), *Central auditory processing disorder: Mostly management* (pp. 131–150). Boston, MA: Allyn and Bacon.

Cunningham, J., Nicol, T., Zecker, S., Bradlow, A., & Kraus, N. (2001). Neurobiologic responses to speech in noise in children with learning problems: Deficits and strategies for improvement. *Clinical Neurophysiology, 112,* 758–767. doi: 10.1016/S1388-2457(01)00465-5

Cunningham, J., Nicol, T., Zecker, S., & Kraus, N. (2000). Speech-evoked neurophysiologic responses in children with learning problems: Development and behavioral correlates of perception. *Ear and Hearing, 21,* 554–568. doi:10.1097/00003446-200012000-00003

Ferre, J. M. (1998). The M3 model for treating central auditory processing disorders. In M. G. Masters, N. A. Stecker, & J. Katz (Eds.), *Central auditory processing disorder: Mostly management* (pp. 103–116). Boston, MA: Allyn & Bacon.

Ferre, J. M. (2002). Behavioral therapeutic approaches for central auditory problems. In J. Katz, R. F. Burkard, & L. Medwetsky (Eds.), *Handbook of clinical audiology* (5th ed., pp. 525–531). Baltimore, MD: Lippincott Williams & Wilkins.

Griffiths, T. D., Bates, D., Rees, A., Witton, C., Gholkar, A., & Green, G. G. (1997). Sound movement detection deficit due to a brainstem lesion. *Journal of Neurology, Neurosurgery, and Psychiatry, 62,* 522–526. doi:10.1136/jnnp.62.5.522

Griffiths, T. D., Dean, J. L., Woods, W., Rees, A., & Green, G. G. R. (2001). The Newcastle Auditory Battery (NAB). A temporal and spatial test battery for use on adult naïve subjects. *Hearing Research, 154,* 165–169. doi: 10.1016/S0378-5955(01)00243-X

Griffiths, T. D., Rees, A., Witton, C., Cross, P. M., Shakir, R. A., & Green, G. G. (1997). Spatial and temporal auditory processing deficits following right hemisphere infarction: A psychophysical study. *Brain, 120*, 785–794. doi:10.1093/brain/120.5.785

Hammill, D. D. (2012). *Helmer Rudolph Myklebust (1910–2008). Hammill Institute Preservation Project.* Retrieved from http://hammill-institute.org/hipp

Hornickel, J., Chandrasekaran, B., Zecker, S. G., & Kraus, N. (2011). Auditory brainstem measures predict reading and speech-in-noise perception in school-aged children. *Behavioural Brain Research, 216*, 597–605. doi:10.1016/j.bbr.2010.08.051

Hornickel, J., Zecker, S., Bradlow, A., & Kraus, N. (2012). Assistive listening devices drive neuroplasticity in children with dyslexia. *Proceedings of the National Academy of Sciences, 109*, [Electronic version]. doi:10.1073/pnas.1206628109. Retrieved from http://www.soc.northwestern.edu/brainvolts/documents/FM_PNAS12.pdf

Houghton Mifflin Harcourt Learning Technology. (2000). *Earobics.* Boston, MA: Author.

Iliadou, V., & Bamiou, D. E. (2012). Psychometric evaluation of children with auditory processing disorder (APD): Comparison to a normal and a clinical non APD group. *Journal of Speech, Language, and Hearing Research, 55*, 791–799. doi:10.1044/1092-4388(2011/11-0035)

Iliadou, V., Bamiou, D. E., Kaprinis, S., Kandylis, D., & Kaprinis, G. (2009). Auditory processing disorders in children suspected of learning disabilities--a need for screening? *International Journal of Pediatric Otorhinolaryngology, 73*, 1029–1034. doi:10.1016/j.ijporl.2009.04.004

Iliadou, V., Bamiou, D. E., Kaprinis, S., Kandylis, D., Vlaikidis, N., Apalla, K., . . . St. Kaprinis, G. (2008). Auditory processing disorder and brain pathology in a preterm child with learning disabilities. *Journal of the American Academy of Audiology, 19*, 557–563. doi:10.3766/jaaa.19.7.5

Jerger, J. (1960). Audiological manifestations of lesions in the auditory nervous system. *Laryngoscope, 70*, 417–425. doi:10.1288/00005537-196004000-00008

Jerger, J. (1970). Diagnostic significance of SSI test procedures: Retrocochlear site. In C. Rojskaer (Ed.), *Speech audiometry* (pp. 163–175). Odense, Denmark: Second Danavox Symposium.

Jerger, J. (2009). *Audiology in the USA.* San Diego, CA: Plural.

Jerger, J. (2011, August 1). *20Q: The right-ear effect: Going strong after 50 years* (G. Mueller, Interviewer). Retrieved from http://www.audiologyonline.com/articles/20q-right-ear-effect-going-818

Jerger, J., & Hayes, D. (1976). The cross-check principle in pediatric audiometry. *Archives of Otolaryngology, 102*, 614–620. doi:10.1001/archotol.1976.00780150082006

Jerger, J., & Jerger, S. (1974). Auditory findings in brainstem disorders. *Archives of Otolaryngology, 99*, 342–350.

Jerger, J., & Jerger, S. (1975a). Clinical validity of central auditory tests. *Scandinavian Audiology, 4*, 147–163. doi:10.3109/14992027509043077

Jerger, J., & Jerger, S. (1975b). Extra- and intra-axial brainstem auditory disorders. *Audiology, 14*, 93–98.

Jerger, J., & Musiek, F. E. (2000). Report of the consensus conference on the diagnosis of auditory processing disorders in children. *Journal of the American Academy of Audiology, 11*, 467–474.

Jerger, J., Speaks, C., & Trammel, J. L. (1968). A new approach to speech audiometry. *Journal of Speech and Hearing Disorders, 33*, 318–328.

Jerger, S. (1987). Validation of the Pediatric Speech Intelligibility Test in children with central nervous system lesions. *Audiology, 26*, 298–311. doi:10.3109/00206098709081557

Jerger, S., & Jerger, J. (1977). Diagnostic value of crossed vs uncrossed acoustic reflexes: Eighth nerve and brain stem disorders. *Archives of Otolaryngology, 103*, 445–453. doi:10.1001/archotol.1977.00780250039002

Jerger, S., & Jerger, J. (1984). *Pediatric Speech Intelligibility Test: Manual for test administration.* St Louis, MO: Auditec.

Jerger, S., Jerger, J., & Abrams, S. (1983). Speech audiometry in the young child. *Ear and Hearing, 4*, 56–66. doi:10.1097/00003446-198301000-00010

Jerger, S., Jerger, J., & Hall, J. W. III. (1979). A new acoustic reflex pattern. *Archives of Otolaryngology, 105*, 24–28. doi:10.1001/archotol.1979.00790130028007

Jerger, S., Johnson, K., & Loiselle, L. (1988). Pediatric central auditory dysfunction: Comparison of children with confirmed lesions versus suspected processing disorders. *American Journal of Otology, 9* 63–71.

Jerger, S., & Zeller, R. S. (1989). Dichotic listening in a child with a cerebral lesion: The "paradoxical" ipsilateral ear effect. *Ear and Hearing, 10*, 167–172.

Johnston, K. N., John, A. B., Kreisman, N. V., Hall, J. W. III., & Crandell, C. C. (2009). Multiple benefits of personal FM system use by children with auditory processing disorder (APD). *International Journal of Audiology, 48*, 371–383. doi:10.1080/14992020802687516

Katz, J. (1962). The use of staggered spondaic words for assessing the integrity of the central auditory nervous system. *Journal of Auditory Research, 2*, 327–337.

Katz, J. (1992). Classification of auditory processing disorders In J. Katz, N. Stecker, & D. Henderson (Eds.), *Central auditory processing: A transdisciplinary view* (pp. 81–92). Chicago, IL: Mosby Yearbook.

Katz, J. (2007). *APD evaluation to therapy: The Buffalo model.* Retrieved from http://www.audiologyonline.com/articles/apd-evaluation-to-therapy-buffalo-945

Katz, J., & Harmon, C. (1981). Phonemic synthesis: Diagnostic and training program. In R. Keith (Ed.), *Central auditory and language disorders in children.* Houston, TX: College-Hill Press.

Katz, J., & Smith, P. S. (1991). The Staggered Spondaic Word Test. A ten-minute look at the central nervous system through the ears. *Annals of the New York Academy of Sciences, 620*, 233–251.

Katz, J., & Wilde, L. (1994). Auditory processing disorders. In J. Katz (Ed.), *Handbook of clinical audiology* (4th ed., pp. 490-502). Baltimore, MD: Williams & Wilkins.

Keith, R. W. (1986). *SCAN: A screening test for auditory processing disorders.* San Antonio, TX: Psychological Corporation, Harcourt Brace Jovanovich.

Keith, R. W. (1994). *ACPT: Auditory Continuous Performance Test (examiner's manual).* San Antonio, TX: Harcourt Brace.

Keith, R. W. (1995). Development and standardization of SCAN-A: Test of Auditory Processing Disorders in adolescents and adults. *Journal of the American Academy of Audiology, 6*, 286–292.

Keith, R. W. (2000a). Development and standardization of the SCAN-C test for auditory processing disorders in children. *Journal of the American Academy of Audiology, 11*, 438–445.

Keith, R. W. (2000b). *Random Gap Detection Test.* St. Louis, MO: Auditec.

Keith, R. W. (2002). Standardization of the Time Compressed Sentence Test. *Journal of Educational Audiology, 10*, 15–20.

Keith, R. W. (Ed.). (1977). *Central auditory dysfunction.* New York: Grune and Stratton.

Kelly, D. A. (1995). *Central auditory processing disorder: Strategies for use with children and adolescents.* San Antonio, TX: Communication Skill Builders.

Kimura, D. (1961a). Cerebral dominance and the perception of verbal stimuli. *Canadian Journal of Psychology, 15*, 166–171. doi:10.1037/h0083219

Kimura, D. (1961b). Some effects of temporal lobe damage on auditory perception. *Canadian Journal of Psychology, 15*, 156–165. doi:10.1037/h0083218

Kimura, D. (1963). Speech lateralization in young children as determined by an auditory test. *Journal of Comparative and Physiological Psychology, 56*, 899–902. doi:10.1037/h0047762

Kimura, D. (1967). Functional asymmetry of the brain in dichotic listening. *Cortex, 22,* 163–178.

Kimura, D. (2011, August 1). *20Q: The right-ear effect: Going strong after 50 years* (G. Mueller, Interviewer). Retrieved from http://www.audiologyonline.com/articles/20q-right-ear-effect-going-818

Lindamood, C., & Lindamood, P. (1971). *Lindamood Auditory Test of Conceptualization (LAC).* Boston, MA: Allyn & Bacon.

Masters, M. G., Stecker, N. A., & Katz, J. (Eds.). (1998). *Central auditory processing disorders: Mostly management.* Boston, MA: Allyn & Bacon.

McCroskey, R. L., & Keith, R. W. (1996). *Auditory Fusion Test-Revised: Instruction and user's manual.* St. Louis, MO: Auditec.

Moncrieff, D. W., & Wilson, R. H. (2009). Recognition of randomly presented one-, two-, and three-pair dichotic digits by children and young adults. *Journal of the American Academy of Audiology, 20,* 58–70. doi:10.3766/jaaa.20.1.6

Musiek, F. E. (1983a). Assessment of central auditory dysfunction: The Dichotic Digit Test revisited. *Ear and Hearing, 4,* 79–83.

Musiek, F. E. (1983b). Results of three dichotic speech tests on subjects with intracranial lesions. *Ear and Hearing, 4,* 318–323. doi:10.1097/00003446-198311000-00010

Musiek, F. E. (1986a). Neuroanatomy, neurophysiology and central auditory assessment. Part II. The cerebrum. *Ear and Hearing, 7,* 283–294.

Musiek, F. E. (1986b). Neuroanatomy, neurophysiology, and central auditory assessment. Part III: Corpus callosum and efferent pathways. *Ear and Hearing, 7,* 349–358.

Musiek, F. E., & Baran, J. A. (1986). Neuroanatomy, neurophysiology, and central auditory assessment. Part I: Brainstem. *Ear and Hearing, 7,* 207–219.

Musiek, F. E., & Baran, J. A. (2006). *The auditory system: Anatomy, physiology and clinical correlates.* Boston, MA: Allyn & Bacon.

Musiek, F. E., Baran, J. A., & Pinheiro, M. L. (1990). Duration pattern recognition in normal subjects and patients with cerebral and cochlear lesions. *Audiology, 29,* 304–313.

Musiek, F. E., Charette, L., Kelly, T., Lee, W., & Musiek, E. (1999). Hit and false-positive rates for the middle latency response in patients with central nervous system involvement. *Journal of the American Academy of Audiology, 10,* 124–132.

Musiek, F. E., & Chermak, G. D. (1994). Three commonly asked questions about central auditory processing disorders: Assessment. *American Journal of Audiology, 3,* 23–27.

Musiek, F. E., & Chermak, G. D. (2009, November). Diagnosis of (central) auditory processing disorder in traumatic brain injury: Psychophysical and electrophysiological approaches. *ASHA Leader.* Retrieved from http://www.asha.org/publications/leader/2009/091124/CAPD.htm

Musiek, F. E., Gollegly, K. M., Kibbe, K. S., & Verkest-Lenz, S. B. (1991). Proposed screening test for central auditory disorders: Follow-up on the Dichotic Digits Test. *American Journal of Otology, 12,* 109–113.

Musiek, F. E., & Pinheiro, M. L. (1985). Dichotic speech tests in the detection of central auditory dysfunction. In *Assessment of central auditory dysfunction: Foundations and clinical correlates* (pp. 201–218). Baltimore, MD: Williams & Wilkins.

Musiek, F. E., & Pinheiro, M. L. (1987). Frequency patterns in cochlear, brainstem and cerebral lesions. *Audiology, 26,* 79–88.

Musiek, F. E., Shinn, J. B., Jirsa, R., Bamiou, D. E., Baran, J. A., & Zaidan, E. (2005). GIN (Gaps-In-Noise) Test performance in subjects with confirmed central auditory nervous system involvement. *Ear and Hearing, 26,* 608–618. doi:10.1097/01.aud.0000188069.80699.41

Musiek, F. E., Weihing, J. A., & Oxholm, V. B. (2007). Anatomy and physiology of the central auditory nervous system: a clinical perspective. In R. J. Roeser, M. Valente, & H. Hosford-Dunn (Eds.), *Audiology: Diagnosis* (Vol. 2, 2nd ed., pp. 37–64). New York, NY: Thieme Medical.

Musiek, F. E., & Wilson, D. H. (1979). SSW and dichotic digit results pre- and post-commissurotomy: A case report. *Journal of Speech and Hearing Disorders, 44,* 528–533.

Myklebust, H. R. (1954). *Auditory disorders in children: A manual for differential diagnosis.* New York, NY: Grune & Stratton.

Myklebust, H. R. (1956). Rh child: deaf or aphasic? 5. Some psychological considerations of the Rh child. *Journal of Speech and Hearing Disorders, 21,* 423–425.

Noffsinger, D., Martinez, C. D., & Wilson, R. H. (1994). Dichotic listening to speech: Background and preliminary data for digits, sentences, and nonsense syllables. *Journal of the American Academy of Audiology, 5,* 248–254.

Noffsinger, D., Wilson, R. H., & Musiek, F. E. (1994). Department of veterans affairs compact disc recordings for auditory perceptual assessment: Background and introduction. *Journal of the American Academy of Audiology, 5,* 231–235.

Russo, N., Nicol, T., Zecker, S. G., Hayes, E., & Kraus, N. (2005). Auditory training improves neural timing in the human brainstem. *Behavioural Brain Research, 156,* 95–103. doi:10.1016/j.bbr.2004.05.012

Schow, R. L., & Chermak, G. D. (1999). Implications from factor analysis for central auditory processing disorders. *American Journal of Audiology, 8,* 137-142. doi:10.1044/1059–0889(1999/012)

Schow, R. L., Seikel, J. A., Chermak, G. D., & Berent, M. (2000). Central auditory processes and test measures: ASHA 1996 revisited. *American Journal of Audiology, 9,* 63–68. doi:10.1044/1059-0889(2000/013)

Scientific Learning Corporation. (1997). *Fast ForWord training program for children. Procedure manual for professionals.* Berkeley, CA: Author.

Sloan, C. (1986). *Treating auditory processing difficulties in children.* London, UK: College-Hill Press.

Strouse, A., & Wilson, R. H. (1999). Recognition of one-, two- and three-pair dichotic digits under free and directed recall. *Journal of the American Academy of Audiology, 10,* 557–571.

Tallal, P., Miller, S. L., Bedi, G., Byma, G., Wang, X., Nagarajan, S. S., . . . Merzenich, M. M. (1996). Language comprehension in language-learning impaired children improved with acoustically modified speech. *Science, 271,* 81–84. doi:10.1126/science.271.5245.81

Warrier, C. M., Johnson, K. L., Hayes, E. A., Nicol, T. G., & Kraus, N. (2004). Learning impaired children exhibit timing deficits and training-related improvements in auditory cortical responses to speech in noise. *Experimental Brain Research, 157,* 431–441. doi: 10.1007/s00221-004-1857-6

Willeford, J. A. (1969). Audiological evaluation of central auditory disorders: Part I. *Maico Audiological Library Series, 6,* 1–4.

Willeford, J. A. (1977). Assessing central auditory behavior in children: A test battery approach. In R. W. Keith (Ed.), *Central auditory dysfunction* (pp. 43–72). New York, NY: Grune and Stratton.

Wilson, R. H., Moncrieff, D. W., Townsend, E. A., & Pillion, A. L. (2003). Development of a 500-Hz masking level difference protocol for clinic use. *Journal of the American Academy of Audiology, 14,* 1–8. doi:10.3766/jaaa.14.1.2

SECTION 2

Interventions

CHAPTER 7

AUDITORY TRAINING

**FRANK E. MUSIEK, GAIL D. CHERMAK, and
JEFFREY WEIHING**

Auditory Training Defined

For many years, auditory training (AT) was associated with rehabilitation efforts directed toward those with peripheral hearing loss. Traditional AT focused on utilizing residual hearing. For example, Goldstein (1939) stated that AT "involved the development and or improvement in the ability to discriminate various properties of speech and nonspeech signals" (Schow & Nerbonne, 1996, p. 95). Carhart (1960) described AT as "the process of teaching the child or adult with hearing impairment to take full advantage of available auditory cues" (Schow & Nerbonne, 2013, p. 137). Erber (1982) viewed AT as "the creation of special communication conditions in which teachers and audiologists help hearing impaired children

acquire many of the auditory perception abilities that normally hearing children acquire naturally without their intervention" (p. 1). Although these traditional definitions of AT are appropriate in the context of peripheral hearing impairment, they do not emphasize the intimate linkage of AT to auditory plasticity and other brain functions and therefore are not particularly relevant to AT for central auditory dysfunction. Indeed, in recent years, AT has been reconceptualized to include treatment for those with central auditory processing disorder (CAPD). We present this reconceptualized perspective and approach to AT in this chapter.

In viewing AT in the context of CAPD, it is imperative to understand that plasticity takes place in the brain, it is a central phenomenon, and it is key to changing auditory performance. In order to expand the definition of AT to include peripheral and central auditory performance, and also to recognize the association between AT and brain function, the following definition is offered. Auditory training is *a set of (acoustic) conditions and or tasks that are designed to activate auditory and related systems in such a manner that their neural base and associated auditory behavior is altered in a positive way*. AT employs repetitive (listening) exercises focused on maximizing the processing of acoustic signals.

Although the most efficient way to promote learning is through active training, perceptual learning occurs to some extent by passive exposure to stimuli (Watanabe, Nanez, & Sasaki, 2001). In some cases, simple (i.e., passive) acoustic stimulation can improve auditory performance. This is often seen in experiments with animals that have been acoustically deprived or experienced damage to their auditory systems. In an all encompassing sense, stimulation alone could be considered a form of AT; however, improving auditory performance is more likely to occur when the subject is actively involved (see Bao, Chang, Woods, & Merzenich, 2004; Musiek & Berge, 1998).

Although passive listening (i.e., stimulation that is not contingent on performing a task) in an acoustically rich environment can enhance auditory skills, active listening (i.e., performing auditory tasks) is much more likely to make a difference (Greenough & Bailey, 1988; Hassmannova, Myslivecek, & Novakova, 1981; Recanzone, Schreiner, & Merzenich, 1993). In reviewing AT methods, the theme that constantly emerges is that the patient, student or participant needs to be engaged and motivated to do the task (Koelsch, 2010). Active participation focuses attention on critical elements, encourages abstraction of procedures, and self-evaluation of understanding, all of which encourage generalization (Singley & Anderson, 1989). This principle and many other important principles in AT are not new; in fact, they have been part of AT's long history.

Significant Events in the History of AT

The concept of AT as sound stimulation has been known for centuries. In Wedenburg's (1951) wonderful review of AT, it was related that in the sixth century doctors used large bells in an attempt to stimulate a hearing response in people who were considered deaf. Though this primitive method was traced back centuries, it really was the initial work of Itard in the 1800s at the Paris school for the deaf that is often considered the beginning of systematic AT. Itard had his students identify and discriminate vowels and consonants, as well as tonal stimuli of different pitches (Hudgins, 1954). It was reported that this training yielded improvements in hearing. In England in the mid to late 1800s, Toynbee and Urbantschitch, two therapists who followed the work of Itard, conducted AT with individuals with hearing impairment. They advanced Itard's work and did much to establish the concept of AT in England (Wedenburg, 1951). Max Goldstein, a student of Urbantschitch, founded the Central Institute for the Deaf (CID) in the United States. Goldstein brought many ideas about AT to the CID and conducted some of the early efficacy studies on AT. Interestingly, over the past 50 years, AT has continued to employ exercises involving identification and discrimination of various sounds, similar to Itard's early approach.

After World War II, audiology was founded in the United States, and because so many soldiers suffered from hearing loss, AT became quite popular. DiCarlo, Carhart, Huizing, Doehring, and Ling were major names associated with rehabilitation and AT. In general, these clinicians focused on identification and discrimination of rhythmic patterns, isolated phonemes, letters, digits, and minimally different words. They also trained intensity and frequency discrimination tasks using pure-tone stimuli (DiCarlo, 1948; Carhart 1960). (See Chapter 6 and Musiek & Berge, 1998 for reviews.)

In the 1950s and 1960s, AT was tied to helping patients fitted with hearing aids accommodate to amplification. During the late 1960s and 1970s, interest in AT began to wane. It was difficult to obtain reimbursement by third party payers, there was little efficacy data, and audiologists and patients felt the procedures were tiring (Musiek & Berge, 1998). In addition, there seemed to be little concern as to the underlying mechanisms that might enhance one's auditory skills and perception. Focus was primarily on peripheral hearing loss and there seemed to be little interest in the role the central auditory nervous system (CANS) and neural plasticity played in AT.

As interest in AT waned, some important events were emerging that would eventually reinvigorate interest in AT —although in a different direction. Webster (1977) showed that auditory deprivation reduced auditory cell volumes in the brainstem. Hassmannova et al. (1981) demonstrated that AT with young mice (which involved passive daily exposure to a wide variety of sounds) enhanced auditory cortex activity as recorded by near-field evoked potentials. These studies showed the effects of peripheral hearing loss (i.e., auditory deprivation) on the CANS and the potential of the CANS to enhance auditory function.

Timing could not have been better because at about the same time clinicians were directing greater attention to children with learning problems who appeared to have CAPD (Willeford, 1977; Pinheiro, 1977). Since CAPD arises from dysfunction in the auditory substrate of the brain (Chermak & Musiek, 2011), it was logical to consider AT, which seemed to be based on brain plasticity, as a possible tool for remediation of CAPD. In the ensuing years, breakthroughs in auditory neuroscience, particularly with regard to plasticity, garnered increasing interest in AT and CAPD, interest that continues to gain momentum today (as discussed below under The Role of Auditory Neuroplasticity). A major finding that emerged from the many animal studies of AT, as well as from other types of behavioral training, is that brain plasticity is critical for successful AT. Also, it became clear that the CANS is plastic and that the peripheral auditory system is not (Lund, 1978). (See Chapter 1 in this Volume and Chapters 1, 3, and 5 in Volume 1 of the Handbook.)

Following the early breakthroughs in auditory neuroscience, AT techniques began to emerge for use with children with language impairments, learning problems, and presumed CAPD. One of the early programs, developed by Katz and Harmon (1982), introduced phonemic synthesis training for CAPD. This program centered on blending sounds into words. At about the same time, Alexander and Frost (1982) introduced an AT program that focused on temporal facets of speech. It was designed to decelerate the speech signal and enhance the perception of transitions by increasing the intensity of these speech segments. In fact, this program was quite similar to the Fast ForWord program introduced many years later. The Alexander and Frost program demonstrated improvements in auditory discrimination in children with language delays—perhaps one of the first extensive efficacy studies on AT. Other AT programs emerged, some commercial and others not. These more modern AT approaches are discussed below. (See Clinical Training of Temporal Processing below.)

Diagnostic Information: Deficit-Specific Intervention

A full central auditory processing diagnostic evaluation must be completed prior to undertaking AT with older children (i.e., ages 7–8 years and older) and adults. The diagnostic test battery should provide information about the patient's particular auditory strengths and weaknesses. Unfortunately, many clinics that perform central auditory processing evaluations today do not have the full range of capabilities, or otherwise choose to assess only a subset of the known auditory processes, thereby often generating an incomplete profile of the patient's auditory strengths and weaknesses (Chermak, Silva, Nye, Hasbrouck, & Musiek, 2007). Most clinics do assess temporal and dichotic processes; therefore, these processes will serve as examples of how diagnostic information can lead to specific interventions. For younger children suspected of CAPD for whom current behavioral tests may be inappropriate

and lead to invalid results (see Chapter 11, Volume 1 of the Handbook), it may be reasonable to introduce listening games similar to those described in the final section of this chapter.

The central auditory test results depicted in Figure 7–1 reveal deficits for frequency pattern recognition, dichotic digits and competing sentences. AT designed to strengthen temporal processing (following from the poor scores on the frequency pattern test) might range from work on the *Simon Game*™ to enrolling the child in the Fast ForWord program. AT exercises directed to improve deficient dichotic listening range from dichotic interaural intensity difference (DIID) training to drilling speech recognition in competition. All of these training procedures, as well as other examples of AT procedures appropriate to specific deficits identified through diagnostic evaluation, are elaborated later in the chapter. (See also Chermak & Musiek, 2002 for additional examples.)

Formal and Informal Approaches to Auditory Training

The concept of formal and informal approaches to AT grew out of an obvious need that was recognized at the Dartmouth Hitchcock Medical Center, which is located in a rural area. It was realized that many patients in need of AT could not travel to the clinic as often as needed to effectively conduct treatment. An attempt was made, therefore, to modify some of the procedures performed in the lab or clinic, in a way that they could be used in everyday training

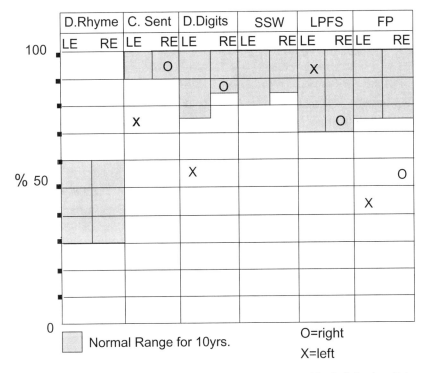

Figure 7–1. Central auditory test battery results with deficits for dichotic listening and frequency pattern perception. Please see discussion in the text. Key: Tests from left to right are: dichotic rhyme, competing sentences, dichotic digits, staggered spondaic words, low-pass filtered speech, and frequency patterns.

environments, such as at school or home (Musiek, 1999). Informal procedures are conducted by school personnel (e.g., speech pathologist, educational audiologist) or in some cases parents.

Formal AT procedures are conducted by audiologically trained personnel in a clinic or lab setting that permits control over stimulus generation and presentation. For example, for formal frequency discrimination AT, tones of slightly different frequency are generated on a computer and the patient is required to judge whether the tones are the same or different. Adaptive approaches also can be employed whereby the stimulus parameters vary on the basis of the patient's performance on preceding trials. The frequency, duration, interstimulus interval and overall intensity are all controlled in formal AT.

Informal AT is used to complement formal AT. Training the patient to discriminate similar sounding notes on a keyboard provides informal AT for temporal processing that complements formal frequency discrimination training. Coupling informal with formal AT offers a more powerful approach, as it provides for more intensive and extensive practice, including in real-world, everyday settings that are functionally significant to the patient. This should maximize generalization and treatment efficacy.

Auditory Training Principles

As conceptualized in the *OPERA hypothesis,* effective AT requires: overlap (O) between the skill trained and the learning outcome sought; tasks that tax the auditory system (P = precision); engagement or emotion (E), since we learn what we care about; repetition (R); and attention (A) (Patel, 2011). These and additional principles are discussed below. See Chapter 11 for additional illustration of the application of the principles discussed below to computerized AT.

Age- and Language-Appropriate Training

One of the primary considerations in AT is to ensure that the materials and the tasks used are age and language appropriate for the patient. If materials and tasks exceed the patient's cognitive, language, or communication skills, interest and progress will be compromised. Conversely, for older children and adults, materials should not be childlike. This latter situation is perhaps more common than the former—primarily because most AT materials have been developed for children. AT materials that are age and communication level appropriate will engage the patient and help the clinician maintain the patient's motivation. Of course, as is well known in rehabilitation science, early intervention is key: The younger the individual is when AT is initiated, the better the chances for improvement. This concept is highlighted by a study on animals with compromised brain (cortex) development that was overcome with early AT training (Threlkeld, Hill, Rosen, & Fitch, 2009).

Developing and Maintaining Motivation

Motivation is perhaps the pivotal factor in AT, as it is for most other behavioral, rehabilitation and learning in general (Danzl, Etter, Andreatta, & Kitzman, 2012; Reagan, 1973). Patients who are not motivated are not likely to be successful in an AT program. In order to maintain motivation, the patient must understand the rationale underlying the AT. Even children need to understand that they are enrolled in AT to improve their listening abilities, which in turn may impact their social and academic success. Teachers, parents, and clinicians should explain to children, using real-world and functional examples (e.g., ability to follow a coach's directions or segment words into syllable), why they are in therapy and how it will help them.

Also heightening motivation is the use of subject matter of interest to the patient. Though it is advantageous to design AT to reinforce the academic curriculum, it is also worthwhile to include other topics of high interest to the child that might not pertain directly to the classroom, but rather to the child's hobbies and social and recreational activities. Encouragement also is crucial to maintaining motivation. Parents and teachers should encourage the child to do his or her best in therapy and in the classroom. Because AT must be intensive and can be quite repetitive, children can lose interest in AT and become bored with the tasks. Tasks must be varied; there is no substitute for variety and innovative approaches to therapy. Computer-assisted AT has grown in use given its ability to engage participants, while providing intensive training with feedback and reinforcement. Positive feedback can facilitate learning through auditory training even when it is not contingent (i.e., randomly presented) on good performance (Amitay, Halliday, Taylor, Sohoglu, & Moore, 2010). Feedback given less frequently (i.e., 10% of the time) appears to be more effective at encouraging learning (perhaps by encouraging self-monitoring and enhancing motivation) than feedback given more frequently (i.e., 90% of the time) (Amitay et al., 2010). Motivation is related to attention. The greater the attention to a given task (such as AT), the more progress is likely to be made: Higher levels of vigilance can be maintained when the individual involved is motivated compared with unmotivated individuals (Tomporowski & Tinsley, 1996). Moreover, top-down processes such as arousal and attention aid perceptual or sensory learning (Alain, Campeanu, & Tremblay, 2009; Amitay, Halliday, Taylor, & Moore, 2006; Amitay et al., 2010; Halliday, Moore, Taylor, & Amitay, 2011). When a child has lost motivation or is poorly motivated at the outset, it is necessary to determine why. Is the child bored with the AT tasks? Are classmates making fun of the fact that the child attends therapy (i.e., peer pressure or ridicule)? Perhaps the child has detected parental discomfort with the therapy program, or perhaps the child has become aware of parental disagreements about the treatment program. These are just a few examples of underlying reasons why motivation toward therapy may be low. Unless these underlying issues are addressed, the effectiveness of AT will be compromised.

Motivation is so important, yet can be so fragile, that at times it may be better, especially when working with adolescents and teenagers, not to enroll the youngster in therapy rather than compromise their self-sense or overall outlook. The adolescent and teenage years are times when most students do not wish to be seen as different—they want to fit in. AT conducted using a pull-out model, which requires students to leave class, often makes this age group feel uncomfortable, especially because they fear they appear *different* to peers. Using computerized AT might offer additional advantages for the student feeling peer-pressure, enabling a less *public* approach to therapy, thereby promoting interest and acceptance of AT, while providing intensive and engaging therapy.

Despite the use of technology, for some students motivation and acceptance of AT is difficult to obtain. In these cases, offering informal approaches using AT software or other exercises that can be done at home may be the best approach. Formal AT could be postponed temporarily until circumstances permit heightened motivation and acceptance. Clearly, there are many complex issues surrounding motivation, a pivotal issue in regard to successful AT.

Varying AT Tasks

As briefly mentioned in regard to motivation, varying AT stimuli and tasks serves to maintain motivation, and should lead to greater performance gains and generalization (Chermak & Musiek, 2002). For example, greater gains in animals' motor skills are seen when motor training tasks vary as opposed to repetitions of the same task or set of tasks (Greenough & Bailey, 1988). An AT program targeting improved temporal resolution should include a variety of tasks, such as click discrimination, gap detection, and backward and forward masking. Each of these training tasks exercises temporal processing, providing more intensive practice while reducing the potential loss of motivation and *burnout*.

Progression of AT Tasks

In addition to varying AT tasks, it has also been shown that the tasks should be graduated in difficulty over time, as a function of the patient's performance (Bailey & Chen, 1988). Tasks should be presented systematically and graduated in difficulty to be challenging and motivating, but not overwhelming. Tasks should be designed to allow patients to work at their skill threshold or edge of competency (Chermak & Musiek, 2002). The clinician can chart patient progress manually or rely on computer software adaptive programming to determine when and by what increment to increase task difficulty. (Adaptive algorithms automatically adjust the progression in task difficulty: As the patient reaches a certain performance criterion level, the program advances to a more demanding level of task difficulty.) The amount or degree of progression is sometimes difficult to determine; most software programs have sufficient flexibility to adjust incremental levels. The issue is the step size of the progression. If the step size is too large, performance will not improve, signaling that a smaller increment in difficulty level should be introduced (see Erber, 1982, pp. 82-102). Appropriate increments in task difficulty have been shown in animal studies to be critical to improvement seen from training (Linkenhoker & Knudsen, 2002).

A Balanced Success-Failure Rate

Another important principle underlying AT is the success/failure criterion ratio to be targeted. This criterion is related to progression (i.e., incremental difficulty level) in that the level of difficulty influences an individual's ability to successfully perform a task. Therapy programs should be designed so that the client experiences success sufficient to maintain motivation at high levels. Success rates approaching 100%, however, usually indicate that the task is too easy and that the patient's auditory system is not sufficiently challenged to elicit optimal change. It may be more appropriate to require 70% accuracy before proceeding to a more demanding task. As noted in several studies, early learning usually is most dramatic, with performance improvements becoming smaller over time (Amitay, Hawkey, & Moore, 2005; Hawkey, Amitay, & Moore, 2004).

One of the few studies that speaks to this issue is the work of Edeline and Weinberger (1993), who measured behavioral and electrophysiologic changes in animals that received two types of AT for frequency discrimination, one considered to be easy and the other highly difficult (i.e., requiring discriminations beyond the capability of the animals). Interestingly, the *easy* AT yielded definite improvements in frequency discrimination measured behaviorally, whereas the *difficult* AT yielded essentially no improvement. Direct measurements at the auditory cortex, however, showed improved receptive field response for both easy and difficult tasks. Based on their findings, training tasks should be designed to maintain motivation; however, difficulty level should not be excessive such that performance plummets and behavioral change is jeopardized.

Also related to training and performance is degree of arousal. As Wingfield (1979) noted, as arousal level progresses along the continuum from sleepiness to boredom, to mild alertness to optimal alertness, performance improves with each successive level until one reaches optimal alertness, which is equated with the highest level of performance. On the other hand, high arousal levels that are associated with stress, anxiety and panic lead to decreased performance; therefore, one must balance task difficulty and arousal level to optimize the benefits of AT. AT tasks must be presented systematically and appropriately graduated in difficulty to ensure persistence on task and challenge, but not overwhelming to the patient.

Sufficient Time Must Be Allotted for Therapy

Sufficient time must be devoted to any therapeutic program, including AT, to induce change. Intensive therapy requires considerable time, which can be distributed in regard to the length of the training session, the number of training sessions, the time intervals between sessions, and the period of time over which training is conducted (Tallal et al., 1996). Duration of the training session can be limited by intrinsic factors such as attention level and performance. Unfortunately, extrinsic factors such as caseload, therapy environment, cost, and schedule conflicts are probably more common issues that frequently reduce therapy time.

Obviously, once the client makes marked improvement to the point where little or no residual problem exists, therapy can be terminated. It is more difficult to decide how long to continue training when little, slow, or no progress is being made. It is important to consider that sometimes progress is not made because insufficient time has been devoted to the training: Therapy sessions are too few

and they have not spanned the necessary time frame. Though much is not known about how much therapy is needed for improvement, and certainly there are many factors that influence this calculation, it does seem based on both experimental and clinical findings and experience that considerable time is needed to evoke change in the nervous system (Delhommeau, Micheyl, Jouvent, & Collet, 2002; Greenough & Bailey, 1988; Recanzone et al., 1993; Tallal et. al., 1996). Although some have recommended five to seven half- to one-hour sessions weekly for at least four to six weeks, neurophysiologic changes have been reported within one to four days and functional changes have been reported as quickly as within 4 days of AT (Tremblay, Kraus & McGee, 1998). The enhanced amplitude of the mismatched negativity potential (MMN) has been seen within a single training session; however, it may have reflected subjects' increased attention to recently learned auditory material or learning per se rather than enhanced auditory abilities (Atienza, Cantero, & Dominguez-Marin, 2002; Gottselig, Brandeis, Hofer-Tinguely, Borberly, & Achermann, 2004).

Recent research suggests that shorter, more frequent training sessions may best foster auditory learning. Molloy, Moore, Sohoglu, and Amitay (2012) trained young adults on a frequency discrimination task for a total of 50 training blocks using several different time schedules: 800 trials a day for two days, 400 trials a day for four days, 200 trials a day for eight days, and 100 trials a day (T100) for eight days. The shortest training sessions were approximately eight minutes and the longest sessions exceeded an hour. While all conditions yielded a similar degree of improvement following the termination of training, the shorter training sessions allowed for more latent learning, or learning that occurred between sessions. Specifically, the T100 group improved most quickly during the early stages of training, which was attributed, in part, to their shorter sessions. As this study was conducted in young adults, it is unknown to what extent the findings might generalize to pediatric populations, though it certainly suggests shorter training sessions, distributed over time, maximize learning efficiency.

Although the specific parameters remain to be delineated, it is fair to say that therapy sessions that last only half-hour and meet only once a week are not sufficient to change the function of the auditory system. Of course, this determination will fluctuate across patients. We do know that the degree to which trained skills generalize will depend on listeners having received a critical amount of exposure to the trained stimulus and task (Delhommeau, Micheyl, & Jouvent, 2005; Grimault, Micheyl, Carlyon, Bacon, & Collet, 2003; Wright & Sabin, 2007). Finally, it is important to recognize the value in setting realistic goals. Unrealistic goals are not likely to be attained no matter the frequency of sessions or the duration of therapy.

Monitoring and Feedback

Careful monitoring of patient progress is important, as it allows the clinician to gauge the appropriateness of the AT program and provides the basis for feedback to the client. Active participation, coupled with salient reinforcement and feedback, motivates, augments attention (both task-specific and general arousal), and maximizes learning (Ahissar, Vaadia, Ahissar, Bergman, Arieli, & Abeles,

1992; Holroyd, Larsen, & Cohen, 2004). Feedback and reinforcement must be included in the design of tasks regardless of the delivery system (i.e., manual vs. computer-assisted) (Erber, 1982). In computer-based AT, feedback is automatic: The adaptive algorithm provides positive feedback as it advances the patient through the program based on successful performance (Tallal et al., 1996). This feedback is also reflected in reward and progress animations.

Monitoring also means using appropriate testing methods to determine if progress is being made (Erber, 1982; Sanders, 1971). Ideally three types of measures should be considered in monitoring auditory changes: (1) psychophysical, (2) electrophysiologic, and (3) questionnaires and scales. These measures should be completed pre- and posttherapy, as well as during the course of treatment. Questionnaires should be completed by the patient where appropriate, as well as by individuals who interact with the client in a variety of settings (e.g., other professionals, parents, teachers). (See Chapter 1 for discussion of outcome measures.)

Acoustical Control

In many cases, it is important to be able to control precisely the acoustic stimulus to achieve the desired type of training, especially when conducting formal AT. Generally, comfortable loudness levels are necessary for most effective training, although for some patients and in some situations, levels slightly above or below comfortable loudness levels (and slower) are needed to achieve best results. For example, certain software increases amplitude and prolongs transitions, and specific level differences between ears are required in the DIID training procedure (as discussed below under Recent Human Studies in Auditory Discrimination Training (Intensity-Frequency). In all cases, however, acoustical control is an important principle guiding effective and safe delivery of AT.

The Role of Auditory Neuroplasticity

Brief Orientation to Neuroplasticity

A brief orientation to auditory plasticity is provided here, with a focus on several particularly relevant aspects of neuroplasticity for AT. The reader is referred to Chapter 1 of this Volume and Chapters 1, 3, and 5 of Volume 1 of the Handbook for in depth discussions.

Auditory plasticity underlies the alteration of the brain subsequent to appropriate AT. Neural plasticity can be defined as the alteration of nerve cells to better conform to immediate environmental influences, with this alteration often associated with behavioral change (Musiek & Berge, 1998). Scheich (1991) described three types of neural plasticity. *Developmental plasticity* results from the maturation of the nervous system as more connections are made between neurons and myelination of neurons progresses. Neural maturation is dependent on stimulation: enriched stimulation increases maturational rate (Kalil, 1989). *Compensatory plasticity* occurs after damage to the nervous system as other areas of the brain assume functions of the damaged areas. The third type of plasticity is *learning related*. Although all three types can play a role in AT, learning-related plastic-

ity is the primary plasticity underlying the success of AT and other behavioral rehabilitative efforts. Plasticity permits changes in the neural substrate that supports performance on a particular task or related tasks. Most importantly, it must be recognized that plasticity is a function of the CANS; plasticity is not a feature of the peripheral auditory system.

Plasticity enables changes in the function of the CANS. For example, Heim, Keil, Choudhury, Thomas Freidman, and Benasich (2013) reported changes in the early oscillatory responses in the auditory cortex following auditory-visual training in children with language-learning impairment, suggesting that training can ameliorate aspects of inefficient sensory cortical processing. Similarly, changes in the speech-evoked auditory brainstem response following auditory-language training of school-aged children diagnosed with CAPD may reflect plasticity of the auditory brainstem (Krishnamurti, Forrester, Rutledge, & Holmes, 2013).

Long-Term Potentiation

Long-term potentiation (LTP) is thought to be the mechanism underlying learning and memory (Hebb, 1949). Specifically, LTP refers to an increase in strength of synaptic transmission related to repetitive use of the neurons involved (Bliss & Lomo, 1973). In a general sense, LTP can be considered a form of plasticity. Exposing an animal (or human) repeatedly to acoustic stimuli should enhance the LTP and also the perception of that repeated stimulus. AT and other behavioral interventions may increase synaptic activity and thereby facilitate behavioral change. Interestingly, LTP has been measured months after repetitive exposure has ended (Greenough & Bailey, 1988). Rogan and LeDoux (1995) showed that LTP was associated with enhanced auditory evoked potentials originating from the neural pathway from the medial geniculate body (MGB) to the amygdala. This increase in the auditory response was maintained for a long duration acoustic stimulation of the MGB and provides evidence of the physiologic underpinnings of AT and bodes well for long-term maintenance of changes observed immediately following treatment.

What Has Been Learned From the Vestibular System?

Perhaps not well known have been the insights suggesting the potential of AT derived from studies and observation of the vestibular system. It is now well known that the human brain accommodates after surgical ablation of the vestibular labyrinth. Immediately following a labyrinthectomy, patients will experience dizziness and feel imbalanced; however, over the course of the next few days, their balance will return due to compensation by central mechanisms, provided the patient is somewhat active during this postsurgical period (Ludman, 2003; Bamiou & Luxon, 2003 for review). Another example of the accommodative capability of central mechanisms can be seen in benign positional vertigo, a condition associated with particular positions or movements. One of the most successful treatments for this condition is repeated movements that actually induce the dizziness. This "vestibular training" forces the central system to accommodate, and in time the dizziness ceases to be a problem (Bamiou & Luxon, 2003). These findings in the vestibular system

reflecting compensation by the central nervous system provide insight as to how training and plasticity work together to improve patients' function. Given the close association between the vestibular system and the auditory system, one would expect that training and plasticity work similarly in the auditory system as observed in the vestibular system.

Results of CANS Stimulation/Training— Selected Animal Models

It has been well established using animal models that auditory stimulation induces changes in the underlying neural substrate of the CANS (Hassmannova et al., 1981; Knudsen, 1988; Likenhoker, von der Ohe, & Knudsen, 2004; Recanzone et al., 1993). CANS plasticity is the basis of these physiologic changes (Salvi & Henderson, 1996). The inference drawn from these animal studies is that if these stimulation paradigms can induce CANS changes in animals, then stimulation delivered through AT of the human auditory system should induce similar neurophysiologic changes. Considered briefly below are some results from selective animal studies that may apply to human AT. (See Chapter 5 in Volume 1 of the Handbook for additional discussion of neurophysiologic changes induced by training.)

Perhaps most directly relevant to AT are the findings of Recanzone and colleagues (1993). In their studies, owl monkeys were trained on an auditory task that required the monkeys to complete a series of frequency discrimination trials using a specific reference frequency. When cortical responses were obtained following training, results indicated that the sharpness of tuning and latency of the evoked response for the trained frequency was greater when compared with untrained controls. Perhaps most importantly, however, was that the amount of cortical tissue that was associated with the trained frequency was greater than that of untrained controls. This indicates substantial cortical reorganization (e.g., plasticity) for stimuli used in the AT paradigm.

Stimulation of the CANS also has been noted as a direct precursor to cell growth. Hassmannova et al. (1981) observed functional and biochemical changes in the juvenile rat cortex following acoustic stimulation with tone pips. Among changes seen was a significant increase in total RNA content in cortical neurons following training relative to the no-stimulation control group. This difference persisted and was maintained up to four weeks after the end of training. Their results suggest that stimulation initiated processes by which new cell division could occur.

Interestingly, the CANS can be modified regardless of whether stimulation increases *or* decreases (Webster & Webster, 1979; Hassmannova et al., 1981). These modifications occur so that the CANS can process acoustic cues optimally when performing a specific function, as seen in the localization research of Knudson and colleagues (Knudsen, 1988; Likenhoker & Knudsen, 2002; Likenhoker et al., 2004).

Knudsen (1988) modified the localization cues presented to barn owls by decreasing the amount of stimulation in one ear (i.e., inserting an ear plug unilaterally). This temporary unilateral loss was created to interfere with the normal binaural localization cues utilized by the owls in hunting. Although localization ability was initially impaired after the loss, performance gradually returned to normal as the CANS adjusted to this new pattern of stimulation. When the ear plug was removed and the unilateral loss corrected, localization performance was again impaired. However, as the CANS again adjusted, this time to increased stimulation, performance returned to normal.

Although training induced localization changes are generally greater in juvenile owls, there is evidence to suggest that adult owls also demonstrate the plasticity necessary for effective AT (Likenhoker et al., 2004; Likenhoker & Knudsen, 2002). For instance, adult barn owls, which learned to localize using incongruent visual-auditory cues as juveniles, showed abnormal anatomical projections in the auditory cortex that were attributed to this early experience. This persistence of the projections may benefit any re-adaptation that may occur later in life (Likenhoker et al., 2004). Additionally, adult barn owls that undergo incremental change, rather than a single large change in visual-auditory cues, learn to adapt better to subsequent large changes in these cues (Linkenhoker & Knudsen, 2002). This finding speaks to the advantage of incremental training in adult subjects (as alluded to earlier under Progression of the Auditory Training Task).

The additional benefits of using training to reorganize the CANS rather than using stimulation alone have been demonstrated by Bao and colleagues (Bao et al., 2004). In this study, rats had to find food in a maze while noise pulses were presented. The rate of noise pulse presentation indicated distance to the food source. As the rats approached the food, the rate of noise pulse presentation increased. The response of auditory cortical neurons to fast rate noise pulses was compared among this group of rats, a second group that received auditory stimulation (i.e., white noise pulses) but were given food freely, and a third control group that did not experience auditory stimulation. Results indicated that greater neural responses were obtained in the trained group. The responses obtained from the second and third groups did not differ significantly. These findings speak to the importance of using structured AT rather than relying on passive stimulation when attempting to induce lasting cortical changes. A recent animal study addresses another important issue in regard to AT: whether AT instituted at some time after auditory deficits occurred (e.g., such as in adulthood) ameliorate auditory deficits incurred much earlier in life (e.g., in childhood) (Pan, Zhang, Cai, Zhou, & Sun, 2011). Pan and associates (2011) showed that deteriorated sound localization resulting from noise exposure in young rats could be improved by intense localization training when the rats reached adulthood. The results of this study suggest the possibility of improving and or restoring appropriate auditory function in the adult long after the initial damage to the auditory cortex. Corroborating these findings is another recent study on rats demonstrating that auditory discrimination deficits that accompany aging can be reversed with intensive auditory training on discrimination tasks (de Villers-Sidani, Alzghoul, Zhou, Simpson, Lin, & Merzenich, 2010). This study demonstrated not only functional changes in auditory discrimination but also structural alterations in the auditory cortex. Both Pan et al. (2011) and de Villers-Sidani et al. (2010) highlight the plasticity in the adult and aging auditory cortex, underscoring the potential of AT for patients of all ages. Indeed, a recent

report reveals the reversal of age-related neural timing delays, as evidenced by greater temporal precision of subcortical processing of speech in noise, following auditory training in older adults (Anderson, White-Schwoch, Parbery-Clark, & Kraus, 2013).

Recent Human Studies in Auditory Discrimination Training (Intensity-Frequency)

One of the most fundamental abilities of the auditory system is discrimination of frequency, intensity, and timing differences within the acoustic signal. The ability to discriminate auditory information is essential for many obvious reasons, including basic orientation and survival. Perhaps the most important use of auditory discrimination for our purposes is its role in the detection and processing of the rapid acoustic changes in speech that underlie language processing and in particular phonological awareness (Tallal et al., 1996). Children with learning disabilities and associated disorders often demonstrate deficits in phonological awareness and abnormal neurophysiologic representation of auditory stimuli in the CANS despite having a normal peripheral auditory system (Hayes, Warrier, Nicol, Zecker, & Kraus, 2003; King, Warrier, Hayes, & Kraus, 2002; Kraus, 1999). Auditory discrimination training can benefit these children, as well as other children and adults demonstrating listening difficulties.

Much of the evidence for the efficacy of auditory discrimination training comes from the work of Kraus, Tremblay, and colleagues (Kraus et al., 1995; Kraus,

1999; Tremblay & Kraus, 2002; Tremblay, Kraus, Carrell, & McGee, 1997; Tremblay, Kraus, & McGee, 1998; Tremblay, Kraus, McGee, Ponton, & Otis, 2001; Tremblay, Shahin, Picton, & Ross, 2009). Kraus et al. (1995) exposed participants with normal peripheral and central hearing to an auditory discrimination protocol and obtained pre- and posttraining behavioral and electrophysiologic measures. The training protocol consisted of discrimination of two synthesized /da/ tokens that differed in the onset frequencies of the second and third formant (F2 and F3) transitions. Training was divided into six one-hour sessions over the course of one week, during which participants determined whether two successive tokens were the same or different. The mismatched negativity response (MMN), an auditory cortical response that occurs as a result of acoustic change in a repetitive sequence of stimuli, served as the electrophysiologic outcome measure.

Efficacy of training was documented in both the behavioral and the electrophysiologic measures. For half the participants, discrimination of /da/ tokens increased from 56% pretraining to 67% posttraining. This behavioral increase persisted one month following the termination of training. Following discrimination training, the duration and amplitude of the MMN was larger for the vast majority of the participants. Interestingly, some of the electrophysiologic changes were not reflected in behavioral change. Whereas only half the sample could behaviorally identify the changes between the two /da/ tokens posttraining, electrophysiologic changes were observed in the large majority of participants following training. Taken together, these findings suggest that training related changes may be below the threshold of conscious detec-

tion in this subset of participants. Additionally, while training requires the attention of the participants, the measurement of training induced physiologic changes can occur in the absence of attention, as indicated by the MMN results.

Tremblay and colleagues (1997) also investigated the efficacy of discrimination training in a manner similar to Kraus et al. (1995) using normal hearing participants. In addition to determining training efficacy, Tremblay et al. (1997) sought to determine to what extent discrimination training with one set of tokens would transfer (i.e., generalize) to another set of tokens not used in training. The training stimuli were two consonant-vowel (CV) continua with voice onset times (VOTs) of different, but similar, durations. The training continuum comprised labial consonants, whereas the posttraining measures utilized both labial and alveolar continua. In addition to discriminating stimulus pairs, participants were asked to identify, from a closed set, which CV (differing by VOT duration) had been presented. Training extended over a five-day period for the experimental group; a second control group did not receive any training. Behavioral outcome measures included measures similar to those used during training. As in the Kraus et al. (1995) study, Tremblay and colleagues recorded the MMN as the electrophysiologic outcome measure. Posttraining results revealed that the trained group, but not the control group, showed increases in behavioral discrimination for both the labial (trained) and alveolar (untrained) CVs. The effect was smaller, however, for the alveolar tokens. For the behavioral identification measure, posttraining improvements were seen for the trained group on the labial (trained) VOTs only; however, MMN responses showed an increase in area and duration for both the labial (trained) and alveolar (untrained) VOTs, although the effect was smaller for the alveolar tokens. An increase in MMN duration was greater over the left frontal lobe.

Similar to the findings of Kraus et al. (1995), the results of Tremblay et al. (1997) speak to the efficacy of AT in improving auditory discrimination ability. In addition, the results demonstrate how the effects of training can generalize beyond the stimuli used during the training session. Although the effects were smaller, improvements in the ability to detect differences in alveolar tokens were noted, even though these tokens were not used during training. The increased MMN duration in the left hemisphere reflects the greater benefit of training to this hemisphere probably due to the greater activity in the left frontal lobe due to the linguistic nature of the stimuli.

Although the MMN response has shown some promise as a research tool, it has yet to show high clinical utility (Tremblay et al., 2001; Tremblay & Kraus, 2002). For this reason, Tremblay and colleagues (2001, 2002) conducted additional AT studies that were similar in nature to those described above, with the exception that the N1–P2 was used as the electrophysiologic outcome measure. It has been suggested that the N1–P2 may be more clinically feasible than the MMN (Tremblay et al, 2001).

Participants were again normal hearing individuals who underwent right ear discrimination and identification training with labial CV tokens (differing by VOT duration) over a period of one week. A similar task was used to obtain posttraining behavioral outcomes. The N1–P2 response was recorded from sev-eral locations on the scalp and separate recordings were made for the two VOT stimuli (e.g., the CV at either end of the continuum). Posttraining, behavioral discrimination performance increased almost 30% (Tremblay et al., 2001). Similarly, posttraining improvements were seen in the amplitude of the N1–P2 complex at Cz when the stimuli were presented at a slow rate (Tremblay et al., 2001). When the amplitudes of P1, N1, and P2 were measured relative to baseline, it was noted that the P1 and the N1 increased over the right frontal lobe only, whereas P2 increases were noted bilaterally (Tremblay & Kraus, 2002). These differences in the late potentials were the same regardless of which CV stimulus was used.

These posttraining improvements are consistent with the MMN trends reported earlier by Kraus et al. (1995) and Tremblay et al. (1997). The N1–P2 potential likely reflects early cortical processes relevant to stimulus encoding and the detection of speech. The MMN likely reflects later processes involving the discrimination of changes in the speech signal (Tremblay et al. 2001; Tremblay & Kraus, 2002). The series of Kraus and Tremblay studies using MMN and N1–P2 suggest that training induced changes using a discrimination paradigm may impact not only auditory processes involved in discrimination, but also the earlier encoding of auditory stimuli as well. The laterality effect noted for P1 and N1 was interpreted by Tremblay & Kraus (2002) to mean that small voicing distinctions are processed as nonlinguistic acoustic cues. This interpretation was suggested since right, not left, hemisphere changes were primarily observed for these potentials. The bilateral P2 changes, on the other hand, may represent a cognitive increase in attention that is necessary for learning to occur.

Similar to some of the studies reported above, Tremblay et al. (2009) trained 13 normal hearing adults on discrimination of VOT continuum ranging from /mba/ to /ba/ for 6 days. Pre- and posttraining auditory late potentials, N1 and P2, evoked using these two stimuli and a control stimulus that was not trained (/a/) were measured at various scalp locations. Improvements in behavioral performance were also examined at these intervals. There was a significant effect of training for both behavioral and electrophysiologic measures that reflected improved discrimination of the stimuli. The electrophysiologic results differed by whether a trained or untrained stimulus was used to evoked the response. When using /mba/ or /ba/, P2 enhancements were noted over the left hemisphere, while when the untrained stimulus was used, enhancements were noted bilaterally. The authors interpreted these findings to indicate that the P2 evoked by the trained stimuli utilized more task dependent attention aimed toward enhancing temporal encoding. Interestingly, the authors noted that subjects with larger pretraining N1 responses tended to show the greatest behavioral benefit from training, suggesting that subjects with larger N1 responses may be better able to synchronize to the onset of stimuli, which would be expected to facilitate performance.

The effects of auditory discrimination training also have been examined using functional magnetic resonance imaging (fMRI). Jancke, Gaab, Wustenberg, Scheich, and Heinze (2001) trained normal hearing participants for a total of nine hours using an oddball paradigm, similar to that used to evoke the MMN. A frequent 950 Hz tone was presented along with a less frequent 952, 954, or 958-Hz tone. Participants were asked to press a button whenever they heard one of the infrequent tones. Functional MRI was conducted pre-, during, and posttraining. A control (C) group also was recruited that did not participate in the training but did participate in imaging for the pre- and postsession. Subsequent analysis revealed that the experimental group could be further divided into one that demonstrated (T+) posttraining improvement and one group that did not show improvements (T−). Compared with the T− and the C groups, following training the T+ group showed a decrease in response from the superior temporal gyrus (bilaterally) and from the planum polare (right hemisphere) for the 954 and 958 Hz tones. Functional MRIs for the T+ group are presented in Figure 7–2. Consistent with Kraus et al. (1995), this research demonstrates that auditory discrimination training can improve behavioral auditory discrimination ability. In addition, Jancke et al. (2001) demonstrated increased discrimination ability paired with a reduction in activation from certain auditory areas within the cortex. Jancke and colleagues suggested that this decrease in activation is consistent with "fast learning theories." These theories suggest that as optimal sensory units are selected for a task, processing becomes more efficient and automatic. As a result, less activation corresponds to a streamlining of auditory processing for optimal performance.

Similar to Tremblay et al.'s (1997) work on generalization of training effects reported in this section, Delhommeau and colleagues (Delhommeau et al., 2002,

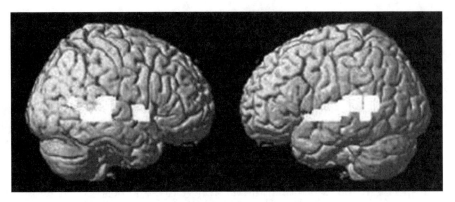

Figure 7–2. White areas reflect significant *decreases* in activation for the T+ group following frequency discrimination training. Decreases in activation may be consistent with "fast learning theories." (Adapted from Jancke, Gaab, Wustenberg, Scheich, & Heinze, 2001).

2005) examined to what extent training generalizes to untrained stimuli. Delhommeau et al. (2002) asked normal hearing participants to determine which of two 1000 Hz tones of variable duration were most similar to a 200 ms 1000 Hz reference tone, thereby establishing a duration discrimination threshold re: 200 ms. This training was conducted using the right ear for eight sessions over a period of four weeks. Baseline and posttraining outcomes were measured using three different durations as a reference (i.e., 40, 100, and 200 ms) to examine transfer of training across different stimulus durations. Following training, participants improved their ability to correctly identify the most similar tone for each of three 1000-Hz duration reference tones, demonstrated that training generalized beyond the trained reference stimulus (i.e., 200 ms). The performance improvement was larger for the 100 and 200-ms duration stimuli than for the 40-ms duration stimulus, perhaps a consequence of reduced temporal integration, although other possibilities were considered by the

researchers (Delhommeau et al., 2002). These results suggest that discrimination training using temporal information is relatively nonduration dependent and generalizes reasonably well.

Delhommeau et al. (2005) also investigated the degree to which frequency discrimination training generalizes to other frequencies. Participants were trained for six sessions in a manner similar to Delhommeau et al. (2002), with the exception that participants were trained on only single reference frequency. The reference frequency varied, however, across participants, and included 750, 1500, 3000, or 6000 Hz. Baseline and posttraining measures included all four frequencies as a reference. Posttraining measures were recorded at three separate times. Organized in this way, the study was able to exam the generalizability of frequency discrimination training to untrained frequencies over a period of time following the termination of training.

Several important findings emerged. Discrimination thresholds improved following training. There was no interaction between session and training frequency, suggesting that the benefit from training was comparable across all frequencies, whether or not they were used in training. However, additional analysis challenged this second finding. When measures from the three posttraining sessions were examined individually, a small difference between the trained and untrained frequencies was observed for the first posttraining session, but not for the later two. The difference between the trained and untrained frequencies disappeared in the later two sessions because performance for untrained frequencies became better, not because performance for the trained frequency deteriorated over time. This finding suggests that a difference in discrimination ability for trained and untrained frequencies may exist immediately following training, even if the difference is very small; however, performance for untrained frequencies quickly improves following exposure to the untrained stimulus.

Delhommeau et al. (2005) explained their findings as evidence of meta-learning, or learning about the basic nature of the discrimination task, which leads to improved performance for untrained frequencies. This notion of meta-learning may also explain the posttraining bilateral P2 increases reported by Tremblay and Kraus (2002). Although both findings might be somewhat incongruous with the findings of Recanzone and colleagues (1993) reported earlier in this chapter (i.e., that the amount of cortical tissue associated with trained frequencies exceeded that for untrained frequencies), utilization of general cognitive resources to enhance task performance is not necessarily mutually exclusive of neurophysiologic changes that are specific to

the central auditory system. (See Chapter 10 for discussion of metacognitive processes and their role in intervention.)

Moore, Rosenberg, and Coleman (2005) looked at the generalization of AT in a broader sense. They used a phoneme continuum discrimination task to examine the affects of AT on receptive language skills, skills that are auditory based, but only indirectly related to the phoneme discrimination task employed. To this end, they recruited normal hearing children and exposed them to four weeks of training (i.e., three days a week for thirty minutes a day) using a computerized discrimination task in which participants were required to determine which of two alternatives were identical to a reference. Each participant was exposed to several different phoneme continua. The procedure was adaptive, becoming more difficult as participants improved. Assessment measures, administered pre- and posttraining, included a phonological assessment battery and a word discrimination test. A second group was recruited that did not participate in the training and was used as a control.

Results provided some evidence for the efficacy of the AT program. Phonologic awareness and word discrimination scores were significantly higher posttraining for the experimental group only and these scores remained high when reassessed some time after the initial posttraining measure. There was no correlation, however, between performance on the training game and improvement in word discrimination and phonologic awareness, suggesting that, although mean differences were found, it was difficult to tease out these effects at the individual level. Moore et al. (2005) mentioned that nonauditory factors (e.g., attention) may have benefited from training and this may complicate interpretation of some analyses. Additionally, since many phoneme continua were used, the amount of training received on any one set may have been too small to produce measurable auditory changes at the individual level. That being said, the mean differences noted for the experimental group on the outcome measures, especially for phonologic awareness, speak to some aggregated affect of the training protocol on the auditory discrimination performance of the participants.

Several additional recent studies from Moore and colleagues have further elucidated the characteristics of auditory frequency discrimination training using their IHR Multicenter Study of Auditory Processing (IMAP) test battery. These studies have included, primarily, normally performing school-aged children with normal hearing. Moore, Ferguson, Halliday, and Riley (2008) observed that children aged 8 to 9 years did not receive significant benefits from one session of training when administered in a laboratory; however, children trained in school did show significant improvements in frequency discrimination training after just one session. In many cases these school-trained participants showed improvements after a single block of training, equivalent to about one minute. The authors attributed this outcome to differences in the school environment, which elicits greater on-task motivation or to the participants comfort level in the more familiar school environment. The lab training also involved more training blocks, which could have been detrimental to attention. The authors observed that younger subjects showed greater variability over time when compared

with older children and adults. Children in the youngest group were more likely to show fluctuating performance over time, which the authors attributed to changes in attention.

Moore and colleagues used the same paradigm in other studies. Halliday, Taylor, Edmonson-Jones, and Moore (2008) trained individuals in several age ranges: 6 to 7 years, 8 to 9 years, 10 to 11 years, and adults 18 to 40 years. In contrast to the findings of Moore et al. (2008), participants in all age groups demonstrated a similar degree of improvement on frequency discrimination tasks following several hours of training in a laboratory setting, although the children's final discrimination ability generally did not approach adultlike levels. Similar to Moore et al, most improvement was witnessed within the first couple of blocks of training. Millward, Hall, Ferguson, and Moore (2011) trained 8- to 10-year-old children on either a frequency discrimination task in quiet or in the presence of modulated noise, or on words in modulated noise. Training occurred in school, in twelve 30-minute sessions administered over the course of four weeks. All trained groups, and even a control group that was untrained, showed some improvements on a words in noise probe; however, frequency discrimination improvements were seen only in subjects who were included in one of the frequency discrimination training groups. The authors conclude that, in general, if the training stimulus shares some dimension with the outcome measure, then training benefits are more likely to be seen. This conclusion was supported by further research showing that learning does not always generalize across stimuli or tasks (Halliday, Taylor, Millward, & Moore, 2012).

Recent Studies in Temporal Processing Training

Like auditory discrimination, temporal processing, or the sequencing, ordering, discrimination, and integration of acoustic events over a period of time, also is integral to auditory processing. Temporal response patterns in the brain have been attributed a very important role as organizing structures that aid in the development and maintenance of unique neural representations, such as speech sounds (Tallal, Merzenich, Miller, & Jenkins, 1998). Temporal processing also has been shown to be important in the normal development of reading. For instance, Kujalaet et al. (2000) found that children with dyslexia often show a fundamental deficit in temporal processing skills. Training temporal processing, therefore, could potentially have many far-reaching, secondary effects, beyond the direct remediation of auditory processes.

To investigate the role of temporal processing in the dyslexic population, Kujala, Ceponiene, Belitz, Turkkila, Tervaniemi, and Naatanen (2001) provided nonverbal AT to a pediatric dyslexic population. Central to this investigation was an attempt to determine the role of an auditory deficit in dyslexia as comorbid or causal. To this end, AT involved stimuli with no linguistic features. Kujala and colleagues reasoned that if training were non-speech-related and still successfully treated the disorder to some degree, then auditory processing must play a causal role in dyslexia at some level.

Training was conducted for 10 minutes twice a week for a total of seven weeks. The training stimuli consisted of sound elements that varied in frequency, intensity, or duration. Participants were asked to match a sound sequence to visual analogs of the sequence on the computer screen (e.g., duration was conveyed by the length of the bar, intensity by the height, etc). Since participants were asked to choose a correct response among several options, this was technically both a temporal processing and a discrimination task. By removing all linguistic elements from the stimuli and the response, the task isolated the fundamental elements of reading that are dependent on temporal processing. The MMN and four measures of reading related skills, including spelling and phonologic awareness measures, were obtained before and after training. A dyslexic group that did not undergo training was used as a control.

Although both the experimental and the control groups showed numerical improvement on the reading skills outcome measures, only the experimental group showed a statistically significant increase in the number of words read correctly and the rate at which words were read. Additionally, the experimental group showed greater amplitude of the MMN following training. Interestingly, the MMN also showed a moderate correlation with some of the behavioral reading measures: as reading scores improved, the amplitude of the MMN tended to increase.

Kujala and colleagues (2001) interpreted this pattern of results to suggest that reading difficulties in dyslexia originate from bottom-up deficits in auditory processing. Their conclusion follows from finding improvements in the MMN, an auditory measure, correlated with reading improvements, in the context of an experimental manipulation that was auditory but nonlinguistic. Their findings suggest the utility of temporal processing training as a treatment for both auditory processing and other processes mediated by auditory processing (e.g., reading). Kujala et al. (2001) emphasized, however, that training also was successful because it was conducted early (children were approximately 7 years of age) and the semantic component was removed from the training paradigm. Training paradigms that do not take such steps may not be as successful.

Foxton, Brown, Chambers, and Griffiths (2004) administered temporal processing training to a normal hearing population using a paradigm very similar to Kujala et al. (2001). Training was conducted over seven sessions for 25 minutes a session with no more than three days separating a session. Participants were included in one of four groups. The visual-auditory contour comparison task (VAC) group was trained using reference stimuli represented both visually and auditorily (e.g., frequency of the reference stimulus was represented aurally, as well as visually by representing the spatial location of bars: the higher the bar, the higher the frequency). Following the reference, participants were required to determine if auditory sequences in a subsequent trial were the same or different than the reference trial. Participants were instructed to attend only to the relative contour of the sequence and not to the actual frequency value. The absolute frequency of tones in a sequence could diverge from the reference; however, if the relative frequency differences between each tone in a sequence were identical to the reference, then the contour was deemed to be identical.

Training for the pitch contour discrimination (PCD) group was identical to that of the VAC group, with the exception that their training included no visual information during the reference trial. Training of the actual pitch discrimination (AD) group was identical to the PCD group with the exception that participants were trained to attend to actual frequency changes in the sequence and not just the contour. The AD group was asked to identify which sequence sounded identical in pitch *and* contour to the reference trial. Finally, a control (C) group was utilized that did not undergo training. Despite different training regimens, each group completed all of the three tasks pre- and posttraining (e.g., the PCD group completed the AD and VAC tasks in addition to the PCD task before and after training).

Significant differences among groups were seen in the amount of improvement on the PCD measure. Specifically, both the PCD and AD groups showed improvement on this measure, with the effect being much bigger for the former group. The VAC and C groups did not show any improvement on this measure. No group showed any improvement on the AD and VAC measures following training. Foxton et al. (2004) explained the finding that frequency discrimination alone (e.g., AD group) aided in contour discrimination by suggesting that proper frequency discrimination also requires proper contour discrimination. The AD group may not have shown a benefit on AD measures because the attended-to tones may have been masked by surrounding tones (i.e., informational masking).

Foxton et al. (2004) interpreted their results as evidence of the importance of contour training. Contour perception is important for frequency and duration pattern tasks, for speech perception and auditory-language processing (conveying many properties such as stress and intonation), for music perception, and for reading (Musiek, Kibbe, & Baran, 1984). Foxton et al. (2004) suggested that AT using contour discrimination tasks and training on a musical instrument may aid in both the improvement of pitch contour perception skills and literacy.

Clinical Training of Temporal Processing

A popular computerized AT program currently used clinically to train temporal processing and phonologic awareness is Fast ForWord (FFW) (Tallal et al., 1996; Merzenich et al., 1996). This program presents training within the context of language (in some ways similar to the approach incorporated in Earobics©, a well-known computerized program discussed below under General and/or Multifaceted Auditory Training Approaches and Auditory-Language Training Approaches); however, the scientific foundation of FFW and the acoustic manipulations introduced lead us to categorize FFW as a temporal processing training program. (See Chapter 11 for discussion of computerized auditory training.)

Several studies have demonstrated the efficacy of FFW. Temple et al. (2003) trained dyslexics on FFW for one hundred minutes a day, five days a week, for almost a month. Pre- and posttraining measures included fMRI. During the fMRI sessions, participants were asked to perform a rhyming task (i.e., push a button if the sounds associated with two letters rhyme, for instance "T" and "D"). A normal nondyslexic control group also completed the rhyming task but did not participate in the training. Increased activation in the left temporoparietal cortex and inferior frontal gyrus were observed following training and these increases were positively correlated with improvements on some nonreading language tasks. Increased activation also was seen in the right inferior and superior frontal gyri and middle temporal gyrus, and these increases were positively correlated with a measure of phonological processing.

Temple et al. (2003) observed changes in activation of cortical areas known to support phonological processing; however, the primary benefits of increased activation in these areas would be expected to be seen for auditory processing. Moreover, cortical activation changes in these areas suggest that treatment exerted both normalizing and compensatory effects. Normalizing effects were seen in the temporoparietal and frontal gyrus regions, where previously depressed activity relative to normal controls increased. Compensatory effects were seen in the remaining cortical areas displaying increased activation, as these are areas that are not typically activated in normal hearing individuals but which nonetheless showed benefit from training. It should be noted that these increases in activation are somewhat inconsistent with the "fast learning theories" described previously in this chapter for discrimination training (Jancke et al., 2001), whereby activation decreases as processing becomes more efficient and automatic. Differences in the direction of activation changes following training may be attributed to the type of training used (frequency discrimination vs. temporal processing training) and/or the clinical status of the participants (normal hearing vs. dyslexic) across the two studies.

FFW also has been investigated in a population with specific language impairment (Agnew, Dorn, & Eden, 2004). This group was trained for 100 minutes a day, five days a week, for four to six weeks. Outcome measures included an auditory duration discrimination task and a visual duration discrimination task. For the auditory duration discrimination task, participants were required to judge whether the duration of a second tone was shorter or longer relative to a preceding 800 ms reference tone. Although technically a discrimination measure, duration discrimination also is an important element in temporal processing and was, therefore, a relevant outcome measure for a study of FFW. The visual task was identical in design to the auditory task, with the exception that pictures were used as stimuli instead of sounds. This visual task was included to determine to what extent AT benefits generalized to other modalities. Two phonological awareness measures were administered to assess reading benefits.

Pre- and posttreatment comparisons revealed significantly improved auditory duration discrimination by almost 15%. No significant improvements were seen on the visual duration discrimination task or the two measures of phonological awareness; hence, AT did not generalize to the visual modality, suggesting the specificity of this type of training to the auditory domain. AT, as administered through FFW, does not appear to benefit nonauditory skills related to learning, such as attention. That is, if attention were influenced, then multimodality effects would have been expected. This contrasts somewhat with the generalizability of auditory discrimination training discussed earlier (Delhommeau et al., 2002, 2005; Tremblay et al., 1997). However, in the auditory discrimination paradigms, generalization was examined within the auditory modality. The Agnew et al. (2004) study suggests that auditory discrimination training may not generalize across modalities.

Marler, Champlin, and Gilliam (2001), using a backward masking paradigm to measure temporal processing ability, showed that FFW improved performance of two children with language problems who initially performed poorly on this specific task. Valintine, Hendrick, and Swanson (2006), also using a backward masking procedure, showed improvement of children with language deficits on this task. Measurements conducted six months after the FFW training showed continued improvement in temporal processing.

Despite the findings of improved performance described above, the overall efficacy of FFW has been challenged for several reasons (Friel-Patti, Loeb, & Gilliam, 2001; Gilliam, Loeb, & Friel-Patti, 2001). For instance, Gilliam et al. (2001) argued that FFW does not truly train temporal processing, noting that no clear relationship has been established between several indirect measures of temporal processing (e.g., perception of backward masked speech) and treatment using FFW. These researchers do not deny, however, that FFW may benefit some aspects of language comprehension and production.

A recent meta-analysis of six studies of FFW with children with reading and oral language problems indicated no significant effect of FFW on any outcome measure in comparison to control groups (Strong, Torgerson, Torgerson, & Hulme, 2011). The few studies that have involved software comparisons have reported little additional benefit for one computerized program over another (Cohen et al., 2005; Gillam et al., 2001, 2008). Fey and colleagues (2009) found no evidence that FFW enhances the response of children with language impairment to conventional language intervention. Based on a review of six studies of FFW training with children diagnosed with language learning impairment or specific reading disorder in which central auditory processing was assessed, Loo, Bamiou, Campbell, and Luxon (2010) reported that four showed improvement in temporal tasks, one showed no change in frequency discrimination, and one showed improvement in speech-evoked cortical potentials (N1–P2). FFW demonstrated some impact on phonological awareness skills, but had little effect on language, spelling, and reading skills of these children.

A training strategy developed at the University of Connecticut (UCONN) Neuroaudiology Lab utilizes the game SIMON™ to treat temporal processing deficits (Musiek, 2005). The training is incremental in difficulty, starting with simple sequencing tasks and progressing to more complicated temporal ordering based on the patient's success. Since the SIMON game provides visual cues, the patient is instructed to perform pertinent tasks without looking at the table-top electronic device. The simplest task requires the patient to label tones. Tones can be labeled in any fashion; for instance, "one" may correspond to the lowest pitch tone and "four" may be assigned to the highest pitch tone. Following success on this simple labeling task, the patient can then be asked to indicate any time a target tone occurs. Similarly, this is followed by the more difficult task of identifying a sequence of target tones (e.g., tone "one" followed by tone "three"). Once proficiency is gained on all of the above

relatively simple tasks, the patient is ready to tackle more complex tasks. In the next phase of training, again without visual cues, the patient plays a tone, to which the device generates a second tone. The patient is required to label the new tone played back by SIMON as higher or lower in frequency than the last tone in the sequence.

Although no efficacy data have yet been collected for this training technique, positive results have been found by Pisoni and colleagues (Cleary, Pisoni, & Geers, 2001; Karpicke & Pisoni, 2004; Pisoni & Cleary, 2004) using a similar paradigm to examine memory. Developed concurrently and independently from the approach used at UCONN, this treatment approach uses a SIMON-like instrument to play verbal stimuli connected to each of four buttons (i.e., labeled either by color or digits) and includes an option to present visual patterns alone without any audio input. Participants are asked to repeat sequences presented by the device. The device has been used successfully to quantify implicit memory differences between a cochlear implant population and normal-hearing controls (Cleary et al., 2001). Additionally, and perhaps more relevant to the present chapter, their approach has been shown to induce learning.

Karpicke and Pisoni (2004) found that when normal hearing participants were trained on sequences that, unbeknown to the participants, followed grammatical rules, they performed better on novel posttraining sequences that followed those grammatical rules than for novel sequences that followed a grammar, but not the one used during training. That is to say, participants' memory was better for sequences that followed ordering rules that they had previously learned during training. Although Karpicke and Pisoni's training objectives and stimuli differ from that of the UCONN SIMON protocol, the use of similar procedures and the reliance on brain plasticity suggest that the SIMON training protocol may also prove to be efficacious.

Other AT paradigms are being developed at UCONN that also focus on temporal processing tasks. One such paradigm utilizes a keyboard or piano to train temporal sequencing abilities. Initially, two different notes are played for the patient in the absence of visual cues. The patient must label them each as high or low pitch in the order that they were played. As the patient improves, task complexity can be increased in at least three ways. First, progressively more notes can be added to the series and labeled by the patient accordingly. Second, the pitch of the notes can be made more similar by selecting keys that are closer together. Third, the interval between each note can be decreased, requiring faster processing of the series in order to provide a correct response. A paradigm that is similar to the piano protocol uses note cadences. The patient is asked to replicate a particular finger tapping cadence, which can be increased in complexity as the task is mastered. Both of the above paradigms train the patient's ability to order a sequence of rapid auditory events.

Dichotic Training

Children with CAPD often demonstrate a left ear deficit on dichotic speech tasks (Musiek et al., 1984). A case study published in 1998 reported significant improvement in binaural listening tasks and academic performance when dich-

otic training tasks were incorporated in the AT program (Musiek & Schochat, 1998). The dichotic interaural intensity difference training (DIID) procedure was used in that case study. See Chapter 9 for extensive discussion of the DIID.

The DIID is derived from research conducted on *split-brain* patients in the late 1970s and throughout the 1980s. These studies demonstrated that split-brain patients are not able to transfer information from the right to left hemisphere due to sectioning of the corpus callosum (Musiek et al., 1984). Kimura (1961) demonstrated suppression of the ipsilateral pathways during dichotic listening, rendering the auditory system a crossed system. This means that during dichotic listening, right ear information is routed to the left cortex and left ear information is routed to the right cortex. Since most people are left hemisphere language dominant, words, numbers, or sentences presented to the right ear are conducted to the speech hemisphere and are easily repeated. Speech stimuli presented to the left ear must cross the corpus callosum to access the language dominant hemisphere in order for the patient to verbally respond. Since the corpus callosum is severed in split-brain patients, this crossover cannot occur and a severe left ear deficit on dichotic listening occurs. Interestingly, Musiek et al. (1984) reported that major left ear deficits also occur in children—especially those with learning disabilities, probably due to delayed myelination of the corpus callosum.

Musiek et al. (1984) found that if dichotic stimuli with greater intensity were presented to the left ear relative to the right ear, scores for the left ear increased and scores for the right ear decreased for both split-brain patients and children with left ear deficits. By training children with various dichotic stimuli using greater intensity to the poorer ear (typically the left ear) to maintain good performance in that ear, the intensity level of the stronger ear could be gradually raised over a period of time and the poorer ear would maintain its high performance. Some children required more training than others; however, a high percentage did improve their left ear performance. Often after training, both ears performed well on subsequent dichotic listening tests. Though the mechanisms underlying this "dichotic improvement" remain under investigation, it appears that greater intensity to the left ear

releases the left auditory pathway from right auditory pathway suppression.

Ongoing research has revealed the DIID to be a highly promising tool for improving left ear deficits in children with CAPD (Figure 7–3). A recent report on a patient with mild head trauma who demonstrated a left ear deficit on dichotic digits and showed marked improvement on dichotic listening after DIID training demonstrated the potential of the DIID to improve dichotic listening across a range of patients, not only children with learning difficulties (Musiek et al., 2004; Wehing and Musiek, 2013). Dichotic listening training has been shown to enhance dichotic listening performance in children

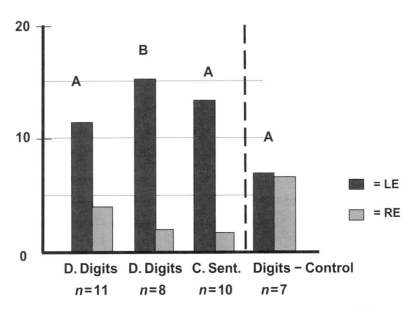

Mean % Dichotic Improvement from DIID Training

Figure 7–3. Mean dichotic listening performance from training on the DIID from two preliminary studies indicated by A (Musiek) and B (Moncrieff & Wertz). Note the improvement primarily for the left ear. Training for study A spanned approximately 3 months, two or three, 20 minute sessions per week. Training for study B spanned four weeks, three 30 minute sessions, three times a week. The tests administered were the dichotic digits (D. Digits) and competing sentences (C. Sent.).

with larger than normal asymmetries in dichotic listening. This improvement in dichotic listening from training also appeared to help language comprehension (Moncrieff & Wertz, 2008). The DIID program was part of a multifaceted auditory training program administered to children diagnosed with CAPD that showed improvement on a number of behavioral and electrophysiologic tests of central auditory function (Schochat, Musiek, Alonso, & Ogata, 2010). Hurley (2011) reported on using dichotic listening training on cases of Landau-Kleffner syndrome. These cases demonstrated marked improvement in dichotic listening as well as improvement in other facets of overall communication. As more research and clinical reports of dichotic listening training are published, this procedure should become an important tool in the remediation of deficits in dichotic processing.

Administering the DIID (and other forms of dichotic training paradigms) is straightforward. A variety of dichotic test materials (e.g., digits, words, sentences, CVs) and a two-channel audiometer are essentially all that is required. The DIID should be applied as both a binaural integration and a separation task. The integration task requires the patient to respond to the stimuli in both ears; the separation task requires the patient to ignore one ear and respond to stimuli presented in the other ear. If the patient shows a greater problem with binaural integration than separation, DIID training should emphasize this aspect of dichotic listening and vice versa. The amount and length of training that is needed is determined by the patient's own progress; however, we generally suggest training 3 to 4 times per week for 20 to 30-minute sessions. Further research, however, may provide more direction in regard to the optimal

intensiveness and frequency of DIID training. The DIID training procedure can be adapted for application in school and at home using modifications of a stereo system and interchangeable earphones. This informal approach is still considered experimental (Musiek et al., 2004).

Speech in Noise Training

Several studies have investigated the impact of a more general approach to auditory training using speech-in-noise as an alternative to a process-specific approach as examined above (e.g., the DIID). Typically these studies employ an auditory discrimination task performed in the presence of acoustic competition, such as noise. Several studies have demonstrated positive outcomes resulting from this more general approach to AT.

Barcroft et al. (2011) had adults with hearing loss perform a word discrimination task in a +2 signal-to-babble ratio. Consonants within words varied in manner, place, or voicing. Participants were exposed to either a single talker, where all words were produced by the same person, or multiple talkers, where one of six different talkers produced the words on any given trial. Words were presented in pairs and participants were asked to identify the picture that depicted the correct combination of words. Following training, participants demonstrated the greatest improvement for stimuli that were most similar to the training stimuli: Subjects trained using a single talker showed the greatest improvement on measures utilizing that single talker, while those in the multitalker group showed the greatest benefit for multitalker stimuli. Regardless, both groups showed some degree of improvement on each group of stimuli (single and multi-talker), and the authors concluded that this transfer of gains indicates that their protocol offers a promising approach to auditory training.

De Boer and Thornton (2008) examined the relationship between discrimination in noise training and efferent activity of the medial olivocochlear bundle (MOCB). Sixteen normal hearing young adults participated in a phoneme discrimination task in noise, in which they were asked to discriminate the consonant portion of a CV. Stimuli fell on a /b/ to /d/ continuum that was created by interpolating the consonant portion of the CV. All CVs were presented monaurally in a 10 dB signal-to-noise ratio. Half of the subjects also had noise presented to the contralateral ear during training, as contralateral noise is more likely to activate the MOCB that might facilitate training effects because of the purported role of the MOCB in suppressing noise. MOCB function was assessed periodically throughout the training by examining suppression of otoacoustic emissions during the presentation of contralateral noise. Subjects were trained over five days, with one hour of training each day. Results showed that individuals who learned to better discriminate the CV stimuli also showed an increase in OAE suppression following training. Effects were uninfluenced by the presence of contralateral noise during testing. The authors concluded that the MOCB plays an important role in yielding improvements during speech-in-noise training.

Cameron and Dillon (2011) investigated the utility of training *spatial hearing in noise*. The training approach is based on the authors' Listening in Spatialized Noise (LiSN) test. Using the LiSN, the authors have identified some children with reported listening difficulties who do not obtain the expected benefit in speech recognition when the location of speech and noise are separated (Cameron & Dillon, 2008). Their program, LiSN and Learn, attempts to improve the listener's ability to make use of spatial separation when listening in noise. See Chapter 8 for elaboration of this training approach. Preliminary data have been encouraging (Cameron & Dillon, 2011).

Using an adaptive training protocol, children (age 6–11 years) who performed below normal limits on the LiSN were required to perform a sentence recognition task in the presence of noise, where sentences are perceived from 0 azimuth and noise from +/−90 degrees. All subjects were trained for 15 minutes a day, 5 days a week, for a total of 12 weeks. Results showed significant improvements in spatial processing immediately following training, which persisted when reassessed 3 months following the end of training. Significant improvements also were noted on some measures of attention and memory, as well as on self-report measures of hearing handicap. The authors attributed some of these improvements to the fact that during the training, subjects had to attend to and remember long sentences in order to respond correctly. Although further research needs to be conducted with proper controls, these initial results seem promising.

Musical Training

In recent years, musical training has become linked with auditory training. Music and speech represent the most cognitively complex use of acoustic information by humans and both take advantage of dynamic modulation of acoustic parameters (Zatorre, Belin, & Benhune, 2002). Musical training has been shown to strengthen cognitive functions (i.e., attention and memory), functions that are known to support auditory functions (Strait, Kraus, Parbery-Clark, & Ashley, 2010). Musicians show more robust and efficient neural responses in subcortical and cortical regions that support language (e.g., Elmer, Meyer, & Jancke, 2012; Meyer et al., 2011; Schon, Magne, & Besson, 2004; Wong, Skoe, Russo, Dees, & Kraus, 2007), demonstrating that musical experience and training may *tune* the brain and facilitate processing of both music and language. One might expect that the neural encoding of speech might be enhanced by interactive auditory training with music. Given the frequently observed difficulty individuals diagnosed with CAPD experience learning songs and nursery rhymes, and their often poor musical and singing skills in general, the potential benefits of musical training and auditory training using musical stimuli is appealing. (Of course, music as a therapy for a number of health and health related conditions has been utilized for many years ["About Music Therapy & AMTA." American Music Therapy Association, 2011. http://www.musictherapy .org/about/quotes/].) Recognizing the potential that musical experience can aid (or induce) neuroplasticity (Herholz & Zatorre, 2012; Kraus & Chandrasekaran, 2010), Chermak (2010) views musical training as a procedure that can enhance auditory function and in particular central auditory function. As noted by Pantev and Herholtz (2011), passive listening to music (not training) may result in some plasticity (and therefore some auditory

enhancement), but training will result in more changes for sophisticated auditory processing.

There are numerous reports relating that musicians perform better than nonmusicians on auditory tasks (see Pantev & Herholtz, 2011 for review). For example there is clear evidence that musicians yield better auditory evoked potentials responses than do nonmusicians (Kraus & Chandrasekaran, 2010; Pantev & Herholtz, 2011; Strait & Kraus, 2011; Trainor, Shahin, & Roberts, 2003). Behavioral measures of musicians versus nonmusicians generally show the same kinds of findings. In research that used dichotic listening paradigms for musical chords, nonmusicians demonstrated a clear left ear advantage, whereas musicians seem to show more symmetrical findings (Morais, Peretz, & Gudanski, 1982; Peretz & Morais, 1979). For dichotically presented violin melodies, musicians showed a right ear advantage and nonmusicians showed a left ear advantage (Johnson, 1977). Similar findings are obtained when popular melodies are presented dichotically to musicians and nonmusicians (Messerli, Pegna, & Sordet, 1995). Superior temporal processing also has been demonstrated for musicians versus nonmusicians for auditory tasks of fusion, rhythm perception, and temporal discrimination (Rammsayer & Altenmuller, 2005). Musicians also were better than nonmusicians for detecting pitch changes in an oddball paradigm using a behavioral assessment (Tervaniemi, Just, Koelsch, Widmann, & Schroger, 2005). See Chapter 7 of Volume 1 of the Handbook for discussion of musicians' more robust encoding of acoustical elements as well as their better perception of speech in noise and other functional enhancements relative to nonmusicians.

It is clear that musicians perform better on various behavioral tests of auditory function than do nonmusicians; however, it is possible that individuals who become musicians already posses greater inherent auditory ability than those who do not study music. Additional study is needed to examine basic auditory function in individuals prior to the start of their musical education. Moreover, studies are needed to examine the potential clinical applications of musical training with nonmusicians. Little research along these lines seems to have been conducted to date. Music is enjoyable and therefore likely to engage participants and allow for more intensive training, and as Patel (2011) noted, music focuses training on specific acoustic dimensions, and does not draw attention to other dimensions (e.g., semantic) as would speech, which means that AT with music might accelerate a patient's progress. Additional research using music as stimulus for auditory training with patients diagnosed with CAPD is needed to determine the true benefits of this approach to AT. In the meantime, Chermak (2010) outlined several formal AT exercises using music as stimulus, including: difference limens for intensity, frequency, and duration; tone glides; contour (e.g., high, low, high vs. low, high, low); rhythm (e.g., short, long, short vs. long, short, long); meter (e.g., waltz vs. march); and timbre (e.g., cello vs. violin).

Pitch discrimination training may be one of the simplest forms of musical training. Pitch discrimination training does not reside exclusively in the musical domain, as it has been used in auditory training programs (with normally hearing subjects?). For example, Menning, Roberts, and Pantev (2000) showed improved frequency discrimination on both behav-ioral and electrophysiologic measures following frequency discrimination training, although a few weeks after cessation of training, auditory evoked potentials returned to pretraining values. Recanzone, Schreiner, and Merzenich (1993) trained monkeys on frequency discrimination tasks and showed improved frequency discrimination after about 2 to 3 weeks of training. In adult humans who underwent frequency discrimination training, improvements also were readily observed regardless of whether right or left ears were trained (Roth, Avrahami, Sabo, & Kishon-Rabin (2004). Melody recognition is another form of musical training. Training on various melodic contours, harmonic complexes, and so forth does improve melody recognition in individuals without musical training (Schulte, Knief, Seither-Preisler, & Pantev, 2002). Questions remain, however, as to whether musical training in the form of voice lessons or singing or more passive listening to a variety of forms of music, and so forth enhances auditory perception—especially in those individuals who present various types of auditory deficits, including CAPD.

General and/or Multifaceted Auditory Training Approaches

Though some AT involves a specific type of training procedure, others report on the use of a multiple procedures used with the same patient. Using a battery of AT procedures has both advantages and disadvantages. Using multiple approaches maximizes the chance that the type of deficit will be *covered* by at least one of the procedures used. Another advantage of multiple procedural AT is that in most cases there will be a variety of therapies utilized that may provide numerous ways to attack the processing deficit (i.e., a *varied* approach, as mentioned earlier). The downside to using multiple procedures is that it is difficult to isolate the specific procedure that might be responsible for any observed improvement, nor is it easy to apportion the degree to which multiple procedures may be responsible for positive change. Finally, one must consider that multiple approaches may be required for patients with multiple auditory deficits.

There have been several studies of AT that have used a multifaceted approach. Sharma, Purdy, and Kelly (2012) employed both top-down and bottom-up AT approaches. Sharma et al. (2012) enrolled children ranging from 7 through 13 years of age and diagnosed with CAPD based on AAA (2010) guidelines either in an auditory training (bottom-up) approach, speech-language (top-down) therapy approach, or in a control group that did not receive any treatment. Although the authors did not report how often each subject failed a specific central auditory processing test, they indicated that their Sharma et al. (2009) paper is characteristic of the distribution encountered in the present sample. All children in Sharma et al. (2009) had difficulty on the frequency patterns test, with a percentage of children also showing difficulty on the dichotic digits and random gap detection tests. The majority of children also had a comorbid reading disorder or language delay. The top-down therapies included language manipulations such as following directions, summarizing short stories, identifying stress patterns, and so forth. Bottom-up auditory training focused on discrimination of intensity and frequency,

gap detection, and pattern identification. Therapy was conducted over a six-week period with weekly one-hour sessions, as well as one to two hours of training by parents at home each week. Both training groups, but not the control group, showed significant improvements on the frequency patterns test and speech-language measures following training. There was no difference in outcomes between the children enrolled in auditory training versus speech-language therapy. It should be noted, however, that it is not clear what percentage of the weekly auditory training actually focused on pattern perception (the main deficit exhibited by most subjects), and since it was likely that some of the children presented dichotic listening deficits, which were not addressed in the therapy provided, it is possible that benefits for the auditory training group may have surpassed the speech-language group if a more process-specific auditory training approach had been implemented. In contrast to the control group who were not trained, trained participants showed improvement using both approaches based on central auditory test measures, as well as language and cognitive measures.

Schochat, Musiek, Alonso, and Ogata (2010) also employed a battery of intervention strategies for a group of children diagnosed with CAPD. This group of children received 8 weeks of AT, approximately 1 hour per week of formal training, and 15 minutes of informal training at home. The formal training included frequency, intensity and temporal discrimination training, as well as the DIID and localization procedures. The informal procedures included following directives, sketching stories told to them, word associations, and so forth. Results showed increased amplitude of the middle latency response (MLR) and improved performance on a central auditory test battery for the trained group but not for the control group.

Putter-Katz, Adi-Bensaid, Feldman, and Hildesheimer (2008) recruited children diagnosed with CAPD ranging in age from 7 through 14 years into an auditory training program that focused on both training auditory processing skills and enhancing top-down processing related to listening. Participants were divided into two groups—one included children who presented only auditory closure deficits, and the second group included children who presented both auditory closure and dichotic processing deficits. Both groups had access to FM systems. A third, control group, did not receive training and presented only auditory closure deficits.

Training was administered once per week for 45 minutes for approximately 4 months. Bottom-up approaches included administration of auditory closure and dichotic exercises, whereas top-down approaches included speech-reading, metacognitive awareness enhancement, and classroom learning strategies. Treatment was adaptive to build upon progress demonstrated by the subject. Posttraining, both the auditory closure and auditory closure-dichotic training groups showed significant improvement on an auditory closure test, while only the auditory closure-dichotic group improved on a dichotic test. The control group did not improve on either the auditory closure or the dichotic measure.

There also have been interesting case studies of patients with CAPD resulting from head trauma. These individuals also have shown improvement utilizing a multifaceted AT approach. In one case of head trauma, the therapies were directed at auditory figure-ground perception, auditory pattern perception, and verbal memory. The patient received eight 40-minute sessions and showed improvement on both behavioral central auditory tests and the P300 event related potentials (Murphy, Fillippini, Palma, Zalcman, Lima, & Schochat, 2011). Similar findings were reported for a patient with a head injury that resulted in a left ear deficit on central auditory tests that improved markedly after informal DIID, and auditory recognition and vigilance training (Musiek, Baran, & Shinn, 2004).

Auditory-Language Training Approaches

Several AT approaches do not fit easily into the categories previously discussed in this chapter. These approaches usually include a variety of AT procedures that are included in one training session or possibly over several sessions. Two such training programs serve as good examples of this general category of AT. One is a workbook-based approach (Sloan, 1986) and the other is Earobics, a well-known computerized program. These two general AT programs focus on basic phonemic awareness, and acoustic discrimination and identification using speech-language tasks. Because these programs cover auditory-language training in broad terms they can be used to treat some of the associated phonologic awareness deficits often presented by individuals diagnosed with CAPD.

The Sloan workbook and the Earobics program incorporated some of the same stimuli and approaches to AT first introduced by Carhart and DiCarlo, mentioned earlier in this chapter. Earobics includes some exercises with time and intensity altered stimuli, which certainly supports temporal training. The focus of this program, however, is directed to phonological awareness training. Several versions of Earobics are available for different age levels (4–7, 7–10, adolescent, and adult), as well as a version for home use. The home version is a valuable tool that allows the clinician to extend training into the home.

Some evidence suggests the efficacy of the Earobics program in improving language processing in children with learning problems. Based on a review of three studies involving children diagnosed with language learning impairment or specific reading disorder, Loo et al. (2010) noted that Earobics training led to improved morphology, amplitudes, and latencies of speech-evoked cortical and subcortical responses in noise. Some positive impact was seen on phonological awareness skills; however, Earobics training had little effect on language, spelling, and reading skills of these children. Increases in the amplitude of evoked responses to speech stimuli related to brainstem and cortical substrate indicated possible improvements in electrophysiologic representation in the CANS following training with Earobics (Russo, Nicole, Zecker, Hayes, & Kraus, 2005; Warrier, Johnson, Hayes, Nicol, & Kraus, 2004).

AT With Preschool Children

Unfortunately, it is not easy to definitively diagnose CAPD in children under 7 years of age due to the difficulty posed by central auditory tests designed to challenge

a redundant CANS. This does not mean, however, that one should not begin AT with younger children deemed at risk for auditory/listening problems (Musiek & Chermak, 1995). Indeed, listening activities typically are part of the preschool curriculum, as they should be since listening activities occupy approximately 75% of a school day (Hubble-Dahlquist, 1998). It is appropriate to involve all young children in listening activities and games, not just those who may be at risk for CAPD. These games can be conducted at home or at school, by parents or teachers. There are a variety of commercial listening games on the market that can be used with preschoolers including Earobics, which has a version for young children (4–7 years) that can be used by parents. With some ingenuity, a number of listening games can be formulated easily. Following are several examples of listening activities for children 4 year of age and older. The reader is referred to Chermak (2010), Chermak and Musiek (2002), Musiek and Chermak (1995) for more expansive discussions of AT for young children, as well as activities for school-age children.

Finding the Target Sound or Word

An adult reads a story to a child or group of children. Before reading, the children are asked to listen for a certain word or sound that occurs in the story. The children are required to raise their hands each time a target word/sound is heard or to keep track of the number of times the target is heard and report at the story's end. The latter variation trains memory as well as selective attention. The former variation might interfere with comprehension;

therefore, it is important to encourage the listener to attend to the story and not only to the individual target.

Localization

The child is blindfolded and asked to point to the location of the person who is speaking while roaming across the room. Task difficulty can be increased by reducing the length or intensity of the speech segment produced at any given location.

Walking and Listening

While accompanying a child on an outdoor field trip, the child is encouraged to listen for sounds and to label these environmental sounds when heard (e.g., a dog barking). This activity can be combined with localization requiring the child to point to the location of the sound after labeling the sound.

Following Directives

The child is asked to follow one, two, or three step motor tasks verbally conveyed by a parent or teacher (e.g., go to the kitchen and turn on the light). The child should be able to easily perform the required motor activity.

Interhemispheric Processing

Practice at transferring information from one hemisphere to another can be a valuable training task—especially with the long maturational course of the corpus callosum (Musiek, Kibbe, & Baran, 1984). Playing "name that tune" likely requires activity between cortices. Also, having children close their eyes and name objects felt with their left hand is an enjoyable game that likely requires information exchange between hemispheres.

Listening to Rhymes

Exposing young children to nursery rhymes, as well as singing songs, helps develop temporal processes that underlie prosody. These activities are enjoyable, employ accessible and varied material, and can be done repetitively without the child tiring or becoming bored.

Musical Chairs

Musical chairs is a game that requires a number of auditory, motor and cognitive processes. Sustained attention is pivotal to the multiple processes and skills trained through this game. Children walk around chairs (equal to the number of children at the outset of the game) set in a circle while music plays in the background. When the music stops, the children must sit in a chair. After each music segment, a chair is removed resulting in one child left standing and eliminated from the game. The game continues until only one chair remains to accommodate one child. The game can be modified to increase the challenge by having the children listen for specific targets within the music (e.g., when the music becomes louder or softer sit down). Also, the time between musical segments can be varied greatly introducing unpredictability and challenge that should exercise the child's ability to maintain attention to the task. See Table 7–1 for additional informal AT activities that incorporate musical stimuli.

Table 7–1. Informal Auditory Training Activities That Incorporate Musical Stimuli

Vigilance & Temporal Resolution	**Interhemispheric Transfer**
Musical Chairs	Dichotic Melodies (also exercises dichotic listening)
Musical Statues	Name That Tune
Red-Light Green-Light	Singing
Auditory Discrimination	Extract Lyrics From Songs
Instrument Same/Different	Link Prosodic & Linguistic Acoustic Features
Chord Discrimination	Link Emotion of Facial Expression to Prosody of Message
Voice Lessons	Playing Instrument Requiring Bimanual Coordination
Patterns/ Rhythm/Prosody	
Keyboard/Cadence Replication	
Nursery Rhymes & Poetry	

Summary

Auditory training (AT) is no longer a rehabilitative approach directed primarily to those with peripheral hearing loss. Recent studies in both animals and humans have demonstrated that AT improves basic central auditory processes and skills. This improvement in auditory capability is linked to plastic changes in the brain. In fact, auditory plasticity underlies the success of AT. To ensure success, however, the principles derived from neuroscience and learning theory reviewed in this chapter must be followed to ensure effectiveness. AT is an essential component of a comprehensive approach to treat CAPD. The reader is referred to Chapters 10 and 12 for elaboration of the other elements (i.e., central resources training and signal enhancement, respectively) of the recommended comprehensive approach to intervention for CAPD.

References

Agnew, J., Dorn, C., & Eden, G. (2004). Effect of intensive training on auditory processing and reading skills. *Brain and Language, 88*, 21–25.

Ahissar, E., Vaadia, E., Ahissar, M., Bergman, H., Arieli, A., & Abeles, M. (1992). Dependence of cortical plasticity on correlated activity of single neurons and on behavioral context. *Science, 257*, 1412–1415.

Alain, C., Campeanu, S., & Tremblay, K. (2009). Changes in sensory evoked responses coincide with rapid improvement in speech identification performance. *Journal of Cognitive Neuroscience, 22*, 392–403.

Alexander, D., & Frost, B. (1982). Decelerated synthesized speech as a means of shaping speed of auditory processing of children with delayed language. *Perceptual and Motor Skills, 55*, 783–792.

Amitay, S., Halliday, L., Taylor, J., & Moore, D. R. (2006). Discrimination learning induced by training with identical stimuli. *Nature Neuroscience, 9*, 1446–1448.

Amitay, S., Halliday, L., Taylor, J., Sohoglu, E., & Moore, D. R. (2010). Motivation and intelligence drive auditory perceptual learning. *PLoS One, 5*, e9816

Amitay, S., Hawkey, D. J. C., & Moore, D. R. (2005). Auditory frequency discrimination learning is affected by stimulus variability. *Perception and Psychophysics, 67*, 691–698.

Anderson, S., & Kraus, N. (2011). Neural encoding of speech and music—implications for hearing speech in noise. *Seminars in Hearing, 32*, 129–139.

Anderson, S., White-Schwoch, T., Parbery-Clark, A., & Kraus, N. (2013, Feb 11). Reversal of age-related neural timing delays with training. *Proceedings of the National Academy of Sciences USA* [Epub ahead of print].

Atienza, M., Cantero, J. L., & Dominguez-Marin, E. (2002). The time course of neural changes in underlying auditory perceptual learning. *Learning and Memory, 9*, 138–150.

Bailey, C., & Chen, M. (1988). Long term memory in aphasia modulates the total number of varicosities of single identified sensory neurons. *Proceeding of the National Academy of Sciences USA, 85*, 2373–2377.

Bamiou, D., & Luxon, L. (2003). Medical management of balance disorders and vestibular rehabilitation. In L. Luxon (Ed.), *Textbook of audiological medicine: Clinical aspects of hearing and balance* (pp. 839–916). London, UK: Martin Dunitz.

Bao, S., Chang, E., Woods, J., & Merzenich, M. (2004). Temporal plasticity in the primary auditory cortex induced by operant perceptual learning. *Nature Neuroscience, 7*, 974–981.

Barcroft, J., Sommers, M., Tye-Murray, N., Mauze, E., Schroy, C., & Spehar, B. (2011). Tailoring auditory training to patient needs with single and multiple talkers: Transfer-appropriate gains on a four-choice discrimination test. *International Journal of Audiology, 50*, 802–808.

Bliss, T., & Lomo, T. (1973). Long-lasting potentiation of synaptic transmission in the dentate area of the anaesthetized rabbit following stimulation of the perforant path. *Journal of Physiology, 232*, 331–356.

Cameron, S., & Dillon, H. (2008). The listening in spatialized noise-sentences test (LISN-S): Comparison to the prototype LISN and results from children with either a suspected (central) auditory processing disorder or a confirmed language disorder. *Journal of the American Academy of Audiology, 19*, 377–391.

Cameron, S., & Dillon, H. (2011). Development and evaluation of the LiSN & Learn auditory training software for deficit-specific remediation of binaural processing deficits in children: Preliminary findings. *Journal of the American Academy of Audiology, 22*, 678–696

Carhart, R. (1960). Auditory training. In H. Davis (Ed.), *Hearing and deafness.* New York, NY: Holt, Rinehart and Winston.

Chermak, G. D. (2010). Music and auditory training. *Hearing Journal, 63*, 57–58.

Chermak, G., & Musiek, F. (2002). Auditory training: Principles and approaches for remediating and managing auditory processing disorders. *Seminars in Hearing, 23*, 297–308.

Chermak, G. D., & Musiek, F.E. (2011). Neurological substrate of central auditory processing deficits in children. *Current Pediatric Reviews, 7*, 241–251.

Chermak, G. D., Silva, M. E., Nye, J., Hasbrouck, J., & Musiek, F. E. (2007). An update on professional education and clinical practices in (central) auditory processing. *Journal of the American Academy of Audiology, 18*, 428–439

Cleary, M., Pisoni, D., & Geers, A. (2001). Some measures of verbal and spatial working memory in eight and nine year old hearing impaired children with cochlear implants. *Ear and Hearing, 22*, 395–411.

Cohen, W., Hodson, A., O'Hare, A., Boyle, J., Durrani, T., McCartney, . . . Watson, J. (2005). Effects of computer-based intervention through acoustically modified speech (Fast ForWord) in severe mixed receptive-expressive language impairment: Outcomes from a randomized controlled trial. *Journal Speech, Language, and Hearing Research, 48,* 715–729.

Danzl, M., Etter, N., Andreatta, R., & Kitzman, P. (2012). Facilitating neurorehabilitation through principles of engagement. *Journal Allied Health, 41,* 35–41.

de Boer, J., & Thornton, A. (2008). Neural correlates of perceptual learning in the auditory brainstem: Efferent activity predicts and reflects improvement at a speech-in-noise discrimination task. *Journal of Neuroscience, 28,* 4929–4937.

de Villers-Sidani, E., Alzghoul, L., Zhou, X., Simpson, K. L., Lin, R. C. S., & Merzenich, M. M. (2010). Recovery of functional and structural age-related changes in the rat primary auditory cortex with operant training. *Proceedings of the National Academy of Sciences of the United States of America, 107,* 13900–13905.

Delhommeau, K., Micheyl, C., & Jouvent, R. (2005). Generalization of frequency discrimination learning across frequencies and ears: implications for underlying neural mechanisms in humans. *Journal of the Association for Research in Otolaryngology, 6,* 171–179.

Delhommeau, K., Micheyl, C., Jouvent, R., & Collet, L. (2002). Transfer of learning across durations and ears in auditory frequency discrimination. *Perception and Psychophysics, 64,* 426–436.

DiCarlo, L. (1948). Auditory training for the adult. *Volta Review, 50,* 490.

Edeline, J., & Weinberger, N. (1993). Receptive field plasticity in the auditory cortex during frequency discrimination training: Selective retuning independent of task difficulty. *Behavioral Neuroscience, 107,* 82–103.

Elmer, S., Meyer, M., & Jancke, L. (2012). Neurofunctional and behavioral correlates of phonetic and temporal categorization in musically trained and untrained subjects. *Cerebral Cortex, 22,* 650–658.

Erber, N. (1982). *Auditory training.* Washington DC: Alexander Graham Bell Association for the Deaf.

Fey, M., Finestack, L., Gajewski, B., Popsecu, M., & Lewine, J. (2009). A preliminary evaluation of Fast-ForWord-Language as an adjuvant treatment in language intervention. *Journal Speech, Language, Hearing Research, 53,* 430–449.

Foxton, J., Brown, A., Chambers, S., & Griffiths, T. (2004). Training improves acoustic pattern perception. *Current Biology, 14,* 322–325.

Friel-Patti, S., Loeb, D., & Gilliam, R. (2001). Looking ahead: An introduction to five exploratory studies in Fast ForWord. *American Journal of Speech-Language Pathology, 10,* 195–202.

Gilliam, R., Loeb, D., & Friel-Patti, S. (2001). Looking back: A summary of five exploratory studies of Fast ForWord. *American Journal of Speech-Language Pathology, 10,* 269–273.

Gillam, R., Loeb, D., Hoffman, L., Bohman, T., Champlin, C., Thibodeau, L., . . . Friel-Patti, S. (2008). The efficacy of Fast ForWord language intervention in school-age children with language impairment: A randomized controlled trial. *Journal of Speech, Language, and Hearing Research, 51,* 97–119.

Goldstein, M. (1939). *The acoustic method.* St Louis, MO: Laryngoscope Press.

Gottselig, J. M., Brandeis, D., Hofer-Tinguely, G., Borberly, A. A., & Achermann, P. (2004). Human central auditory plasticity associated with tone sequence learning. *Learning and Memory, 11,* 151–171.

Greenough, W., & Bailey, C. (1988). Anatomy of a memory: Convergence of results across a diversity of tests. *Trends in Neuroscience, 11,* 142–146.

Grimault, N., Micheyl, C., Carlyon, R. P., Bacon, S. P., & Collet, L. (2003). Learning in discrimination of frequency or modulation rate: Generalization to fundamental frequency discrimination. *Hearing Research, 184,* 41–50.

Halliday, L., Moore, D., Taylor, J., & Amitay, S. (2011). Dimension-specific attention directs learning and listening on auditory training tasks. *Attention Perception Psychophysics, 73,* 1329–1335.

Halliday, L., Taylor, J., Edmonson-Jones, A., & Moore, D. (2008). Frequency discrimination learning in children. *Journal of the Acoustical Society of American, 123,* 4393–4402.

Halliday, L., Taylor, J., Millward, K., & Moore, D. (2012). Lack of generalization of auditory learning in typically developing children. *Journal Speech, Language, Hearing Research, 55,* 168–181.

Hassmannova, J., Myslivecek, J., & Novakova, V. (1981). Effects of early auditory stimulation on cortical centers. In J. Syka & L. Aitkin (Eds.), *Neuronal mechanisms of hearing* (pp. 355–359). New York, NY: Plenum.

Hawkey, D., Amitay, S., & Moore, D. R. (2004). Early and rapid perceptual learning. *Nature Neuroscience, 7,* 1055–1056.

Hayes, E., Warrier, C., Nicol, T., Zecker, S., & Kraus, N. (2003). Neural plasticity following auditory training in children with learning problems. *Clinical Neurophysiology, 114,* 673–684.

Hebb, D. O. (1949). *The organization of behavior.* New York, NY: John Wiley & Sons.

Heim, S., Keil. A., Choudhury, N., Thomas Friedman, J., & Benasich, A. (2013). Early gamma oscillations during rapid auditory processing in children with a language-learning impairment: Changes in neural mass activity after training. *Neuropsychologica* [Epub ahead of print].

Herholz, S., & Zatorre, R. (2012). Musical training as a framework for brain plasticity: Behavior, function, and structure. *Neuron, 76,* 486–502.

Holroyd, C. B., Larsen, J. T., & Cohen, J. D. (2004). Context dependence of the event-related brain potential associated with reward and punishment. *Psychophysiology, 41,* 245–253.

Hubble-Dahlquist, L. (1998). *Classroom amplification: Not just for the hearing impaired anymore.* CSUN '98 Papers [online]. Retrieved from http://www.dimf.ne.jp/doc/english/Us_Eu/conf/csun_98/csun98_124.htm

Hudgins, C. V. (1954). Auditory training: Its possibilities and limitations. *Volta Review, 56,* 339.

Hurley, A. (2011, April 7) Central auditory processing remediation for patients with Landau-Kleffner syndrome. *ASHA Leader.*

Jancke, L., Gaab, N., Wustenberg, H., Scheich, H., & Heinze, H. (2001). Short-term functional plasticity in the human auditory cortex: An fMRI study. *Cognitive Brain Research, 12,* 479–485.

Jenkins, W., & Merzenich, M. (1996). Language comprehension in language-learning impaired children improved with acoustically modified speech. *Science, 271,* 81–84.

Johnson, P. (1977). Dichotically stimulated ear differences in musicians and nonmusicians. *Cortex, 13,* 385–389.

Kalil, R. (1989). Synapse formation in the developing brain. *Scientific American, 261,* 76–87.

Karpicke, J., & Pisoni, D. (2004). Using immediate memory span to measure implicit learning. *Memory & Cognition, 32,* 956–964.

Katz, J., & Harmon, C. (1982). *Phonemic synthesis: Blending sounds into words.* Allen, TX: Developmental Learning Materials.

Kimura D. (1961). Some effects of temporal lobe damage on auditory perception. *Canadian Journal of Psychology, 15,* 157–165.

King, C., Warrier, C., Hayes, E., & Kraus, N. (2002). Deficits in auditory brainstem pathway encoding of speech sounds in children with learning problems. *Neuroscience Letters, 319,* 111–115.

Knudsen, E. (1988). Experience shapes sound localization and auditory unit properties during development in the barn owl. In G. Edleman, W. Gall, & W. Cowan (Eds.), *Auditory function: Neurological bases of hearing.* New York, NY: John Wiley & Sons.

Koelsch, S. (2010). Towards a neural basis of music-evoked emotions. *Trends in Cognitive Science, 14,* 131–137.

Kraus, N. (1999). Speech sound perception, neurophysiology, and plasticity. *Pediatric Otorhinolaryngology, 47,* 123–129.

Kraus, N., & Chandrasekaran, B. (2010). Music training for the development of auditory skills. *Nature Reviews Neuroscience, 11,* 599–605.

Kraus, N., McGee, T., Carrell, T., King, C., Tremblay, K., & Nicol, T. (1995). Central auditory system plasticity associated with speech discrimination training. *Journal of Cognitive Neuroscience, 7,* 25–32.

Krishnamurti, S., Forrester, J., Rutledge, C., & Holmes, G. (2013). A case study of the changes in the speech-evoked auditory brainstem response associated with auditory training in children with auditory processing disorders. *International Journal Pediatric Otorhinolaryngology* [Epub ahead of print].

Kujala, T., Karma, K., Ceponiene, R., Belitz, S., Turkkila, P., Tervaniemi, M., & Naatanen, R. (2001). Plastic neural changes and reading improvement caused by audiovisual training in reading-impaired children. *Proceedings of the National Academy of Sciences of the USA, 98,* 10509–10514.

Kujala, T., Myllyviita, K., Tervaniemi, M., Alho, K., Kallio, J., & Naatanen, R. (2000). Basic auditory dysfunction in dyslexia as demonstrated by brain activity measurements. *Psychophysiology, 37,* 262–266.

Linkenhoker, B., & Knudsen, E. (2002). Incremental training increases the plasticity of the auditory space map in adult barn owls. *Nature, 419,* 293–296.

Linkenhoker, B., von der Ohe, C., & Knudsen E. (2004). Anatomical traces of juvenile learning in the auditory system of adult barn owls. *Nature Neuroscience, 8,* 93–98.

Loo, J., Bamiou, D., Campbell, N., & Luxon, L. (2010). Computer-based auditory training (CBAT): Benefits for children with language- and reading-related learning difficulties. *Developmental Medicine and Child Neurology, 52,* 708–717.

Ludman, H. (2003). The role of surgery in the management of the dizzy patient. In L. Luxon (Ed.), *Textbook of audiological medicine: Clinical aspects of hearing and balance* (pp. 917–928). London, UK: Martin Dunitz.

Lund, R. (1978). *Development and plasticity of the brain: An introduction.* New York, NY: Oxford University Press.

Marler, J., Champlin, C., & Gilliam, R. (2001) Backward and simultaneous masking measured in children with language learning impairments who received intervention with Fast ForWord or Laureate Learning Systems software. *American Journal of Speech-Language Pathology, 10,* 258–269.

Menning, H., Roberts, L. E., & Pantev, C. (2000). Plastic changes in the auditory cortex induced by intensive frequency discrimination training. *NeuroReport, 11,* 817–822.

Merzenich, M., Jenkins, W., Johnston, P., Schreiner, C., Miller, S., & Tallal, P. (1996). Temporal processing deficits of language-learning impaired children ameliorated by training. *Science, 271,* 77–81.

Messerli, P., Pegna, A., & Sordet, N. (1995). Hemispheric dominance for melody recognition in musicians and non-musicians. *Neuropsychologia, 33,* 395–405.

Meyer, M., Elmer, S., Ringli, M., Oechslin, M., Baumann, S., & Jancke, L. (2011). Long-term exposure to music enhances the sensitivity of the auditory system in children. *European Journal Neuroscience, 34,* 755–765.

Millward, K., Hall, R., Ferguson, M., & Moore, D. (2011). Training speech-in-noise perception in mainstream school children. *International Journal Pediatric Otorhinolaryngology, 75,* 1408–1417.

Molloy, K., Moore, D., Sohoglu, E. & Amitay, S. (2012). Less is more: Latent learning is maximized by shorter training sessions in auditory perceptual learning. *PLoS One, 7,* e36929.

Moncrieff, D., & Wertz, D. (2008). Auditory rehabilitation for interaural asymmetry: Preliminary evidence of improved dichotic listening performance following intensive training. *International Journal of Audiology, 47,* 84–97.

Moore, D., Ferguson, M., Halliday, L., & Riley, A. (2008). Frequency discrimination in children: Perception, learning, and attention. *Hearing Research, 238,* 147–154.

Moore, D., Rosenberg, J., & Coleman, J. (2004). Discrimination training of phonemic contrasts enhances phonological processing in mainstream school children. *Brain and Language, 94,* 72–85.

Morais, J., Peretz, I., & Gudanski, M. (1982). Ear asymmetry for chord recognition in musicians and non-muscians. *Neuropsychologia, 20,* 351–354.

Murphy, C. F. B., Fillippini, R., Palma, D., Zalcman, T. E., Lima, J. P., & Schochat, E. (2011). Auditory training and cognitive functioning in adult with traumatic brain injury. *Clinics, 66,* 713–715.

Musiek F. E. (1999) Habilitation and management of auditory processing disorders: Overview of selected procedures. *Journal of the American Academy of Audiology, 10,* 329–342

Musiek, F. (2005). Temporal (auditory) training for (C)APD. *Hearing Journal, 58,* 46.

Musiek, F., Baran, J., & Shinn, J. (2004). Assessment and remediation of an auditory processing disorder associated with head trauma. *Journal of the American Academy of Audiology, 15,* 133–151.

Musiek, F., & Berge, B. (1998). A neuroscience view of auditory training/stimulation and central auditory processing disorders. In M. Masters, N. Stecker, & J. Katz (Eds.). *Central auditory processing disorders: Mostly management* (pp 15–32). Boston, MA: Allyn & Bacon.

Musiek, F. E., & Chermak, G. D. (1995). Three commonly asked questions about central auditory processing disorders: Management. *American Journal of Audiology, 4,* 15–18.

Musiek, F., Gollegly, K., & Baran, J. (1984). Myelination of the corpus callosum and auditory processing problems in children: Theoretical and clinical correlates. *Seminars in Hearing, 5,* 231–241.

Musiek, F., Kibbe, K., & Baran, J. (1984). Neuroaudiological results from split-brain patients. *Seminars in Hearing, 5,* 219–229.

Musiek F., & Schochat, E. (1998). Auditory training and central auditory processing disorders. *Seminars in Hearing, 9,* 357–366.

Musiek, F., Shinn, J., & Hare, C. (2002). Plasticity, auditory training, and auditory processing disorders. *Seminars in Hearing, 23,* 263–275.

Pan, Y., Zhang, J., Cai, R., Zhou, X., & Sun, X. (2011). Developmentally degraded directional selectivity of the auditory cortex can be restored by auditory discrimination training. *Behavior Brain Research, 225,* 596–602.

Pantev, C., & Herholz, S. C. (2011). Plasticity of the human auditory cortex related to musical training. *Neuroscience Biobehavioral Reviews, 35,* 2140–2154.

Peretz, I., & Morais, J. (1979). A left ear advantage for chords in non-musicians. *Perceptual and Motor Skills, 49,* 957–958.

Parbery-Clark, A., Skoe, E., & Kraus, N. (2009). Musical experience limits the degradative effects of background noise on the neural processing of sound. *Journal of Neuroscience, 29,* 14100–14107.

Parbery-Clark, A., Skoe, E., Lam, C., & Kraus, N. (2009). Musician enhancement for speech-in-noise. *Ear and Hearing, 30,* 653–661.

Patel, A. (2011). Why would musical training benefit the neural encoding of speech? The OPERA hypothesis. *Frontiers in Psychology, 2,* 1–12.

Pinheiro, M. (1977). Tests of central auditory function in children with learning disabilities. In R. Keith (Ed.), *Central auditory dysfunction* (pp. 223–256). New York, NY: Grune & Stratton.

Pisoni, D., & Cleary, M. (2004). Learning, memory, and cognitive processes in deaf children following cochlear implantation. In F. Zeng, A. Popper, & R. Fay (Eds.), *Cochlear implants: Auditory prostheses and electric hearing* (pp. 407–418). New York, NY: Springer.

Putter-Katz, H., Adi-Bensaid, L., Feldman, I., & Hildesheimer, M. (2008). Effects of speech in noise and dichotic listening intervention programs on central auditory processing disorders. *Journal of Basic and Clinical Physiology and Pharmacology, 19*, 301–316.

Rammsayer, T., & Altenmuller, E. (2006). Temporal information processing in musicians and non-musicians. *Music Perception, 24*, 37–48.

Recanzone, G., Schreiner, C., & Merzenich, M. (1993). Plasticity in the frequency representation of primary auditory cortex following discrimination training in adult owl monkeys. *Journal of Neuroscience, 13*, 97–103.

Reagan, C. (1973). *Handbook of auditory perceptual training* (pp. 11, 30, 65–66). Springfield, IL: Charles C. Thomas.

Rogan, M. T., & LeDoux, J. E. (1995). LTP is accompanied by commensurate enhancement of auditory-evoked responses in a fear conditioning circuit. *Neuron, 15*, 127–136.

Roth, D., Avrahami, T., & Sabo, Y. (2004). Frequency discrimination training: Is there ear symmetry? *Journal Basic Clinical Physiology Pharmacolology, 15*, 15–27.

Russo, N., Nicole, T., Zecker, S., Hayes, E., & Kraus, N. (2005). Auditory training improves neural timing in the human brainstem. *Behavioural Brain Research, 156*, 95–103.

Salvi, R., & Henderson, D. (1996). *Auditory system plasticity and regeneration*. New York, NY: Thieme Medical.

Sanders, D. A. (1971). *Aural rehabilitation*. Englewood Cliffs, NJ: Prentice-Hall.

Scheich, H. (1991). Auditory cortex: Comparative aspects of maps and plasticity. *Current Opinion in Neurobiology, 1*, 236–247.

Schochat, E., Musiek, F. E., Alonso, R., & Ogata, J. (2010). Effect of auditory training on the middle latency response in children with (central) auditory processing disorder. *Brazilian Journal of Medical and Biological Research, 43*, 777–785.

Schon, D., Magne, C., & Besson, M. (2004). The music of speech: Music training facilitates pitch processing in both music and language. *Psychophysiology, 41*, 341–349.

Schow, R., Balsara, N., Smedley, T., & Whitcomb, C. (1993). Aural rehabilitation by ASHA audiologists: 1980-1990. *American Journal of Audiology, 2*, 28–37.

Schow, R., & Nerbonne, M. (1996). *Introduction to audiological rehabilitation* (3rd ed.). Boston, MA: Pearson.

Schow, R., & Nerbonne, M. (2013). *Introduction to audiological rehabilitation* (6th ed.). Boston, MA: Pearson.

Schulte, M., Knief, A., Seither-Preisler, A., & Pantev, C. (2002). Different modes of pitch perception and learning-induced neuronal plasticity of the human auditory cortex. *Neural plasticity, 9*, 161–175.

Sharma, M., Purdy, S., & Kelly, A. (2009). Comorbidity of auditory processing, language, and reading disorders. *Journal of Speech, Language, and Hearing Research, 52*, 706–722.

Sharma, M., Purdy, S. C., & Kelly, A. S. (2012). A randomized control trial of interventions in school-aged children with auditory processing disorders. *International Journal of Audiology, 51*, 506–518.

Singly, K., & Anderson, J. (1989). *The transfer of cognitive skill*. Cambridge, MA: Harvard University Press.

Sloan, C. (1986). *Treating auditory processing difficulties in children*. San Diego, CA: College-Hill Press.

Strait, D. L., & Kraus, N. (2011). Can you hear me now? Musical training shapes functional brain networks for selective auditory attention and hearing speech in noise. *Frontiers in Psychology, 2*, 113.

Strait. D. L., Kraus, N., Parbery-Clark, A., & Ashley, R. (2010). Musical experience shapes top-down auditory mechanisms: Evidence from masking and auditory attention performance. *Hearing Research, 261*, 22–29.

Strong, G., Torgerson, C., Torgerson, D., & Hulme, C. (2011). A systematic meta-analytic review of evidence for the effectiveness of the "Fast ForWord" language intervention program. *Journal Child Psychology and Psychiatry, 52*, 224–235.

Tallal, P., Merzenich, M., Miller, S., & Jenkins, W. (1998). Language learning impairments: Integrating basic science, technology, and remediation. *Experimental Brain Research, 123,* 210–219.

Tallal, P., Miller, S. L., Bedi, G., Byma, G., Wang, X., Nagarajan, S., . . . Merzenich, M. (1996). Language comprehension in language-learning impaired children improved with acoustically modified speech. *Science, 271,* 81–84.

Temple, E., Deutsch, G., Poldrack, R., Miller, S., Tallal, P., Merzenich, M., & Gabrieli, J. (2003). Neural deficits in children with dyslexia ameliorated by behavioral remediation: evidence from functional MRI. *Proceedings of the National Academy of Sciences of the United States of America, 100,* 2860–2865.

Tervaniemi, M., Just, V., Koelsch, S., Widman, A., & Schroger, E. (2005). Pitch discrimination accuracy in musicians vs. nonmusicians: An event-related potential and behavioral study. *Experimental Brain Research, 161,* 1–10.

Threlkeld, S., Hill, C., Rosen, G., & Fitch, R. (2009). Early acoustic discrimination experience ameliorates auditory processing deficits in male rats with cortical developmental disruption. *International Journal Developmental Neuroscience, 27,* 321–328.

Tomporowski, P. D., & Tinsley, V. F. (1996). Effects of memory demand and motivation on sustained attention in young and older adults. *American Journal of Psychology, 109,* 187–204.

Trainor, L. J., Shahin, A., & Roberts, L. (2003). Effects of musical training on the auditory cortex in children. *Annals of the New York Academy of Sciences, 999,* 506–513.

Tremblay, K., & Kraus, N. (2002). Auditory training induces asymmetrical changes in cortical neural activity. *Journal of Speech, Language, and Hearing Research, 45,* 564–572.

Tremblay, K., Kraus, N., Carrell, T., & McGee, T. (1997). Central auditory system plasticity: generalization to novel stimuli following listening training. *Journal of Acoustical Society of America, 102,* 3762–3773.

Tremblay, K., Kraus, N., & McGee, T. (1998). The time course of auditory perceptual learning: neurophysiological changes during speech-sound training. *NeuroReport, 16,* 3557–3560.

Tremblay, K., Kraus, N., McGee, T., Ponton, C., & Otis, B. (2001). Central auditory plasticity: changes in the N1-P2 complex after speech-sound training. *Ear and Hearing, 22,* 79–90.

Tremblay, K., Shahin, A., Picton, T., & Ross, B. (2009). Auditory training alters the physiological detection of stimulus-specific cues in humans. *Clinical Neurophysiology, 120,* 128–135.

Valentine, D., Hendrick, M., & Swanson, L. (2006). Effect of an auditory training program on reading, phoneme awareness and language. *Perception and Motor Skills, 103,* 183–196.

Warrier, C., Johnson, K., Hayes, E., Nicol, T., & Kraus, N. (2004). Learning-impaired children exhibit timing deficits and training-related improvements in auditory cortical responses to speech and noise. *Experimental Brain Research, 157,* 431–441.

Watanabe, T., Nanez, J., & Sasaki, Y. (2001). Perceptual learning without perception. *Nature, 413,* 844–848.

Webster, D., & Webster, M. (1977) Neonatal sound deprivation affects brainstem auditory nuclei. *Archives of Otolaryngology, 103,* 392–396.

Wedenburg, E. (1951). Auditory training of the deaf and hard of hearing children. *Acta Otolaryngologica, 94*(Suppl.), 1–29.

Weihing, J., & Musiek, F. (2013). Dichotic interaural intensity difference DIID training. In D. Geffner & D. Ross-Swain (Eds.), *Auditory processing disorders: Assessment, management, and treatment* (2nd ed., pp. 447–468). San Diego, CA: Plural.

Willeford, J. (1977). Assessing central auditory behavior in children: A test battery approach. In R. Keith (Ed.), *Central audi-*

tory dysfunction (pp. 43–72). New York, NY: Grune & Stratton.

Wingfield, A. (1979). *Human learning and memory*. New York, NY: Harper & Row.

Wong, P., Skoe, E., Russo, N., Dees, T., & Kraus, N. (2007). Musical experience shapes human brainstem encoding of linguistic pitch patterns. *Nature Neuroscience, 10,* 420–422.

Wright, B., & Sabin, A. (2007). Perceptual learning: How much daily training is enough? *Experimental Brain Research, 180,* 727–736.

Zatorre, R. J., Belin, B., & Benhune, V. B. (2002). Structure and function of auditory cortex: Music and speech. *Trends in Cognitive Sciences, 6,* 37–46.

CHAPTER 8

REMEDIATION OF SPATIAL PROCESSING ISSUES IN CENTRAL AUDITORY PROCESSING DISORDER

SHARON CAMERON and HARVEY DILLON

Spatial Processing

When we are trying to listen to speech in noisy environments, auditory processes in the brain help us to focus on the person we want to hear while simultaneously suppressing competing sounds coming from different locations. The target speech appears to *pop out* from the competition, so to speak. The technical term for this process is spatial release from masking—or spatial processing—and it allows us to take in the vital information we need to be able to comprehend speech and participate in conversations. But what if we didn't have this ability? What if we when we were listening to speech in noise nothing seemed to *pop out*, but instead all we could hear was a jumble of sounds? We would most likely

fail to hear key information, limiting our ability to communicate effectively. This is exactly what happens to children and adults with spatial processing disorder (SPD).

In this chapter we discuss how spatial processing assists in communication and the underlying mechanisms involved. We also discuss how deficits in spatial processing ability impact listeners, particularly children who, despite normal hearing thresholds and cognitive ability, have difficulty understanding speech in the classroom when background noise is present. Difficulty understanding speech when there is competing speech or other types of background noise is a commonly reported symptom of central auditory processing disorder (CAPD) (Bamiou, Musiek, & Luxon, 2001; Jerger & Musiek, 2000; Vanniasegaram, Cohen, & Rosen,

2004). We are certainly not suggesting that spatial processing disorder is the only cause of difficulty understanding speech in background noise for children with normal hearing thresholds, but it is an important cause. For many children, it is the only cause. The main focus of the chapter involves the remediation of spatial processing disorder using the LiSN & Learn, a deficit-specific computer-based auditory training program.

Spatial Processing and Communication

Normal hearing listeners effortlessly communicate in very complex acoustic environments that may contain multiple sound sources, as well as room reverberation. In such adverse conditions, the auditory system takes advantage of the temporal-spectral dynamics of the acoustic input at the two ears to analyze the spatial acoustic scene and thus, to understand speech. For example, listeners can use differences in sound source directions to perceptually separate target speech from one or more interfering sources (Cherry, 1953; Hirsch, 1950). This can result in a significant improvement in speech intelligibility.

As previously mentioned, the benefit gained from spatially separating distracting noise from a target signal is known as spatial release from masking (SRM), or alternatively *spatial advantage* (Bronkhorst, 2000; Cameron, Dillon, & Newall, 2006a; Darwin, 2008; Yost, 1997; Zurek, 1993). Spatial advantage is particularly large (as much as 14 dB depending on age) when maskers are also speech signals (Behrens, Neher, & Johannesson, 2008; Cameron & Dillon, 2007a; Jones & Litovski, 2011; Marrone, Mason, & Kidd

2008a). As shown in Figure 8–1, spatial advantage improves with increasing age until late adolescence and remains stable until at least age 60 (Brown, Cameron, Martin, Watson, & Dillon, 2010; Cameron & Dillon, 2007a; Cameron, Dillon, & Newall, 2006b; Cameron et al., 2009; Cameron, Glyde, & Dillon, 2011; Glyde, Cameron, Dillon, Hickson, & Seeto, 2013).

Crandell and Smaldino (1995) reported that the accurate perception of speech—which is essential for academic achievement—is particularly degraded by noises with spectra similar to the speech spectrum, as these are most effective at masking speech cues (although this effectiveness is influenced by fluctuations in the intensity of the noise over time). Noise generated within a classroom, including children talking, is said to be the most detrimental to a child's ability to perceive speech, because the frequency content of the noise is spectrally similar to the teacher's voice. Thus, the ability of children to utilize spatial processing mechanisms to separate their teacher's voice from background noise is critical to their ability to understand speech in the classroom.

Mechanisms Underlying Spatial Processing

Sensing sounds in two ears is referred to as binaural hearing. Binaural hearing makes it possible for a person to locate the source of sounds in the horizontal plane (Dillon, 2012). However, the main benefit of binaural hearing to humans is to aid the detection of sounds in noisy environments (Moore, 1991). Accurate horizontal localization of sounds coming from a particular location is made

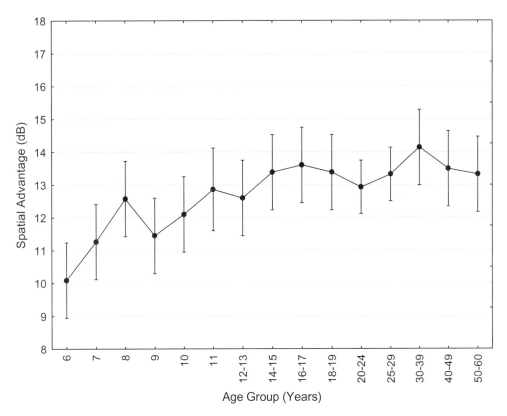

Figure 8–1. Normative data for the spatial advantage measure of the LiSN-S (*n* = 202). Error bars represent the 95% confidence intervals from the mean. (Adapted from Cameron et al., 2011, with permission.)

possible by analysis of differences in the arrival time and the intensity of such sound between the two ears. Sounds arrive at the ear closer to the source before they arrive at the ear farther away. The resulting difference in arrival time at the two ears is called the interaural time difference (ITD). ITD is zero for sounds located directly in front of the listener (i.e., 0° aximuth) and increases to a maximum of about 0.7 ms for sounds coming from 90°, relative to the front. Because any time delay leads to a phase delay, an ITD results in an interaural phase delay. Furthermore, head diffraction produces an attenuation of sound on the side of the

head farther from the sound source and a boost on the side of the head nearer to the sound source, referred to as interaural level differences (ILDs).

The initial detection of interaural time and intensity differences occurs at the superior olivary complex (SOC; Reuss, 2000), which is located bilaterally at the base of the brainstem in the caudal portion of the pons, ventral and medial to the cochlear nuclei (CN). Neurons within the medial superior olivary nuclei (MSO) receive phase-locked excitatory input to low-frequency stimuli (and the envelopes of high-frequency stimuli) bilaterally from the CN. Responses to ITD similar to those recorded at the MSO are also recorded in the lateral superior olivary nuclei (LSO), except that the input from the contralateral CN is changed from excitatory to inhibitory at the trapezoid body (Fitzpatrick, Kuwada, & Batra, 2002). The LSO also is implicated in the detection of ILDs (Grothe, 2000). Inhibitory and excitatory responses from the CN that are used to code ITD in the MSO and LSO of the SOC are preserved in the inferior colliculus (IC). Cohen and Knudsen (1999) stated that a *space map* is formed in the nontonotopic subdivisions of the IC, where information about spatial cues is combined across frequency channels, yielding neurons that are broadly tuned for frequency and finely tuned for sound source location. Afferents from the IC are relayed to the primary (A1) and secondary (A2) auditory cortex via the medial geniculate body (MGB) (Pickles, 1988). Animal research has shown that the locations of sound sources are represented in a distributed fashion within individual auditory cortical areas and among multiple cortical areas with similar degrees of location sensitivity, including A1 and A2 (Middlebrooks, Xu, Furukawa, & Macpherson, 2002). However, these authors suggest that the special role of the auditory cortex is only in distributing preprocessed information about sound-source location to appropriate perceptual and motor stations, not actual computation of source locations. Other cortical areas might utilize auditory spatial information from A1 and A2 to perform functions that are not overtly spatial, but the spatial information might assist those functions by helping to segregate multiple sound sources.

Thus, although both localization and spatial release from masking rely on intensity and time differences between the two ears, there is no reason to believe that the two phenomena rely on the same brain processes using these cues. Based on observations of patients with damage to specific brain regions, it seems unlikely that the same brain processes are responsible for both abilities (Litovsky, Fligor, & Tramo, 2002; Thiran & Clarke, 2003). When the task of a listener is to understand a speech signal presented in noise, the improvement in speech reception threshold (SRT) relative to diotic stimulation is referred to as the binaural intelligibility level difference (BILD). Whereas both ITDs and ILDs contribute to BILD, recent studies have shown that in people with normal hearing, ILDs are the dominant mechanism enabling spatial release from masking when speech maskers are symmetrically positioned around the listener and a target talker is in front of the listener (Glyde, Buchholz, Dillon, Cameron, & Hickson, 2013). Moment-by-moment fluctuations in the amplitude and spectrum of each masker cause one masker to dominate over the other at each specific frequency and point in time. At that frequency and point in time, the ear on the side of the head opposite to the dominant masker has a better signal-to-noise ratio (SNR) than the ear closer to the dominant masker. Referred to as *cross-ear dip listening* (Brungart & Iyer, 2012; Glyde et al., in press), this dynamic process, originally hypothesized by Zurek (1993), involves integrating information across the two ears, by selecting, separately for each frequency band, the signal from the ear with the better SNR at each point in time. Cross-ear dip listening effectively creates an optimal signal that has a better SNR than that available at either ear.

Diagnosing Deficits in Spatial Processing

As for other types of CAPD, it is essential that any test of SPD not spuriously indicate the presence of SPD as a consequence of the child having a memory, attention, or language disorder. The LiSN-S is an adaptive speech-in-noise test conducted under headphones that has been designed to avoid such confusions. The target and distracter (i.e., masker) sounds are speech materials that have been synthesized with head-related transfer functions in order to create a three-dimensional effect (Brown et al., 2009; Cameron & Dillon, 2007; Cameron et al., 2011a). A simple repetition-response protocol is used to assess a listener's speech reception threshold (SRT), which is defined as the SNR that yields 50% intelligibility. The target stimuli (sentences) are spoken by a female speaker and always appear to emanate from 0° azimuth (directly in front of the listener). The distracters (looped children's stories) are manipulated so that they appear to come from either 0° azimuth (collocated) or ±90° azimuth simultaneously (spatially separated). The distracter stories are spoken by either the same female speaker as the target sentences or two different female speakers. This test configuration results in four listening conditions: same voice at 0° (or low cue SRT); same voice at ±90°; different voices at 0°; and different voices at ±90° (or high cue SRT), as shown in Figure 8–2.

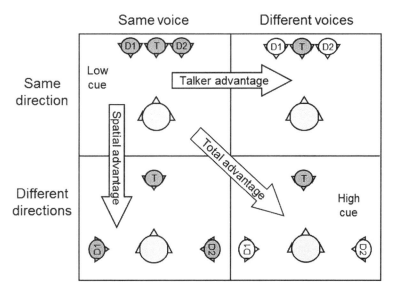

Figure 8–2. The four subtests of the LiSN-S test, and the three difference scores (advantage measures) that can be derived from them. The target speech, T, always comes from the front, whereas the two distracter stories, D1 and D2, come from the front or the sides, in different conditions. D1 and D2 can be the same voice as T or different voices. (Adapted from Cameron et al., 2011, with permission.)

Performance on the LiSN-S is evaluated on the low and high cue SRT conditions, as well as on three derived *advantage* measures. These advantage measures represent the benefit in decibels (dB) gained when either talker (pitch), spatial, or both talker and spatial cues are incorporated in the maskers, compared with the baseline (low cue SRT) condition where no talker or spatial cues are present in the maskers. It is the use of these advantage measures that avoids any chance of an attention, memory or language disorder leading to a false designation of a SPD. Any of these conditions could lead to elevated (i.e., poorer) SRTs, but there is no reason why they would consistently increase the SRTs more in the spatially separated conditions than in the collocated conditions. The impact of higher order processes on diagnosis of CAPD is discussed further in the following section.

Spatial Processing Deficits in Children With Normal Hearing Thresholds

The LiSN-S test can detect spatial processing deficits in children with suspected CAPD (SusCAPD) whose primary difficulties in the classroom stem from poor listening behavior, despite having normal hearing thresholds. Cameron, Dillon, and Newall (2006c) used a prototype of the LiSN-S test, to assess a group of 10 children who presented with difficulties hearing in the classroom but who tested as having no routine audiological or language, learning, or attention deficits. The spatial advantage measure for the 10 children was significantly poorer (p <.000001) than for a group of 48 normally hearing, age-matched controls. Nine of the 10 children were outside normal lim-

its on this task (on average by 5 standard deviations). In contrast, none of the 10 children were outside normal limits on the baseline condition where the maskers were co-located (low-cue SRT measure).

Cameron and Dillon (2008) assessed a group of 9 children (SusCAPD group) on both the LiSN-S and a traditional CAPD test battery (Pitch Pattern Test, Dichotic Digits, Random Gap Detection Test, and Masking Level Difference Test). The SusCAPD group presented with difficulties hearing in the classroom in the absence of any routine audiological or language, learning, or attention deficits to explain such a difficulty. In order to study the effect of higher order deficits on the LiSN-S, a group of 11 children (LD group) were also included in the study who presented with a range of documented learning or attention disorders, such as auditory memory deficits, dyslexia, specific language impairments, and attention deficit hyperactivity disorder. There were no significant differences on any LiSN-S performance measure between the LD group and 70 age-matched controls (p ranging from .983 to .136). There were, however, significant differences between the SusCAPD group and the controls, but only on the LiSN-S conditions where the physical location of the maskers was different from that of the target speaker (high cue SRT, p = .001; spatial advantage, p <.0001; and total advantage, p <.0001). These results support Jerger's (1998) hypothesis that a high proportion of children with suspected CAPD have a deficit in the mechanisms that normally use the spatial distribution of sources to suppress unwanted signals. (Note, however, that the proportion will be distorted if the assessment process ascertains the presence of memory, attention, and language deficits that may co-occur with CAPD.)

The LiSN-S did not correlate significantly with any test in the traditional central auditory test battery, nor were the nonspatial and spatial performance measures of the LiSN-S correlated. This is the result one would expect if the only problem these children had involved spatial processing, and the only test conditions affected by spatial processing were the spatially separated conditions of the LiSN-S. The average spatial advantage score for the SusCAPD group was 2.0 standard deviations below the age-appropriate mean score, whereas the average for the LD group was only 0.1 standard deviation below the age-appropriate mean. All the children in the SusCAPD group performed within normal limits on the traditional central auditory test battery, except for one participant who was just outside normal limits on the dichotic digit test. One child in the LD group (who presented with an auditory memory deficit) was outside normal limits on both the left and right ear conditions of the dichotic digit test. Two other participants in the LD group were outside the normal range on the pitch pattern test. All other children in the LD group performed within normal limits on the traditional battery.

Some readers might wonder how the children in the SusCAPD group could have such a deficit in spatial processing ability and yet pass a commonly used CAPD test battery. This should not be a surprise when one realizes that none of the tests in the standard battery attempt to test the same auditory skills as those assessed in spatially separated condition of the LiSN-S. This pattern is therefore precisely what would be expected for children who had reduced ability to separate a target sound from competing sounds on the basis of their direction of

arrival but had no other deficit in their auditory processing ability.

Finally, as noted by Chermak, Bellis, and Musiek (2007), the clinician must be aware that a difficulty understanding spoken language in the presence of competing noise can be caused by deficits other than a CAPD. Inadequate language resources may prevent the child from using linguistic knowledge to compensate for the degraded signal. Similarly, attention-based deficits can interfere with the child's ability to selectively attend to a target signal. To mitigate the impact of higher order functions on LiSN-S performance, spatial processing is quantified by calculating the difference in dB between two test conditions where only one variable (spatial location) is manipulated. As such, it is expected that the child's higher order processing ability will equally affect the SRT when the distracters are presented at 0° and when they are spatially separated at ±90°. Language and executive functioning should have minimal effect on the difference in dB between the SRTs in these two conditions (see the spatial advantage measure in Figure 8–2). Thus, the differences that inevitably exist between individuals in such functions is controlled for, allowing for clearer evaluation of their abilities to use spatial cues to aid speech understanding (Brown et al., 2010; Cameron et al., 2011).

Spatial Processing Disorder— Diagnosis, Prevalence, and Management Options

Children who present with a pattern of depressed scores on the spatially separated conditions of the LiSN-S (high cue SRT, spatial advantage and total advantage) combined with near-normal scores on the co-located conditions (low cue SRT and talker advantage) are said to have a spatial processing disorder, or SPD (Cameron & Dillon, 2011; Cameron, Glyde & Dillon, 2012). In other words, SPD is diagnosed by looking at the individual's pattern of results on the LiSN-S. However there are many small variations to this typical scenario, such as performance just inside normal limits on spatial advantage or performance well above normal limits on another measure (such as low cue SRT and/or talker advantage), and these can be more difficult for a clinician to interpret. To minimize any error in the interpretation of LiSN-S results caused by these other scenarios, the LiSN-S relies on a *spatial pattern measure*, as described in Cameron and Dillon (2011), which is equal to the release from masking provided by spatial separation, averaged across both the same voice and different voice contexts. The spatial pattern measure is therefore a better indicator of whether a set of LiSN-S results is indicative of a spatial processing disorder. The pattern measure score, which is calculated automatically by the LiSN-S software, is more reliable than just observing the spatial advantage score alone, as it uses all four LiSN-S condition scores in its calculation. Like the other measures, the spatial pattern measure score is described as being outside normal limits if the result is more than two standard deviations from the age-adjusted mean. This criterion has some degree of arbitrariness: Deviations much greater than this indicate a deficit more serious than deviations only slightly greater than two standard deviations. Similarly, deviations between one and two standard deviations below the mean may still be associated with greater than average difficulty in communicating in noise.

Dillon, Cameron, Glyde, Wilson, and Tomlin (2012) reported that 17% of children referred for assessment for CAPD across various studies have been diagnosed with SPD. A large proportion of the children in these studies presented with a history of chronic otitis media. Reduced transmission through the middle ear can disturb interaural differences in two ways. First, asymmetrical attenuation in the two ears will change the usual interaural level differences by the amount of the asymmetry. Second, if the attenuation is sufficiently great that the transmission path through bone conduction induced by the incoming sound field vibrating the whole skull is comparable to the transmission path through the impaired middle ear system, interaural time differences may also be disturbed. This is because the time differences applicable to the bone conduction path are much less than those for the air conduction path (Stenfelt, 2005). It may be hypothesized that fluctuating access to the normal binaural cues may negatively influence the development of spatial processing mechanisms within the central auditory nervous system.

SPD might be managed through the provision of an assistive listening device, such as an FM system or other remote-microphone hearing aid, in order to improve the signal-to-noise ratio in the classroom. In addition, a child with SPD can be seated at the front of the class. Central resources training can also be provided to help the child to compensate for their disorder by utilizing high-order cognitive skills to deduce the meaning implied from fragmented information received (see Chapter 10 for Chermak's overview of intervention incorporating cognitive, metacognitive, and metalinguistic skills and strategies). However, as mentioned by Dawes and Bishop (2009), the aim of such approaches is to lessen the impact of the impairment, rather than attempting to ameliorate the auditory problems directly. Below we discuss auditory training to ameliorate SPD.

Spatial Processing Deficits in People With Hearing Impairment

Spatial processing ability is often reduced in listeners with hearing impairment who commonly report difficulty in understanding speech in background noise despite amplification (Gelfand, Ross & Miller, 1988; Helfer & Freyman, 2008; Glyde et al., 2013; Marrone, Mason & Kidd., 2008b). Glyde et al. (2013) assessed 80 adults and children aged 7 to 89 years, with a wide range of hearing thresholds. They were tested on a version of the Listening in Spatialized Noise–Sentences Test (LiSN-S; Cameron & Dillon, 2009) that incorporated individually prescribed frequency-dependent amplification of the target and distracter stimuli. Those with a hearing impairment were less able than normal hearers to use spatial cues to help them understand speech in noise. In fact, even very mild hearing losses were associated with spatial processing deficits and as hearing loss worsened so did spatial processing ability. This result was not significantly correlated with age or cognition.

In people with hearing impairment, reduced audibility (which effectively lessens access to the weaker speech sounds that remain unmasked in the ear

closer to the momentarily weaker distracter) explains most of their observed spatial processing deficits (Glyde et al., manuscript in preparation). The remaining deficit may perhaps be explained by reduced ability to use cross-ear dip listening mechanisms, most likely due to widened auditory bands in the cochlea, and/or by reduced temporal processing that restricts the ability to use ITD information to differentiate the frontal target from the nonfrontal distracters (Glyde et al., in preparation b).

Overview of the LiSN & Learn Auditory Training Software

The LiSN & Learn software was developed as an at-home training system to specifically remediate SPD (Cameron & Dillon, 2011; Cameron et al., 2012). As such, this training is intended to remedy the deficit observed in children who perform outside the normal range on the LiSN-S. It is therefore training the ability to hear in spatially separated noise, not the ability to localize the direction from which individual sounds emanate. The LiSN & Learn software produces a three-dimensional auditory environment under headphones (Sennheiser HD215) on a personal computer. There were four training games in the research software: Listening House, Listening Ladder, Goal Game, and Answer Alley. An additional game, Space Maze, was added to the commercial version of the software (Cameron & Dillon, 2012), along with various motivational and reward features as described below.

Speech Stimuli and Spatialization

In the four standard LiSN & Learn games the child's task is to identify a single word from a target sentence presented in background noise (two looped children's stories). All the target sentences are six words in length (e.g., The clown dropped three red cars). A total of 136 semantic items were used to develop a base list of 324 sentences. The sentences were recorded, synthesized with head related transfer functions (HRTFs), and edited into individual words (with each word maintaining its coarticulation). An algorithm was developed to generate natural-sounding target sentences from these individual words. In total, 131,220 unique sentences can be generated by the software. Ninety of the 136 semantic items (nouns, verbs, and adjectives) were utilized as the target words that the listener was required to identify. All the target words are acquired by 30 months of age (Fenson et al., 1992).

Akin to the Same Voice 90° condition of the LiSN-S, the LiSN & Learn target sentences appear to come from directly in front of the listener (at 0° azimuth), whereas the competing speech appears to come from either side of the listener simultaneously (+ and −90° azimuth). The sentences and competing stories are all spoken by the same female speaker, so the child must rely on spatial cues (i.e., differences in the physical location of the speech streams) to be able to distinguish the sentence (and hence the target word) from the distracting speech. A tone burst is presented before each sentence to alert the child that a sentence will be presented.

In the four standard games, four images and a question mark appear at the top of the screen immediately following the presentation of the sentence. In a five-alternative, forced-choice, adaptive method, the child uses the computer mouse to select either one of the images that matches a word from the sentence he or she had just heard or to make an *unsure* response by selecting an image of a question mark (Figure 8–3).

As previously noted, an additional game, Space Maze, was added when the commercial version of the software was released. In this game the child hears an instruction (e.g., *move up three spaces*) and must use the computer mouse to select a direction (up, down, left, right) and a number (from 1 to 10) in order to move around the maze. The direction and number buttons remain on the screen throughout the game. When the child gets four instructions correct, the maze graphical user interface (GUI) changes so that the child remains entertained by the visual properties of the game (Figure 8–4).

Training Hierarchy and Adaptive Difficulty Levels

The starting level of 7 dB SNR utilized in the LiSN-S diagnostic test is also used in the LiSN & Learn training program. This starting level was chosen to ensure that the child could begin training with relatively high success. A weighted up-down adaptive procedure is used to adjust the signal level of the target based on the child's response. The advantage of an adaptive program is that the task can continually adjust to more difficult levels as the listener answers correctly. Specifically, the target sentence is decreased when the child correctly identifies the target image and increased if the wrong

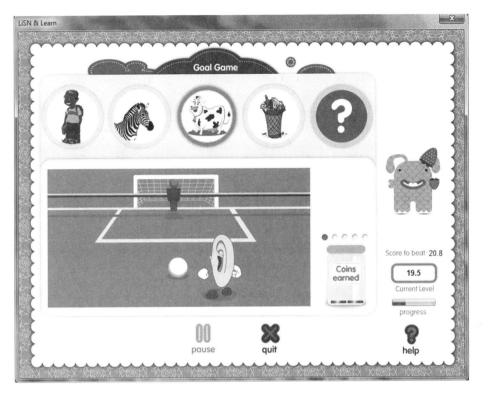

Figure 8–3. Image of a LiSN & Learn training game from Cameron and Dillon (2012).

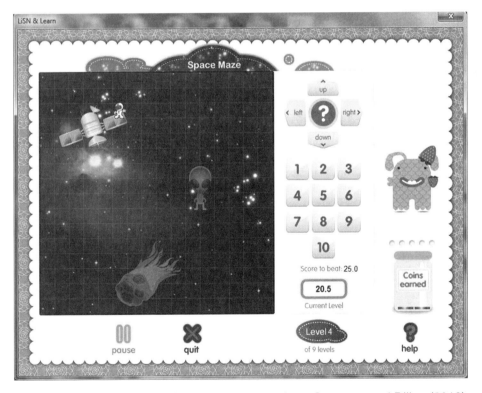

Figure 8–4. Image of the Space Maze game from Cameron and Dillon (2012).

image or an "unsure" (question mark) response is made. Thus, after an incorrect response, the difficulty level is lowered so that the next trial is more likely to be completed correctly. Such a tracking rule may be considered more enjoyable by some children (Bamiou, Campbell, & Sirimanna, 2006; Thibodeau, 2007) and therefore contribute to program completion.

A minimum of five sentences are provided as practice; however, practice continues until one upward reversal in performance has been recorded. There are 40 sentences in any game. The child's SRT for each game is measured as the average SNR over all sentences, excluding the practice.

Calibration is undertaken at startup using a reference signal (whooshing sound) that is adjusted by the child using a slider bar. The child is instructed to move the slider bar until he or she can barely hear the whooshing sound. The reference signal is level normalized so that its rms level is 40 dB less than the rms level of the combined distracters. Thus, when presented, the sensation level of the combined distracters is at least 40 dB SL.

Feedback, Positive Reinforcement, and Motivation

In line with the principles of learning theory (Wolfle, 1951), information regarding a child's performance during a game is provided following each response and this feedback is tailored to the GUI used for each particular game. For example, when the child makes a correct response in Answer Alley, the LiSN & Learn Ear knocks over the all the bowling pins and the word "strike" is heard over the headphones. This type of positive reinforcement encourages the child to persist with the training despite increasing difficulty (Thibodeau, 2007). In a review of research on computer-aided auditory rehabilitation, Sweetow and Henderson Sabes (2010) stipulated that measurement and feedback to the user should be provided regarding progress or lack of progress. As such, feedback is also provided by presenting the child's score at any point in the LiSN & Learn game in the "Current Level" box following each response. A progress bar shows the child how far through the game they have progressed.

As well as providing engaging graphics, feedback, positive reinforcement, and progress indicators, external motivators are incorporated in the commercial version of the software to motivate the child to continue training over the course of the treatment schedule. When the software is installed, the user is prompted to create a "buddy," who provides additional feedback during the game in the form of speech bubbles, such as "well done." The buddy is an avatar that the child designs from a number of options, including the buddy's shape, color, and facial features. Additional motivators are provided in the form of "LiSN & Learn currency" that children earn for identifying correct target words and for beating their best game score. LiSN & Learn currency can be used by the child in the LiSN & Learn Reward Shop to play nontraining games incorporated in the software and to buy accessories for their buddy (Figure 8–5).

Some children may require additional motivators in the form of physical rewards. Reward charts can be downloaded from the LiSN & Learn Additional Resources section of the National Acoustic Laboratories

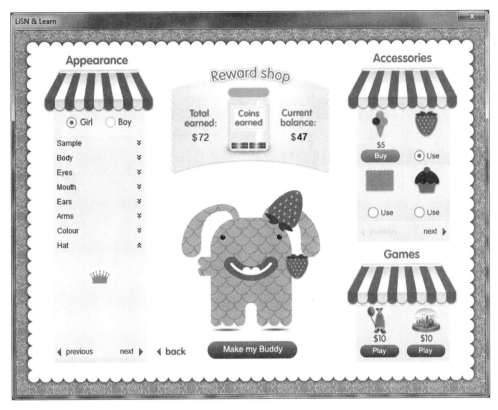

Figure 8–5. Image of the LiSN & Learn Reward Shop from Cameron and Dillon (2012).

CAPD website (http://capd.nal.gov.au/). It is also suggested that a caregiver be present during each training session to motivate the child to focus and do their best while training.

LiSN & Learn Research Studies

According to Chermak et al. (2007), the effectiveness of deficit-specific auditory intervention should be gauged, primarily, by improvements seen on central auditory tests, as well as concomitant improvement in functional listening skills. In a preliminary study, Cameron and Dillon (2011) aimed to evaluate the effectiveness of the

LiSN & Learn to remediate SPD based on the abovementioned principles. A second study (Cameron et al., 2012) aimed to determine whether improvements in the ability to understand speech in noise in children diagnosed with SPD following training with the LiSN & Learn were specific to that training program, or if such improvements might occur following exposure to *any* computer-based auditory training software. Both studies were conducted using the research version of the software (i.e., without the Space Maze game and reward shop). All training occurred in the client's own home, except for one child in the Cameron and Dillon (2011) study, who trained for part of the time at school under his teacher's supervision.

Preliminary Study

Nine children aged between 6 and 11 years with normal peripheral hearing took part in the Cameron and Dillon (2011) study. All participants were diagnosed with SPD using the LiSN-S. The participants trained on the LiSN & Learn for 15 minutes a day, five days a week for three months, until they had completed 120 games. Participants were assessed on the LiSN-S, as well as on the auditory subtests of Test of Variables of Attention (TOVA; Greenberg, Kindschi, Dupuy, & Hughes, 2007), the memory subtest of the Test of Auditory Processing Skills–3 (TAPS-3; Martin & Brownell, 2005) and a version of the Speech, Spatial and Qualities of Hearing Scale questionnaire (SSQ; Noble & Gatehouse 2004) developed by Flinders University in South Australia specifically for children with CAPD. In order to determine whether any improvements in performance were maintained, performance on all tasks was reassessed after three months posttraining.

It was found that SRTs on the LiSN & Learn improved on average by 10 dB over the course of training (Figure 8–6). At the end of the training period, there

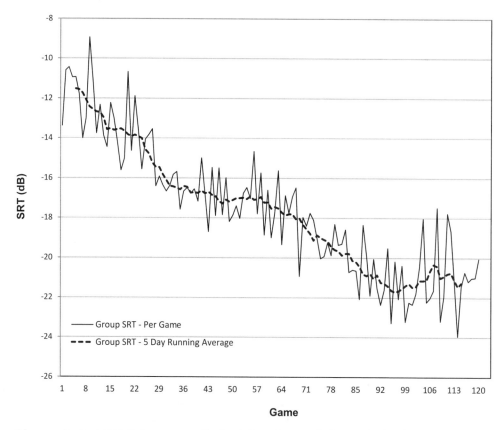

Figure 8–6. LiSN & Learn results from the start until the end of training, averaged across the nine children from the Cameron and Dillon (2011) study. Performance is measured as the speech reception threshold (SRT) in decibels achieved over the 120 games played. (Adapted from Cameron & Dillon, 2011, with permission.)

was no significant improvement on the two control conditions of the LiSN-S (low cue SRT and talker advantage) where the target and distracters all emanated from 0° azimuth (p ranging from .07 to .86, η^2 ranging from 0.362 to 0.004). In contrast, all of the children improved significantly on the three conditions of the LiSN-S that evaluate spatial processing (p ranging from <.003 to .0001, η^2 ranged from 0.694 to 0.873) and were all performing within normal limits (Figure 8–7). SRTs in the high cue condition (which is the condition most similar to real life listening) improved by an average of 2.4 standard deviations (3.9 dB). For all but one of the children these improvements were

maintained after a three-month period without any further training.

Significant improvements were also found posttraining on the memory subtest of the TAPS-3 and in commission errors on the TOVA. These improvements were not seen as being specific to the LiSN & Learn spatial discrimination training. Rather, we attributed improvements in the memory tests to the nature of the LiSN & Learn task, which required remembering a sentence while selecting a matching image. We attributed improvements in attention to increased auditory vigilance attained from playing the LiSN & Learn games five days a week over the three-month training period. Importantly

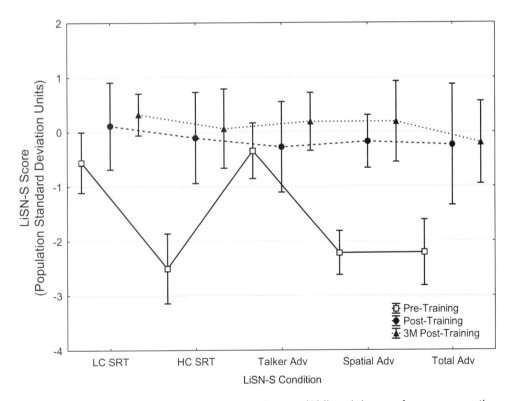

Figure 8–7. Pre-, post-, and three-month post-(3M) training performance on the LiSN-S for the nine children in the Cameron and Dillon (2011) study. Performance is expressed in population standard deviation units from the mean. Error bars represent 95% confidence intervals. (Adapted from Cameron & Dillon, 2011, with permission.)

though, participants reported a very significant improvement posttraining in their ability to understand speech in noisy environments ($p = .000007$, $\eta^2 = 0.930$). The average rating on a modified version of the SSQ developed for children with CAPD improved from 3.10 (between "hard" and "very hard") to 1.78 (between "easy" and "OK"). There were no significant differences between post- and three-month posttraining scores on any of the assessment tools. It was concluded that the initial LiSN & Learn study showed that children as young as 6 years of age were able to complete the training (although some coaxing was needed in a minority of cases) and that training led to significant improvements in spatial processing ability.

Randomized Blinded Controlled Study

Cameron et al. (2012) utilized a randomized blinded controlled design to evaluate whether posttraining improvements in spatial processing ability in children diagnosed with SPD were specific to LiSN & Learn or if training with nonspatially separated stimuli could also result in improvements in this ability as measured with the LiSN-S. Participants were 10 children between 6 and 9 years of age who were diagnosed as having SPD with the LiSN-S. The children were randomly allocated to train with either the LiSN & Learn or another auditory training program—Earobics Home Version (Cognitive Concepts, 2008)—for approximately 15 minutes per day for 12 weeks. The Earobics software provides training on phonological awareness, auditory processing, and language processing skills through a number of interactive com-

puter games. Specifically, the program consists of audiovisual exercises, presented either in quiet or in nonspatialized noise, that incorporate training in phoneme discrimination, auditory memory, auditory sequencing, auditory attention, rhyming, and sound blending skills (Hayes, Warrier, Nichol, Zecker, & Kraus, 2003). Participant, parent, and teacher questionnaires as detailed below were administered to determine the real-life listening benefit of the training. The children and their parents and teachers were blinded as to whether the participant was in the experimental or control group.

Over the course of training, the experimental group improved on average by 10.9 dB in respect to their SRT on the LiSN & Learn. As expected, based on the 2011 preliminary study, there were no significant improvements posttraining by either the LiSN & Learn or Earobics group on the control conditions of the LiSN-S where the target and distracter stimuli were co-located. Also, as expected, there was a significant improvement posttraining on the LiSN-S scores that were affected by spatial processing ability for the LiSN & Learn group ($p = .03$ to $.0008$, $\eta^2 = 0.75$ to 0.95, $n = 5$). As hypothesized, there was no significant improvement on these scores for the children who had trained with the Earobics software ($p = .5$ to $.7$, $\eta^2 = 0.1$ to 0.04, $n = 5$), as shown in Figure 8–8. SRT in the high cue condition (the condition most similar to real-life listening condition) improved on average by 2.7 standard deviations (4.4 dB) for the LiSN & Learn group but only by 0.4 standard deviations (1.0 dB) for the Earobics group.

In respect to measures of real-world listening ability, group results of posttraining listening performance by children, parents, and teachers also reflected

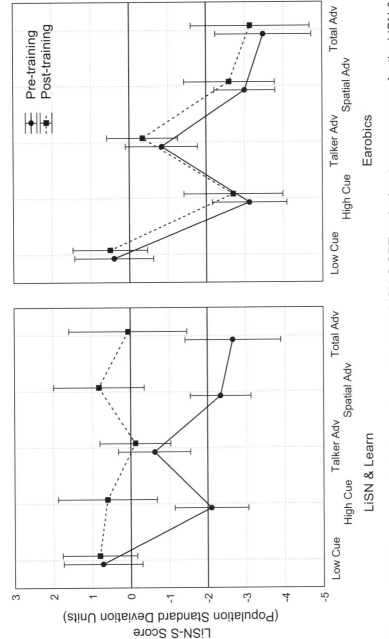

Figure 8–8. Pre- and posttraining performance on the LiSN-S SRT and advantage measures for the LiSN & Learn group compared with the Earobics group for the 10 children in the Cameron et al. (2012) study. Performance is expressed in population standard deviation units from the mean. Error bars represent 95% confidence intervals. (Adapted from Cameron et al., 2012, with permission.)

posttraining LiSN-S performance in the two groups. On the self-reported questionnaire, the Listening Inventory For Education (LIFE)–Student (Anderson & Smaldino, 1998a), the children in the LiSN & Learn group rated their own listening skills as improving by 22% posttraining compared with 9% in the Earobics group. The teacher questionnaire was the LIFE-Teacher (Anderson & Smaldino, 1998b), which utilizes an incremental listening improvement rating scale from −35 to +35, where 0 is considered "No Change: Benefit of Use Not Identified" and 17 is considered "Support for Positive Change: Use is Beneficial." The LiSN & Learn group showed a mean posttraining improvement rating of 15.8 compared with 6.6 for the Earobics group. Using Fisher's Auditory Problems Checklist (Fisher, 2008), parents reported that the listening skills of children in the LiSN & Learn group had improved on average by 31% following training, compared with 8% for the children in the Earobics group. The increase in parent-reported scores for the experimental group was significantly larger than for the controls (p = .028).

It was concluded that LiSN & Learn training improved binaural processing ability in children with SPD, enhancing their ability to understand speech in noise, as directly measured in the spatially separated conditions of the LiSN-S test. These results were specific to the LiSN & Learn training protocol, as expected. Exposure to nonspatialized auditory training did not produce similar outcomes, emphasizing the importance of deficit-specific remediation.

Improvements in academic performance following training were not specifically measured in either the preliminary LiSN & Learn study or the randomized

blinded control study. A child with SPD characteristically presents as not understanding speech in the classroom as well as his or her peers, most notably when background noise is present. It should be noted that the typical presenting profile of a child with SPD is a history of chronic otitis media, not a language or learning disorder (Cameron & Dillon, 2008). The SPD itself may result in auditory fatigue. The child may also miss important information during lessons if the listening environment is noisy. Following training, a general improvement in listening ability in the classroom and reductions in auditory fatigue that will benefit general classroom performance over time is expected, as found from posttraining self-report, parent, and teacher questionnaires (Cameron & Dillon, 2011; Cameron et al., 2012). Improvements in any academic area that had suffered due to a child's difficulties hearing in noise over time due to SPD would likely take some time to reverse, possibly requiring additional, specialized tutoring if the child was seriously behind his or her peers.

Other Considerations

System Requirements and Headphones

The LiSN & Learn software is designed for use in the child's home, avoiding the need for daily trips to a clinic. Version 3.0.0 of the software can be installed on any PC running Windows XP, Vista, 7 or 8. It is recommended that Sennheiser HD215 headphones, provided with the software, be used during playback as the stimuli have been filtered to correct for the response of these specific headphones (Cameron & Dillon, 2011).

Treatment Schedule and Environment

The recommended training schedule is for the child to play 2 LiSN & Learn games per day, five days per week, until at least 100 games have been completed. As each game takes about 5 to 10 minutes to complete, this program can generally be completed by training for 15 minutes per day for 10 weeks. Chermak and Musiek (2002) stipulate that auditory training should be conducted in an intensive manner, and suggest five to seven sessions be scheduled weekly. The authors further noted that research has shown that regular and consistent training for as little as 10 to 15 minutes a day over a number of weeks provides the intensity needed to maximize success in the training task.

Bellis (2002) points out that because therapy is costly in terms of time and money, research is needed to determine the frequency and intensity of a particular therapy that is necessary but sufficient to achieve desired results. A total of 120 games were played in the Cameron and Dillon (2011) and Cameron et al. (2012) studies. However, as can be seen from Figure 8–6, maximum improvement in SRT (around 10 dB) is achieved by around game 95. Once children achieve their maximum improvement, it becomes more challenging to continue training, as they are less likely to beat a previous high score, and as a consequence reward currency is earned less frequently. At this point the child should be encouraged to

continue playing until the minimum 100 game level has been reached in order to consolidate the improvements in skills already achieved.

A graph of the child's progress over time can be accessed by the parent from the main menu by selecting the *Progress Report* button. The parent is also able to generate progress reports that can be forwarded to any professional involved in the child's management program.

Of course, training can be conducted in any environment, including schools, as long as the training can occur on a daily basis, the environment is quiet, and the child is not distracted by other children or nearby activities. It is recommended that, particularly for younger children, an adult supervise training to ensure that the child stays on task throughout each training session (Figure 8–9).

Whereas the software was designed for children aged between 6 and 11 years, it could be used with older children as long as he or she is prepared to accept that the software is tailored for younger children and does not become disheartened with the GUI. It should be noted that research has not be conducted to determine the efficacy of training with anyone over the age of 12 years.

Finally, Cameron and Dillon (2011) found that spatial processing ability was maintained three months posttraining with no further use of the LiSN & Learn. However, once a child has completed the recommended number of training games, he or she may wish to use the software occasionally to check that their spatial processing, measured as an SRT on the various LiSN & Learn games, has not deteriorated. Simple real-world listening strategies should also be practiced, such as maintaining eye contact with the

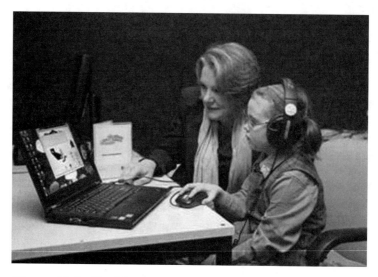

Figure 8–9. Sophie, age 7, using the LiSN & Learn software with her mother, Sonia. July 2012. (Used with permission.)

target speaker and avoiding any activity, such as fidgeting, that diverts attention from the speaker.

Summary

In this chapter, we have discussed the diagnosis and remediation of spatial processing disorder (SPD), which is a specific type of CAPD. SPD presents as a markedly reduced ability to selectively attend to sounds coming from one direction and suppress sounds coming from other directions. The disorder likely results from an inability to utilize binaural cues, such as variances in interaural time and intensity differences between speech streams, and consequent differences in target-to-masker SNRs at the two ears, to separate a target auditory stimulus from distracting auditory stimuli. As is common in CAPD, SPD leads to difficulty in understanding speech in noisy situations. The exact cause of SPD in children with

normal hearing thresholds is not known; however, we believe that it is much more likely to be present in children who have had prolonged or repeated bouts of otitis media during childhood.

SPD is differentially diagnosed by presenting target stimuli with and without spatial separation from competing signals. The Listening in Spatialized Noise–Sentences Test (LiSN-S) accomplishes this using speech processed through head-related transfer functions presented under headphones. Our research, presented in this chapter, demonstrates the potential to treat SPD successfully by giving children practice at listening to frontally oriented speech in the presence of competing signals coming from other directions. The LiSN & Learn auditory training program achieves this using sounds processed through head-related transfer functions and presented over headphones on the child's home computer. Research studies such as Cameron and Dillon (2011) have shown that 10 weeks' training at home (15 minutes per day, 5 days per week) is sufficient to remove all signs of SPD and results in improvements in spatial processing that are maintained without further training. Further, in a randomized blinded controlled study, Cameron et al. (2012) found that improvements in ability to understand speech in noise following training were specific to the LiSN & Learn training protocol and that exposure to nonspatialized auditory training does not produce similar outcomes. This research emphasizes the importance of deficit-specific remediation for SPD. The effect of the remediation in both studies was evident as improved speech in noise scores on LiSN-S test. The changes were also evident from the progressive improvement in SRT over the three months of training with the LiSN & Learn. Further changes were reflected in questionnaires addressing listening ability in real life.

References

Anderson, K. L., & Smaldino, J. J. (1998a). *The Listening Inventory for Education: An efficacy tool. Student appraisal of listening difficulty.* Tampa, FL: Educational Audiology Association.

Anderson, K. L., & Smaldino, J. J. (1998b). *The Listening Inventory for Education: An efficacy tool. Teacher appraisal of listening difficulty.* Tampa, FL: Educational Audiology Association.

Bamiou, D-E., Campbell, N., & Sirimanna, T. (2006). Management of auditory processing disorders. *Audiological Medicine, 4,* 46–56.

Bamiou, D-E., Musiek, F .E., & Luxon, L. M. (2001). Aetiology and clinical presentations of auditory processing disorders—a review. *Archives of Disease in Childhood, 85,* 361–365.

Behrens, T., Neher, T., & Johannesson, R. B. (2008). Evaluation of speech corpus for assessment of spatial release from masking. In T. Dau, J. M. Buchholz, J. Harte, & T. U. Christiansen (Eds.), *Auditory signal processing in hearing-impaired listeners* (pp. 449–457). Copenhagen, Denmark: Centertryk A/S.

Bellis, T. J. (2002). Auditory training: Principles and approaches for remediating and managing auditory processing disorders. *Seminars in Hearing, 23,* 297–308.

Bronkhorst, A. (2000). The cocktail party phenomenon: A review of research on speech intelligibility in multiple-talker conditions. *Acoustica, 86,* 117–128.

Brown, D., Cameron, S. Martin, J., Watson, C., & Dillon, H. (2010). The North American Listening in Spatialized Noise–Sentences Test (NA LiSN-S): Normative data and test-retest reliability studies for adolescents and young adults. *Journal of the American Academy of Audiology, 21,* 629–641.

Brungart, D. S., & Iyer, N. (2012). Better-ear glimpsing efficiency with symmetrically-placed interfering talkers. *Journal of the Acoustical Society of America, 132,* 2545–2556.

Cameron, S., Brown, D., Keith, R., Martin, J., Watson, C., & Dillon, H. (2009). Development of the North American Listening in Spatialized Noise–Sentences Test (NA LISN-S): Sentence equivalence, normative data and test-retest reliability studies. *Journal of the American Academy of Audiology, 20,* 128–146.

Cameron, S., & Dillon, H. (2008). The Listening in Spatialized Noise–Sentences Test: Comparison to prototype LISN test and results from children with either a suspected (central) auditory processing disorder of a confirmed language disorder. *Journal of the American Academy of Audiology, 19,* 377–391.

Cameron, S., & Dillon, H. (2009) *Listening in Spatialized Noise–Sentences test (LISN-S)* (Version 2.003) [Computer software]. Murten, Switzerland: Phonak Communications AG.

Cameron, S., & Dillon, H. (2011). Development and evaluation of the LiSN & Learn auditory training software for deficit-specific remediation of binaural processing deficits in children: Preliminary findings. *Journal of the American Academy of Audiology, 22,* 678–696.

Cameron, S., & Dillon, H. (2012). *LiSN & Learn Auditory Training Software* (Version 3.0.0) [Computer software]. Sydney, NSW, Australia: National Acoustic Laboratories.

Cameron, S., Dillon, H., & Newall, P. (2006a). Development and evaluation of the Listening in Spatialized Noise Test. *Ear and Hearing, 27,* 30–42.

Cameron, S., Dillon, H., & Newall, P. (2006b). Listening in Spatialized Noise Test: Normative data for children. *International Journal of Audiology, 45,* 99–108.

Cameron, S., Dillon, H., & Newall, P. (2006c). The Listening in Spatialized Noise Test: An auditory processing disorder study. *Journal of the American Academy of Audiology, 17,* 306–320.

Cameron, S., Glyde, H., & Dillon, H. (2011). Listening in Spatialized Noise–Sentences Test (LiSN-S): Normative and retest reliability data for adolescents and adults up to 60 years of age. *Journal of the American Academy of Audiology, 22,* 697–709.

Cameron, S., Glyde, H., & Dillon, H. (2012). Efficacy of the LiSN & Learn auditory training software: Randomized blinded controlled study. *Audiology Research, 2,* 86–93. doi:10.4081/68

Chermak, G. D. (2007). Central resources training. Cognitive, metacognitive, and metalinguistic skills and strategies. In G. D. Chermak & F. E. Musiek (Eds.), *Handbook of (central) auditory processing disorder. Comprehensive intervention* (Vol. II, pp. 107–166). San Diego, CA: Plural.

Chermak, G. D., Bellis, T. J., & Musiek, F. E. (2007). Neurobiology, cognitive science, and intervention. In G. D. Chermak & F. E. Musiek (Eds.), *Handbook of (central) auditory processing disorder. Comprehensive intervention* (Vol. II, pp. 3–28). San Diego, CA: Plural.

Chermak, G. D., & Musiek, F. E. (2002). Auditory training: Principles and approaches for remediating and managing auditory processing disorders. *Seminars in Hearing, 23,* 297–308.

Cherry, E. C. (1953). Some experiments on the recognition of speech, with one and with two ears. *Journal of the Acoustical Society of America, 25,* 975–979.

Cognitive Concepts. (2008). *Earobics* [CD-ROM]. Boston, MA: Houghton Mifflin Harcourt.

Cohen, Y. E., & Knudsen, E. I. (1999). Maps versus clusters: Different representations of auditory space in the midbrain and forebrain. *Trends in Neuroscience, 22,* 128–135.

Crandell, C. C., & Smaldino, J. J. (1995). Classroom acoustics. In R. J. Roeser & M. P. Downs (Eds.), *Auditory disorders in school children* (pp. 219–234). New York, NY: Thieme Medical.

Darwin, C. J. (2008). Listening to speech in the presence of other sounds. *Philosophical Transactions of the Royal Society B: Biological Sciences, 363,* 1011–1021.

Dawes, P., & Bishop, D. (2009). Auditory processing disorder in relation to developmental disorders of language, communication and attention: A review and critique. *International Journal of Language and Communication Disorders, 44,* 440–465.

Dillon, H. (2012). *Hearing aids.* Turramurra, NSW, Australia: Boomerang Press.

Dillon, H., Cameron, S., Glyde, H., Wilson, W., & Tomlin, D. (2012). Opinion: Redesigning the process of assessing people suspected of having central auditory processing disorders. *Journal of the American Academy of Audiology, 23,* 97–105.

Fenson, L., Dale, P., Reznick, J. S., Thal, D., Bates, E., Hartung, J., Pethick, S., & Reilly, J. (1992). *The MacArthur-Bates Communicative Development Inventories.* Baltimore, MD: Paul H. Brookes.

Fisher, L. I. (2008). *Fisher's auditory problems checklist.* Tampa, FL: Educational Audiology Association.

Fitzpatrick, D. C., Kuwada, S., & Batra, R. (2002). Transformations in processing interaural time differences between the superior olivary complex and inferior colliculus: Beyond the Jeffress model. *Hearing Research, 168*, 79–89.

Gelfand, S. A., Ross, L., & Miller, S. (1988). Sentence reception in noise from one versus two sources: effects of aging and hearing loss. *Journal of the Acoustical Society of America, 83*, 248–256.

Glyde, H., Buchholz, J., Dillon, H., Best, V., Hickson, L., & Cameron, S. (in press). The effect of better-ear glimpsing on spatial release from masking. *Journal of the Acoustical Society of America.*

Glyde, H., Buchholz, J., Dillon, H., Cameron, S., & Hickson, L. (2013). The importance of interaural time differences and level differences in spatial release from masking. *Journal of the Acoustical Society of America Express Letters, 134*(2), EL147–EL152.

Glyde, H., Buchholz, J., Dillon, H., Cameron, S., Hickson, L., & Best, V. (manuscript in preparation). The effect of audibility on spatial release from masking for speech-on-speech paradigms.

Glyde, H., Cameron, S., Dillon, H., Hickson, L., & Seeto, M. (2013). The effects of hearing impairment and aging on spatial processing. *Ear and Hearing, 34*, 15–28.

Greenberg, L. M., Kindschi, C. L., Dupuy, T. R., & Hughes, S. J. (2007). *TOVA 7.3 Clinical Manual.* Los Alamitos, CA: Tova Company.

Grothe, B. (2000). The evolution of temporal processing in the medial superior olive, and auditory brainstem structure. *Progress in Neurobiology, 61*, 581–610.

Hayes, E. A., Warrier, C. M., Nichol, T. G., Zecker, S. G., & Kraus, N. (2003). Neural plasticity following auditory training in children with learning problems. *Clinical Neurophysiology, 114*, 673–684.

Helfer, K. S., & Freyman, R. L. (2008). Aging and speech-on-speech masking. *Ear and Hearing, 29*, 87–98.

Hirsch, I. J. (1950). The relation between localization and intelligibility. *Journal of the Acoustical Society of America, 22,* 196–200.

Jerger, J. (1998) Controversial issues in central auditory processing disorders. *Seminars in Hearing, 19*, 393–398.

Jerger, J., & Musiek, F. (2000) Report of the consensus conference on the diagnosis of auditory processing disorders in school-aged children. *Journal of the American Academy of Audiology, 11*, 467–474.

Jones, G. L., & Litovsky, R. Y. (2011). A cocktail party model of spatial release from masking by both noise and speech interferers. *Journal of the Acoustical Society of America, 130*, 1463–1474.

Litovsky, R. Y., Fligor, B. J., & Tramo, M. J. (2002) Functional role of the human inferior colliculus in binaural hearing. *Hearing Research, 165*, 177–188.

Marrone, N. L., Mason, C. R., & Kidd, G. Jr. (2008a). Tuning in the spatial dimension: Evidence from a masked speech identification task. *Journal of the Acoustical Society of America, 124*, 1146–1158.

Marrone, N. L., Mason, C. R., & Kidd, G. Jr. (2008b). The effects of hearing loss and age on the benefit of spatial separation between multiple talkers in reverberant rooms. *Journal of the Acoustical Society of America, 124*, 3064–3075.

Martin, N., & Brownell, R. (2005). *Test of Auditory Processing Skills* (3rd ed.). Novato, CA: Academic Therapy.

Middlebrooks, J. C., Xu, L., Furukawa, S., & Macpherson, E. A. (2002). Cortical neurons that localize sounds. *Neuroscientist, 8*, 73–83.

Moore, D. R. (1991). Anatomy and physiology of binaural hearing. *Audiology, 30*, 125–134.

Noble, W., & Gatehouse, S. (2004). The speech, spatial and qualities of hearing scale (SSQ). *International Journal of Audiology, 43*, 85–99.

Pickles, J. O. (1988). *An introduction to the physiology of hearing.* London, UK: Academic Press.

Reuss, S. (2000). Introduction to the superior olivary complex. *Microscopy Research and Technique, 51*, 303–306.

Stenfelt, S. (2005). Bilateral fitting of BAHAs and BAHA® fitted in unilateral deaf persons: Acoustical aspects. *International Journal of Audiology, 44,* 178–189.

Sweetow, R. W., & Jenderson Sabes, J. (2010). Auditory training and challenges associated with participation and compliance. *Journal of the American Academy of Audiology, 21,* 586–593.

Thibodeau, L. M. (2007). Computer-based auditory training (CBAT) for (central) auditory processing disorders. In G. D. Chermak & F. E. Musiek (Eds.), *Handbook of (central) auditory processing disorder. Comprehensive intervention* (Vol. II, pp. 167–206). San Diego, CA: Plural.

Thiran, A. B., & Clarke, S. (2003). Preserved use of spatial cues for sound segregation in a case of spatial deafness. *Neuropsychologia, 41,* 1254–1261.

Vanniasegaram, I., Cohen, M., & Rosen, S. (2004). Evaluation of selected auditory tests in school-age children suspected of auditory processing disorders. *Ear and Hearing, 25,* 586–597.

Wolfle, D. (1951). Training. In S. S. Stephens (Ed.), *Handbook of experimental psychology.* New York, NY: John Wiley.

Yost, W. A. (1997). The cocktail party problem: Forty years later. In R. Gilkey & T. Anderson (Eds.), *Binaural and spatial hearing in real and virtual environments* (pp. 329–348). Mahwah, NJ: Erlbaum.

Zurek, P. M. (1993). Binaural advantages and directional effects in speech intelligibility. In G. A. Studebaker & I. Hochberg (Eds.), *Acoustical factors affectings hearing aid performance* (pp. 255–276). Boston, MA: Allyn & Bacon.

CHAPTER 9

DICHOTIC INTERAURAL INTENSITY DIFFERENCE (DIID) TRAINING

JEFFREY WEIHING and FRANK E. MUSIEK

Introduction

Dichotic Interaural Intensity Difference (DIID) training, first introduced by Musiek and Schochat (1998), is an auditory rehabilitation procedure for children and adults with central auditory processing disorder (CAPD). It is based in part on the study of dichotic processing in adults with neurological lesions of the corpus callosum (e.g., "split-brain" patients) and in children with suspected maturational delays of these same regions. Notably, individuals in these groups demonstrate an alleviation of this dichotic deficit when the interaural intensity difference between the ears is manipulated (Musiek & Wilson, 1979). That is, if sound is made less intense in one ear, performance in the other ear tends to improve. This chapter discusses the conceptual and physiological foundations of the DIID, in addition to detailing how the procedure can be conducted in the clinic. Although research is still ongoing, initial studies suggest the DIID is an efficacious auditory training procedure.

Dichotic Processing

Background

The DIID is a form of auditory training that addresses central auditory deficits in dichotic processing (Baran, Shinn, & Musiek, 2006; Musiek & Schochat, 1998; Musiek, Shinn, & Hare, 2002). The procedure relies on neuroplasticity in an attempt to establish beneficial, long-term changes in the central auditory system (Musiek et al., 2002). As the DIID specifically targets dichotic processing, it is necessary to consider the nature and measurement of this process before providing a detailed discussion of the training. Although the DIID may generalize to other types of auditory deficits, it was designed to address this specific mechanism.

The concept of dichotic processing, first introduced by Broadbent (1954), refers to a paradigm in which a different stimulus is presented to each ear simultaneously and is distinguished from diotic tasks, in which the same stimulus is presented to both ears at the same time, and monotic tasks, in which a stimulus is presented to only one ear. In a clinical dichotic paradigm, a patient is asked to recall one or both the auditory stimuli being presented. If both left and right ear stimuli are asked to be recalled, then the task is one of binaural integration. If the stimulus from only ear is to be recalled, and the other ignored, then the task is one of binaural separation (Musiek, 1999; Musiek & Pinheiro, 1985; Musiek et al., 2002). For example, in a binaural integration paradigm, if the word "hot dog" were presented to the left ear and "pancake" were presented to the right ear, the expected response would be "hot dog, pancake." In a binaural separation paradigm, the patient might be asked to repeat the right ear stimulus only and would say "pancake." Although both binaural integration and separation tasks are similar in execution, the physiological mechanisms underlying these two tasks vary somewhat (Jancke & Shah, 2002).

A variety of tests can be used to diagnose dichotic processing deficits in the clinic. Most of these tests utilize single words or utterances, although several tests have been developed that make use of sentence material. Table 9–1 summarizes some of the dichotic tests more commonly used in clinical practice. For reasons that are discussed below, the left ear is often the "weaker" ear, showing performance below normal limits in cases of dichotic processing deficits (Musiek et al., 2002; Musiek & Schochat, 1998). Therefore, a patient with this deficit might score 50% in the weaker ear and 90% in the stronger ear on the dichotic digits. These scores would indicate that, while the right is performing normally, the left ear performance is below normal limits. It is ultimately the goal of the DIID to bring the performance of the weaker ear up into the normal range while retaining the stronger ear's performance.

Clinicians are encouraged to establish their own normative values for each of the dichotic tests in the population that they treat. As unpredictable variations in performance may occur with certain populations, clinic-specific norms are very important. However, most of the dichotic tests in Table 9–1 have had normative values published, and these can be used as a guideline for testing in the absence of other norms. Special consideration should be given to the patient with hearing loss, as this will undoubtedly affect test performance. For instance, dichotic digits normative values of 90% for both the left and right ears have been suggested for normal hearing individuals; however, 80% is a more reasonable norm for individuals with hearing loss (Musiek, Gollegly, Kibbe, & Verkest-Lenz, 1991).

There is a neuromaturational time course to dichotic processing that must also be taken into consideration when interpreting test results (Musiek & Gollegly, 1988). This time course applies more to left than right ear performance, since

Table 9–1. Dichotic Tests

Test	Stimulus Example	Citation
Dichotic Digits	Left Ear—1,2 Right Ear—5, 8	Musiek, F. E. (1983). Assessment of central auditory dysfunction: The dichotic digit test revisited. *Ear and Hearing, 4,* 79–83.
Dichotic Rhyme	Left Ear—pill Right Ear—bill	Wexler, B., & Halwes, T. (1983). Increasing the power of dichotic methods: the fused rhymed words test. *Neuropsychologia, 21,* 59–66.
Dichotic CVs	Left Ear—ta Right Ear—da	Berlin, C. I., Lowe-Bell, S. S., Jannetta, P. J., & Kline, D. G. (1972). Central auditory deficits after temporal lobectomy. *Archives of Otolaryngology, 96,* 4–10.
Staggered Spondaic Words (SSW)	Left Ear—wash**tub** Right Ear—**black**board (bold portions are simultaneous)	Katz, J. (1962). The use of staggered spondaic words for assessing the integrity of the central auditory system. *Journal of Auditory Research, 2,* 327–337.
Competing Sentences Test	Left Ear—I'm expecting a phone call. Right Ear—Please answer the doorbell.	Willeford, J. (1978). Sentence tests of central auditory function. In J. Katz (Ed.), *Handbook of clinical audiology.* Baltimore, MD: Williams & Wilkins.
SSI	Left Ear—A small boat with a picture has become. Right Ear—"a competing passage about 'Davy Crockett'"	Jerger, J. F., & Jerger, S. W. (1974). Auditory findings in brainstem disorders. *Archives of Otolaryngology, 99,* 342–349.

right ear performance is usually high even at a young age. For left ear performance, the age of maturation can be as late as 10 to 12 years, especially for more linguistically loaded dichotic tasks (e.g., sentence material) (Musiek & Gollegly, 1988). Therefore, consideration of age-related variations in normative values is important for the pediatric patient.

Regardless of the age of the patient, it should be noted that lesions that contribute to dichotic processing deficits can also lead to abnormal performance on other types of central auditory processing tests. For instance, scores on some temporal processing tests (e.g., frequency and duration patterns) often will be below normal limits in cases of dichotic processing deficits due in part to shared reliance on the corpus callosum (Musiek, Pinheiro, & Wilson, 1980). These tests can be used in conjunction with dichotic tests to assist in diagnosis of dichotic listening deficits. Further, some studies have shown a relationship between dichotic listening and speech understanding in noise ability, with speech understanding ability becoming poorer concurrently with dichotic deficits (Bamiou et al., 2007; Walden & Walden, 2005).

Physiological Mechanisms

The current application of the DIID is built on what is known about the physiological mechanisms underlying dichotic processing (for a review, see Musiek & Weihing, 2011). In the central auditory nervous system (CANS), there are two main pathways that extend from the periphery (e.g., cochlea) to the auditory cortex. The stronger of these two pathways are the contralateral tracts that ultimately connect the left periphery to the right hemisphere and the right periphery to the left hemisphere. The weaker ipsilateral tracts course from the left periphery to the left hemisphere (Pickles, 1982). As research findings using animal models have demonstrated, the ipsilateral connections may be weaker, in part, because there are more contralateral connections in the central nervous system (Rosenzweig, 1951; Tunturi, 1946).

Utilization of these two pathways depends on the mode of stimulation. When a stimulus is presented monotically, the signal is directed toward the cerebrum via both the contralateral and ipsilateral pathways. For instance, if "hot dog" is presented to the right ear, the ipsilateral connections will bring the signal to the right hemisphere, whereas the contralateral connections will bring the signal to the left hemisphere. The situation changes, however, when stimuli are presented dichotically at equal sensation levels. The contralateral connections will still carry the signal, but the ipsilateral connections will now be suppressed to some degree (Hall & Goldstein, 1968; Rosenzweig, 1951). This means that under dichotic conditions, the pathways contributing to auditory processing are mainly the stronger contralateral connections. Presumably, this suppression of the ipsilateral connections occurs because of overlap between the two pathways at some point along the ascending route (Kimura, 1961). Competition by the two pathways for critical neural substrate may also contribute to suppression of the ipsilateral connections.

The conditions described above assume passive stimulation without requiring the patient to make a response. How does the situation change when the patient is asked to repeat back what is heard in a dichotic task? Figure 9–1 depicts this scenario. Both speech signals, again presented at equal sensation levels, must reach the language areas in the left cerebral hemisphere in order to be perceived as speech. The right ear stimulus can reach this area directly along the contralateral pathway. However, the left ear cannot directly reach the left hemisphere because the ipsilateral pathway is suppressed during dichotic listening. Instead, the left ear signal first must go to the right hemisphere via the contralateral connections, and then travel to the

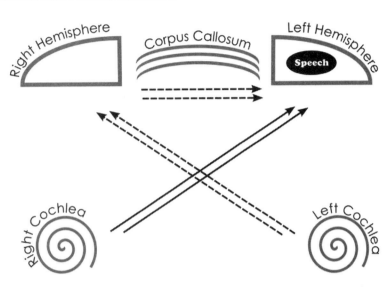

Figure 9–1. Left and right ear pathways during dichotic listening. Note that the left ear pathway must cross the corpus callosum to reach the left hemisphere speech areas.

left hemisphere via the interhemispheric connections (i.e., corpus callosum).

The ability to respond to stimuli in a dichotic task, therefore, requires different neurologic substrate depending on which ear is being considered. For the right ear, the contralateral pathway and language areas in the left hemisphere need to be uncompromised. For the left ear, the contralateral pathway, the right hemisphere, the corpus callosum, and the language areas in the left hemisphere must be uncompromised. In a healthy auditory system, both of these routes are able to function appropriately and dichotic stimuli can be repeated verbally. However, this ability to perform dichotically becomes compromised in the presence of central auditory dysfunction. Of interest is the effect of a callosotomy (e.g., "split-brain" procedure), which is sometimes used to treat intractable epilepsy. When the auditory (posterior) region of the corpus callosum is sectioned, the result is an often drastic decrease in performance on tests that require inter-

hemispheric interaction (Milner, Taylor, & Sperry, 1968; Sparks & Geschwind, 1968). Specifically, the patient has considerable difficulty repeating back stimuli that are presented to the left ear. This has been shown using dichotic digits and/or words (Damasio & Damasio, 1979; Damasio, Damasio, Castro-Caldas, & Ferro, 1976; Musiek, Wilson, & Pinheiro, 1979), the Dichotic Rhyme Test (Musiek et al., 1989), the Staggered Spondaic Word Test (Musiek & Wilson, 1979; Musiek, Wilson, & Reeves, 1981), competing sentence tests (Musiek et al., 1979, 1981), and the Frequency Patterns Test (Musiek et al., 1980). When a lesion is created in the corpus callosum, the neural signal can no longer travel between hemispheres because of the damaged fibers. Hence, the right and left auditory cortices have become "disconnected."

Consider again the dichotic scenario presented above in which the patient must repeat back all stimuli that are heard. If the corpus callosum is damaged, the right ear pathway likely will be unaffected. The signal will travel from the right ear, along the contralateral connections, to the language areas in the left hemisphere. The left ear pathway, however, will no longer behave normally. The signal will travel to the right hemisphere via the contralateral connections. However, upon reaching the right hemisphere, the signal can no longer be transmitted to the left hemisphere language areas. This is because the route of transmission, the corpus callosum, is no longer functioning properly. Therefore, the patient with a callosotomy will be able to say the right ear stimulus but not the left ear stimulus when the stimuli are presented dichotically. This is why callosal lesions typically yield a left ear deficit.

Although asymmetric dichotic performance is noted in these neurological cases when stimuli are presented at equal sensation levels in both ears, an important change in performance occurs when stimuli are presented at *unequal* sensation levels (e.g., when there is an interaural presentation level difference). Specifically, when the intensity level in the better ear (i.e., usually right ear) is decreased, whereas the level in the poorer ear (i.e., usually left ear) is kept constant, the patient can respond more easily to poorer ear stimuli. This was observed by Musiek et al. (1979), who reported that patients with callosal lesions could correctly identify more left ear stimuli when the right ear presentation level was decreased (i.e., creating an interaural difference of about 25 to 30 dB). Figure 9–2 demonstrates this principle. The specific mechanism underlying the improvement in the performance of the poorer ear is not entirely clear; however, it is thought

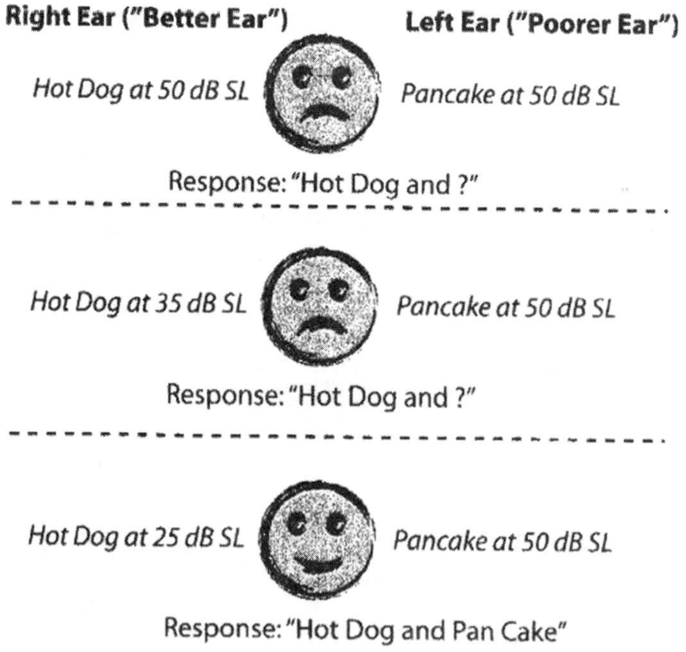

Right Ear ("Better Ear")   **Left Ear ("Poorer Ear")**

Hot Dog at 50 dB SL   *Pancake at 50 dB SL*

Response: "Hot Dog and ?"

Hot Dog at 35 dB SL   *Pancake at 50 dB SL*

Response: "Hot Dog and ?"

Hot Dog at 25 dB SL   *Pancake at 50 dB SL*

Response: "Hot Dog and Pan Cake"

Figure 9–2. Improved performance of left ear stimuli in DIID paradigm achieved by decreasing the intensity of the stimulus in the right ear. Notable increases in left ear performance usually begin to appear at IIDs between 25 and 30 dB.

that decreasing the better ear presentation level releases other pathways, including the left ear ipsilateral pathway, from suppression. This occurs because the greater the intensity of a stimulus, the greater the amount of neural substrate that is activated (Langers, van Dijik, Shoenmaker, & Backus, 2007). As a result, utilization of this ipsilateral pathway allows the left ear signal to reach the left hemisphere language areas with greater ease. As discussed in the sections that follow, it is this interaural intensity difference phenomenon upon which the DIID is based. See Chapter 6 of Volume 1 of the Handbook for additional discussion of the neurophysiology of dichotic processing.

Learning Disabilities and the Corpus Callosum

Due to the relatively high prevalence of learning disabilities (Boyle, Decoufle, & Yeargin-Allsopp, 1994; Brown et al., 2001) and the increasing awareness of auditory involvement in this disorder (Chandrasekaran, Hornickel, Skoe, Nicol, & Kraus, 2009; Hornickel, Skoe, Nicol, Zecker, & Kraus, 2009; Song, Banai, & Kraus, 2008), the DIID has considerable potential as a treatment in this population. In some cases, it is suspected that the delayed corpus callosum development may impede the interhemispheric transfer of auditory information. This is a similar end-result as is encountered with adults who have neurological lesions of the corpus callosum. In patients with neurologically based callosal lesions, this impediment arises from direct damage to the corpus callosum. In some children with learning disabilities, it has been theorized that a similar reduction in cor-

pus callosum function arise from a maturational delay in myelin development (Musiek, Gollegly, & Baran, 1984).

Myelin is a fatty substance that surrounds axons. Axons transmit the neural signal between neuron groups. The greater the amount of myelin surrounding an axon, the faster the signal can travel within the cerebrum and the more efficient processing may become (Waxman & Bennett, 1972). Relative to other parts of the central nervous system, the corpus callosum is especially highly myelinated and requires this myelin in order to perform optimally (Bear, Connors, & Paradiso, 2007; Musiek et al., 1984). Unlike some other components of the central nervous system, myelin is not completely developed at birth and takes time to fully mature. For instance, myelination of some auditory regions of the cerebrum may not be completed until the child is 10 to 12 years of age or older (Giedd et al, 1996; Salamy, 1978; Yakovlev & LeCours, 1967). Probably not coincidentally, left ear performance on dichotic processing tests shares a similar maturational time course (Musiek & Gollegly, 1988).

It should be noted that the 10- to 12-year maturational milestone for myelin development is not, however, a time course that applies to all children. There is considerable variability in myelin development across individuals. Salamy (1978) reported that the age at which adult levels of myelin are reached can vary between 10 and 20 years. Therefore, there is potential for considerable delays in myelin maturation. It is for those children who exhibit these delays that a reduction in callosal efficiency becomes noteworthy (Musiek et al., 1984).

The fact that myelin maturation varies across individuals is central to the similarities witnessed between patients with callosal lesions and those with learning disabilities. Incomplete myelin production in children with learning disabilities may lead to a temporary developmental delay that would manifest similarly on measures of dichotic processing to that of the neurologically induced lesion of split-brain patients. In both cases there is an inability to transfer the neural signal from the right to the left hemisphere efficiently, and left ear deficits would be expected as a result.

The connection between myelin delays and learning disabilities has thus far been one of inference. Indirect evidence includes the fact that similar dichotic deficits are also witnessed in cases of neurological callosal lesions (Milner et al., 1968; Musiek et al., 1979; Musiek, Geurkink, & Kietel,1982; Musiek et al., 1984; Sparks & Geschwind, 1968) and that a similar neuromaturational time course is observed for both left ear performance on dichotic processing tasks and myelin development. However, does there exist any direct evidence that can link corpus callosum abnormalities to children with learning disabilities? Although the research is somewhat inconsistent concerning this relationship, there are some reports documenting differences in the corpus callosum of the child with learning disabilities. Hynd et al. (1991) and Semrud-Clikeman et al. (1994) used magnetic resonance imaging (MRI) to compare the structure of the corpus callosum in children with learning disabilities and/or attention deficit disorder (ADD) to normal controls. It was found in both cases that the auditory region of the corpus callosum (i.e., isthmus/sulcus) was significantly smaller in the experimental group than in the control group. The researchers suggested that this smaller posterior region may negatively affect modulation of cerebral activity in the experimental group (Hynd et al., 1991). Additionally, the number of fibers in the posterior region may be smaller in the experimental group (Semrud-Clikeman et al., 1994).

Animal models have also provided indirect evidence for callosal involvement in cases of learning disabilities. Specifically, it has been suggested that lesions created in the corpus callosum can produce behaviors not dissimilar to those exhibited by children with learning disabilities and/or ADD. Sechzer, Folstein, Geiger, and Mervis (1977) completely sectioned the corpus callosum in a group of neonatal cats and compared their behavioral development to normal controls. It was found that the experimental group tended to be more hyperactive than the control group. For instance, whereas control cats huddled around the parent and slept, the experimental group continually roamed around the cage and over the parent's body. The experimental group also had difficulties with a memory task. When having to learn which of two patterns signified food, it took the experimental group almost twice the number of trials compared with controls to reach a 90% correct criterion. Both of these behaviors, hyperactivity and difficulties with memory, are often exhibited by children with learning disabilities and suggest a possible link between structure and behavior.

Dichotic Interaural Intensity Difference Training

Procedure

The DIID makes use of the physiological principles delineated above to train the neural connections involved in dichotic processing. Specifically, patients involved in DIID training participate in a variety of dichotic tasks, not unlike the clinical dichotic tasks that are used diagnostically. However, unlike diagnostic dichotic tests, which are presented at equal sensation levels bilaterally, the DIID stimuli are presented at various interaural intensity differences (IID). The purpose of the procedure is to, first, reduce the amount that the weaker connections are suppressed by the stronger connections and, second, to strengthen the weaker connections under progressively more challenging listening conditions. To reduce the amount of suppression, the presentation level in the better ear (typically the right ear) is decreased until the left ear performs normally. To then strengthen the weaker connections under challenging conditions, the presentation level in the better ear is gradually increased over time. The ultimate goal of DIID training is to have the poorer ear perform normally when the IID is zero.[1] Conceptually, DIID training is similar to the research conducted by Wiesel and Hubel (1965) and Hubel and Wiesel (1970), who examined the effects of visual deprivation and subsequent rehabilitation in the cat.

The first step in conducting the DIID is to establish that a dichotic processing deficit is present. Considerations for this have already been discussed in previous sections. Again, the left ear typically will be the poorer ear on these tasks. Following diagnosis, the crossover point should be established. The "crossover point" is the IID at which performance in the poorer ear exceeds performance in the better ear. If performance never "crosses over," then the patient will likely not benefit from the DIID. Stimuli are presented to both ears at equal sensation levels re: speech recognition threshold, generally at 50 dB SL. The presentation level in the better ear is then systematically decreased before beginning each dichotically presented list of stimuli. We generally recommend decreasing in 7 dB increments, although other increments may work just as well. When the poorer ear performance exceeds the better ear performance, crossover has been reached. This is typically accomplished at 20 to 30 dB IID.

When establishing crossover, it is important to take two criteria into consideration. The first criterion is that performance in the poorer ear should be close to normal limits when stimuli are presented at the crossover levels. For instance, consider the case where a patient scores 20% in the better ear and 30% in the poorer ear at crossover. This patient may have achieved crossover, but the performance in the poorer ear is still considerably below normal limits. If patients are unable to achieve near normal levels in the poorer ear when stimuli are presented at crossover levels, they may not be a good candidates for the DIID procedure. The second criterion is that the stimulus presented to the better ear should never be presented below the level of audibility. Although performance in the better ear will become poorer as the presentation level in that ear is decreased, performance should never extinguish completely. In order for this to remain a dichotic task, both stimuli need to be audible.

Once the crossover point has been properly established, training can begin. The initial session should begin at an IID

---

[1] It has also been suggested that making the onset of the two stimuli progressively less synchronous can also accomplish the same end. For a review of this method, the interested reader should refer to Musiek et al., 2008.

that is slightly larger than that needed for crossover. Typically, the initial IID used is 3 to 5 dB greater than the crossover level. In other words, if crossover is obtained when the sensation level is 30 dB in the better ear and 50 dB in the poorer ear, then the presentation level for the better ear during the initial session should be approximately 25 dB SL. At this IID, the patient should be administered a variety of dichotic tasks. The tasks should be conducted using both binaural integration and binaural separation paradigms, and different types of stimuli should be presented (e.g., words, digits, CVs, sentences). Depending on the task and stimuli used, varying degrees of auditory and cognitive resources will be recruited (see discussions of binaural integration and binaural separation in Chapters 21 of this Volume and Chapters 6 and 18 of Volume 1 of the Handbook). Thus, by using a wide range of tasks and stimuli, it is expected that training will target both auditory and cognitive abilities important for listening. In general, it may be preferable to employ binaural separation tasks, as many of the DIID stimuli described below are longer words and sentences that would impose undue burden on memory unless completed in the binaural separation mode; performing binaural integration tasks with these stimuli would be difficult even for individuals with normal CANS function. It is essential to maintain a log of what types of tasks were conducted, which stimuli were used, what the presentation level was in each ear, and how the patient performed. This log will be used to document the patient's progress over the course of training. An illustrative log is provided in Table 9–2.

A typical formal training schedule is to have the patient complete the DIID in the clinic for 15 to 30 minutes, three to four times a week. Informal training can be used to supplement formal training, and is discussed in greater detail below. Following the initial week of training, an attempt should be made to make the task more challenging by decreasing the IID. This is accomplished by increasing the level in the stronger ear. In the first attempt, the IID should be decreased by 5 dB (e.g., raise the level in the stronger ear by 5 dB). From our example above, if the presentation level is 25 dB SL in the better ear, it should be raised to 30 dB SL at the beginning of the second week. If performance in the poorer ear is 80% or greater at this smaller IID, then training should continue for the next week at this presentation level. If not, then a second attempt should be made in which the IID is decreased in 1 dB increments. If the patient performance is 80% or greater in the poorer ear with even a 1 dB decrease in the IID, this new presentation level should be used. If the patient is unable to tolerate even a 1 dB change in the IID, then training for the week should continue with the IID unchanged. However, another attempt should be made to modify the IID at the beginning of the following week. It is important to realize that it can take several weeks for a patient to tolerate any change in the initial IID; sometimes improvement in auditory processing happens in an incremental, and not a continuous, fashion.

Subsequent weeks should continue in the manner described, with each week beginning with an attempt to decrease the IID. If the patient begins to show a rapid increase in improvement, decrements in the IID can be attempted at the beginning of each session. For the patient who benefits from the DIID, the log should demonstrate a decrease in the IID

Table 9–2. A Sample Progress Log for the DIID*

Date	9/1/10					
Task 1	Binaural Separation					
Stimuli	Words					
Instructions	Directed Report/ Attend Left					
IID	20 dB					
% LE	70					
% RE	Not Applicable: since the task is binaural separation and the patient is attending to left ear only					
Task 2	Binaural Integration					
Stimuli	CV					
Instructions	Free Report/ Both Ears					
IID	20					
% LE	75					
% RE	50					
Task 3	Binaural Separation					
Stimuli	Sentences					
Instructions	Directed Report/ Attend Left					
IID	20					
% LE	70					
% RE	Not Applicable: since the task is binaural separation and the patient is attending to left ear only					

*Each column represents a different DIID session, with the date increasing chronologically from left to right. The log allows for multiple exercises on a given date. This particular example is for an individual with a left ear deficit.

over the course of the training period. As previously stated, the ultimate goal of the training protocol is to have the patient perform dichotic processing tasks within normal limits bilaterally when stimuli are presented at equal sensation levels. However, it has been our experience that if this goal has not been achieved by approximately 3 months time, then it is unlikely the patient will receive any further benefit from the procedure.

As part of the current DIID protocol, patients are typically retested approximately one year following the completion of training. This posttreatment testing is done in order to determine how well the effects of training have been maintained. Although not essential, a reevaluation has the obvious benefit of long-term monitoring of the patient's condition and can address the efficacy of the DIID training. To achieve the best outcomes, it is important when administering the DIID that the clinician be somewhat flexible in administration guidelines to accommodate clinical constraints. Although we have outlined here some basic guidelines to follow in applying the DIID, for any given patient it may be necessary to modify these guidelines somewhat to achieve the best result.

Special Considerations

Hardware

No additional hardware is needed beyond a calibrated two channel device to conduct DIID training. In the clinic, the most common of these devices would be a two-channel audiometer that can receive an external input from a compact disc player or a tape deck and is calibrated to ANSI standards. However, if such equipment is unavailable, then a good substitute is a laptop that is able to present a stereo signal and can be calibrated. The bottom line is that it is not necessary to have a high-tech clinic in order to conduct the DIID. In fact, perhaps one of the greatest advantages of this procedure is that it can be administered using equipment and materials that most audiologists already own.

It is beneficial to also have the patient conduct informal training at home to supplement the formal clinical training. Such informal training can be accomplished in a variety of ways. For instance, if the patient owns a portable audio device that has a balance between left and right stereo channels, this balance can be adjusted to create an IID. If the left ear is the poorer ear, then the balance can be turned toward the left channel so that the signal emitted from that channel is stronger. Alternatively, a laptop could be used in the same manner. Most computer operating systems allow the user to adjust the output balance. Again, the signal will become stronger on the channel toward which the balance is shifted. Of course, it is difficult to determine precisely at what IID the stimuli are being presented using this equipment. The patient should simply be instructed to modify the balance until the stimulus becomes just easy enough to understand in the poorer ear without removing the better ear stimulus entirely.

There are still many informal training procedures that can be conducted in addition to those described above. Almost any activity or task that can create an IID is acceptable. For example, a patient had been completing a binaural separation task by listening to words through a portable compact disc (CD) player with one ear and exposing himself to a competing signal through a television speaker with his other ear. He used a television channel that broadcast mostly talk programming (e.g., a news station). He then adjusted the presentation level of the CD player until his performance repeating back the CD words was approximately 70 to 80%, and trained at this level for approximately 20 minutes. It should be noted that when performing the DIID informally, there needs to be some flexibility so as to accommodate the patient's technical ability and home environment. Maintaining reasonable task difficulty while keeping patient motivation high should be the primary goal.

The DIID has been conducted both over headphones and through speakers in the sound field. Although the headphones create a more controlled environment, presenting stimuli in the sound field may create a more challenging listening situation since the two stimuli are mixed at the ear level (Musiek & Schochat, 1998). In other words, the left ear will still receive the majority of the left stimulus, but the right stimulus will reach the left ear as well, albeit to a lesser degree. Certainly, training in the sound field can provide an ecologically valid alternative to headphones, and may benefit the patient if done in moderation or if it is the only transducer available. However, the majority of training should be conducted over headphones as it is important to maintain a specific IID.

Stimuli

As mentioned previously, it is important to use a variety of stimuli when formally conducting the DIID. For formal training, any material that can be calibrated and

has a different stimulus on each channel can be used. The onsets of the stimuli should be relatively aligned; however, precise alignment is not essential. Any combination of stimulus types can be used. For instance, patients could also be asked to repeat back words from the poorer ear while sentences in the better ear are ignored, or they can be asked to repeat back a CV from one ear and a digit in the other ear. The most important point is that dichotic tasks be completed and that they are done so with a variety of stimulus types. There are several materials that can be used to this end: Constraint Induced Auditory Training (CIAT) (Hurley & Davis, 2012); Auditory Rehabilitation for Interaural Asymmetry (ARIA) (Moncrieff & Wertz, 2008); Qualitone (Q/MASS), Speech Audiometry Volume 1 (Qualitone, 1988); Department of Veterans Affairs, Speech Recognition and Identification Materials (Wilson, 1993); and Department of Veterans Affairs Tonal and Speech Materials (Wilson, 1993). Recently, two software-based versions of dichotic training have been developed, Sound Auditory Training ([SAT]; Chermak, Musiek, & Weihing) and Integrated Werks ([IW]; Lau, 2012). The former program, SAT, utilizes IIDs whereas the latter, IW, utilizes interaural timing differences instead of IIDs to achieve the same effect (Integrated Werks, 2012). Both programs adaptively adjust the difficulty of the tasks, and use some combination of digits, CVs, and/or words in the exercises.

When training the patient, it is important to limit the use of diagnostic tests as training materials. Tests that will be used as pre- and posttraining measures should mostly be reserved for the evaluation sessions only. Obviously, if these tests are overused during the training, the patient may become familiar with the stimuli.

The list then becomes a closed-set and demands placed on the auditory system are decreased. Additionally, as a post-training measure, the test may become invalid. Although it may not always be possible to limit use of these tests entirely during training, special attention should be given to nondiagnostic stimulus sets for DIID training.

Behavioral Tasks

The majority of DIID training requires the patient to complete binaural integration and binaural separation type tasks. There are, however, other types of tasks the patient can be asked to complete. It is thought that the more varied the tasks, the greater the area of the central nervous system that will be trained. Cognitive-based approaches, for instance, can tap neural substrate beyond that used for central auditory processing and may increase the generalization of training. These more cognitive approaches to DIID training involve having patients make some sort of decision about the stimuli that are presented. For instance, four numbers could be presented to each ear and they could be asked to repeat back only the first and third numbers in each ear, thereby tapping working memory. They might also be asked to label each word that is heard as a person, place, or thing, thereby tapping into semantic categories.

Efficacy

Although efficacy data for the DIID continue to be collected, several studies and preliminary data have shown the DIID to provide benefit to patients experienc-

ing weak dichotic listening skills. In a sample of children with CAPD, Musiek (unpublished manuscript) examined performance on the Dichotic Digits Test (Musiek, 1983) pre- and post-DIID training. The degree of improvement noted was compared with a control group with a similar diagnosis who participated in speech-language therapy and/or a non-dichotic auditory task (e.g., auditory discrimination). It was observed that improvement for the weaker ear in the experimental group (30%) was significantly greater than that seen in the control group (7%). Musiek et al. (2008) administered a variant of the DIID that utilizes interaural timing instead of intensity differences to children with dichotic deficits. They too noted an increase of approximately 30% in poorer ear performance following DIID therapy. Moncrieff and Wertz (2008) conducted a similar study, comparing the improvement on dichotic tests in a group of children with CAPD pre- and posttraining. Left ear improvement was approximately 15 to 25% following training. These benefits were related to significant improvements in listening ability, as determined by listening comprehension and word recognition measures. Additionally, 38% of subjects showed improved phonological awareness ability following training. The authors determined the same amount of dichotic benefit was received regardless of whether the subject participated in 12, 16, or 24 sessions.

Case studies that incorporate behavioral measures have also shown evidence of DIID benefits. Musiek and Schochat (1998) administered the DIID as part of an auditory training battery to a 15-year-old boy with learning disabilities. Pre-training, the patient showed a bilateral deficit on dichotic digits with poorer performance in the left ear. Following 6 weeks of training, performance on this measure returned to normal limits in both ears. Improvements were also reflected on speech-language measures and in academic performance; however, it is unclear whether these secondary benefits could be attributed to the DIID (Musiek & Schochat, 1998). Musiek, Baran, and Shinn (2004) also administered the DIID as part of an informal auditory training protocol for an adult who had sustained a closed head injury. Prior to beginning the training protocol, the patient demonstrated a left ear deficit for dichotic digits and competing sentences. At the end of training, the left ear performance for dichotic digits was within normal limits and was borderline normal for competing sentences. This patient also reported that she was now able to engage in activities she previously had not been able to do (e.g., listen on the phone with her left ear), although her ability to complete these activities had still not returned to premorbid state. Hurley (2005) administered the DIID to a child diagnosed with Landau-Kleffner syndrome and who had received only mild benefit from computer-based auditory training. Results indicated improved dichotic processing performance following several weeks of training, as well as parent report that the child was showing improved "speech-language skills" after involvement in the protocol.

Effects of the DIID have also been investigated electrophysiologically. Schochat, Musiek, Alonso, and Ogata (2010) administered an auditory training protocol, in which the DIID was a component, to thirty children with CAPD, as well as a control group. Results confirmed that not only did the children demonstrate benefits behaviorally, but that their evoked potentials improved as well. Specifically, the middle latency response Na-Pa amplitude at the C3 electrode (i.e., electrode over the left hemisphere) was greater in the CAPD group following training, but not in a control group. These results demonstrate that changes induced by an auditory training protocol that includes the DIID may be measured electrophysiologically as well as behaviorally.

Finally, there is some evidence to indicate that DIID training may transfer to reflect benefits in natural listening situations. Musiek et al. (2008) asked parents and teachers to rate children's communication and academic performance following participation in DIID training. Questions probed communication ability, academic performance, attention, and the ability to hear in noise. Each area was rated from 0 to 5, with 0 indicating no improvement and 5 indicating 100% improvement. Following DIID training, parents and teachers assigned all dimensions scores of at least a 3 on average, with some, including academic performance, scoring a 4 on average. This suggests that the auditory processing benefits of DIID training may generalize to other areas, although this study did not demonstrate with certainty that gains in these related areas are auditorily based.

Summary

This chapter detailed the nature of dichotic processing deficits and how the DIID can be used to treat dichotic processing/listening deficits. Neurophysiological and conceptual foundations were provided and detailed procedural details were elaborated for DIID training. Although results from initial efficacy studies have been encouraging, further research using double-blind and randomized group designs are needed to further demonstrate the potential of DIID training to improve dichotic listening in individuals with CAPD and related diagnoses. Additional research also is needed to elucidate the specific auditory mechanisms that are strengthened as a result of DIID training. Since myelin takes longer than three months to develop, it seems unlikely that more myelin is being generated as a result of DIID training. The underlying cause of improved performance may be biochemical, or may simply involve an increase in the number of usable neurons along the weaker ipsilateral pathways. It is conceivable that by stimulating the weaker connections the number of viable neuron groups and/or the number of connections amongsuch groups increases (Musiek et al., 2002). Regardless of the source of change, that the DIID provides benefit is the ultimate criterion and initial research seems promising in this regard. Additional research is needed to demonstrate the long-term efficacy of the procedure.

References

Bamiou, D., Free, S., Sisodiya, S., Chong, W., Musiek, F., Williamson, K., . . . Luxon, L. (2007). Auditory interhemispheric transfer deficits, hearing difficulties, and brain magnetic resonance imaging abnormalities in children with congenital aniridia due to PAX6 mutations. *Archives of Pediatric and Adolescent Medicine, 161,* 463–469.

Baran, J., Shinn, J., & Musiek, F. (2006). New developments in the assessment and management of auditory processing disorders. *Audiological Medicine, 4,* 35–45.

Bear, M., Connors, B., & Paradiso, M. (2007). *Neuroscience—exploring the brain* (3rd ed.). New York, NY: Lippincott, Williams, & Wilkins.

Boyle, C., Decoufle, P., & Yeargin-Allsopp, M. (1994). Prevalence and health impact of developmental disabilities in U.S. children. *Pediatrics, 93,* 399–403.

Broadbent, D. E. (1954). The role of auditory localization in attention and memory span. *Journal of Experimental Psychology, 47,* 191–196.

Brown, R., Freeman, W., Perrin, J., Stein, M., Amler, R., Feldman, H., . . . Wolraich, M. (2001). Prevalence and assessment of attention deficit/hyperactivity disorder in primary care settings. *Pediatrics, 107,* 43–53.

Chandrasekaran, B., Hornickel, J., Skoe, E., Nicol, T., & Kraus, N. (2009). Context dependent encoding in the human auditory auditory brainstem relates to hearing speech in noise: Implications for developmental dyslexia. *Neuron, 64,* 311–319.

Damasio, H., & Damasio, A. (1979). Paradoxic ear extinction in dichotic listening: Possible anatomical significance. *Neurology, 29,* 644–653.

Damasio, H., Damasio, A., Castro-Caldas, A., & Ferro, J. (1976). Dichotic listening pattern in relation to inerhemispheric disconnection. *Neuropsychologia, 14,* 247–250.

Giedd, J. N., Rumsey, J. M., Castellanos, F. X., Rajapakse, J. C., Kaysen, D., Vaituzis, A. C., . . . Rapoport, J. L. (1996). A quantitative MRI study of the corpus callosum in children and adolescents. *Developmental Brain Research, 91,* 274–280.

Hall, J., & Goldstein, M. (1968). Representations of binaural stimuli by single units in primary auditory cortex of unanesthetized cats. *Journal of the Acoustical Society of America, 43,* 456–561.

Hornickel, J., Skoe, E., Nicol, T., Zecker, S., & Kraus, N. (2009). Subcortical differentiation of stop consonants relates to reading and speech-in-noise perception. *Proceedings of the National Academy of Sciences of the USA, 106,* 13022–13027.

Hubel, D., & Wiesel, T. (1970). The period of susceptibility to the physiological effects of unilateral eye closure in kittens. *Journal of Physiology, 206*, 419–436.

Hurley, A. (2005). *Auditory remediation for patients with Landau-Kleffner syndrome.* Retrieved from http://www.asha.org/Publications/leader/2011/110405/Auditory-Remediation-for-Patients-With-Landau-Kleffner-Syndrome.htm

Hurley, A., & Davis, D. (2011). *Constraint induced auditory therapy (CIAT): A dichotic listening auditory therapy.* St. Louis, MO: AudiTec.

Hynd, G., Semrud-Clikeman, M., Lorys, A., Novey, E., Eliopulos, D., & Lyytinen, H. (1991). Corpus callosum morphology in attention deficit-hyperactivity disorder: Morphometric analysis of MRI. *Journal of Learning Disabilities, 24*, 141–146.

Jancke, L., & Shah, N. (2002). Does dichotic listening probe temporal lobe functions? *Neurology, 58*, 736–743.

Kimura, D. (1961). Some effects of temporal-lobe damage on auditory perception. *Canadian Journal of Psychology, 15*, 156–165.

Langers, D., van Dijik, P., Shoemaker, E., & Backus, W. (2007). fMRI activation in relation to sound intensity and loudness. *NeuroImage, 35*, 709–718.

Milner, B., Taylor, S., & Sperry, R. (1968). Lateralized suppression of dichotically presented digits after commissural section in man. *Science, 161*, 184–185.

Moncrieff, D., & Wertz, D. (2008). Auditory rehabilitation for interaural asymmetry: Preliminary evidence of improved dichotic listening performance following intensive training. *International Journal of Audiology, 47*, 84–97.

Musiek, F. (unpublished data). Dichotic interaural intensity difference training.

Musiek, F. (1983). Assessment of central auditory function: The dichotic digits test revisited. *Ear and Hearing, 4*, 79–83.

Musiek, F. (1999). Central auditory tests. *Scandinavian Audiology, 28*(Suppl. 51), 33–46.

Musiek, F., Baran, J., & Shinn, J. (2004). Assessment and remediation of an auditory processing disorder associated with head trauma. *Journal of the American Academy of Audiology, 15*, 117–132.

Musiek, F., Geurkink, N., & Kietel, S. (1982). Test battery assessment of auditory perceptual dysfunction in children. *Laryngoscope, 92*, 251–257.

Musiek, F., & Gollegly, K. (1988). Maturational considerations in the neuroauditory evaluation of children. In H. Bess (Ed.), *Hearing impairment in children.* Parkton, MD: York Press.

Musiek, F., Gollegly, K., & Baran, J. (1984). Myelination of the corpus callosum and auditory processing problems in children: Theoretical and clinical correlates. *Seminars in Hearing, 5*, 231–241.

Musiek, F., Gollegly, K., Kibbe, K., & Verkest-Lenz, S. (1991). Proposed screening test for central auditory disorders: Follow-up on the Dichotic Digits Test. *American Journal of Otology, 12*, 109–113.

Musiek, F., Kurdziel-Schwan, S., Kibbe, K., Gollegly, K., Baran, J., & Rintelmann, W. (1989). *Ear and Hearing, 10*, 33–39.

Musiek, F., & Pinheiro, M. (1985). Dichotic speech tests in the detection of central auditory dysfunction. In M. Pinheiro & F. Musiek (Eds.), *Assessment of central auditory dysfunction: Foundations and clinical correlates.* Baltimore, MD: Williams & Wilkins.

Musiek, F., Pinheiro, M., & Wilson, D. (1980). Auditory pattern perception in "split brain" patients. *Archives of Otolaryngology, 106*, 610–612.

Musiek, F., & Schochat, E. (1998). Auditory training and central auditory processing disorders—a case study. *Seminars in Hearing, 19*, 357–366.

Musiek, F., Shinn,. J., & Hare, C. (2002). Plasticity, auditory training, and auditory processing disorders. *Seminars in Hearing, 23*, 263–275.

Musiek, F., & Weihing, J. (2011). Perspectives on dichotic listening and the corpus callosum. *Brain and Cognition, 76*, 225–232.

Musiek, F., Weihing, J., & Lau, C. (2008). Dichotic interaural intensity difference (DIID) training: A review of existing literature and future directions. *Journal of the Academy of Rehabilitative Audiology, 41,* 51–65.

Musiek, F., & Wilson, D. (1979). SSW and dichotic digit results pre- and post-commissurotomy: A case report. *Journal of Speech, Language, and Hearing Disorders, 44,* 528–533.

Musiek, F., Wilson, D., & Pinheiro, M. (1979). Audiological manifestations in "split brain" patients. *Journal of the American Auditory Society, 5,* 25–29.

Musiek, F., Wilson, D., & Reeves, G. (1981). Staged commissurotomy and central auditory function. *Archives of Otolaryngology, 107,* 233–236.

Pickles, J. O. (1982). *An introduction to the physiology of hearing.* London, UK: Academic Press.

Qualitone. (1988). *Q/MASS speech audiometry.* Minneapolis, MN: Author.

Rosenzweig, M. (1951). Representations of two ears at the auditory cortex. *American Journal of Physiology, 167,* 147–158.

Salamy, A. (1978). Commissural transmission: Maturational changes in humans. *Science, 200,* 1409–1410.

Schochat, E., Musiek, F., Alonso, R., & Ogata, J. (2010). Effects of auditory training on the middle latency response in children with (central) auditory processing disorder. *Brazilian Journal of Medical and Biological Research, 43,* 777–785.

Sechzer. J., Folstein, S., Geiger, E., & Mervis, D. (1977). Effects of neonatal hemispheric disconnection in kittens. In S. Harnard, R. Doty, L. Goldstein, J. Jaynes, & G. Krauthamer (Eds.), *Lateralization in the nervous system.* New York, NY: Academic Press.

Semrud-Clikeman, M., Filipek, P., Biederman, J., Steingard, R., Kennedy, D., Renshaw, P., & Bekken, K. (1994). Attention-deficit hyperactivity disorder: Magnetic resonance imaging morphometric analysis of the corpus callosum. *Journal of the American Academy of Child and Adolescent Psychiatry, 33,* 875–881.

Song, J., Banai, K., & Kraus, N. (2008). Brainstem timing deficits in children with learning impairment may result from corticofugal origins. *Audiology and Neurootology, 13,* 335–344.

Sparks, R., & Geschwind, N. (1968). Dichotic listening in man after section of neocortical commissures. *Cortex, 4,* 3–16.

Tunturi, A. (1946). A study of the pathway from the medial geniculate body to the acoustic cortex in the dog. *American Journal of Physiology, 147,* 311–319.

Walden, T., & Walden, B. (2005). Unilateral versus bilateral amplification for adults with impaired hearing. *Journal of the American Academy of Audiology, 16,* 574–584.

Waxman, S., & Bennett, M. (1972). Relative conduction velocity of small myelinated and non-myelinated fibres in the central nervous system. *Nature New Biology, 238,* 217–219.

Wiesel, T., & Hubel, D. (1965). Extent of recovery from the effects of visual deprivation in kittens. *Journal of Neurophysiology, 28,* 1060–1072.

Wilson, R. (1993). Development and use of auditory compact discs in auditory evaluation. *Journal of Rehabilitation Research and Development, 30,* 342–351.

Yakovlev, P., & LeCours, A. (1967). Myelogenetic cycles of regional maturation of the brain. In A. Minkowski (Ed.), *Regional development of the brain in early life.* Philadelphia, PA: F. A. Davis.

CHAPTER 10

CENTRAL RESOURCES TRAINING: COGNITIVE, METACOGNITIVE, AND METALINGUISTIC SKILLS AND STRATEGIES

GAIL D. CHERMAK

Intervention for central auditory processing disorder (CAPD) should commence as soon as possible following diagnosis to take advantage of the plasticity of the central nervous system and thereby maximize therapeutic effectiveness and minimize functional deficits (AAA, 2010; ASHA, 2005; Chermak, 2007; Chermak & Musiek, 1997). Intervention should be comprehensive and multidisciplinary, given the potential impact of CAPD on listening, communication, and learning, as well as the frequent comorbidity of CAPD with language, learning, attention and related disorders (Chermak, Hall, & Musiek, 1999; Chermak & Musiek, 1992, 1997; Iliadou, Bamiou, Kaprinis, Kandylis, & Kaprinis, 2009; Musiek, Bellis, & Chermak, 2005; Sharma, Purdy, & Kelly, 2009). The influence of higher order, non-modality-specific processes such as attention, executive control, memory, and decision making on all auditory tasks further underscores the need for comprehensive intervention (Ciccia, Meulenbroek, & Turkstra, 2009; Musiek et al., 2005; Salvi, Lockwood, Frisina, Coad, Wack, & Frisina, 2002). This undergirding of basic perceptual events by supramodal cognitive processes is demonstrated, for example, by the integral role of working memory in numerous auditory processes, including localization, temporal resolution, dichotic listening, speech recognition in noise, and pattern recognition (Akeroyd, 2008; Jancke & Shah, 2002; Marler, Champlin, Gillam, 2002; Martin, Jerger, & Mehta, 2007; Martinkauppi,

Rama, Aronen, Korvenoja, & Carolson, 2002; Salvi, Lockwood, Frisina, Coad, Wack, & Frisina, 2002; Wong et al., 2009; Zattore, 2001; Zatorre, Belin, & Benhune, 2002). Notwithstanding the primacy of auditory processing deficits in CAPD, comorbid supramodal cognitive, attention, language, and related deficits can compound auditory processing deficits and exacerbate the adverse impact of CAPD for listening, communication, and learning (Chermak, 2007; Chermak & Musiek, 1997). Indeed, links between inefficient auditory processing and language or learning problems have been documented both behaviorally and electrophysiologically (e.g., Bellis & Ferre, 1999; Boscariol et al., 2011; Cunningham, Nicol, Zecker, Bradlow, & Kraus, 2001; Gomez & Condon, 1999; Hornickel, Skoe, Nicol, Zecker, & Kraus, 2009; Iliadou et al., 2009; Kraus et al., 1996; Moncrieff & Musiek, 2002; Pillsbury, Grose, Coleman, Conners, & Hall, 1995; Purdy, Kelly, & Davies, 2002; Riccio, Hynd, Cohen, Hall, & Molt, 1994; Sharma et al., 2009; Sharma, Purdy, Newall, Wheldall, Beaman, & Dillon, 2006; Tillery, Katz, & Keller, 2000; Wible, Nicol, & Kraus, 2002, 2005; Warrier, Johnson, Hayes, Nicol, & Kraus, 2004; Wright et al., 1997). Similarly, even though CAPD is not posited as a direct cause of all or even most cases of academic failure, learning disability, or reading disability, CAPD certainly can exacerbate academic challenge (e.g., listening in noisy classroom environments) (Musiek, Bellis, & Chermak, 2005). Comorbid deficits can impede generalization of strategic listening behaviors across settings and may jeopardize treatment effectiveness and efficacy (Borkowski & Burke, 1996; Chermak, 2007; Chermak & Musiek, 1997). Intervention to address the clinical and functional deficit profile that accompanies CAPD must be comprehensive in scope. Comprehensive, mulitidsciplinary intervention builds listening skills and strategies, provides compensatory techniques to minimize functional listening deficits, and promotes efficient allocation of perceptual and higher order central resources. The effectiveness and efficacy of CAPD intervention should not be gauged, primarily, however, by academic outcomes or social skills, but rather by improvements in auditory function. These, in turn, will support improvements in those functions (e.g., listening and spoken language processing) that are dependent upon audition (Musiek et al., 2005). See Chapter 1.

While the complex organization of the brain, involving interactive and interfacing sensory, cognitive, and linguistic networks may underlie comorbidity and compound the impact of CAPD, that same complex organization presents opportunities to benefit intervention (Chermak, 2007; Chermak & Musiek, 1997; Kauramaki, Jaaskelainen, & Sams, 2009; Merzenich, Schreiner, Jenkins, & Wang, 1993; Poremba et al., 2003; Price, Thierry, & Griffiths, 2005). Central resources, comprised of cognitive (i.e., processes involved in *knowing*), metacognitive (i.e., use of knowledge), and language resources, can be engaged to buttress central auditory processing and complement direct auditory skills training, thereby minimizing the functional consequences of CAPD (Chermak, 2007; Chermak & Musiek, 1997). This chapter focuses on the role of central resources training in comprehensive intervention to enhance central auditory processing, listening and spoken language understanding.

Brain Organization and Neuroplasticity

A comprehensive approach to intervention capitalizes on the complex organization of the brain and its neuroplasticity. The neural substrate of the auditory system is extensive, interfacing with other sensory, language, cognitive, motor control, and linguistic networks (Bayazit, Oniz, Hahn, Gunturkun, & Ozgoren, 2009; Ciccia et al., 2009; Petacchi, Kaernbach, Ratnam, & Bower, 2011; Poldrack et al., 2001; Poremba et al., 2003; Wong et al., 2009; Salvi et al., 2002). Conversely, widespread cortical networks spanning temporal, frontal, and parietal lobes sustain cognitive processes (e.g., attention and memory) that support auditory processing (Gaffan, 2005; Lopez-Aranda et al., 2009; Thiebaut de Schotten et al., 2005).

Consistent with a network model, emphasizing the distributed nature of information processing within the nervous system, perceptual responses to sensory stimuli are mediated across a large number of brain regions involving multiple serial, parallel, and dispersed neural networks (AAA, 2010; ASHA, 1996; Bushman & Miller, 2007; Masterton, 1992; Price et al., 2005; Ungerleider, 1995). Neuroplasticity is induced through experience and stimulation and leads to reorganization (i.e., remapping) of the cortex (and brainstem) and cognitive and behavioral change (de Boer &Thornton, 2008; Elbert, Pantev, Wienbruch, Rockstroh, & Taub, 1995; Johnson et al., 2008;

Nicol & Kraus, 2005; Knudsen, 1998; Merzenich, Schreiner, Jenkins, & Wang, 1993; Moore, 1993; Recanzone, Schreiner, & Merzenich, 1993; Robertson & Irvine, 1989; Russo, Nicol, Zecker, Hayes, & Kraus, 2005; Snyder, Bonham, & Sinex, 2008; Song, Skoe, Wong, & Kraus, 2008; Weinberger & Diamond, 1987; Willott, Aiken, & McFadden, 1993). Even mature sensory systems retain the potential for extensive plasticity induced by stimulation and behavioral demands (Pienkowski & Eggermont, 2011; see Feldman & Brecht, 2005 and Ohl & Scheich, 2005 for reviews). An array of plastic changes underlie cortical reorganization, including the potential for enlargement of a region's function (i.e., map expansion), compensatory allocation (i.e., novel allocation of particular process to another brain region), cross-modal reassignment (i.e., region of the brain accepting input from a new sensory modality), and homologous area adaptation (i.e., same area in opposite hemisphere assuming processing responsibility) (Grafman & Litvan, 1999). Since all auditory skills are affected by higher order, non-modality-specific factors (e.g., attention, memory, motivation, and decision processes) and the underlying multimodal, cross-modal, and supramodal neural interfaces that support performance, the array of potential neuroplastic changes bodes well for successful outcomes when intervention is undertaken comprehensively and broadly.

The plasticity of the central auditory nervous system (CANS) provides tremendous opportunity to improve central auditory processes and skills through direct treatment (i.e., auditory training). This neuroplasticity also compels us to undertake central resources training to engage related systems that interface with the

CANS and can, through those interactions, potentially reduce the functional impact of CAPD and enhance listening, communication, social and learning outcomes. (See Chapter 1 of this volume and Chapters 1, 4, and 5 of Volume 1 of the Handbook for additional discussion of neuroplasticity.)

Modeling Central Auditory Processing: Information Processing

Recent developments in cognitive neuroscience underscore the highly complex, multistage, interactive, and integrative nature of central auditory processing and the complementary interplay of both bottom-up and top-down information processing strategies (Chermak, 2007; Chermak & Musiek, 1992, 1997; Massaro, 1987; Peele, Troiani, Grossman, & Wingfield, 2011). Also becoming clear is the essential role of neurotransmitters and molecular mechanisms, triggered by sensory stimulation, in facilitating central auditory processing (Altschuler & Shore, 2010; Aoki & Siekevitz, 1988; Gopal, Bishop, & Carney, 2004a, 2004b; Kalil, 1989; Morley & Happe, 2000; Musiek & Hoffman, 1990; Pickles, 2008; Sahley, Musiek, & Nodar, 1996; Sahley & Nodar, 1994; Syka, 2002; Wu & Kelly, 1992).

The emerging conceptualization of central auditory processing views information processing as neither exclusively bottom-up nor top-down (Chermak, 2007; Chermak & Musiek, 1997). Bottom-up processing encompasses data-driven strategies in which the listener is alerted to novel or incompatible information. Complementary top-down strategies emphasize context and assimilation of lower order information within the experience and expectations of the listener (Chermak, 2007; Chermak & Musiek, 1992; Neisser, 1976; Rumelhart, 1984). According to information processing theory, an active listener selectively attends, processes data, and imposes higher level constraints to construct the signal or message (Borkowski & Burke, 1996; Flavell, 1981; Gibson, 1966; Watson & Foyle, 1985). Listeners assign meaning to audible discourse based on the extraction of information through various interactions among central auditory processing and cognitive, language, and metacognitive functions (Chermak, 2007; Chermak & Musiek, 1997; Massaro, 1975a, 1975b, 1976). Skilled listeners are actively engaged in discovering the speaker's message. They orchestrate various bottom-up (e.g., segmenting, discriminating, and sequencing) and top-down strategies (e.g., question formulation, paraphrasing, mnemonics, note-taking, drawing, verbal rehearsal, mental imaging, and summarizing) to monitor listening and extract information from the spoken message (Chermak, 2007; Chermak & Musiek, 1997).

The relative contribution of bottom-up and top-down processes is driven by the changing demands of the listening situation. The influence of top-down processes is more substantial when stimuli are presented in degraded form, including noisy environments and linguistically ambiguous contexts (Marslen-Wilson & Tyler, 1980; Neisser, 1976; Rumelhart, 1980, 1984; Warren & Warren, 1970). For persons with CAPD who routinely confront internal distortions that degrade the signal, top-down processing exerts a more significant influence in all listening situations, especially in noisy and reverberant environments and when coupled with complex linguistic and cognitive demands (e.g., in classrooms).

Comprehensive intervention for CAPD is structured consistent with information processing models that involve the complementary interplay of both bottom-up and top-down strategies (Chermak, 2007; Chermak & Musiek, 1997). Skilled listeners, actively engaged in discovering what speakers are communicating, rely on central auditory processes to segment, discriminate, integrate, and organize the acoustic information inherent to the auditory signal, as well as various executive strategies to monitor their listening and extract meaningful information from the spoken message (Chermak, 2007; Chermak & Musiek, 1997). They must organize and elaborate information and deploy executive strategies and self-regulatory processes to guide the flow of information processing and coordinate knowledge sources (Borkowski & Burke, 1996; Flavell, 1981; Gibson, 1966). Conceptualized within this framework in which processes at various sensory and central levels influence information processing, CAPD resulting from specific, sensory processing deficiencies may be exacerbated by higher order (i.e., top-down) deficiencies in regulating or coordinating central auditory and cognitive and linguistic processes (AAA, 2010; ASHA, 1996; Chermak, 2007; Chermak & Musiek, 1992, 1997; Swanson, 1987). In addition to deficits in specific central auditory processes (e.g., auditory discrimination, temporal processing, performance with competing or degraded acoustic signals), individuals with CAPD may lack listening strategies or employ inappropriate strategies and fail to engage in self-monitoring behavior (Chermak, 2007; Chermak & Musiek, 1997).

Consistent with information processing theory, bottom-up and top-down approaches form two complementary components of a comprehensive intervention program for CAPD (Table 10–1). Bottom-up approaches for CAPD focus

Table 10–1. Components of Comprehensive Intervention for Central Auditory Processing Disorder

Bottom-Up Treatment
Environmental Modifications: Control Noise & Enhance Acoustics (i.e., Increase Clarity of Signal & Listening Environment, Assistive Listening Systems, Clear Speech, Improved Room Acoustics, etc.)
Auditory Training (i.e., Direct [Auditory] Skills Remediation to Reorganize the CANS)
Top-Down Management: Compensatory and Accommodative Approaches
Central Resources/Compensatory Training (i.e., Language Strategies, Cognitive Strategies, & Metacognitive Strategies)
Educational Accommodations (i.e., Instructional Modifications & Learning Strategies)
Workplace, Recreational & Home Accommodations (e.g., Written directives such as memos, e-mails; post chores on white board)

on auditory training and enhancement of the acoustic signal and the listening environment. Top-down approaches focus on central resources, including cognitive skills (e.g., attention, working memory); metacognitive knowledge and skills (e.g., monitoring, coordinating, and deploying strategies); language (e.g., metalinguistic) skills and strategies; classroom, instructional, and learning strategies; and workplace, recreational, and home accommodations (ASHA, 2005; Chermak, 2002, 2007; Chermak & Musiek, 1997, 2002). See Chapter 1 for additional discussion of bottom-up and top-down processing.

Systems Theory

The tenets of systems theory support a collaborative and ecological or context-based approach to intervention (Chermak, 2007; Chermak & Musiek, 1997). The study of systems as entities rather than a conglomeration of parts has received broad application across disciplines, including in the social sciences, education, and health and rehabilitation sciences (Bartoli & Botel, 1988; Damico, Augustine, & Hayes, 1996; Duranti & Goodwin, 1990; Weaver, 1993). A systems perspective considers an individual as a system of interacting cognitive, affective, and physiological subsystems and as a part of larger social systems, including the family, school, workplace, and community. Environmental events are seen as directly impacting the individual's function. In contrast to a medical model in which behavioral problems are attributed solely to the neurobiological problems of the individual, a systems approach encompasses a broad perspective whereby factors external to the individual are seen as interacting with internal neurobiological predispositions, thereby contributing

to behavioral deficits (Chermak, 2007; Chermak & Musiek, 1997). In effect, an individual's behavior is the culmination of numerous transactional interactions between the individual and his or her context (i.e., environment, culture, society) (Chermak, 2007; Chermak & Musiek, 1997). Notwithstanding the neurobiologic basis of CAPD, environmental expectations and demands (e.g., listening to sophisticated language in a noisy classroom) exacerbate the mismatch between internal capacity and external structure and lead to communication dysfunction and academic underachievement (Chermak, 2007; Chermak & Musiek, 1997).

The assumptions of systems theory reinforce the importance of collaboration and empowerment for successful intervention. These assumptions translate into interventions that include attention to interacting internal and external factors, interventions directed toward the individual, including central resources training, as well as environmental interventions, in the classroom, workplace, and recreational settings (Bartoli & Botel, 1988; Chermak & Musiek, 1997; Gibson, 1966; Maag & Reid, 1996; Poplin, 1988a, 1988b; Weaver, 1985, 1993).

Central Resources Utilization Strategy

A central resources utilization strategy is derived from a processing model in which resources are finite and must be efficiently allocated across sensory and central systems (McCoy et al., 2005; Pichora-Fuller, Schneider, & Daneman, 1995; Piquado, Cousins, Wingfield, & Miller, 2010). Emerging from that *finite pie* model, a comprehensive intervention approach develops auditory perceptual skills and fortifies central systems to efficiently and effectively allocate resources across sensory and central systems proportionate to the demands of a particular listening task. In so doing, resources are available *downstream* (i.e., peripheral) or *upstream* (i.e., central) to most efficiently and accurately execute the task (Chermak, 2007).

Strengthening central resources does not target central auditory processes directly; however, augmenting central resources complements and supplements direct treatment provided through auditory training (described in Chapters 7 and 9) and signal enhancement (discussed in Chapter 12), providing a more thorough and encompassing approach to remediating and minimizing CAPD and related functional deficits. Moreover, neuroscience-based learning primciples support extensive training to: (1) exploit the large, shared and overlapping auditory, cognitive, and language systems; (2) buttress the auditory system and reduce functional deficits; (3) emphasize interactions between bottom-up and top-down processing, and supramodal, crossmodal, and multimodal interfaces; and (4) maximize generalization and effectiveness (Chermak, 2007). Although a growing number of published reports document improved psychophysical performance, neurophysiologic representation of acoustic stimuli, and listening and related function in children and adults following auditory training (e.g., Bao, Chang, Woods, & Merzenich, 2004; deVillers-Sidani et al., 2010; Hayes, Warrier, Nicol, Zecker, & Kraus, 2003; Jirsa, 1992; Kraus & Disterhoft, 1982; Kraus et al., 1995; Merzenich, Grajski, Jenkins, Recanzone, & Peterson, 1991; Merzenich et al., 1996; Miller & Knudsen, 2003; Millward, Hall, Ferguson, & Moore, 2011; Moncrieff & Wertz, 2008; Murphy & Schochat, 2011;

Musiek, Baran, & Pinheiro, 1992; Musiek, Baran, & Shinn, 2004; Pan, Zhang, Cai, Zhou, & Sun, 2011; Pinheiro, & Capellini, 2010; Russo, Nicol, Zecker, Hayes, & Kraus, 2005; Schochat, Musiek, Alonso, & Ogata, 2010; Strait & Kraus, 2011; Tallal et al., 1996; Tremblay & Kraus, 2002; Tremblay, Kraus, Carrell, & McGee, 1997; Tremblay, Kraus, & McGee, 1998; Tremblay, Kraus, McGee, Ponton, & Otis, 2001; Warrier, Johnson, Hayes, Nicol, & Kraus, 2004; also see Chapter 3), central resources training complements these remedial efforts, providing buttressing and compensatory techniques (e.g., bolstered metacognitive knowledge and strategies to strengthen self-regulation of spoken language processing) to more effectively address functional deficits (Chermak, 2007). These techniques also will mitigate auditory processing deficits more resistant to treatment. Components of central resources training are listed in Table 10–2.

Fortified central resources (i.e., cognitive, metacognitive, linguistic and metalinguistic skills and knowledge) promote improved listening and spoken language comprehension (Chermak, 2007; Chermak & Musiek, 1997). To the extent central resource augmentation improves listening and reading comprehension, such augmentation also may reduce learning problems. For example, training in deducing word meaning from context should benefit both listening and reading comprehension, given the robust correlations among vocabulary, reading comprehension, and listening comprehension (Perfetti, 1985; Samuels, 1987; Stanovich, 1993; Sticht & James, 1984; Wiig, Semel, & Crouse, 1973). Similarly, therapy to increase phonological awareness and segmentation skills should aid both reading and listening comprehension (Agnew, Dorn, & Eden, 2003; Ehri et al.,

Table 10–2. Components of Central Resources Training for Central Auditory Processing Disorder (CAPD)

Metacogntive Resources: Skills and Strategies	Cognitive Resources: Skills & Strategies
Attribution Retraining	Sustained Auditory Attention (Auditory Vigilance)
Self-Instruction	
Cognitive Problem Solving	Memory
Self-Control (Self-Regulation)	Mnemonics
Cognitive Strategy Training	Auditory Memory Enhancement (AME)
Cognitive Style and Reasoning	Mind Mapping
Reciprocal Teaching	Working Memory
Assertiveness Training	
Metalinguistic Resources: Skills and Strategies	
Schema Induction and Discourse Cohesion Devices	Phonological Awareness (Phonemic Analysis and Synthesis)
Auditory-Verbal Closure	Prosody (Temporal Processing)
Vocabulary Building and Semantic Network Expansion	Listening Strategies

2001; Gillon, 2005; Liberman, Cooper, Shankweiler, & Studdert-Kennedy, 1967; Mann, 1991; Mattingly, 1972; Perfetti & McCutchen, 1982; Swanson, Hodson, & Schommer-Aikins, 2005).

Pivotal Role of Metacognition and Executive Function in Central Resources Training

Metacognition refers to the active monitoring and consequent regulation and orchestration of attention, memory, learning, and language processes in the service of some goal (Flavell, 1976). Executive function, a component of metacognition, refers to the self-directed actions of an individual that are used to self-regulate to accomplish self-control and goal-directed behavior and maximize future outcomes (Barkley, 1997). Executive function involves involves judgment, planning, and organization. These general control processes coordinate knowledge (i.e., cognition) and metacognitive knowledge, transforming such knowledge into behavioral strategies, which ensure that an individual's behavior is adaptive, consistent with some goal, and beneficial to the individual (Chermak, 2007; Chermak & Musiek, 1997). Because listening takes place within the multiple contexts of the acoustic, phonetic, linguistic, and social domains, simultaneous and integrated orchestration of multiple knowledge bases and skills is required for spoken language comprehension (Chermak, 2007; Chermak & Musiek,

1997). Metacognition drives this coordinated effort and is, therefore, pivotal to central resources training.

Listening with a compromised CANS requires a disproportionate allocation of processing resources to the auditory system, potentially rendering insufficient resources available "upstream" to support spoken language comprehension (Pichora-Fuller, Schneider, & Daneman, 1995). Cognitive areas can be recruited, however, to compensate for the reduction in CANS efficiency (e.g., Sarampalis, Edwards, Kalluri, & Hafter, 2009; Wong, Ettlinger, Sheppard, Gunasekera, & Dhar, 2010). Metacognition directs the allocation of central resources for self-regulation of skills and strategies, maximizing the efficient allocation of resources across sensory and cognitive systems (Chermak, 2007; Chermak & Musiek, 1997; McCoy et al., 2005; Piquado et al., 2010; Tun, Williams, Small, & Hafter, 2012). Moreover, by directing the allocation of central resources, metacognition indirectly influences bottom-up perceptual events (Ahissar & Hochstein, 1993). The observation that listeners require a larger interval of silence (i.e., gap) to perform a *between-channel* versus a *within-channel* gap detection task demonstrates how central resource allocation influences auditory perception (Phillips, Hall, Harrington, & Taylor, 1998; Phillips, Taylor, Hall, Carr, & Mossop, 1997). By engaging metacognitive processes, we encourage our clients to reflect on the demands inherent in a situation, as well as the skills and the actions needed to achieve their goals, thereby promoting a client-centered approach to therapy that should maximize intervention efficiency as a self-regulating client generalizes skills and strategies to everyday settings, including the classroom, workplace, and home. Active engagement reduces feelings of helplessness, facilitates development of self-esteem, and is likely to enhance the success of intervention (Danzl, Etter, Andreatta, & Kitzman, 2012). Extending skills and strategies across settings provides considerable practice opportunities, which optimizes plasticity (Hassamannova, Myslivecek, & Novakova, 1981; Rumbaugh & Washburn, 1996) and encourages generalization (Singley & Anderson, 1989). Metacognition is key to central resources training and ultimately to successful rehabilitation outcomes.

Metacognition and CAPD

Although CAPD, by definition, is not a metacognitive disorder, the experiential deficit incurred by individuals with CAPD in processing the auditory signal can lead to metacognitive deficits, since metacognition develops through experience in a skill-based context, such as spoken language processing (Harris, Reid, & Graham, 2004; Wong, 1991). Although much of the evidence documenting metacognitive strategy deficits has been collected from subjects who were described as learning disabled, subject selection criteria and histories indicate the likelihood that these subjects also presented central auditory processing deficits (Bos & Filip, 1982; Gerber, 1993b; Hallahan & Kneedler, 1979; Kotsonis & Patterson, 1980; Paris & Myers, 1981; Pressley & Levin, 1987; Suiter & Potter, 1978; Swanson, 1989, 1993; Torgesen, 1979; Torgesen & Houck, 1980; Wiens, 1983; Wong, 1987; Wong & Jones, 1982). The evidence reveals that these individuals present a passive and inefficient approach to problem solving (Swanson, 1989; Torgesen,

1979), a lack of metacognitive awareness (Brown, Bransford, Ferrara, & Campione, 1983; Hallahan & Kneedler, 1979; Paris & Myers, 1981; Swanson, 1993; Wiens, 1983), and difficulty monitoring comprehension (Bos & Filip, 1982; Kotsonis & Patterson, 1980; Wong & Jones, 1982). They tend not to deploy strategies spontaneously, often requiring external prompting to mobilize a strategy, and have difficulty choosing appropriate problem solving devices (Chermak, 2007; Chermak & Musiek, 1997). Less likely to activate schematic knowledge, they do not elaborate and construct information that guides comprehension (Gerber, 1993b).

This evidence coupled with clinical experience suggests that individuals with CAPD may not always exert executive control in deploying strategies to aid in organizing, monitoring, and understanding the acoustic signal, strategies that might facilitate information processing and enable them to compensate to some extent for the deficient central auditory processes that characterize the disorder (Chermak & Musiek, 1992, 1997; Gerber, 1993b; Harris, Reid, & Graham, 2004; Pressley & Levin, 1987; Suiter & Potter, 1978; Torgesen & Houck, 1980; Wong, 1987). As passive or inactive listeners, they may fail to attend selectively, organize input, deploy listening comprehension strategies, maintain on-task behavior, or employ task-approach skills, including the ability to focus on relevant task information (Chermak, 2007; Chermak & Musiek, 1997).

Metacognitive deficits in individuals with CAPD are secondary deficits resulting from repeated failure and lack of task persistence, limited use of executive function, inadequate experience with successful listening strategies, and low motivation (Chermak, 2007; Chermak &

Musiek, 1997). Fortunately, metacognitive deficits are responsive to intervention directed toward informed strategy use (Borkowski, Weyhing, & Carr, 1988; Brown et al., 1983; Fabricus & Hagen, 1984; Kendall & Braswell, 1982; Moynahan, 1978; Paris, Newman, & McVey, 1982; Reid & Borkowski, 1987). If left untreated, metacognitive deficits can exacerbate the impact of CAPD for spoken language understanding; with treatment, individuals with CAPD can become skilled listeners who actively engage in discovering what speakers are communicating. To achieve this goal they must be trained to use their metacognitive knowledge and strategies (i.e., executive function) to regulate and guide their listening and extraction of information from the spoken message (Chermak & Musiek, 1992). Comprehensive treatment of CAPD demands attention to both first-order problems of deficient central auditory processes and second-order metacognitive deficits.

Metacognition Promotes Generalization

Generalization of newly learned skills and strategies to contexts not employed during treatment is requisite to documenting change in function and treatment efficacy (Olswang & Bain, 1994). Failure to generalize may reflect metacognitive deficits and/or limitations of the treatment program (Borkowski, Johnston, & Reid, 1987; McReynolds, 1989). As argued by Borkowski, Estrada, Milstead, and Hale (1989), generalization of even ingrained strategy-specific knowledge to new stimuli and novel situations requires intact executive processing to guide selection and monitoring of strategies. Further, to achieve generalization, specific strategy knowledge and executive processes must be coupled with appropriate attributional beliefs of the likelihood of success (Borkowski et al., 1989). The metacognitive fulcrum of central resources training reinforces a number of generalization strategies.

Generalization Strategies

Consistent with the neuroscience-based training principles discussed above, extensive training, increased practice and rehearsal promote mastery of skills and automaticity of function (Chermak & Musiek, 1997). Role-playing and simulation provide opportunities to practice skills in contexts that are meaningful and relevant to the individual. Such activities also serve to reduce the differences between the treatment and natural environments, a strategy that has been identified as important to generalization (Stokes & Baer, 1977). Training that allows the client to explore the use of the target skill in multiple and diverse contexts expands the client's focus and is among the practices most often suggested to promote generalization of skills (Griffiths & Craighead, 1972; McReynolds, 1989; Murdock, Garcia, & Hardman, 1977; Rumbaugh & Washburn, 1996). Training in diverse contexts, with focus on multiple treatment settings and naturalistic settings including the home, school, and workplace, also underscores the importance of collaboration among professionals and families (Chermak & Musiek, 1997). Active client involvement in the therapy process through self-monitoring and ultimately self-regulation motivates the client to consider the use of a particular

skill or strategy and is of great value in promoting generalization of behaviors (Guevremont, 1990; Koegel, Koegel, & Ingham, 1986). (See Chapter 1 for additional discussion of collaboration, and Chermak and Musiek (1997) for other suggestions to promote generalization.)

Using Feedback to Promote Executive Control and Generalization

Salient reinfocrcement and feedback motivate, augment attention (both task-specific and general arousal) and maximize learning (Merzenich & Jenkins, 1999; Moore et al., 2009; Swanson & Cooney, 1991). Strong feedback is both positive and corrective (Chermak & Musiek, 1997). Effective feedback statements recognize effort and convey specific suggestions for improvement (Brophy, 1981). Moreover, feedback regarding the value of a strategy yields positive effects on strategy use and generalization (Ellis, Lenz, & Sabornie, 1987; Kennedy & Miller, 1976; Lenz, 1984; Ringel & Springer, 1980). Feedback need not avoid mention of errors. In fact, specific suggestions concerning how one might avoid particular errors further strengthens feedback (Ellis & Friend, 1991). Engaging clients in self-monitoring and recording their performance using charts, logs, or other devices is probably more reinforcing than providing extrinsic rewards (e.g., tokens, points, or prizes) (Ellis & Friend, 1991). Self-monitoring renders feedback more effective and develops executive control (Chermak & Musiek, 1997). Similarly, giving clients an opportunity to elaborate on the clinician's feedback, explaining the shortcomings of their strategies and steps that might be taken to improve their performance, also strengthens feedback, motivates clients, and promotes self-regulation (Adelman & Taylor, 1983; Ellis & Friend, 1991; Pressley, Johnson, & Symons, 1987). Hence, feedback serves an important function in promoting executive control.

As the client demonstrates greater skill level, the clinician should shift more responsibility for monitoring and adjusting behavior to the client, moving away from directive feedback statements and toward feedback that is more mediative (Ellis & Friend, 1991). Such mediative feedback provides cues to help clients discover and elaborate their own strategies and solutions rather than providing them directly to the client (Ellis & Friend, 1991; Ellis, Lenz, & Sabornie, 1987; Stone & Wertsch, 1984). Encouraging clients to monitor and track their progress through maintenance of a diary or log of reflections on strategy successes and failures increases the effectiveness of mediative feedback and promotes executive control (Chermak & Musiek, 1997). Moreover, encouraging clients to reestablish goals on the basis of feedback strengthens motivation. The reader is referred to Chermak and Musiek (1997) for additional discussion of feedback and goal structuring.

Central Resources: Knowledge, Strategies, and Skills

Metacognitive Knowledge and Strategies

Improved spoken language comprehension may be achieved through the development of listening strategies (Aarnou-tse, Van Den Bos, Kees, & Brand-Gruwel, 1998; Brand-Gruwel, Aarnoutse, & Van Den Bos, 1998; Graham & Harris, 2003; Harris, Reid, & Graham, 2004; Harris & Sipay, 1990; McKenzie, McKenzie, Neilson & Braun, 1981; Palincsar & Klenk, 1992; Pearson & Fielding, 1982; Reid, 1992; Pratt & Bates, 1982; Wong, 1993). Similar to the gains in memory seen with increasing age that are attributed to the development of mnemonic strategies (discussed below) rather than capacity (Pressley, 1982), improved spoken language comprehension may be achieved through self-regulation of listening strategies (Chermak & Musiek, 1997; Harris, Reid, & Graham, 2004; Reid, 1992). Interventions combining performance strategies (e.g., metalinguistic strategies that make use of context to derive meaning or invoke schemata to guide interpretation) with self-regulation training are more successful than either approach in isolation (Brown, Campione, & Day, 1981; Graham & Harris, 2003). Moreover, the prospects for transfer or generalization of strategy use to other appropriate situations are excellent since metacognitive strategies (i.e., planning, checking, and monitoring) are not task specific, but rather constitute a general approach to problem solving (Brown, Campione, & Barclay, 1979; Lodico, Ghatala, Levin, Pressley, & Bell, 1983). Implementing executive or metacognitive strategies training in conjunction with other top-down and bottom-up approaches, particularly auditory training (e.g., auditory discrimination, temporal processing), provides a powerful intervention approach.

Metacognitive Knowledge

Regulation and deployment of metacognitive strategies require a motivated individual in control of certain executive knowledge and functions (Chermak & Musiek, 1997). In particular, three types of knowledge (i.e., declarative, procedural, and conditional) are needed to effectively implement metacognitive strategies.

Declarative knowledge refers to knowledge that is known in a propositional manner. For example, prior knowledge of the topic and pertinent vocabulary facilitate message comprehension. Procedural knowledge refers to awareness of the processes underlying effective listening and spoken language comprehension. An effective listener, for instance, knows how to scan the message for main ideas, how to paraphrase the message, and how to incorporate context to facilitate message comprehension (Chermak & Musiek, 1997).

Declarative and procedural knowledge are necessary but not sufficient for effective listening unless employed in conjunction with conditional knowledge (Chermak & Musiek, 1997). Being aware of conditions that affect listening is integral to conditional knowledge, as well as knowing why particular strategies work and when to use them. Conditional knowledge would enable an effective listener to parse a message for facts when precise detail is required in response, rather than to paraphrase it. Conversely, deficient conditional knowledge would be evident in giving undue attention to a political theme of a message about voting irregularities at the expense of honing in on percentages and demographics detailed in the message.

Informal assessment of metacognitive strategies, prior to and during the therapy process, can reveal a client's metacognitive knowledge and processes and better prepare the clinician to train metacognitive strategy use. Items of a metacognitive knowledge and strategies assessment developed for reading (*Index of*

Reading Awareness) by Jacob and Paris (1987) can be adapted relatively easily to evaluate clients' awareness of the listening process (Chermak & Musiek, 1997).

Self-regulation is key to converting knowledge into practice. A skilled listener selectively deploys and coordinates resources and strategies using the executive processes of planning, evaluation, and regulation to achieve spoken language comprehension (Chermak & Musiek, 1997). Failed comprehension can be recognized through ongoing self-monitoring, after which the listener can modify strategies to meet the changing demands of the listening task, and ultimately enjoy successful message comprehension.

Metacognitive Strategies

Metacognitive strategies used for listening comprehension rely on the following skills and processes: (1) understanding task demands, (2) appropriately allocating attention, (3) identifying important parts of the message, (4) self-monitoring, (5) self-questioning, and (6) deployment of debugging strategies (Chermak & Musiek, 1997). Although skilled listeners use many of these processes automatically and tacitly, individuals with CAPD may require direct instruction and opportunities for application and reinforcement. These practice opportunities will encourage individuals with CAPD take deliberate actions to enhance listening through conscious, metacognition (Chermak & Musiek, 1997).

CAPD intervention programs may incorporate several metacognitive approaches, all of which promote active self-regulation and share several distinguishing features (Chermak & Musiek, 1997). Notwithstanding their differences, these approaches typically provide explicit and detailed instruction regarding the goals of strategies and their application to tasks, as well as training self-regulation and self-monitoring of strategy deployment and outcomes of that deployment (Palinscar & Brown, 1987). They encourage self-identification of strategies employed and the rationale for their use, as well as feedback about the efficacy of strategies for particular tasks (Palinscar & Brown, 1987; Pressley, Borkowski, & O'Sullivan, 1984).

Elements of one metacognitive approach often reinforce aspects of another, a good reason to combine several metacognitive approaches in an intervention program (Chermak & Musiek, 1997). For instance, motivation underlies assertiveness training, and attribution training strengthens motivation. Similarly, self-instruction can be used to model cognitive problem solving. Also demonstrating the reinforcing linkages among metacognitive approaches, reciprocal teaching instills self-esteem and self-regulation and is highly motivating. The explosion in mobile technology provides access to preinstalled smartphone calendars and numerous applications that can be downloaded to mobile phones and tablets (e.g., myHomework) that can provide metacognitive rehabilitation "on the go." Eight metacognitive approaches useful in managing CAPD are discussed below.

Attribution Training

Chronic listening problems and the often associated academic or workplace failures, as well as the social frustrations inherent in the inability to integrate fully within the family or peer group, places individuals with CAPD at risk for developing motivational problems (Chermak & Musiek, 1997). Some individuals with CAPD become reconciled to the belief that their listening abilities (and perhaps intellectual abilities as well) are poor and cannot be improved and that their efforts to succeed are futile (Chermak & Musiek, 1997). These beliefs lead to poor motivation and deterioration in task persistence, and paradoxically, these beliefs often infiltrate their perception of their successes as well as their failures (Torgesen, 1980). Attribution problems occur, then, when these individuals attribute successes to luck, an easy task, or the benevolence of a teacher, coworker, or employer (Bryan, 1991; Butkowsky & Willows, 1980; Pearl, 1982; Torgesen, 1980).

Dysfunctional attributional patterns in which success is attributed to external factors (e.g., luck, a *nice* teacher) develop concurrent with an eroded motivation to learn, with failure being attributed to internal factors such as inability (Pearl, 1982). Academic failure underscores the futility of effortful learning, and results in low self-concept. These faulty beliefs and attributions engender low self-esteem and self-efficacy. Not unexpectedly, these individuals may avoid the challenging task of listening, particularly in competing backgrounds or when the message is otherwise degraded or difficult to sort. Moreover, they will fatigue and give up prematurely under these circumstances, failing to invoke listening strategies to meet task demands and achieve success. Because deployment of self-regulatory behavior depends on motivation, this sequence of events leads to deficits in executive functions and a passive approach to listening (Chermak & Musiek, 1997). Passivity and inactivity, therefore, can be traced to a compromised self-system, a system that comprises self-efficacy, self-esteem, and attributions.

Rather than slide into passivity and low motivation, some maintain confidence by erroneously attributing their failings to teachers, parents, employers, or other external agents or circumstances. Others attribute difficulties to insufficient effort, an attribution tending to increase motivation (Licht, Kistner, Ozkaragoz, Shapiro, & Clausen, 1985; Speece, McKinney, & Applebaum, 1985). Attributions of failure to insufficient effort have, in fact, been shown to correlate with academic success (Kistner, Osborne, & LeVerrier, 1988).

Attribution retraining provides a direct approach to develop persistence and reestablish self-confidence in individuals who demonstrate a maladaptive motivational pattern (Licht & Kistner, 1986). Instilling causal attributions for failure to factors that are under the individual's control (e.g., insufficient effort) rather than to sensory or intellectual incapacity is a goal of attribution retraining, which should increase both self-esteem and persistence when individuals confront challenging listening tasks and conditions (Chermak & Musiek, 1997; Medway & Venino, 1982; Thomas & Pashley, 1982). Incorporating attribution training in therapy programs for young children with CAPD offers a preventive approach to motivational problems (Chermak & Musiek, 1997).

Components of Attribution Training. Attribution (re)training is a two-step procedure. As outlined by Chermak and Musiek (1997), the client is confronted with some failure (e.g., an incorrect response to a question posed following an oral-aural story presentation). The key component involves teaching the client to attribute the failure to insufficient effort. The clinician might tell the client that his or her answer was not correct, that he or she is working hard but should listen even more carefully. In a parallel manner,

the clinician should attribute successes to effort, providing feedback that communicates that the response was correct and acknowledging that the client was listening carefully and trying hard.

Clients tend to be motivated to improve their performance and experience success when the wording of attributional statements (i.e., feedback) acknowledges hard work while urging even greater effort (Miller, Brickman, & Bolen, 1975; Schunk, 1982). Feedback that fails to recognize efforts already expended, indicating that the clinician perceived no effort or that the client was not indeed already working hard, are less likely to be effective (Miller et al., 1975; Schunk, 1982).

In addition to the specific wording of the attributional statements, the effectiveness of attribution retraining also depends on the proportion of successes and failures and scheduling of failures (Chermak & Musiek, 1997). Although confronting failure is integral to attribution retraining, some success is necessary to cultivate the self-efficacy needed to trust the method's premise that increased effort will lead to increased success (Clifford, 1978; Dweck, 1975). Tasks must be structured to allow that degree of success. Moreover, persistence is fostered by varying the number of difficult items, which demand increased effort, within an activity (Chapin & Dyck, 1976).

Payoff—improved performance resulting from increased effort—establishes the validity of attribution retraining. Treatment effects will not persist or generalize without this validation or payoff (Dweck, 1977; Licht & Kistner, 1986). The client must be able to deploy appropriate metacognitive, cognitive, and metalinguistic strategies to maximize the chances that additional effort will lead to improved performance (Reid & Borkowski, 1987).

Improved auditory skills developed through direct auditory training also are crucial to improved listening and hence the validation of attribution training. Knowing how to work harder, through sustained effort coupled with listening strategies, is more likely to lead to permanent improvements in performance and spontaneous deployment of these strategies (Borkowski, Weyhing, & Carr, 1988; Fabricus & Hagen, 1984; Kendall & Braswell, 1982; Moynahan, 1978; Paris et al., 1982). As stated by Reid and Borkowski (1987), "self-attributions about the importance of effort in producing success serve an energizing function in the deployment of available strategies and sustain the cognitive search for alternative strategies in the face of learning obstacles" (p. 306).

Cognitive Behavior Modification

Cognitive behavior modification depends on a client's planful use of strategies, notably executive and task-specific strategies (Lloyd, 1980). With the goal of self-control through a reflexive processing and response style, a client instructed in cognitive behavior modification employs, monitors, checks, and evaluates behavioral strategies (Brown et al., 1981). Critical to this approach is the informed and active client.

Cognitive behavior modification is classified into four categories: self-instruction, problem solving, cognitive strategy training, and self-regulation (Whitman, Burgio, & Johnson, 1984). Although cognitive behavior modification methods fall into categories with distinct emphases and procedures, the commonality across methods is fundamental (Meichenbaum, 1986; Whitman et al., 1984). All cognitive behavior modification procedures include: (1) client involvement as active collabora-

tors; (2) target strategies modeled during training; (3) a reflective processing and response style; and (4) analysis of the relationship between the client's actions and the task outcome (Lloyd, 1980; Meichenbaum, 1986). Also shared across the procedures is the use of daily logs or diaries. Encouraging the client to maintain a daily log exploring difficult listening situations and the relative value of strategies deployed to enhance listening promotes self-monitoring of the effectiveness of listening comprehension strategies (Chermak & Musiek, 1997). The use of diaries and logs as homework also benefits generalization of executive and task-specific strategies and skills (Guevremont, 1990).

Self-instruction, problem solving, self-regulation, and cognitive strategy training denote separate, but often interdependent, approaches in cognitive behavior modification. Demonstrating this overlap, self-instruction uses directive self-statements to train task specific strategies and self-control, which are the foci of cognitive strategy training and self-regulation, respectively (Chermak & Musiek, 1997). Cognitive problem solving, while using self-instruction and self-regulation techniques, taps into a different aspect of the cognitive domain: reducing uncertainty and resolving problems (Chermak & Musiek, 1997). Clearly, combining procedures from more than one approach can increase training effectiveness (Whitman et al., 1984).

Self-Instruction. Self-instruction methods train clients to formulate adaptive and self-directing verbal cues before and during a task or situation (Chermak & Musiek, 1997). In addition to listening training, self-instruction is particularly useful in addressing academic difficulties, including reading comprehension problems, and impulsive and hyperactive behaviors (Hart & Morgan, 1993; Wong, 1993). Five sequential steps of self-instruction, outlined by Meichenbaum and Goodman (1971), promote the inculcation and generalization of the self-instructional routine: (1) the clinician performs the task while self-verbalizing aloud; (2) the client performs the task while the clinician verbalizes; (3) the client performs while self-instructing aloud; (4) the client performs while whispering; and (5) the client performs while self-instructing covertly (i.e., silently).

Several problem-solving skills are incorporated in self-instruction (Chermak & Musiek, 1997). The client must approach the listening situation with a planful and reflective attitude, self-monitoring for any signs of inattention or distraction and assessing the purpose of the message. Next, the listener must focus on key words, examine context, make predictions, and draw inferences. The clinician may encourage general or more specific problem-solving instructions depending on the nature of the task. Drawing on the classification system of the cognitive domain developed by Bloom (1956) (i.e., knowledge, comprehension, application, analysis, synthesis, and evaluation), clients should be encouraged to pose more critical questions demanding higher level thinking commensurate with the message content and task requirements (Wilson, Lanza, & Barton, 1988). The clinician may find it helpful to move problem-solving instructions from the specific to more general as the client's skills increase (Chermak & Musiek, 1997). Self-monitoring continues throughout the task, culminating in self-evaluation and feedback. Self-reinforcement, the final step in the self-instruction procedure, establishes a sense of pride and accomplishment and should increase the client's motivation to transfer the self-instructional technique to novel situations (Chermak & Musiek, 1997). If the client is not successful, the clinician should offer some guidance for coping with failure. As discussed in the preceding section, coping with failure may be best handled by self-attributions of failure to something under the client's control (e.g., improper strategy selection, insufficient effort).

Cognitive Problem Solving. Cognitive problem solving offers clients opportunities to resolve problems through systematic analysis and self-regulation. In basically a five-stage process, the clinician serves as a consultant as the client learns to reconceive the potentially anxiety-producing listening situation as a problem to be solved (Chermak & Musiek, 1997). Clients are taught to deploy executive processes in conjunction with the requisite auditory and language skills to resolve the message. They are instructed to analyze situations and generate a variety of potentially viable responses, recognizing and implementing the most effective response. Further, they are helped to confront cognitive distortions (e.g., catastrophizing, jumping to conclusions), which may be sustaining unnecessary anxiety or fear (Hart & Morgan, 1993). Self-regulation procedures (described in the next section) are used to maintain and generalize the productive response (Goldfried & Davison, 1976). Cognitive problem solving is especially therapeutic when working with individuals with anxiety, fear, or phobias (Hart & Morgan, 1993) and has been used successfully in management of patients with tinnitus (Sweetow, 1986).

In perhaps the most important stage of problem solving, the process begins by familiarizing oneself with the nature of the problem (D'Zurilla, 1986). The second stage requires the generation of hypotheses regarding solutions to the problem. In the third stage, one evaluates the solution options, considers their utility and predicts possible costs or consequences, and selects the best one. The fourth stage is bifurcated. If a viable solution is found, it is implemented; if no solution is deemed tenable, the incubation phase begins during which no active effort is expended toward solving the problem (Halpern, 1984). Ironically, it is during this incubation phase that solutions often appear as an epiphany or *out of the blue* (Halpern, 1984, p. 163). A fifth stage in the process involves the monitoring and evaluation of one's performance in relation to solving the problem. Self-monitoring homework assignments are useful in measuring progress. Self-reinforcement for successful problem solving (e.g., spoken language understanding) should lead to enhanced self-efficacy and generalization of the process (Haaga & Davison, 1986). A flowchart illustrating cognitive problem solving in spoken language comprehension is presented in Figure 10–1.

In addition to self-instruction and self-monitoring, cognitive rehearsal is another useful problem solving technique (Haaga & Davison, 1986). Mentally reviewing the listening task prior to completing it provides an opportunity to identify potential obstacles, solutions, and preventative steps so that listening may be successful (Chermak & Musiek, 1997).

Cognitive Strategy Training. Cognitive strategy training helps clients become more aware of their own cognitive processes and gain skills in deploying specific task strategies underlying effective performance (Brown & French, 1979; Whitman et al., 1984). Cognitive strategies may be taught following Meichenbaum and Goodman's (1971) five-step self-instruction program. Extended training of the strategy and feedback on the strategy's effectiveness are crucial to successful implementation of cognitive strategy training (Whitman et al., 1984).

Self-Regulation Procedures. Self-regulation training leads clients toward self-control through self-monitoring, self-evaluation, and self-reinforcement (Brown et al., 1981; Kanfer & Gaelick, 1991; Whitman et al., 1984). Training begins by increasing awareness of the behavior targeted for control and proceeds by teaching goal setting and self-monitoring skills for behavioral change (Whitman et al., 1984). Qualitative monitoring of performance involves the client noting factors such as attitude and emotional state, whereas quantitative monitoring measures successful performance (Chermak & Musiek, 1997). The client self-evaluates favorably if information obtained through self-monitoring matches his or her standards or listening comprehension goals. Self-reinforcement ensues, primarily from internal satisfaction and heightened motivation rather than self-administered reward (Kanfer & Gaelick, 1991).

Self-regulation training promotes effective listening by encouraging the listener to monitor comprehension processes to determine whether they are meeting his or her comprehension needs (Chermak & Musiek, 1997). When comprehension errors, disruptions, or inadequacies are detected, the listener learns to modify strategies to handle ambiguities, inconsistencies, or complexities that might

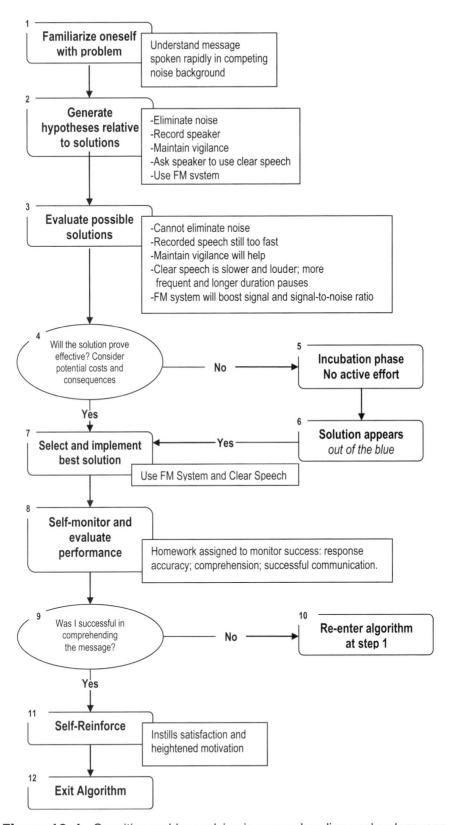

Figure 10–1. Cognitive problem solving in comprehending spoken language.

otherwise compromise spoken language understanding (Danks & End, 1987).

Active Listening. Active listening emerges from information processing theory that suggests that skilled listeners actively deploy various bottom-up (e.g., segmenting, discriminating, and sequencing) and top-down strategies to monitor listening and extract information from the spoken message in discovering the speaker's message (Chermak & Musiek, 1997). Active listening training combines the techniques of essentially all of the metacognitive strategies discussed above. The elements of active listening must be made explicit and practice opportunities provided for clients with CAPD. These elements include: listening intently; showing interest through the use of eye contact, body language and posture; listening empathetically (i.e., placing yourself in the other's "shoes"); using closure, inferencing, deducing, and predicting skills; using communication repair strategies (e.g., requesting repetition, rephrasing, confirmations); ignoring background noise; and not giving up prematurely. It is important to teach young children "how" to listen, including emphasis on attending behaviors (e.g., be still and quiet) and readiness to listen (e.g., sit tall and flat in chair), as discussed below under Listening Tactics (Truesdale, 1990).

Reciprocal Teaching

The client and clinician alternate roles in reciprocal teaching, allowing the client to take the role of teacher as well as student (Casanova, 1989; Chermak, Curtis, & Seikel, 1996; Palincsar & Brown, 1984). Reciprocal teaching lets clients anchor their knowledge of their executive processes by making explicit their knowledge and use of strategies; in addition, most clients enjoy heightened self-esteem and self-efficacy in reciprocal role playing (Chermak & Musiek, 1997). Reciprocal teaching promotes analysis and problem solving and allows the clinician to ascertain the client's understanding and mastery of skills and strategies. Reciprocal teaching has produced demonstrated gains in reading comprehension, self-monitoring, memory, and health education, including hearing conservation (Aarnoutse et al., 1998; Brand-Gruwel et al., 1998; Chermak et al., 1996; Clarke, MacPherson, Holmes, & Jones, 1986; Palincsar & Brown, 1984, 1986; Palincsar & Klenk, 1992; Paris, Wixson, & Palincsar, 1986).

The following principles and procedures underlie reciprocal teaching: (1) modeling of the target behavior by the clinician-teacher, making the processing strategies overt, explicit, and concrete; (2) contextual modeling of strategies; (3) verbal analysis of the strategies used by the client to comprehend the message, as well as corroboration of the message's content (4) clinician feedback; and (5) transfer of responsibility for comprehension from the clinician to the client once competence is demonstrated by the client (Harris & Sipay, 1990).

Cognitive Style and Reasoning

Selecting the appropriate cognitive style is necessary to meet diverse processing demands and listening tasks (Chermak & Musiek, 1997). Skillfully matching the cognitive style with changing tasks requires reasoning: critically evaluating arguments, drawing inferences and conclusions, and generating and testing hypotheses (Nickerson, 1986). Effective listening requires reasoning to critically evaluate and ultimately reconstruct the messages we hear, as well as the flexibility to invoke the cognitive style that best meets changing task demands (Chermak & Musiek, 1997). Inflexible reasoning and sole reliance on any one cognitive style is ineffective in meeting the diverse processing demands of a complex linguistic signal often presented in challenging (and unfavorable) listening environments (e.g., noisy and reverberant). Dependence on a single cognitive style, such as overreliance on literal interpretation, could lead to failure to comprehend figurative language such as metaphors, idioms, and proverbs (Bard, Shillcock, & Altmann, 1988; Marslen-Wilson & Tyler, 1980; Warren & Warren, 1970). Overreliance on the cognitive style of bottom-up processing could lead to failure to discern multiple meaning words (e.g., homonyms and heteronyms) and misunderstanding a message's content. Similarly, overreliance on top-down processing may cause schema inflexibility, biasing interpretation, and impeding comprehension. (See Schema Theory and Use below.)

Spoken language is most efficiently comprehended through complementary cognitive styles. The model of central auditory processing outlined earlier in this chapter illustrates the necessity for the operation of complementary cognitive styles for spoken language comprehension. Accessing multiple cognitive styles is amplified for individuals with CAPD whose deficient auditory processes render them less able to cope with degraded acoustic signals and for whom sole reliance on bottom-up processing would leave them extremely vulnerable to comprehension problems (Chermak & Musiek, 1997). Individuals with CAPD should be trained to take advantage of specific information revealed through bottom-up processing (e.g., auditory segmentation,

auditory discrimination, pattern recognition), as well as more global information extracted from top-down processes that facilitate auditory and grammatic closure, inferencing, and recognition of conceptual nuances (Chermak & Musiek, 1997).

Although skilled listeners often unconsciously and automatically adjust their cognitive style to meet the processing demands of the task, less skilled listeners must be instructed to make these seamless transitions and reach a level of automaticity (Chermak & Musiek, 1997). Fortunately, cognitive style can be changed through training. For example, children become more reflective following training in the use of a verbal self-control strategy (Craighead, Wilcoxon-Craighead, & Meyers, 1978). Individuals with CAPD may benefit from exercises that reveal the advantages of analysis and reflection prior to synthesizing information and converging on an interpretation of a complex message. Given the importance of cognitive style flexibility for spoken language comprehension, training individuals with CAPD to vary their cognitive styles provides them the opportunity to become appropriately responsive listeners (Chermak & Musiek, 1997).

Deductive and Inductive Inferencing. Effective listening requires use of the full range of cognitive approaches to information processing and reasoning, including both deduction and induction and analysis and synthesis (Chermak & Musiek, 1997). Inductive inferencing involves generalization, reasoning from the particulars to the general; deductive inferencing involves reasoning from the general to the particular (Nickerson, 1986). Spoken language comprehension often requires that individuals infer information not specifically presented in the message but that may be implied and induced or deduced from the available patterns of information. Inferencing skills can be developed through the context-derived vocabulary building technique described later in this chapter. Also useful are short stories requiring inferencing on the basis of perceptual information, logic, and/or evidence (see Gerber, 1993b). Attention to the appropriate use of diverse cognitive styles (e.g., divergent/convergent, impulsive/reflective, adaptive/innovative, synthetic/analytic, field dependent/field independent) should also be introduced in therapy (Chermak & Musiek, 1997).

Assertiveness Training

Assertiveness training empowers individuals and advances all intervention goals. Assertion can be defined as "self-expression through which one stands up for one's own basic human rights without violating the basic human rights of others" (Kelley, 1979, p. 14). Command of basic interpersonal and communication skills is necessary to assert effectively; however, motivation drives assertiveness, for without a desire to succeed and a positive cognitive *mindset*, one is not likely to assume the personal responsibility inherent to assertiveness (Chermak & Musiek, 1997). The goal of assertion is to attain personal effectiveness by communicating what one feels, thinks, and wants (Chermak & Musiek, 1997). Assertive behavior is self-enhancing and empowering, engendering good feelings about one's self, as well as furthering attainment of one's desired goals (Alberti & Emmons, 1978). Assertiveness can be learned (Bornstein, Bellack, & Hersen, 1977; Rehm, Fuchs, Roth, Kornblith, & Romano, 1979); how-

ever, self-confidence and self-esteem are prerequisite (Kelley, 1979).

Clinical experience indicates that successful treatment outcomes are correlated with a client's assertiveness (Chermak & Musiek, 1997). Because assertive clients tend to be more actively involved in planning and directing their own therapy, they tend to derive greater gains. Moreover, their higher motivation and positive mindset lead assertive clients to generalize new strategies and skills to everyday life contexts (Chermak & Musiek, 1997).

Assertion typically involves a verbal exchange, whereby the individual formulates and delivers an assertive message (Kelley, 1979). Nonverbal skills also influence message impact: The effectiveness of the assertion is influenced by the nonverbal aspects of the message's delivery, including paralinguistic elements (e.g., vocal intensity, intonation, rhythm), kinesics (e.g., facial expression, posture, gestures), and proxemics (e.g., distance between parties, seating arrangements) (Chermak & Musiek, 1997). Nonverbal cues can reinforce the verbal message and strengthen the effectiveness of that message. Assertiveness training techniques may involve modeling, guided practice, coaching, homework and self-management, readings, and small group discussion (Kelley, 1979).

Metacognition in the Classroom

Access to the communication in the classroom is crucial to academic success. In addition to the specific metacognitive strategies discussed above, audiologists and speech-language pathologists should alert teachers and students with CAPD to the role of particular words (many of which are formal schemata) and phrases often used in the classroom that like schemata carry organizational, integrational and predictive value. Ellis (1989) referred to these words as *alert words* and encouraged educators to make obvious to students their power to augment listening and participation in class discussions. The four word classes signal: (1) reasons (e.g., because, reasons, since, therefore); (2) examples (e.g., example, instance, sample, type, model); (3) comparisons (e.g., associated, contrast, differences, similarities, in relation to, opposite, parallel, on the other hand); (4) main idea (e.g., basically, in essence, in conclusion, in summary, key point, the most important, the gist is); and (5) lists of important information (e.g., categories, characteristics, divisions, features, groups, kinds, parts, members, stages, ways).

Cognitive Training

Cognition refers to the automatic and unconscious processes (e.g., perceiving, recognizing, conceiving, judging, sensing, reasoning) that underlie the activity of knowing (Nickerson, 1986). Cognition encompasses the acquisition, organization, and use of knowledge (Neisser, 1976). Cognitive processes allow the listener to transform, reduce, elaborate, store, recover, and use sensory input. Attention and memory are two primary and highly interdependent and interactive cognitive resources (de Fockert, Rees, Frith, & Lavie, 2001; Sorqvist, Stenfelt, & Ronnberg, 2012). Demonstrating increased reaction times, greater distracter interference, and increased activity in the prefrontal cortex under high working memory loads, de Fockert et al. (2001) concluded that working memory maintains prioritization of relevant information, reduces distraction, and modulates attention (Sorqvist et al., 2012). In the same way, attention to a stimulus or task is essential to memory. Clearly, alerting a child in a classroom to *follow along* or *listen carefully* is an important first step toward improving a child's memory of the classroom presentation.

Attention

Attention is a multidimensional psychological construct, which when viewed from an information processing point of view includes sustained attention or vigilance, selective attention, and divided attention. Attention is fundamental to the coordination, organization, and execution of human behavior (Sergeant, 1996). Attention is ubiquitous in perception, cognition, and learning. Demonstrating the powerful role of attention for learning, Solan, Shelley-Tremblay, Silverman, and Larson (2003) reported that 12 one-hour sessions of computer-assisted attention therapy improved reading comprehension in a group of adolescents with reading disabilities compared with the control group that showed no significant improvement in reading comprehension scores. The capacity for selective attention is fully developed in children by age 7 years of age, while sustained attention (i.e., vigilance) continues to develop throughout adolescence (McKay, Halperin, Schwartz, & Sharma, 1994).

Vigilance is a higher order, supramodal process that serves acoustic signal processing (Farah, Wong, Monheit, & Morrow,

1989). Vigilance can be trained using procedures much like those employed in auditory or continuous performance tasks (Keith, 1994; Riccio, Reynolds, & Lowe, 2001). The individual is required to sustain attention to a continuous stream of auditory stimuli, such as environmental sounds, syllables, or words, and to respond (e.g., by raising a hand, tapping a table) when a particular stimulus is heard. Failure to detect the target stimulus reflects inattention. False positive errors (i.e., responding to a stimulus other than the target stimulus) may reflect impulsivity. Training auditory attention is discussed further in Chapter 7.

Memory

Exercises to strengthen memory should benefit individuals with CAPD given the essential role of memory for spoken language processing and learning. Metamemory, or knowledge and awareness of one's own memory systems and strategies (Flavell & Wellman, 1977), provides one focus for memory improvement (Chermak & Musiek, 1997). A number of direct memory enhancement techniques provide a second group of approaches. Although some drugs have been shown to improve memory losses associated with neurodegenerative diseases such as Alzheimer's disease (Howard et al., 2012; Lopez et al., 2009) by regulating the activity of glutamate or increasing the amount of acetylcholine in the brain, pharmacological therapies are not available yet nor recommended to enhance memory in individuals with CAPD (Chermak & Musiek, 1997; Musiek & Hoffman, 1990). Given our still limited understanding of the neurochemistry of the auditory system (AAA, 2010; ASHA,

2005; Musiek & Oxholm, 2003) and the absence of a pharmacological treatment for CAPD, it is appropriate to consider the full range of behavioral interventions. (See Chapter 22 for emerging and future trends in intervention.)

Certainly, adults demonstrate a substantial understanding of metamemory (Flavell & Wellman, 1977). Children, however, gradually acquire knowledge and appreciation of retrieval cues and effective strategies for coding, organizing, and retrieving items in memory (Howe & Ceci, 1978). Most children begin to demonstrate some awareness of the limitations of memory and of factors affecting memory (e.g., realizing that they cannot remember all information with equal ease) by age 6 years (Kreutzer, Leonard, & Flavell, 1975); and by age 8 to 10 years, children demonstrate a planful approach to encoding and retrieval, including becoming aware of mnemonics and their benefits (Cavanaugh & Perlmutter, 1982; Harris, 1978; Harris & Terwogt, 1978; Kail, 1990; Kreutzer et al., 1975). Memory enhancement techniques and strategies discussed in this section include: mnemonics, auditory memory enhancement (AME), and mind mapping. Also discussed is a variety of specific approaches to target working memory, a specific and pervasive component of memory.

External compensatory aids (e.g., prosthetic devices, cognitive orthotic devices) offer a relatively powerful and immediate means to augment memory; however, external devices should not be used to the exclusion of internal aids and repetitive practice (Chermak & Musiek, 1997). Internal strategies and repetitive practice are preferable to external aids because they require an individual's active control and self-regulation and are therefore more likely to be applied across settings and maintained over time (Borkowski et al., 1989; Guevremont, 1990). The reader is referred to Chermak and Musiek (1997), Harrell, Parente, Bellingrath, and Lisicia (1992), and Harris (1992) for discussion of external devices. In addition to the strategies and techniques presented here, the reader is reminded that memory can be enhanced through the influence of executive functions. (See Metacognitive Strategies above.)

Mnemonics

Mnemonics are *artificial* or contrived memory aids for organizing information that operate through the application of basic learning principles (e.g., association, organization, meaningfulness, attention) (Harris, 1992; Loftus & Loftus, 1976). Mnemonics can employ acronyms, rhymes, verbal mediators, visual imagery, and drawing, among other devices.

They are consciously learned and used, and the majority is language based. Mnemonic techniques and systems have been shown to improve memory in subjects of various ages, including preschool-age children (Levin, 1976) and older adults (Treat, Poon, Fozard, & Popkin, 1977). Described below are elaboration, transformation, chunking, and coding, probably the four most frequently used mnemonic devices (Chermak & Musiek, 1997).

Elaboration entails assigning meaning to items to be remembered by recasting them in meaningful sentences, analogies, or acronyms. For example, the sentence "Richard Of York Gained Battles In Vain" is an example of elaboration in which the first letter of each word represents the first letter of the colors of the spectrum of light (i.e., red, orange, yellow, green, blue, indigo, and violet) (Chermak &

Musiek, 1997). Another common example of an elaboration mnemonic is the sentence "Every Good Boy Does Fine," used to recall the notes on the treble staff lines (Chermak & Musiek, 1997). First-letter cueing to form acronyms aids memory for sequences. The acronym TORCH (i.e., toxoplasmosis, rubella, syphilis, cytomegalovirus, and herpes) represents the most common perinatal infections that raise the risk of morbidity, especially auditory morbidity. In the same manner, verbal chaining, or assembling items into sentences, may facilitate memory for otherwise unrelated items. The use of rhymes, such as the one beginning "Thirty days hath September. . . . " also demonstrates the power of elaboration to benefit memory for the odd distribution of days across the various months. Finally, paraphrasing and summarizing are two additional examples of elaborative techniques (Chermak & Musiek, 1997).

Transformation involves reconstituting complicated material into a more basic form that can be more easily remembered. For example, transforming Pythagoras' theorem regarding the relationships among the three sides of a right triangle into a simple equation ($a^2 + b^2 = c^2$) gives the trigonometry student a concise means for storing complicated mathematical relationships. Some types of paraphrasing also may be considered transformations, and thus benefit memory (Chermak & Musiek, 1997).

Chunking entails organizing items into categories. Organizing a mental *to-do* list into office, home, and weekend is an example of chunking. In the same way, grouping telephone numbers into parts, a three-digit area code, three-digit exchange, and the final four digits into a calendar year also reflects a chunking operation (Chermak & Musiek, 1997).

Coding involves recasting the form in which information is presented. Creating mental images (e.g., real scenes or diagrams) or drawing pictures to capture information presented auditorily are examples of coding (Chermak & Musiek, 1997). Drawing may be a particularly useful coding technique for individuals experiencing spoken language processing difficulties because as a nonlinguistic mnemonic drawing activates the primary motor cortex of the right hemisphere and thereby applies bihemispheric processing to a verbal memory task (Musiek & Chermak, 1995).

Auditory Memory Enhancement (AME)

Musiek (1999) described the auditory memory enhancement procedure as an expansion and modification of the early work of Wittrock (1974). The frequent encouragement to *listen carefully* may inadvertently cause children with CAPD to rely excessively on analytic processing such that they may not develop the complementary gestalt processing strategy (Musiek, 1999). Supporting this observation are findings that individuals with CAPD have poor contour recognition, a gestalt feature, which is needed in acoustic pattern perception (Pinheiro & Musiek, 1985). The AME method stimulates the analytic-gestalt interface by encouraging imagery and spatial elaboration, as well as analytical listening (Musiek, 1999). The AME procedure promotes concept development and listening (reading) comprehension through the use of generative processes, interhemispheric transfer, and multimodal integration. The AME also provides a useful strategy for note-taking and for interpreting complex auditory information and in this regard is similar to mind mapping techniques (discussed below), which employ drawings supplemented by words to enhance relationships and anchor concepts.

The three key steps in the AME procedure are: listening or reading (verbal/analytic), sketching (spatial/gestalt), and discussing or writing (Musiek, 1999). The choice of modality depends upon the individual's age and reading and writing capability. After listening (or reading) to several paragraphs or pages of information, the client is asked to sketch (within no more than 2–3 minutes) the main concept(s) presented (Musiek, 1999). The imposition of a time limit is key to the success of the procedure, as it forces the individual to reduce the main concept into its basic form and transfer from a verbal/analytic representation to a spatial/gestalt representation (Musiek, 1999). This transfer supports retention and access (Ashcraft, 1989; Wittrock, 1974). This process may be repeated until the entire story or other written material (e.g., journal article, newspaper article) is reviewed and sketched. In the final stage of this procedure, the client is asked to review the sketches and convey to the clinician, either orally or in writing, the entire story, including all of the main concepts. Musiek (1999) described remedial steps if the individual experiences difficulty with the procedure. For example, if the client's sketch does not reflect the main concept, the clinician discusses the story with the client to help make the concept salient to the client. Following this discussion, the client is asked to resketch the story's main concept.

Engaging clients in sketching, a generative process, promotes retention of information (Wittrock, 1977). Transferring the analytic/verbal representation into a gestalt/spatial representation aids access and recall, since a gestalt representation promotes the formulation of general concepts that are easier to remember than large quantities of analytic information (Hergenhan & Olsen, 1993). Also aiding memory is the involvement of multiple modalities, including the motor system (Musiek, 1999). Sketching activates the *visual-spatial sketch pad,* a subsystem of working memory, while the verbal information in its analytic form activates another working memory subsystem, the *phonologic loop* (Schacter & Tulving, 1994). The multiple representations (i.e., verbal, spatial, auditory, visual, somatic, and motor) should improve memory processes (Massaro, 1987). The transfer of analytic, verbal-based information (i.e., primarily left hemisphere) to a more gestalt representation (i.e., primarily right hemisphere) depends on the use of mental imagery, which has been shown to enhance recall and information processing (as discussed above under Mnemonics) (MacInnis & Price, 1987; Miller, 1956; Wittrock, 1974). The concurrent activation of analytic/verbal, gestalt/spatial, and motor processes galvanizes a larger neural network, with the attendant interactions, redundancies, and opportunities to guide memory and comprehension (Ashcraft, 1989).

Mind Mapping

Mind mapping is a visually based approach, involving the drawing of pictures, usually supplemented by words, as an alternative to note-taking or outlining (Margulies, 1991). These maps provide a nonlinear means of recording information and reflecting relationships among concepts and ideas. Like the AME procedure described above, mind mapping fosters retention and comprehension though the concurrent interplay of auditory, visual, somatic, and motor modalities, as well as activation of analytic/verbal and gestalt/spatial processes and representations.

Encouraging students to use visual and auditory input for better comprehension is central to academic success; however, note-taking precludes watching the teacher, forcing students with CAPD to rely solely on their compromised auditory system for all information. Because these youngsters are often poor writers, their pedestrian note-taking skills exacerbate an already difficult situation as their transcription lags behind the spoken message (Chermak & Musiek, 1992). The resulting antagonism between writing and listening leads to division of attention; instead of summating information across auditory and visual modes, confusion ensues as attention is diverted from the already less than adequate auditory system (Chermak & Musiek, 1997). Providing lecture notes to youngsters with CAPD prior to the class presentation, having another student take notes for them, or using a tape recorder for later transcription enables students with CAPD to attend to and process both auditory and visual information (Chermak & Musiek, 1992). Similarly, supplementing verbal instructions with visual instructions and using computer-aided instruction and other audiovisual equipment benefits students with CAPD. Concurrently, audiologists, speech-language pathologists, and teachers can collaborate to improve note-taking skills by encouraging students' use of prosodic cues and formal schemata both discussed below), and metamemory strategies to gauge the relative importance of information, guide organization and outlining, and enhance retention. (See Chapter 13 for additional discussion of classroom and instructional modifications for students with CAPD.)

Working Memory

Working memory involves the temporary storage of information used during reasoning and planning (Baddeley, 1995). It requires the storage of some information during processing of other information. Holding an address in mind while simultaneously retaining a sequence of travel directions or listening to a sequence of events while trying to understand the meaning are everyday examples of working memory. In contrast to short-term memory, working memory involves executive processing and manipulation in addition to simple storage of information. Working memory supports executive control and is crucial to problem solving (i.e., analysis and synthesis) (Barkley, 1997). Working memory perceptually organizes sounds, segregating and integrating spectral and temporal attributes that occur simultaneously and sequentially. It functions similarly in segmenting and integrating tones into melodies and parsing harmonies (Schon et al., 2004). Working memory modulates attention (de Fockert et al., 2001; Sorqvist et al., 2012) and supports auditory processing, including auditory localization (Martinkauppi et al., 2002), auditory pattern processing (Zatorre, 2001; Zatorre et al., 2002), speech recognition in noise (Akeroyd, 2008; Salvi et al., 2002; Wong et al., 2009), and dichotic listening (Janco & Shah, 2002; Martin et al., 2007) . Working memory is key to understanding spoken language, especially as the signal is degraded by background noise (Pichora-

Fuller et al., 1995; Ronnberg, 2003). Not unexpectedly, working memory demonstrates strong correlations with academics and language, including vocabulary, language acquisition, listening comprehension, reading comprehension, problem solving, and mathematics (Daneman & Blennerhasett, 1984; Daneman & Merikle, 1996).

Working memory deficits have been documented in individuals diagnosed with attention deficit hyperactivity disorder (ADHD), language impairment, learning disability, and those with histories of chronic otitis media (Daneman & Merikle, 1996). Cases of working memory deficits in children diagnosed with CAPD also have been reported. Bamiou et al. (2007) described working memory deficits and central auditory processing (dichotic digit and pitch pattern) deficits in a child with congenital aniridia and abnormalities of the interhemispheric pathway due to PAX 6 mutation. Mody, Schwartz, Gravel, and Ruben (1999) found poorer retention and recall of consonant-vowel syllables among subjects with positive histories of otitis media, which they attributed to underspecified coding of phonetic features in working memory. Working memory deficits likely result in difficulties maintaining relevant information simultaneously and integrating information, inefficient resource allocation, and listening comprehension deficits (Daneman & Blennerhasett, 1984). Additional research is needed to explore the degree to which working memory deficits exacerbate CAPD.

Working memory can be exercised through a variety of activities, including formulating sentences, sentence combining or assembly, sentence completion (which also trains auditory closure, as discussed below and in Chapter 7), word associations, trail making, digit span, and verbal fluency. Daneman and Carpenter (1980) designed a working memory span paradigm in which subjects listen to increasingly longer sets of sentences, and at the end of the set, they attempt to recall the final word of each sentence in the set. Ellis Weismer, Evans, and Hesketh (1999) described a rather standard approach to working memory in which subjects demonstrate comprehension by answering questions following a sentence, and demonstrate working memory by recalling the last word of each sentence after all the sentences in the series have been presented. Another common task that exercises working memory requires a client to answer a question about the set of rhyming words before reciting those words. For example, the clinician would present a series of rhyming words (e.g., fun, run, sun) and ask the client to recognize whether one or more words were among those on the list (e.g., was bun or sun presented) before recalling and reciting the rhyming words. Similarly, a client might be asked to order and recall a phoneme-number span (e.g., 4, /r/, 2, /m/) beginning with digits and following with the phonemes (e.g., 2, 4, /m/, /r/) (Baddeley 1986; Shallice & Vallar, 1990). Listening span exercises also exercise working memory. After a client indicates whether each of a series of sentences is absurd (e.g., The cream is black), the client is asked to recall either the first or final word of all the sentences in correct serial order.

As mentioned below (under Central Resources Training With Young Children), music can be incorporated to train self-control (e.g., musical chairs, which also exercises vigilance). So too, music can be used to used to train working memory. For example, clients can be required to repeat the word that appears prior to a target word in line from a song, with the target word not identified until after the line is sung. One may also present similar melodies dichotically (e.g., *Here Comes The Bride* and *Hail to the Chief*), requiring the listener to identify, sing, or hum both melodies. Applications can be downloaded to mobile phones and tablets to exercise memory (e.g., *Sound Match*).

A number of auditory training approaches can be used to exercise working memory as well, including speech recognition in noise, time compressed speech recognition, following auditory directives, and reverse digit span recall (Chermak & Musiek, 1997). (See Chapters 7 and 9.)

Metalinguistic Strategies

Metalinguistic strategies comprise the final type of central resources training approaches. Metalinguistic strategies involve: discourse cohesion devices, schema induction, auditory-verbal closure, segmentation (i.e., phonemic analysis and synthesis), prosody, and listening tactics.

Discourse Cohesion Devices

Discourse cohesion devices are linguistic forms that connect propositions into more complex messages (Halliday & Hasan, 1976; van Dijk, 1985). These devices allow speakers and listeners to more efficiently formulate and resolve messages. Cohesive devices establish relationships between ideas (e.g., causal relationships denoted by *because* or *so*) and build cohesive chains through the use of devices that are either explicit (e.g., pronouns and conjunctions) or must be inferred (e.g., ellipsis) (Chermak & Musiek, 1997). As illustrated in Table 10–3, discourse cohesion devices include referents (e.g., pronouns), substitution (e.g., use of different terminology as co-referent), ellipsis (i.e., deleting rather than reiterating part of a message that can be inferred), definiteness (e.g., activating known versus new information), and conjunctions (e.g., words that connect and specify relationships across a message). In contrast to other cohesive devices, conjunctions specify relationships within and across propositions without presupposing other elements in the preceding or subsequent text.

Although discourse cohesion devices typically reduce verbiage and therefore increase efficiency of message transfer, they do so by placing additional cognitive (e.g., memory) and linguistic processing demands on the listener (Chermak & Musiek, 1997). Listeners must grasp precisely the relationships signaled by the cohesive devices to discern subtle

Table 10–3. Discourse Cohesion Devices[a]

Referents	
Pronouns	Isaac prepared dinner. *He* prepared *it*.
Pro-verbs	The blizzard enveloped the city. When it *did*, electrical lines were downed.
Comparatives	Alina dances with grace. *Similarly,* Isaac skis with agility and balance.
Substitution	The orchestra played a marvelous concert. The audience was surprised by the *musicians'* artistry.
Ellipsis	Isaac enjoys practicing his instrument. Alina does too. (Alina enjoys practicing too.)
Definiteness	The computer controlling the hybrid engine would not re-boot. The technician's utilities failed to correct *the* problem.
Conjunctions[b]	
Additive	A democratic nation must ensure security *and* freedom.
Adversative	*Although* he applied to many schools, none accepted him.
Causal	The CEO violated securities law; *therefore,* she was convicted and sent to prison.
Disjunctive	She chose to learn French *instead* of Spanish, despite Spanish being more useful.
Temporal	One should think *before* one speaks.

[a]This table provides examples of the major cohesion signaling devices. It is not an exhaustive listing of the various subtypes.

[b]In contrast to the other cohesive devices, conjunctions do not presuppose other elements in the preceding or subsequent text. Rather, they specify relationships within and across propositions.

semantic differences. Notwithstanding these additional demands, improved use of discourse cohesion devices should benefit listening and spoken language processing (Chermak & Musiek, 1997; McKenzie et al., 1981).

Schema Theory and Use

A schema is a metacognitive construct used to explain knowledge organization that is accessed when undertaking behavioral or cognitive tasks (Kintsch, 1988; Rumelhart, 1980). A schema is defined as "a structured cluster of concepts, a set of expectations, as well as an abstract and generic knowledge structure stored in memory that preserves the relations among constituent concepts and generalized knowledge about a text, event, message, situation, or object, thereby providing a framework to guide interpretation" (Chermak & Musiek, 1997, p. 194). A schema functions as a conceptual framework connecting interrelated ideas (Chermak & Musiek, 1997). Schema theory provides an explanation as to how knowledge and experience are mapped in the *mind* and how those representations facilitate comprehension and learning (Rumelhart, 1980, 1984).

Schemata have been invoked to explain one's ability to theorize, predict, infer, and make default assumptions about unmentioned aspects of a situation (Chermak & Musiek, 1997). "Schemata are employed in the process of interpreting sensory data (both linguistic and nonlinguistic), in retrieving information from memory, in organizing actions, in determining goals and subgoals, in allocating resources, and generally, in guiding the flow of processing in the system" (Rumelhart, 1980, pp. 33–34). By guiding processing, schemata serve an

executive function (Chermak & Musiek, 1997). Although deploying schemata maximizes the best fit between data and structure, it does not guarantee message understanding (Rumelhart, 1980, 1984).

Schema activation demonstrates the complementary function of bottom-up (i.e., data-driven and top-down (i.e., concept-driven) processing (Rumelhart, 1980). A schema provides top-down guidance to the listener; however, its activation is dependent on a match between its criterial features and descriptions yielded by lower level (i.e., bottom-up) analysis (Rumelhart, 1980). Through top-down processes the listener recognizes patterns and evidence supporting a schema and upholds the interpretation supported by the schema (Chermak & Musiek, 1997).

Children as young as 2 to 3 years demonstrate the use of formal schemata (e.g., *and*, *then*, *because*) in their language as they develop awareness of spatial, temporal, and causal relationships (French & Nelson, 1985; Nippold, 1988). Development continues through adolescence to include more complex conjunctions (Nippold, 1988).

Content Schemata

Schemata function at two different levels. Formal schemata (discussed below) involve knowledge of discourse conventions and "give form or structure to experience" (Dillon, 1981, p. 51). Content or contextual schemata provide a generalized interpretation of the content of experience (Dillon, 1981). Also referred to as scripts, content schemata facilitate interpretation by organize facts and establishing a framework that allows listeners to impose certain constraints on events, precepts, situations, and objects (Rumelhart, 1980).

Listeners use content schemata to interpret spoken messages (Chermak & Musiek, 1997). For example, listeners employ particular content schemata that stipulate the sequential stages of a common event. For example, having accessed a particular script, the listener anticipates that the story setting should precede the major actions of the characters, with a closing following the denouement (Chermak & Musiek, 1997).

Formal Schemata

Formal schemata are linguistic markers that organize, integrate, and predict relationships across propositions and thereby foster the cohesiveness and coherence of messages (Dillon, 1981). Formal schemata include conjunctions (i.e., additive [e.g., *and, furthermore*], adversative [e.g., *although, nevertheless, however*], causal [e.g., *because, therefore, accordingly*], disjunctive [e.g., *but, instead, on the contrary*], and temporal conjunctions [e.g., *before, after, subsequently*], as well as patterns of parallelism and correlative pairs [e.g., *not only/but also; neither/nor*]).

Formal schemata do not specify meaning. As recurring patterns, however, they induce certain expectations, narrowing the range of possibilities and providing the skilled listener with direction in constructing meaning (Chermak & Musiek, 1997). By instantiating formal schemata, listeners gain insight as to the probable message structure and they use that knowledge as a framework to generate expectations about the organization and relationships among the content (Chermak & Musiek, 1997). Listeners must still construct the specific detail to fully understand the message.

The organizing function of formal schemata is most salient at the global level. This more global organizing function is represented by expressions such as the *first point, and finally*, and *in summary* (Chermak & Musiek, 1997). The addition of paralinguistic cues, including speaking rate, pauses, repetitions, and inflection, and nonverbal cues such as body posture, eye contact, facial expression, and hand gestures further potentiates the organizing function of these phrases for the listener (Buttrill, Niizawa, Biemer, Takahashi, & Hearn, 1989).

The integrative and predictive functions of formal schemata operate at local levels (Dillon, 1981). They focus listeners' attention on patterns that fuse and presage ideas and facilitate the construction of relationships between the ideas (Chermak & Musiek, 1992). For example, the causal conjunction *because* integrates two propositions and predicts the relationship between them (Chermak & Musiek, 1997). Similarly, *if-then* constructions activate schemata depicting either causation (prediction) or speculation (via the subjunctive conditional), thereby facilitating comprehension (Chermak & Musiek, 1997). The integrative function of formal schemata also reduces the processing required to comprehend complex sentences (Chermak & Musiek, 1997). For example, the suspensive construction in the sentence "Children listen more effectively, despite the challenges imposed by competing noise, when deploying central resource strategies" is less likely to disrupt comprehension if a listener employs formal schematic knowledge. Finally, given their predictive function, formal schemata assist both literal and figurative interpretation, including inferencing, as discussed above under Cognitive Style and Reasoning.

In summary, formal schemata provide frameworks that facilitate the organization, integration, and ultimately the comprehension of information. By providing extensive networks that link new stimuli with stored knowledge and expectation, they render particular perspectives salient, allow for efficient resource allocation and processing, and facilitate comprehension (Chermak & Musiek, 1997).

Clinical Application

Schemata influence listening comprehension. The ability to select and deploy appropriate schemata may account in part for differences between effective and ineffective listeners (Chermak & Musiek, 1992). Individuals with CAPD and learning disabilities may experience difficulty processing schemata and other discourse cohesion devices (Liles, 1985, 1987; Wren, 1983). Lack of familiarity with the linguistic structure of a message leads to difficulty in determining what is important and relevant, as well as in deciphering the interrelationships among the information presented (Chermak & Musiek, 1997). This in turn leads to less efficient allocation of resources and to difficulties guiding the flow of processing in the system, both of which compromise message comprehension (Rumelhart, 1980). Since schema deployment depends not only on linguistic facility and cognition (e.g., memory), but also on executive functions (e.g., self-regulation and self-monitoring) and cognitive flexibility as well (Rumelhart, 1984), clinical approaches (discussed above) that enhance metacognitive knowledge and skills will also benefit schema use (Chermak & Musiek, 1997).

Exercises that emphasize recognizing and interpreting formal schemata should benefit individuals with CAPD (Chermak & Musiek, 1992). Better able to elicit the appropriate formal schemata, the listener with CAPD would invoke a generic framework that exposes relationships across propositions and thereby assist listening comprehension (Chermak & Musiek, 1997). In addition, because formal schemata often occur at phrase boundaries, they may help the listener parse larger and more complex messages into smaller units, promoting both comprehension and retention (Chermak & Musiek, 1997).

Schema Induction

Induction learning emphasizes the central role of discovery for learning and presupposes that induction is natural and that learners approach the learning situation with a predeveloped, perhaps innate, induction capability (Connell, 1988). As illustrated in Table 10–4, the induction procedure provides clients the opportunity to discover the functions and advantages of formal schemata for listening comprehension. The clinician's goal is to facilitate the client's recognition of the patterns that exist in the message and to explain these patterns so that they may be used to support message comprehension, as well as message formulation (Chermak & Musiek, 1997). To achieve these outcomes, the clinician structures the message so that information necessary to induce the rules governing the patterns are salient to the listener (Connell, 1988).

Although the discovery aspect of the inductive method can be engaging and effective, it may be too difficult for some clients. Even the most basic conjunctions (e.g., *and, then, because*) may prove too difficult to decipher when presented in the context of the inductive method to young clients, those with more severe

Table 10–4. Clinical Illustration of Schema Induction

Objectives: To identify and produce causal conjunctions and constructions.[a]	

Step 1   *Clinician:* "It snowed a lot last night. School was canceled. Why do you think school was canceled?"

Client: "Because the roads are snowy. It's dangerous. If you drive on the road, you will have an accident."

Step 2   *Clinician:* "Yes, now let's listen to (look at[b]) what you said." (Clinician plays back client's response.) "Tell me which words tell you why school was canceled."

Client: "Because I said *because.* I said *if* you drive on the road, you could have an accident."

Clinician: "Yes, you are correct. *If* and *because* are the important words which prepare us for the reasons, the answers to the question *why.*"

Step 3   *Clinician:* "Listen to this short story and tell me if you recognize any of the same important words you just told me about."

Mom and Dad tell me that I should sleep well every night. They say that if I sleep well, then I will be more alert in school. If I am more alert, then I will earn better grades. If I earn better grades, then I will be more successful. I will sleep well because I want to be successful.

Step 4   *Clinician:* "Did you recognize any of the important words?"

Client: "You said that mom and dad said *if* I sleep well and *if* I am alert."

Clinician: "Yes. You are correct. Did you hear any other important key words?" (Clinician may play back the story if the client has difficulty recalling additional words.)

Client: "Yes, the boy said he will sleep well *because* he wants to be successful."

Step 5   *Clinician:* "Now, I want you to tell me a short story using these important key words and I will try to identify them and explain their function to you.[c]

Objectives: To produce and identify temporal conjunctions.[d]	

Step 1   *Clinician:* "Tell me what you do when you get up in the morning."

Client: "First I get out of bed. Then I brush my teeth. Finally, I get dressed.

Step 2   *Clinician:* "Now, let us listen to (look at) what you said." (Clinician plays back client's description.) "Tell me the important key words you said to let me know that you began by getting out of bed."

Client: "I said, *first* I get out of bed."

Clinician: "Yes, that word *first* certainly gave me a big clue. Now tell me which important word you said so that I would know what happened in the end."

Table 10–4. *continued*

Client: "I said *finally*, I get dressed."
Clinician: "Yes, that is correct."

[a]The reader will note variations in the sequence of activities supporting the two different objectives. For the first objective (to identify and produce causal conjunctions and constructions), clients listen to a story that is likely to lead them to produce causal conjunctions and constructions. The clinician then asks the client to identify the causal conjunctions/ constructions and explain their function. The last step, illustrating reciprocal teaching, requires that the client generate a story which the clinician then analyzes. In the second series of steps supporting the production and identification of temporal conjunctions, the client first produces the organizational words and then identifies them and explains their function. The clinician may then proceed to tell the client a story and ask the client to identify the temporal conjunctions and explain their function. The reader will recognize yet other variations on this induction sequence.

[b]The clinician may wish to exploit the advantage of bisensory processing by using audiovisual presentations. Audiotaping and visual aids (e.g., pictures for younger children and written transcripts for older clients) should improve the effectiveness of this procedure.

[c]This step begins a reciprocal teaching sequence wherein the client assumes the teacher's role and thereby promotes metacognitive control.

[d]This truncated sequence begins with the client generating a story. The clinician may expand this sequence by generating stories for the client to examine.

CAPD, and those with associated cognitive, language, or peripheral hearing problems (Chermak & Musiek, 1997). If prompting, rephrasing, and modeling prove ineffective, it may be necessary to suspend the strict inductive approach and revert to an approach that more directly draws the client's attention to the formal schemata (Chermak & Musiek, 1997). Chermak and Musiek (1997) offered several modifications of the approach outlined in Table 10–4 for clients who cannot contextually extract the meaning of formal schemata. One alternative approach to underscoring schematic contrast is to focus on minimal pairs—for example, (1) *I eat because I am hungry* contrasted with *I eat because I am satisfied*; (2) *I sleep because I am tired versus I sleep, but I am tired*; (3) *Before I go to school, I get dressed versus Before I go to school, I eat dinner*; (4) *I sleep because*

I am tired versus I sleep, but I am awake; *(5) I get dressed before I go to school versus I get dressed after I go to school*. Sentence pairs that contrast conjunctions (#2, #5) present greater challenge than pairs involving only one conjunction (#1, #3). Pairs with contrasting conjunctions also serve to transition to another conjunction in a training sequence. Sentence pairs in which both the conjunction and the predicate phrase vary concurrently (#4) are inherently more difficult than sentence pairs in which either the conjunction (#5) or the predicate phrase is altered (#1, #3). The semantic absurdities resulting from inappropriate use of a conjunction (and/ or predicate phrase) intrigues youngsters while providing an opportunity to examine the rule and then return to the induction approach with more confidence and knowledge at some later time (Chermak & Musiek, 1997). Another alternative to the direct induction approach involves asking clients to paraphrase conjoined sentences by incorporating conjunctions —for example, *The exams were graded./ Scores were posted* is conjoined as *After the exams were graded, the scores were posted* or *Before the scores were posted, the exams were graded.*

Closure

Listeners employ several levels of closure to complete and make whole an incomplete message. Auditory closure refers to the most basic type of closure in which a listener recognizes a whole word despite the absence of certain elements. Listeners achieve auditory closure by filling in the gaps in the acoustic sound stream, in part by taking advantage of the inherent acoustic redundancies due to coarticulation and parallel transmission of the acoustic-phonetic information (Liberman et al., 1967). Auditory-verbal closure refers to the ability to use spoken contextual (i.e., primarily semantic) information to facilitate message recognition. Grammatic closure, perhaps the most sophisticated type of closure, denotes the ability to invoke syntactic rules to complete phrases or sentences despite missing words or morphemes (e.g., filling in the verb form *is* versus *are* to conjugate with the subject *he*). Listeners use context and language knowledge, inductive and deductive reasoning, and auditory and grammatic closure to derive the meaning of words and messages.

Practice recognizing (low-redundancy) speech that is distorted or degraded (filtered, compressed, interrupted, or presented in noise, competing messages, or reverberation) offers a direct approach to developing auditory and auditory-verbal closure skills. This approach is elaborated as a component of auditory training in Chapter 7.

Vocabulary Building and Construction of Meaning

Deficits in word knowledge have been reported in individuals with CAPD and learning disabilities, including limited vocabulary, restrictions in word meaning, difficulties with multiple meaning words, difficulties with comprehension of conjunctions, and deficits in interpreting figurative language (Ferre & Wilber, 1986; Gajar, 1989; Hoskins, 1983; Houck & Billingsley, 1989; Johnson & Myklebust, 1967; Keith & Novak, 1984; Mann, 1991; Matkin & Hook, 1983; Snider, 1989; Willeford & Burleigh, 1985; Wren, 1983). Given the central role vocabulary serves in spoken language comprehension (Anderson & Freebody, 1981; Beck et al., 2002; Biemiller & Boote, 2006; Perfetti, 1985; Samuels, 1987; Stanovich, 1993; Sticht & James, 1984; Wiig, Semel, & Crouse, 1973), central resources training for CAPD should incorporate vocabulary building from both a quantitative and a qualitative or semantic network perspective. By focusing on semantic relationships as well as lexicon, the network perspective broadens vocabulary building to foster the larger goal of the construction of meaning (Chermak & Musiek, 1997). Context-derived vocabulary building, word derivation, flexibility with multiple meaning words, and inferencing are among the procedures recommended for extending the breadth and depth of vocabulary knowledge. Concurrently, several of these procedures also promote auditory closure skills that are especially important to resolving messages in unfavorable listening environments.

Context-Derived Vocabulary Building

Linguistic context reduces uncertainty and can be used to derive word meaning and thereby expand vocabulary and enhance message comprehension (Miller & Gildea, 1987). The listener must invoke auditory-verbal, as well as grammatic closure in some instances, to resolve vocabulary (Chermak & Musiek, 1992). Like sentence completion tasks, as well as the Cloze procedure employed in reading instruction, context-derived vocabulary building encourages listeners to delve into their linguistic and world knowledge to ascertain specific word meaning and ultimately comprehend the auditory message (Gerber, 1981).

In many cases context establishes word meaning; however, relying on context may not always prove effective because some contexts are ambiguous, misleading, or simply uninformative (Miller & Gildea, 1987). For example, the context surrounding the unknown word *alighted* in the sentence "The bird alighted on the perch" is sufficiently informative to enable a listener with basic vocabulary knowledge to derive its meaning. In contrast, the relatively uninformative context preceding the unknown word *magnanimity* in the sentence "The man spoke about magnanimity" does not provide sufficient information to clarify meaning. Nonetheless, deducing word meaning from context may be more effective than consulting a dictionary, which requires considerable sophistication if the user is to select the intended meaning from the multiple listings of alternative meanings in dictionaries (Miller & Gildea, 1987).

In constructing sentences for context-derived vocabulary building, the clinician imbeds an unknown word in the context of rather concrete, known vocabulary that provides sufficient contextual cues to enable the client to deduce the meaning of the new vocabulary word. Task difficulty can be modified by altering the number and quality of contextual cues.

Developing auditory-verbal closure skills while emphasizing the important comprehension cues provided by context also may be accomplished through the use of sentence material like that incorporated in the Speech Perception in Noise (SPIN) Test (Bilger, Neutzel, Rabinowitz, & Rzeczkowski, 1984; Kalikow, Stevens, & Elliott, 1977). The listener is required to identify the final word of sentences that are preceded by phrases providing high or low test word predictability. High predicatability sentences contain high levels of context or *clue words* (e.g., *The watchdog gave a warning growl.*). Low predictability sentences contain little context from which the final target word can be deduced (e.g., *I had not thought about the growl.*).

Construction of Meaning

Examining the relationship between root words and derivations (e.g., able/disability, know/knowledge, spirit/inspire, revise/revision) fosters word knowledge and vocabulary expansion (Chermak & Musiek, 1997). Multiple meaning words (e.g., block, fly, hard, menu, spring), homophones/homonyms (e.g., night/knight, fowl/foul, muscle/mussel, medal/meddle), and homographs (e.g., sow [female pig] and sow [seeds]; bow [in hair or of an instrument], bow [of a ship], and bow [gesture]) encourage facility and flexibility in comprehension (Gerber, 1993a) while providing opportunities to expand semantic networks and increase vocabulary (Chermak & Musiek, 1997). Multiple meaning words placed in context can also serve as material for context-derived vocabulary building. For example, the sentence "When *spring* arrives, I *spring* to my feet to walk leisurely along the *spring* that flows beside the trail" serves several instructional goals: to learn word meaning, expand semantic networks, and use context to determine meaning (Chermak & Musiek, 1997). In the same way, heteronyms (e.g., project/project, object/object, record/record, digest/digest), words spelled identically but pronounced with different stress patterns, afford an excellent vehicle for building vocabulary while also focusing on the role of prosody (i.e., temporal distinctions cued by stress) in spoken language comprehension (Musiek & Chermak, 1995). Finally, in addition to exercises directed toward construction of literal meaning, efforts also may be focused on expanding figurative language. Use of metaphors, similes, slang, sarcasm, idioms, and proverbs provide additional opportunities to build semantic networks (Nippold, 1991; Nippold & Fey, 1983).

Segmentation

Phonological awareness, the explicit awareness of the sound structure of language, includes the recognition that words are comprised of syllables and phonemes (Catts, 1991). Listeners use phonologic awareness to segment words into their constituent sound elements (Lewkowitz, 1980). Segmentation training (i.e., phonemic analysis) exercises temporal processing, albeit within the context of phonological awareness, and as such is an example of informatl auditory training (see Chapter 7). Beyond temporal processing, such training should benefit reading and language processing, given the increasing evidence of the

causal linkages between phonological processing ability and reading skill, as well as spoken language comprehension (Adams, 1990; Ball & Blachman, 1991; Stanovich, 1993; Wagner & Torgesen, 1987). The cognitive and linguistic demands inherent to phonological awareness activities must be considered carefully, however, since the development of phonological awareness varies among children (Bradley & Bryant, 1985; Catts, 1991). Other metalinguistic approaches that dually train temporal processing within the context of central resources training (i.e., following directives and resolving prosodic cues) are discussed below.

Auditory Discrimination

Auditory discrimination is one of most fundamental central auditory processing skills underlying spoken language comprehension (Chermak & Musiek, 2002). The ability to perceive acoustic similarities and differences between sounds is essential to segmentation skills, which require the listener to recognize the acoustic contrasts among contiguous phonemes (Chermak & Musiek, 1997). In this way, auditory discrimination is fundamental to phonemic analysis and phonemic synthesis. Auditory discrimination and phonemic segmentation are so crucial to spoken language comprehension that treatment programs for CAPD have been designed around them (Sloan, 1986). (See Chapter 7 for additional discussion of auditory discrimination.)

Phonemic Analysis and Phonemic Synthesis

Phonemic analysis and phonemic synthesis (i.e., sound blending) provide two reciprocal approaches to phonological awareness and segmentation training (Chermak & Musiek, 1997). The primary goal of phonemic analysis is to develop phonemic encoding and decoding skills using either multisyllabic nonsense sequences (Lindamood & Lindamood, 1975) or single syllables and multisyllabic words (Sloan, 1986). The listener identifies which sound is heard and its position in the syllable or word.

Several commercially available treatment programs provide extensive activities to strengthen auditory discrimination and phonemic analysis, including Sloan's (1986) treatment program and the Lindamood Phoneme Sequencing Program for Reading, Spelling, and Speech (LiPS), formerly Auditory Discrimination in Depth (ADD) (Lindamood & Lindamood, 1975). Recognizing the linkage among central auditory processing, language learning, and language use, Sloan's (1986) four-part program develops skills in auditory discrimination, sound analysis, and sound-symbol (phoneme-grapheme) association and applies these skills to reading and spelling words. Similarly, the LiPS program develops auditory discrimination for sameness, difference, number, and order of speech sounds, as well as sound-symbol association encoding (spelling) and decoding (reading) skills as prerequisite, and complementary, to reading programs.

Other programs targeting phonemic synthesis stress the blending of discrete phonemes into the correctly sequenced, coarticulated sound patterns. The Phonemic Synthesis program developed by Katz and Harmon (1982) is an example of a program designed to promote mastery of sequential phoneme blending skills. (See Chermak & Musiek, 1997 and Chapter 17 for additional discussion of approaches to syllabic segmentation and blending.) Finally, as noted above under metacognition and memory, applications can be downloaded to mobile phones and tablets to exercise metalinguistic skills (e.g., abc Pocket Phonics to drill sound segmentation, sound-symbol association, and sound blending).

Prosody

In contrast to segmental analysis, prosody involves the suprasegmental aspects of spoken language. Like segementation, prosody training builds central resources as well as providing opportunities for informal auditory training. Prosody refers to the dynamic melody, timing, rhythm, and amplitude fluctuations of fluent speech. Prosodic information is integral to spoken language processing at a number of levels. Prosody links phonetic segments (Goldinger, Pisoni, & Luce, 1996). Prosody guides attention to the more instructive parts of a message (Cutler & Fodor, 1979; Cutler & Foss, 1977). Further, prosody provides information about the lexical, semantic, and syntactic content of the spoken message (Goldinger, Pisoni, & Luce, 1996; Studdert-Kennedy, 1980).

A number of approaches may be useful in targeting perception of prosody in the context of spoken language (Chermak & Musiek, 1997). As mentioned above in the section on vocabulary building and the construction of meaning, heteronyms require focus on prosody (specifically accent or stress pattern) to resolve semantic distinctions. Ambiguous phrases also can be used to draw attention to prosodic detail while training context-derived vocabulary building skills (Chermak & Musiek, 1992). For example, durational contrasts and context allow the listener to disambiguate sentences with identical surface structure (e.g., *The girl saw the boy with the binoculars* that she purchased for a bird watching expedition./*The girl saw the boy with the binoculars* that she hoped to purchase for herself some day.).

Intonation is used as an aid to resolve ambiguous messages where prosody changes meaning. As illustrated by Musiek and Chermak (1995), the sentence "Look out the window," can be parsed and interpreted differently depending on the speaker's intonation and timing. It could mean "Look out! The window," Look! Out the window," or simply the simple imperative statement "Look out the window." In a similar manner, temporally cued sentences (e.g., "The judge went to the fairgounds for a divorce" vs. "The judge said he saw fair grounds for a divorce) (Cole & Jakimik, 1980, p. 159) also may serve to instill an appreciation in the listener for the use of prosody and segmentation knowledge (as well as context) in resolving messages (Chermak & Musiek, 1997). Parsing of words and phrases based on duration and juncture (e.g., nitrate vs. night rate, it sprays vs. it's praise) and reading poetry and noting the location of the emphasis and stress in sentences and words also promote this appreciation and may improve perception of prosody (Chermak & Musiek, 1997). (The reader is referred to Cole and Jakimik (1980) who present a series of temporally cued sentence pairs that contrast one- versus two-word segmentation of the same phoneme sequence.)

Listening Tactics

While it is essential that clients *practice* listening, it is often pivotal for clinicians to first teach clients *how* to listen, emphasizing attending behaviors (e.g., be still, quiet, think about listening, pay atten-

tion to sounds), and that when we try hard to listen, we also listen with our brain and our eyes (Truesdale, 1990). Strategies used to monitor listening and extract information include: question formulation, paraphrasing, mnemonics, note-taking, drawing, verbal rehearsal, mental imaging, and summarizing. Clients must be introduced and trained to practice active listening that involves: listening intently and taking responsibility for listening success; physical adjustments that demonstrate interest through eye contact, body language, and posture; empathetic listening (i.e., placing oneself in the *other's shoes*); using closure, inferencing, deducing, and predicting skills; using communication repair strategies (e.g., requesting repetition, rephrasing, confirmations, etc.); ignoring background noise and competing messages; and not giving up prematurely.

Central Resources Training With Young Children

Early identification and diagnosis of CAPD in children is crucial given the potential adverse impact of CAPD for communication, academic achievement, and social function (AAA, 2010; ASHA, 2005; Bellis, 2003; Bellis & Ferre, 1999; Musiek & Chermak, 1995; Willeford, 1985). Unfortunately, few tests with sufficiently documented sensitivity and specificity for CAPD are available for young children (i.e., under age 7–8 years), rendering diagnosis of CAPD difficult at best (Chermak & Musiek, 1997). Nonetheless, it is prudent to involve young children suspected of, or at risk for, CAPD (e.g., children with histories of recurrent and persistent otitis media with effusion; prematurity and low birth weight; prenatal drug exposure; associated developmental disorders) in programs designed to promote development of auditory perceptual skills. (See Chapters 10 and 11 of Volume 1 of this Handbook for discussion of screening for CAPD, and considerations when testing young children, respectively.)

Central resource training for children at-risk for and suspected of CAPD should emphasize the principles of natural language learning (Norris & Damico, 1990). An enriched language environment involving activities that engage young children and provide natural opportunities for listening and communication fosters the development of auditory perceptual and auditory-language skills (Chermak & Musiek, 1997). For example, repetition of daily routines creates a sense of familiarity, allowing the child to focus attention on new auditory information. Collaboration between speech and hearing professionals, preschool teachers, and families maximizes the transfer of skills to daily routines and other settings (Chermak, 1993).

Since listening supports learning, providing optimal listening environments is pivotal to the success of early intervention (or prevention) efforts (Chermak & Musiek, 1997). Strategies used to enhance the acoustic signal and the listening environment for individuals with hearing impairment also are appropriate for children suspected of, or at risk for, CAPD. In addition to auditory strategies, maximizing access to visual information (e.g., pictures, facial expression, gestures and other nonverbal cues) supports and reinforces auditory information and thereby enhances the saliency of the acoustic

signal (Chermak & Musiek, 1997). Strategies to enhance the acoustic signal and the listening environment, including personal FM and sound-field technology are described in Chapters 4, 12, and 13.

A number of activities are outlined below that provide opportunities to reinforce good listening skills through bottom-up (e.g., discriminating sounds) and top-down processes (e.g., being read to) and may be used with older children, as well as with children as young as 3 to 5 years. Activities are described that promote a number of emerging processes and skills, including selective attention, metalinguistic skills (e.g., auditory-verbal closure), resolution of prosodic cues, multisensory integration, vocabulary building, following directions, inferencing skills, executive function (e.g., planning, self-regulation), and comprehension. (See Chapter 7 for discussion of additional activities that develop listening skills in young children.)

Listening to Stories

Reading aloud to children promotes concept learning, vocabulary building, and practice in vigilance and selective listening (Musiek & Chermak, 1995). If one's focus is to encourage selective listening, target words, for which the child is instructed to monitor and signal the occurrence (e.g., by raising their hands each time a word is read that represents an animal), should be designated before beginning the story. The child might also be encouraged to listen for subtle prosodic cues (e.g., intonation, stress), while focusing on target words. Posing comprehension questions at the end of the story promotes listening for meaning (i.e., comprehension) while still exercising targeted or selective listening (Chermak & Musiek, 1997). Questions can be formulated around a story grammar (e.g., where and when did events in the story take place [setting]; what did the main character do [action]; what happened as a result of the main character's action [consequences]). A combination of questions that require tracking of the story context as well as the designated target words promotes auditory closure and comprehension (Chermak & Musiek, 1997). Concurrently, multisensory integration can be encouraged by allowing the child to examine the accompanying pictures and words as the story is read aloud (Chermak & Musiek, 1997). Having the caregiver and the child jointly elaborate on the pictures in a book or sections of the text that are of particular interest to the child fosters vocabulary development and reading skills (Ninio, 1980; Teale, 1984, Wells, 1985).

Following Directions

Following directions engages a number of central resources, including attention and working memory, as well as basic central auditory processes, most notably temporal processing. In addition to providing real, everyday functional contexts in which the child must follow sequenced directives to successfully complete a task, games can be organized that require the child to follow directions presented auditorily (e.g., Simon Says) (Musiek & Chermak, 1995). To augment reauditorization and transference to a motor activity (for directives requiring some motor task), the child can be required to repeat the directive before acting (Chermak & Musiek, 1997). A variety of other games (e.g., *Telephone*) requiring children to repeat

(in sequence) what they have heard to other people, as well as barrier games in which the child must follow directions presented auditorily to create something (e.g., building or drawing) or to replicate a configuration of objects on the other side of the barrier without the benefit of visual cues also are effective activities to promote listening.

Chermak and Musiek (1997) outlined a range of directives of varying complexity and difficulty. Oral directives may be made more complex by inserting adjective sequences, prepositions, and a number of facts, or by using more sophisticated linguistic concepts (e.g., use of *suspensive* phrasing such as "Point to the pictures of animals, but only if they live on farms, after you point to the pictures of toys").

Inferencing

Activities that require the drawing of inferences can be entertaining and appropriate for younger clients. The context-derived vocabulary building technique (discussed above) can be used to develop inferencing skills, as well as build vocabulary and develop auditory-verbal closure skills (Chermak & Musiek, 1997). Young children can be encouraged to draw inferences on the basis of information (i.e., *clues*) presented in stories and in poetry read aloud. Clinicians should discuss with children their inferences and the processes they deployed to externalize and strengthen their reasoning strategies (Chermak & Musiek, 1997). In addition to promoting cognitive style flexibility, inferencing also challenges memory, as stored knowledge is essential to the inferencing process (Chermak & Musiek, 1997).

Executive Function

By age 5 years, children have begun to develop metacognitive knowledge and executive strategies (Kreitler & Kreitler, 1987). Since these strategies underlie attention and listening comprehension, activities to reinforce and cultivate these strategies is worthwhile (Chermak & Musiek, 1997). Preschool-age children have developed metacognitive message evaluation skills and respond well to self-regulation training that involves asking questions and evaluating message ambiguity (Pratt & Bates, 1982). Role playing affords children the opportunity to gain experience with emotional control and the rules that guide interactions. Similarly, childhood games such as Musical Chairs and freezing when the music stops, also exercise self-regulation, as well as working memory and auditory vigilance. Some research suggests that executive function (and underlying prefrontal cortical function) can be trained through a variety of methods, including direct practice of activities requiring attention, inhibition, and memory (Tamm, Nakonezny, & Hughes, 2012), computerized working memory training (Holmes, Gathercole, & Dunning, 2009; Holmes et al., 2010; Klingberg et al., 2005; Thorell, Lindqvist, Bergman, Bohlin, & Klingberg, 2009; aerobic exercise (Hillman, Erickson, & Kramer, 2008; Chaddock, Pontifex, Hillman, & Kramer, 2011); musical training that requires bimanual coordination (Budde, Voelcker-Rehage, Pietrabyk-Kendziorra, Ribeiro, & Tidow, 2008; Rauscher et al., 1997; Uhrick & Swalm, 2007); and mindfulness practice (e.g., martial arts and meditation) that demand focus and perseverance (Lakes & Hoyt, 2004; Flook et al., 2010; Manjunath & Telles, 2001). Efforts can be directed to developing skills that underlie problem solving, such as reasoning skills. For instance, philosophical questioning helps develop reasoning skills (as well as ethics). Leading children in a discussion about how we should treat nature, environmental ethics, respect, etc. promotes reasoning skills (Wartenberg, 2009), as do discussions of children's books that raise deep philosophical issues (e.g., *The Giving Tree by* Shel Silverstein, in which a tree surrenders its shade, fruit, branches, and finally its trunk to a boy it befriended).

Short scenarios can provide contexts for follow-up questions that require planning knowledge and thereby develop executive strategies (Kreitler & Kreitler, 1987), as illustrated in the following scenario.

Isaac and Alina were both planning birthday parties for the same day. Both children wanted their parties at the arts and crafts center in the local mall. The management agreed to allow both parties to run concurrently; however, the children would have to share the facilities. If you were Alina or Isaac, how would you plan your party so that you did not interfere with the other child's celebration?

Metalinguistic Skills and Vocabulary Building

A number of activities promote the development of metalinguistic skills in preschool age children, including rhyme play and *knock-knock* jokes (van Kleeck, 1994). For example, emerging metalinguistic skills enable preschool-age children to appreciate the word play (duration and juncture variations) and humor of the following *knock-knock* jokes:

"Knock, knock. Who's there? Pasture. Pasture who? It's *past your* bedtime." and "Knock, knock. Who's there? Gladys. Gladys who? *Gladys we can be* to wish you a happy birthday!" In the same way, auditory-verbal closure skills can be developed in young children by omitting phrase and sentence final words in familiar nursery rhymes and songs (e.g., "Twinkle, twinkle little *star*," "Little Bo Peep has lost her *sheep*"). Word games (e.g., Mad Gab™) that involve duration, juncture, and segmentation skills (e.g., resegment "amen ask hurt" to form a meaningful phase "a mini skirt") engage the young child while training central resources. Other classic word games (e.g., Password™) take advantage of semantic relationships to build vocabulary.

Central Resources Training for Adults and Older Adults

Age is one of the most significant sources of individual variability. The individual's response to the variety of developmental, situational, environmental, social, and economic factors influencing that individual at various periods throughout life is dynamic (Chermak & Musiek, 1997). Just as children experience increasing and more complex central auditory processing demands as they face more intellectually and linguistically challenging academic and social situations, the central auditory processing demands facing the older adult in retirement differ from the demands he or she confronted as a young, ambitious professional (Chermak & Musiek, 1997). However, in contrast to children with CAPD who may never have developed efficient processing skills,

older adults with CAPD are experiencing loss or disruption of processing functions that were previously intact (Chermak & Musiek, 1997). Moreover, the older adult with CAPD typically presents a complex clinical profile due to the difficulties caused by comorbid conditions, including peripheral hearing loss and cognitive deficits, as well as the diminished plasticity of the central nervous system. Older adults also may present differences in cognitive style that may affect processing outcomes. For example, finding that older adults required longer duration segments to correctly identify monosyllabic word targets, Craig, Kim, Rhyner, and Chirillo (1993) concluded that older adults may impose greater lexical restraint than younger adults, displaying less flexible lexical searching behavior. Also exacerbating older adults' difficulties understanding spoken language are differences in decision-making strategies and reduction in the overall speed of processing (Craig et al., 1993). All of the aforementioned factors may complicate efforts to alleviate the central auditory processing deficits experienced by older adults. (The reader is referred to Bellis and Jorgensen's Chapter 18 in Volume I of this Handbook for an indepth review of the aging auditory system and factors contributing to older adults' speech understanding difficulties.)

Clinical Profile

Estimates of CAPD in older adults range from 23% to 76% (Cooper & Gates, 1991; Golding, Carter, Mitchell, & Hood, 2004; Stach, Spretnjak, & Jerger, 1990). CAPD is seen in older adults due to aging, or associated with neurological diseases, disorders and insults, including neurodegenerative diseases (Baran & Musiek, 1991; Bellis, Nicol, & Kraus, 2000; Jerger, Moncrieff, Greenwald, Wambacq, & Seipel, 2000; Musiek & Gollegly, 1988; Musiek, Gollegly, Lamb, & Lamb, 1990; Pichora-Fuller & Souza, 2003; Tremblay, Piskosz, & Souza, 2003; Willott, 1999; Woods & Clayworth, 1986). Approximately 1 in 3 older adults 65 years of age and older present with peripheral hearing loss (Ries, 1994).

Although peripheral hearing loss, particularly at the high frequencies, accounts for some of the difficulties older adults experience understanding speech in competing noise backgrounds, other factors including CANS changes and/or senescent changes in cognition may also contribute to reduced speech understanding in noise among older adults (CHABA Working Group on Speech Understanding and Aging, 1988; Pichora-Fuller & Souza, 2003). A substantial body of research has demonstrated that age-related decline in spoken language comprehension cannot be explained on the basis of peripheral hearing loss or cognitive decline alone (Chmiel & Jerger, 1996; Chmiel, Jerger, Murphy, Pirozzolo, & Tooley-Young, 1997; Jerger, 1992; Jerger, Jerger, Oliver, & Pirozzolo, 1989; Jerger, Jerger, & Pirozzolo, 1991; Jerger, Stach, Pruitt, Harper, & Kirby, 1989). CAPD may account for the decline in spoken language comprehension unexplained by these other peripheral and cognitive factors (Chermak & Musiek, 1997).

Following an extensive literature review, Bellis and Jorgensen (Chapter 18, Volume I of the Handbook) conclude that older adults experience a variety of central auditory processing deficits due to aging that exacerbate the speech understanding difficulties attributed to peripheral auditory dysfunction and that can lead to speech understanding difficulties even in the absence of peripheral hearing loss. Moreover, noting the absence of correlation between degree of cognitive deficit and perceived self-assessment of hearing handicap in older listeners, Bellis and Jorgensen also conclude that the speech understanding difficulties of older adults can not be explained completely or even primarily by cognitive decline. In contrast, positive correlations between perceived degree of hearing handicap and CANS status (Fire, Lesner, & Newman, 1991) underscore both the impact of CAPD in compromising spoken language understanding and the value of intervention to improve central processing function.

Neurophysiology of CAPD in Older Adults

A neurobiological disorder is suspected in the majority of youngsters with CAPD, possibly involving inefficient interhemispheric transfer of auditory information and/or lack of appropriate hemispheric lateralization, atypical hemispheric asymmetries, imprecise synchrony of neural firing, or other factors (Jerger et al., 2002; Kraus et al., 1996; Moncrieff, Jerger, Wambacq, Greenwald, & Black, 2004). In contrast, the central auditory processing deficits of older adults are acquired, resulting from accumulated damage or deterioration to the CANS due to neurological diseases, disorders and insults, including neurodegenerative diseases, which may or may not involve fairly circumscribed and identifiable lesions of the CANS (Baran & Musiek, 1991; Musiek & Gollegly, 1988; Musiek et al., 1990), or from the aging process (e.g., less synchrony and time-locking, slower refractory periods, decreased central inhibition, and interhemispheric transfer deficits) (Bellis et al., 2000; Jerger et al., 2000; Pichora-Fuller & Souza, 2003; Tremblay et al., 2003; Willott, 1999; Woods & Clayworth, 1986).

Neuroplasticity and Aging

Neural reorganization and recovery of function following injury or disease is less likely in older adults due to the reduction in brain plasticity associated with aging, as well as the slow, but sustained loss of neurons that begins in adolescence and continues throughout the aging process (Kolb, 1995). In fact, neural reorganization (e.g., tonotopic reorganization of frequency maps) may actually *cause* or exacerbate perceptual difficulties for some older adults (Willott, 1999). Although young children may benefit from a great degree of brain plasticity, they do not present the wealth of language and world knowledge or the metacognitive knowledge acquired by the older adult, all of which, if intact, can mitigate the impact of CAPD (Chermak & Musiek, 1997). Conversely, decline in an older adult's central resources can exacerbate the impact of the CAPD.

Implications for Intervention

Intervention to alleviate some of the central auditory processing deficits common to the aging process often is complicated by several factors, including diminished plasticity and comorbid peripheral hearing loss and cognitive deficits. There is little doubt that peripheral deficits and cognitive decline or differences potentially exacerbate the effects of CAPD

(Chermak & Musiek, 1997). Management must begin by considering amplification, since the primary complaint of the older adult with CAPD is difficulty understanding spoken language in the presence of background noise, as well as the frequent co-occurrence of peripheral hearing loss in this population (Chmiel & Jerger, 1996; Stach et al., 1990). Hearing aids and personal hearing assistive technology (e.g., personal frequency modulation [FM] systems) should be fitted in advance of intervention directed toward the CAPD. The remote microphone technology employed in FM systems is more effective than hearing aids in reducing background competition, which interferes with the older adult's ability to understand spoken language (Stach et al., 1990; Stach, Loiselle, Jerger, Mintz, & Taylor, 1987). When fitting hearing aids to older adults with mixed peripheral and central hearing problems, consideration should be given to the possibility that a monaural fitting may be more effective than a binaural fitting due to interhemispheric transfer problems (Bellis et al., 2000; Jerger et al., 2000; Strouse Carter, Noe, & Wilson, 2001).

The intervention program should also include communication repair strategies and auditory-visual speech perception training (i.e., speech-reading), particularly when the older adults presents with both peripheral and central auditory disorders. Home-based therapy programs may be particularly appropriate for older adults. One such program designed specifically for adults with peripheral hearing impairment, LACE™ (Listening and Communication Enhancement), trains auditory-visual communication via an interactive computer program (Sweetow & Henderson-Sabes, 2004). The development of strategies to enhance utilization of central (i.e., compensatory) resources discussed in this chapter is essential to ensure that the older adult takes optimum advantage of linguistic and other top-down skills and strategies during listening. Intact, central resources provide tremendous opportunity to mitigate the consequences of the CAPD in the older adult.

Remedial efforts to acquire or recover normal (or equivalent) function in children should prove successful due to the inherent plasticity of their developing brains. In contrast, due to the reduced plasticity inherent to their mature central nervous system, intervention for older adults (and adults) often focuses more (although not exclusively) on compensation rather than recovery of function (ASHA, 1996). Nonetheless, remedial approaches may still succeed—for example, with adults and older adults who have sustained acute brain insults where opportunity presents for spontaneous recovery and stimulation-induced recovery of function (ASHA, 1996). Likewise, as elaborated earlier in this chapter, intervention for children should be comprehensive, including central resources (i.e., compensatory strategies) training to scaffold skills not completely responsive to treatment or remediation, as well as to provide bridging strategies during periods of (re)learning (Chermak & Musiek, 1997).

The prognosis for effective implementation of compensatory or remedial strategies is determined in large part by the source of the CAPD (i.e., circumscribed lesion or pervasive and diffuse neuropathology). An older adult suffering from aphasia is likely to benefit less from CAPD therapies than an otherwise normal older adult with presbycusis who is experiencing CAPD as a result of an aging CANS (ASHA, 1996). Differences in intellectual, cognitive, linguistic, and psychosocial state will influence treatment outcomes across individuals and must therefore be taken into consideration in planning and delivering intervention. Key to successful outcomes with older adults, as with children, is the collaborative involvement of family, other communicative partners, and related professionals in the comprehensive intervention program. See Chapter 15 in this volume and Chapter 18 in Volume 1 of the Handbook for additional discussion of intervention with older adults with CAPD.

Summary

Given the pivotal role of audition for communication and learning, as well as the frequent comorbidity of CAPD with cognitive, attention, and language and related deficits, comprehensive intervention is essential to address the clinical and functional deficit profile frequently associated with CAPD. Although the complex organization of the brain, involving interactive and interfacing sensory, cognitive, and linguistic networks leads to more heterogeneous deficit profiles, that organization also provides treatment and management opportunities. To achieve the ultimate goals of improved listening ability and spoken language comprehension, comprehensive intervention must include central resources training with an emphasis on self-regulation of listening strategies. Coupling auditory training with central resources knowledge, skills, and strategies training helps listeners structure auditory input and orchestrate information processing. Moreover, coupling direct auditory skills training with central resources training empowers clients to invoke complementary strategies to meet the variety of processing demands and listening tasks. This approach should provide a powerful intervention program likely to lead to generalization of skills across settings. A growing body of research has demonstrated the effectiveness of auditory training (see Chapters 3 and 7) and the potential of metacognitive training to improve listening and reduce spoken language comprehension deficits. Nonetheless, additional research is needed to confirm these encouraging findings. Such research should involve subjects diagnosed with CAPD (rather than learning disabilities or language impairment with characteristics suggestive of CAPD) and employ a robust battery of tests to obtain the high levels of evidence (e.g., randomized controlled trials; meta-analysis of randomized controlled trials) needed to demonstrate intervention effectiveness and efficacy.

References

AAA (American Academy of Audiology). (2010). *Guidelines for the diagnosis, treatment, and management of children and adults with central auditory processing disorder.* Retrieved from http://www.audiology.org/resources/documentlibrary/Documents/CAPD%20Guidelines%208-2010.pdf

Aarnoutse, C. A. J., Van Den Bos, K.P., Kees, P., & Brand-Gruwel, S. (1998). Effects of listening comprehension training on listening and reading. *Journal of Special Education, 32,* 115–126.

Adams, M. J. (1990). *Beginning to read: Thinking and learning about print.* Cambridge, MA: MIT Press.

Adelman, H. S., & Taylor, L. (1983). Enhancing motivation for overcoming learning and behavior problems. *Journal of Learning Disabilities, 16,* 384–392.

Agnew, J. A., Dorn, C., & Eden, G. F. (2003). Effect of intensive training on auditory processing and reading skills. *Brain and Language, 88,* 21–25.

Ahissar, M., & Hochstein, S. (1993). Attentional control of early perceptual learning. *Proceedings of the National Academy of Science, 90,* 5718–5722.

Akeroyd, M. (2008). Are individual differences in speech reception related to individual differences in cognitive ability? A survey of twenty experimental studies with normal and hearing impaired adults. *International Journal of Audiology, 47*(Suppl.), S53–S71.

Alberti, R. E., & Emmons, M. L. (1978). *Your perfect right* (3rd ed.). San Luis Obispo, CA: Impact.

Altschuler, R. A., & Shore, S. E. (2010). Central auditory neurotransmitters. In A. Rees & A. Palmer (Eds.), *The auditory brain* (pp. 65–92). Oxford, UK: Oxford University Press.

Anderson, R. C., & Freebody, P. (1981). Vocabulary knowledge. In J. T. Guthrie (Ed.), *Comprehension and teaching: Research reviews* (pp. 77–117). Newark, DE: International Reading Association.

Aoki, C., & Siekevitz, P. (1988). Plasticity in brain development. *Scientific American, 259,* 56–64.

ASHA (American Speech-Language-Hearing Association). (1996). Central auditory processing: Current status of research and implications for clinical practice. *American Journal of Audiology, 5,* 41–54.

ASHA. (2005). *(Central) auditory processing disorders.* Retrieved from http://www.asha.org/members/deskref-journals/deskref/default.

Ashcraft, M. H. (1989). *Human memory and cognition.* Glenview, IL: Scott, Foresman.

Baddeley, A. (1986). *Working memory.* Oxford, UK: Oxford University Press.

Baddeley, A. (1995). Working memory. In M. Gazzaniga (Ed.), *The cognitive neurosciences* (pp. 755–764). Cambridge, MA: MIT Press.

Ball, E. W., & Blachman, B. A. (1991). Does phoneme segmentation training in kindergarten make a difference in early word recognition and developmental spelling. *Reading Research Quarterly, 26*, 49–66.

Bamiou, D., Free, S. L., Sisodiya, S. M., Chong, W. K., Musiek, F., Williamson, K. A., . . . Luxon, L. M. (2007). Auditory interhemispheric transfer deficitis, hearing difficities, and brain magnetic resonance imaging abnormalities in children with congenital anaridia due to PAX6 mutations. *Archives of Pediatric and Adolescent Medicine, 161*, 463–469.

Bao, S., Chang, E. F., Woods, J., & Merzenich, M. M. (2004). Temporal plasticity in the primary auditory cortex induced by operant perceptual learning. *Nature Neuroscience, 7*, 974–981.

Baran, J. A., & Musiek, F. E. (1991). Behavioral assessment of the central auditory nervous system. In W. F. Rintelmann (Ed.), *Hearing assessment* (pp. 549–602). Austin, TX: Pro-Ed.

Bard, E. G., Schillcock, R. C., & Altmann, G. T. M. (1988). The recognition of words after their acoustic offsets in spontaneous speech: Effects of subsequent context. *Perception and Psychophysics, 44*, 395–408.

Barkley, R. A. (1997). Behavioral inhibition, sustained attention, and executive functions: Constructing a unifying theory of ADHD. *Psychological Bulletin, 121*, 65–94.

Barkley, R. A. (1997). *ADHD and the nature of self-control.* New York, NY: Guilford Press.

Bartoli, J., & Botel, M. (1988). *Reading/learning disability: An ecological approach.* New York, NY: Teachers College Press.

Bayazit, O., Oniz, A., Hahn, C., Gunturkun, O., & Ozgoren, M. (2009). Dichotic listening revisited: Trial-by-trial ERP analyses reveal intra- and inter-hemispheric differences. *Neuropsychologia, 47*, 536–545.

Beck, I., McKeown, M., & Kucan, L. (2002). *Bringing words to life: Robust vocabulary instruction.* New York, NY: Guilford Press.

Bellis, T. J. (2003). *Assessment and management of central auditory processing disorders in the educational setting* (2nd ed.). Clifton Park, NY: Delmar Learning.

Bellis, T. J., & Ferre, J. M. (1999). Multidimensional approach to the different diagnosis of central auditory processing disorders in children. *Journal of the American Academy of Audiology, 10*, 319–328.

Bellis, T. J., Nicol, T., & Kraus, N. (2000). Aging affects hemispheric asymmetry in the neural representation of speech sounds. *Journal of Neuroscience, 20*, 791–797.

Biemiller, A., & Boote, C. (2006). An effective method for building meaning vocabulary in primary grades. *Journal of Educational Psychology, 98*, 44–62.

Bilger, R. C., Neutzel, J. M., Rabinowitz, W. M., & Rzeczkowski, C. (1984). Standardization of a test of speech perception in noise. *Journal of Speech and Hearing Research, 27*, 32–48.

Bloom, B. (1956). *Taxonomy of educational objectives handbook I: Cognitive domain.* New York, NY: McKay.

Borkowski, J. G., & Burke, J. E. (1996). Theories, models, and measurement of executive functioning: An information processing perspective. In G. R. Lyon & N. A. Krasnegor (Eds.), *Attention, memory, and executive function* (pp. 235–261). Baltimore, MD: Paul H. Brookes.

Borkowski, J. G., Estrada, M. T., Milstead, M., & Hale, C. (1989). General problem-solving skills: Relations between metacognition and strategic processing. *Learning Disability Quarterly, 12*, 57–70.

Borkowski, J. G., Johnston, M. B., & Reid, M. K. (1987). Metacognition, motivation, and controlled performance. In S. J. Ceci (Ed.), *Handbook of cognitive, social, and neuropsychological aspects of learning disabilities* (Vol. 2, pp. 147–174). Hillsdale, NJ: Lawrence Erlbaum.

Borkowski, J. G., Weyhing, R. S., & Carr, M. (1988). Effects of attributional retraining on strategy-based reading comprehension in learning-disabled students. *Journal of Educational Psychology, 80*, 46–53.

Bornstein, M. R., Bellack, A. S., & Hersen, M. (1977). Social-skills training for unassertive children: A multiple-baseline analysis. *Journal of Applied Behavior Analysis, 10,* 183–195.

Bos, C., & Filip, D. (1982). Comprehension monitoring skills in learning disabled and average students. *Topics in Learning Disabilities, 2,* 79–85.

Boscariol, M., Guimarães, C., Hage, S., Garcia, V., Schmutzler, K., Cendes, F., & Guerreiro, M. (2011). Auditory processing disorder in patients with language-learning impairment and correlation with malformation of cortical development. *Brain Development, 33,* 824–831.

Bradley, L., & Bryant, P. (1985). Rhyme and reason in reading and spelling. *International Academy for Research in Learning Disabilities Monograph Series, No. 1.* Ann Arbor, MI: University of Michigan Press.

Brand-Gruwel, S., Aarnoutse, C. A. J., & Van Den Bos, K. P. (1998). Improving text comprehension strategies in reading and listening settings. *Learning and Instruction, 8,* 63–81.

Brophy, J. E. (1981). Teacher praise: A functional analysis. *Review of Educational Research, 51,* 5–32.

Brown, A. L., Bransford, J., Ferrara, R. A., & Campione, J. C. (1983). Learning, remembering, and understanding. In J. Flavell & E. M. Markman (Eds.), *Carmichael's manual of child psychology* (Vol. 1, pp. 77–166). New York, NY: John Wiley & Sons.

Brown, A. L., Campione, J., & Barclay, C. R. (1979). Training self-checking routines for estimating test readiness: Generalization for list learning to prose recall. *Child Development, 50,* 501–512.

Brown, A. L., Campione, J. C., & Day, J. D. (1981). Learning to learn: On training students to learn from texts. *Educational Researcher, 10,* 14–21.

Brown, A. L., & French, L. (1979). The zone of potential development: Implications for intelligence testing in the year 2000. *Intelligence, 2,* 46–53.

Bryan, T. (1991). Social problems and learning disabilities. In B. Y. L. Wong (Ed.), *Learning about learning disabilities* (pp. 195–229). San Diego, CA: Academic Press.

Budde, H., Voelcker-Rehage, C., Pietrabyk-Kendziorra, S., Ribeiro, P., & Tidow, G. (2008). Acute coordinative exercise improves attentional performance in adolescents. *Neuroscience Letters, 441*(2), 219–223.

Buschman, T., & Miller, E. (2007). Top-down versus bottom-up control of attention in the prefrontal and posterior parietal cortices. *Science, 315,* 1860–1862.

Butkowski, I. S., & Willows, D. M. (1980). Cognitive-motivational characteristics of children varying in reading ability: Evidence for learned helplessness in poor readers. *Journal of Educational Psychology, 72,* 408–422.

Buttrill, J., Niizawa, J., Biemer, C., Takahashi, C., & Hearn, S. (1989). Serving the language learning disabled adolescent: A strategies-based model. *Language, Speech, and Hearing Services in Schools, 20,* 185–203.

Casanova, U. (1989). Being the teacher helps students learn. *Instructor, 98,* 12–13.

Catts, H. W. (1991). Facilitating phonological awareness: Role of speech-language pathologists. *Language, Speech, and Hearing Services in Schools, 22,* 196–203.

Cavanaugh, J. C., & Perlmutter, M. (1982). Metamemory: A critical examination. *Child Development, 53,* 11–28.

Chaddock, L., Pontifex, M., Hillman, C., & Kramer, A. (2011). A review of the relation of aerobic fitness and physical activity to brain structure and function in children. *Journal of the International Neuropsychological Society, 17,* 975–985.

Chermak, G. D. (1993). Dynamics of collaborative consultation with families. *American Journal of Audiology, 2,* 38–43.

Chermak, G. D. (Ed.) (2002). Management of auditory processing disorders. *Seminars in Hearing, 23*(4).

Chermak, G. D. (2007). Central resources training: Cognitive, metacognitive, and metalinguistic skills and strategies. In G. D. Chermak & F. E. Musiek (Eds.), *Hand-*

book of central auditory processing disorder (pp. 107–166). San Diego, CA: Plural.

Chermak, G. D., Curtis, L., & Seikel, J. A. (1996). The effectiveness of an interactive hearing conservation program for elementary school children. *Language, Speech, and Hearing Services in Schools, 27*, 29–39.

Chermak, G. D., Hall, J. W., & Musiek, F. E. (1999). Differential diagnosis and management of central auditory processing disorder and attention deficit hyperactivity disorder. *Journal of the American Academy of Audiology, 10*, 289–303.

Chermak, G. D., & Musiek, F. E. (1992). Managing central auditory processing disorders in children and youth. *American Journal of Audiology, 1*, 61–65.

Chermak, G. D., & Musiek, F. E. (1997). *Central auditory processing disorders: New perspectives.* San Diego, CA: Singular.

Chermak, G. D., & Musiek, F. E. (2002). Auditory training: Principles and approaches for remediating and managing auditory processing disorders. *Seminars in Hearing, 23*, 297–308.

Chmiel, R., & Jerger, J. (1996). Hearing aid use, central auditory disorder, and hearing handicap in elderly persons. *Journal of the American Academy of Audiology, 7*, 190–202.

Chmiel, R., Jerger, J., Murphy, E., Pirozzolo, G., & Tooley-Young, C. (1997). Unsuccessful use of binaural amplification by an elderly person. *Journal of the American Academy of Audiology, 8*, 1–10.

Ciccia, A. H., Meulenbroek, P., & Turkstra, L. S. (2009). Adolescent brain and cognitive developments. Implications for clinical assessment in traumatic brain injury. *Topics in Language Disorders, 29*, 249–265.

Clarke, J., MacPherson, B., Holmes, D., & Jones, R. (1986). Reducing adolescent smoking: A comparison of peer-led, teacher-led, and expert interventions. *Journal of School Health, 98*, 92–96.

Clifford, M. M. (1978). Have we underestimated the facilitative effects of failure? *Canadian Journal of Behavioral Science, 10*, 308–316.

Cole, R., & Jakimik, J. (1980). A model of speech perception. In R. Cole (Ed.), *Perception and prediction of fluent speech* (pp. 133–160). Englewood Cliffs, NJ: Lawrence Erlbaum.

Committee on Hearing, Bioacoustics, and Biomechanics (CHABA). (1988). Working Group on Speech Understanding and Aging. Speech understanding and aging. *Journal of the Acoustical Society of America, 83*, 859–893.

Connell, P. J. (1988). Induction, generalization, and deduction: Models for defining language generalization. *Language, Speech, and Hearing Services in Schools, 19*, 282–291.

Cooper, J. C. Jr., & Gates, G. A. (1991). Hearing in the elderly—the Framingham Cohort, 1983–1985: Part II. Prevalence of central auditory processing disorders. *Ear and Hearing, 12*, 304–311.

Craig, C. H., Kim, B. W., Rhyner, P. M. P., & Chirillo, T. K. B. (1993). Effects of word predictability, child development, and aging on time-gated speech recognition performance. *Journal of Speech and Hearing Research, 36*, 832–841.

Craighead, W. E., Wilcoxon-Craighead, L., & Meyers, A. (1978). New directions in behavior modification with children. In M. Hersen, R. Eisler, & P. Miller (Eds.), *Progress in behavior modification* (Vol. 6, pp. 159–201). New York, NY: Academic Press.

Cunningham, J., Nicol, T., Zecker, S. G., Bradlow, A., & Kraus, N. (2001). Neurobiologic responses to speech in noise in children with learning problems: Deficits and strategies for improvement. *Clinical Neurophysiology, 112*, 758–767.

Cutler, A., & Foder, J. A. (1979). Semantic focus and sentence comprehension. *Cognition, 7*, 49–59.

Cutler, A., & Foss, D. J. (1977). On the role of sentence stress in sentence processing. *Language and Speech, 20*, 1–10.

Damico, J. S., Augustine, L. E., & Hayes, P. A. (1996). Formulating a functional model of attention deficit hyperactivity disorder for the practicing speech-language pathologist. *Seminars in Speech and Language, 17*, 5–20.

Daneman, M., & Blennerhasset, A. (1984). How to assess the listening comprehension skills of prereaders. *Journal of Educational Psychology, 76*, 1372–1381.

Daneman, M., & Carpenter, P. A. (1980). Individual differences in working memory and reading. *Journal of Verbal Learning and Verbal Behavior, 19*, 450–466.

Daneman, M., & Merikle, P. (1996). Working memory and language comprehension: A meta-analysis. *Psychonomic Bulletin and Review, 3*, 422–433.

Danks, J. H., & End, L. J. (1987). Processing strategies for reading and listening. In R. Horowitz & S. J. Samuels (Eds.), *Comprehending oral and written language* (pp. 271–294). San Diego, CA: Academic Press.

Danzl, M., Etter, N., Andreatta, R., & Kitzman, P. (2012). Facilitating neurorehabilitation through principles of engagement. *Journal Allied Health, 41*, 35–41.

de Boer, J., & Thornton, A. R. D. (2008). Neural correlates of perceptual learning in the auditory brainstem: Efferent activity predicts and reflects improvement at a speech-in-noise discrimination task. *Journal of Neuroscience, 28*, 4929–4937.

de Fockert, J., Rees, G., Frith, C., & Lavie, N. (2001). The role of working memory in visual selective attention. *Science, 291*, 1803–1806.

deVillers-Sidani, E., Alzghoul, L., Zhou, X., Simpson, K., Lin, R., & Merzenich, M. (2010). Recovery of functional and structural age-related changes in the rat primary auditory cortex with operant training. *Proceedings of the National Academy of Sciences, 107*, 13900–13905.

Dillon, G. L. (1981). *Constructing texts*. Bloomington, IN: Indiana University Press.

Duranti, A., & Goodwin, C. (1990). *Rethinking context: Language as an interactive phenomenon*. Cambridge, UK: Cambridge University Press.

Dweck, C. S. (1975). The role of expectations and attributions in the alleviation of learned helplessness. *Journal of Personality and Social Psychology, 31*, 674–685.

D'Zurilla, T. J. (1986). *Problem-solving therapy: A social competence approach to clinical intervention*. New York, NY: Springer.

Ehri, L. C., Nunes, S. R., Willows, D. M., Schuster, B. V., Yaghoub-Zadeh, Z., & Shanahan, T. (2001). Phonemic awareness instruction helps children learn to read: Evidence from the National Reading Panel's meta-analysis. *Reading Research Quarterly, 36*, 250–287.

Elbert, T., Pantev, C., Wienbruch, C., Rockstroh, B., & Taub, E. (1995). Increased cortical representation of the fingers of the left hand in string players. *Science, 270*, 305–306.

Ellis, E. (1989). A metacognitive intervention for increasing class participation. *Learning Disabilities Focus, 5*, 36–46.

Ellis, E. S., & Friend, P. (1991). Adolescents with learning disabilities. In B. Y. L. Wong (Ed.), *Learning about learning disabilities* (pp. 506–561). San Diego, CA: Academic Press.

Ellis, E. S., Lenz, B. K., & Sabornie, E. J. (1987). Generalization and adaptation of learning strategies to natural environments—Part 2: Research into practice. *Remedial and Special Education, 8*, 6–23.

Ellis Weismer, S., Evans, J., & Hesketh, L. J. (1999). An examination of verbal working memory capacity in children with specific language impairment. *Journal of Speech, Language, and Hearing Research, 42*, 1249–1260.

Fabricius, W. V., & Hagen, J. W. (1984). Use of causal attributions about recall performance to assess metameory and predict strategic memory behavior in young children. *Developmental Psychology, 20*, 975–987.

Farah, M. J., Wong, A. B., Monheit, M. A., & Morrow, L. A. (1989). Parietal lobe mechanisms of spatial attention: Modality-specific or supramodal? *Neuropsychologia,* *27,* 461–470.

Feldman, D. E., & Brecht, M. (2005). Map plasticity in somatosensory cortex. *Science,* *310,* 810–815.

Ferre, J. M., & Wilber, L. A. (1986). Normal and learning disabled children's central auditory processing skills: An experimental test battery. *Ear and Hearing, 7,* 336–343.

Fire, K.M., Lesner, S.A., & Newman, C. (1991). Hearing handicap as a function of central auditory abilities in the elderly. *American Journal of Otolaryngology, 122,* 105–108.

Flavell, J. H. (1976). Metacognitive aspects of problem solving. In L. B. Resnick (Ed.), *The nature of intelligence* (pp. 231–235). Hillsdale, NJ: Lawrence Erlbaum Associates.

Flavell, J. H. (1981). Cognitive monitoring. In W. P. Dickson (Ed.), *Children's oral communication skills* (pp. 35–60). New York, NY: Academic Press.

Flavell, J. H., & Wellman, H. M. (1977). Metamemory. In R. V. Kail & J. W. Hagan (Eds.), *Perspectives on the development of memory and cognition* (pp. 3–33). Hillsdale, NJ: Lawrence Erlbaum.

Flook, L., Smalley, S., Kitil, M., Galla, B., Kaiser-Greenland, S., Locke, J., . . . Kasari, C. (2010). Effects of mindful awareness practices on executive functions in elementary school children. *Journal of Applied School Psychology, 26,* 70–95.

French, L., & Nelson, K. (1985). *Young children's knowledge of relational terms.* New York, NY: Springer-Verlag.

Gaffan, D. (2005). Widespread cortical networks underlie memory and attention. *Science, 309,* 2172–2173.

Gajar, A. H. (1989). A computer analysis of written language variables and a comparison of compositions written by university students with and without learning disabilities. *Journal of Learning Disabilities, 22,* 125–130.

Gerber, A. (1981). Remediation of language processing problems of the school-age child. In A. Gerber & D. N. Bryen (Eds.), *Language and learning disabilities* (pp.

159–215). Baltimore, MD: University Park Press.

Gerber, A. (1993a). Intervention: Preventing or reversing the failure cycle. In A. Gerber (Ed.), *Language-related learning disabilities: Their nature and treatment* (pp. 323–393). Baltimore, MD: Paul H. Brookes.

Gerber, A. (Ed.). (1993b). *Language-related learning disabilities: Their nature and treatment.* Baltimore, MD: Paul H. Brookes.

Gibson, J. J. (1966). *The senses considered as perceptual systems.* Boston, MA: Houghton Mifflin.

Gillon, G. T. (2005). Facilitating phoneme awareness development in 3 and 4-year-old children with speech impairment. *Language, Speech, and Hearing Services in Schools, 36,* 308–324.

Goldfried, M. R., & Davison, G. C. (1976). *Clinical behavior therapy.* New York, NY: Holt, Rinehart & Winston.

Golding, M., Carter, N., Mitchell, P., & Hood, L. (2004). Prevalence of central auditory processing (CAP) abnormality in an older Australian population: The Blue Mountains Hearing Study. *Journal of the American Academy of Audiology, 15,* 633–642.

Goldinger, S. D., Pisoni, D. B., & Luce, P. A. (1996). Speech perception and spoken word recognition: Research and theory. In N. J. Lass (Ed.), *Principles of experimental phonetics* (pp. 277–327). St. Louis, MO: Mosby.

Gomez, R., & Condon, M. (1999). Central auditory processing ability in children with ADHD with and without learning disabilities. *Journal of Learning Disabilities, 32,* 150–158.

Gopal, K., Bishop, C., & Carney, L. (2004a). Auditory measures in clinically depressed individuals. II. Auditory evoked potentials and behavioral speech tests. *International Journal of Audiology, 43,* 499–505.

Gopal, K., Carney, L., & Bishop, C. (2004b). Auditory measures in clinically depressed individuals. I. Basic measures and transient otoacoustic emissions. *International Journal of Audiology, 43,* 493–498.

Grafman, J., & Litvan, I. (1999). Evidence for four forms of neuroplasticity. In J. Grafman & Y. Christen (Eds.), *Neuronal plasticity: Building a bridge from the laboratory to the clinic* (pp. 131–139). New York, NY: Springer-Verlag.

Graham, S., & Harris, K. R. (2003). Students with LD and the process of writing: A meta-analysis of SRSD studies. In L. Swanson, K. R. Harris, & S. Graham (Eds.), *Handbook of research on learning disabilities* (pp. 323–344). New York, NY: Guilford Press.

Griffiths, H., & Craighead, E. W. (1972). Generalization in operant speech therapy for misarticulation. *Journal of Speech and Hearing Disorders, 37,* 485–492.

Guevremont, D. (1990). Social skills and peer relationship training. In R. A. Barkley (Ed.), *Attention-deficit hyperactivity disorder: A handbook for diagnosis and treatment* (pp. 540–572). New York, NY: Guilford Press.

Haaga, D. A., & Davison, G. C. (1986). Cognitive change methods. In F. H. Kanfer & A. P. Goldstein (Eds.), *Helping people change: A textbook of methods* (pp. 236–282). New York, NY: Pergamon Press.

Hallahan, D. P., & Kneedler, R. D. (1979). *Strategy deficits in the information processing of learning-disabled children.* Charlottesville, IN: University of Virginia Learning Disabilities Research Institute, Technical Report, No. 6.

Halliday, M. A. K., & Hasan, R. (1976). *Cohesion in English.* London, UK: Longman.

Halpern, D. F. (1984). *Thought and knowledge: An introduction to critical thinking.* Hillsdale, NJ: Lawrence Erlbaum.

Harrell, M., Parente, F., Bellingrath, E. G., & Lisicia, K. A. (1992). *Cognitive rehabilitation of memory: A practical guide.* Gaithersburg, MD: Aspen.

Harris, A. J., & Sipay, E. R. (1990). *How to increase reading ability* (9th ed.). New York, NY: Longman.

Harris, J. E. (1992). Ways to help memory. In B. Wilson & N. Moffat (Eds.), *Clinical management of memory problems* (pp. 56–82). San Diego, CA: Singular.

Harris, K., Reid, R., & Graham, S. (2004). Self-regulation among students with LD and ADHD. In B. Y. L. Wong (Ed.), *Learning about learning disabilities* (3rd ed., pp.167–195). San Diego, CA: Elsevier Academic Press.

Harris, P. L. (1978). Developmental aspects of memory: A review. In M. M. Gruneberg, P. E. Morris, & R. N. Sykes (Eds.), *Practical aspects of memory* (pp. 369–377). London, UK: Academic Press.

Harris, P. L., & Terwogt, M. M. (1978). How does memory write a synnopsis. In M. M. Gruneberg, P. E. Morris, & R. N. Sykes (Eds.), *Practical aspects of memory* (pp. 385–392). London, UK: Academic Press.

Hart, K. J., & Morgan, J. R. (1993). Cognitive-behavioral procedures with children: Historical context and current status. In A. J. Finch, W. M. Nelson, & E. S. Ott (Eds.), *Cognitive-behavioral procedures with children and adolescents* (pp. 1–24). Boston, MA: Allyn & Bacon.

Hassamannova, J., Myslivecek, J., & Novakova, V. (1981). Effects of early auditory stimulation on cortical areas. In J. Syka & L. Aitkin (Eds.), *Neuronal mechanisms of hearing* (pp. 355–359). New York, NY: Plenum Press.

Hayes, E. A., Warrier, C. M., Nichol, T. G., Zecker, S. G., & Kraus, N. (2003). Neural plasticity following auditory training in children with learning problems. *Clinical Neurophysiology, 114,* 673–684.

Hergenhahn, B. R., & Olson, M. H. (1993). *An introduction to theories of learning.* Englewood Cliffs, NJ: Prentice-Hall.

Hillman, C., Erickson, K., & Kramer, A. (2008). Be smart, exercise your heart: Exercise effects on brain and cognition. *Nature Reviews Neuroscience, 9,* 58–65.

Holmes, J., Gathercole, S., & Dunning, D. (2009). Adaptive training leads to sustained enhancement of poor working memory in children. *Developmental Science, 12,* 9–15.

Holmes, J., Gathercole, S., Place, M., Dunning, D., Hilton, K., & Elliott, J. (2010). Working memory deficits can be overcome: Impacts of training and medication on working memory of children with ADHD. *Applied Cognitive Psychology, 24,* 827–836

Hornickel, J., Skoe, E., Nicol, T., Zecker, S., & Kraus, N. (2009). Subcortical differentiation of stop consonants relates to reading and speech-in-noise perception. *PNAS, 106,* 13022–13027.

Hoskins, B. (1983). Semantics. In C. Wren (Ed.), *Language learning disabilities* (pp. 85–111). Rockville, MD: Aspen Systems.

Houck, C. K., & Billingsley, B. S. (1989). Written expression of students with and without learning disabilities: Differences across the grades. *Journal of Learning Disabilities, 22,* 561–572.

Howard, R., McShane, R., Lindesay, J., Ritchie, C., Baldwin, A., Barber, R., . . . Phillips, P. (2012). Donepezil and memantine for moderate-to-severe Alzheimer's disease. *New England Journal of Medicine, 366,* 893–903.

Howe, M. J. A., & Ceci, S. J. (1978). Why older children remember more: Contributions of strategies and existing knowledge of developmental changes in memory. In M. M. Gruneberg, P. E. Morris, & R. N. Sykes (Eds.), *Practical aspects of memory* (pp. 393–400). London, UK: Academic Press.

Iliadou, V., Bamiou, D-E., Kaprinis, S., Kandylis, D., & Kaprinis, G. (2009). Auditory processing disorders in children suspected of learning disabilities—a need for screening. *International Journal of Pediatric Otorhinolaryngology, 73,* 1029–1034.

Jacob, J. E., & Paris, S. G. (1987). Children's metacognition about reading: Issues in definition, measurement and instruction. *Educational Psychology, 22,* 255–278.

Jancke, L., & Shah, N. (2002). Does dichotic listening probe temporal lobe function? *Neurology, 58,* 736–743.

Jerger, J. (1992). Can age-related decline in speech understanding be explained by peripheral hearing loss? *Journal of the American Academy of Audiology, 3,* 33–38.

Jerger, J., Jerger, S., Oliver, T., & Pirozzolo, F. (1989). Speech understanding in the elderly. *Ear and Hearing, 10,* 79–89.

Jerger, J., Jerger, S., & Pirozzolo, F. (1991). Correlational analysis of speech audiometric scores, hearing loss, age, and cognitive abilities in the elderly. *Ear and Hearing, 12,* 103–109.

Jerger, J., Moncrieff, D., Greenwald, R., Wambacq, I., & Seipel, A. (2000). Effect of age on interaural asymmetry of event-related potentials in a dichotic listening task. *Journal of the American Academy of Audiology, 11,* 383–389.

Jerger, J., Stach, B., Pruitt, J., Harper, R., & Kirby, H. (1989). Comments on "Speech understanding and aging." *Journal of the Acoustical Society of America, 85,* 1352–1354.

Jerger, J., Thibodeau, L., Martin, J., Mehta, J., Tillman, G., Greenwald, R., . . . Overson, G. (2002). Behavioral and electrophysiologic evidence of auditory processing disorder: A twin study. *Journal of the American Academy of Audiology, 13,* 438–460.

Jirsa, R. E. (1992). The clinical utility of the P3 AERP in children with auditory processing disorders. *Journal of Speech and Hearing Research, 35,* 903–912.

Johnson, D. J., & Myklebust, H. R. (1967). *Learning disabilities: Educational principles and practices.* New York, NY: Grune & Stratton.

Johnson, K. L., Nicol, T., Zecker, S. G., & Kraus, N. (2008). Developmental plasticity in the human auditory brainstem. *The Journal of Neuroscience, 28,* 4000–4007.

Kail, R. V. (1990). *The development of memory in children.* New York, NY: W. H. Freeman.

Kalikow, D. N., Stevens, K. N., & Elliott, L. L. (1977). Development of a test of speech intelligibility in noise using sentence materials with controlled word predictability. *Journal of Acoustical Society of America, 61,* 1337–1351.

Kalil, R. E. (1989). Synapse formation in the developing brain. *Scientific American, 261,* 76–85.

Kanfer, F. H., & Gaelick, L. (1991). Self-management methods. In F. H. Kanfer & A. P. Goldstein (Eds.), *Helping people change: A textbook of methods* (4th ed., pp. 305–360). Needham Heights, MA: Allyn & Bacon.

Katz, J., & Harmon, C. (1982). *Phonemic synthesis*. Allen, TX: Developmental Learning Materials.

Kauramaki, J., Jaaskelainen, I. P., & Sams, M. (2007). Selective attention increases both gain and feature selectivity of the human auditory cortex. *PLoS ONE*, Issue 9, e909.

Keith, R. W. (1994). *ACPT: Auditory continuous performance test*. San Antonio, TX: Psychological Corporation.

Keith, R. W., & Novak, K. K. (1984). Relationships between tests of central auditory function and receptive language. *Seminars in Hearing, 5*, 243–250.

Kelley, C. (1979). *Assertion training: A facilitator's guide*. San Diego, CA: University Associates.

Kendall, P. C., & Braswell, L. (1982). Cognitive-behavioral self-control therapy for children. A components analysis. *Journal of Consulting and Clinical Psychology, 50*, 672–689.

Kennedy, B. A., & Miller, D. J. (1976). Persistent use of verbal rehearsal as a function of information about its value. *Child Development, 47*, 566–569.

Kintsch, W. (1988). The role of knowledge in discourse comprehension: A construction-integration model. *Psychological Review, 95*, 163–182.

Kistner, J. A., Osborne, M., & LeVerrier, L. (1988). Causal attributions of learning-disabled children: Developmental patterns and relation to academic progress. *Journal of Educational Psychology, 80*, 82–89.

Klingberg, T., Fernell, E., Olesen, P. J., Johnson, M., Gustafsson, P., Dahlstrom, K., . . . Westerberg, H. (2005). Computerized training of working memory in children with ADHD—a randomized, controlled, trial. *Journal of the American Academy Child and Adolescent Psychiatry, 44*, 177–186.

Knudsen, E. (1998). Capacity for plasticity in the adult owl auditory system expanded by juvenile experience. *Science, 279*, 1531–1533.

Koegel, L. K., Koegel, R. L., & Ingham, J. C. (1986). Programming rapid generalization of correct articulation through self-monitoring procedures. *Journal of Speech and Hearing Disorders, 51*, 24–32.

Kolb, B. (1995). *Brain plasticity and behavior*. Mahwah, NJ: Lawrence Erlbaum.

Kotsonis, M. E., & Patterson, C. J. (1980). Comprehension monitoring skills in learning disabled children. *Developmental Psychology, 16*, 541–542.

Kraus, N., & Disterhoff, J. F. (1982). Response plasticity of single neurons in rabbit auditory association cortex during tone-signalled learning. *Brain Research, 246*, 205–215.

Kraus, N., McGee, T., Carrell, T., King, C., Tremblay, K., & Nicol, T. (1995). Central auditory system plasticity associated with speech discrimination training. *Journal of Cognitive Neuroscience, 7*, 25–32.

Kraus, N., McGee, T. J., Carrell, T. D., Zecker, S. D., Nicol, T. G., & Koch, D. B. (1996). Auditory neurophysiologic responses and discrimination deficits in children with learning problems. *Science, 273*, 971–973.

Kreitler, S., & Kreitler, H. (1987). Plans and planning: Their motivational and cognitive antecedents. In S. L. Friedman, E. K. Scholnick, & R. R. Cocking (Eds.), *Blueprints for thinking: The role of planning in cognitive development* (pp. 110–178). New York, NY: Cambridge University.

Kreutzer, M. A., Leonard, C., & Flavell, J. H. (1975). An interview study of children's knowledge about memory. *Monographs of the Society for Research in Child Development, 40* (Serial No. 159), 1–58.

Lakes, K., & Hoyt, W. (2004). Promoting self-regulation through school-based martial arts training. *Journal of Applied Developmental Psychology, 25*, 283–302.

Lenz, B. K. (1984). *The effect of advance organizers on the learning and retention of learning disabled adolescents within the context of a cooperative planning model*. Final research report submitted to the U.S. Department of Education, Special

Education Services. Lawrence: University of Kansas.

Levin, J. R. (1976). What have we learned about maximizing what children learn? In J. R. Levin & V. L. Allen (Eds.), *Cognitive learning in children* (pp. 105–134). New York, NY: Academic Press.

Lewkowitz, N. (1980). Phonemic awareness training: What to teach and how to teach it. *Journal of Educational Psychology, 72,* 686–700.

Liberman, A. M., Cooper, F. S., Shankweiler, D., & Studdert-Kennedy, M. (1967). Perception of the speech code. *Psychological Review, 74,* 431–461.

Licht, B., & Kistner, J. A. (1986). Motivational problems of learning-disabled children: Individual differences and their implications for treatment. In J. K. Torgesen & B. Y. L. Wong (Eds.), *Psychological and educational perspectives on learning disabilities* (pp. 225–255). San Diego, CA: Academic Press.

Licht, B., Kistner, J., Ozkaragoz, T., Shapiro, S., & Clausen, L. (1985). Causal attributions of learning disabled children: Individual differences and their implications for persistence. *Journal of Educational Psychology, 77,* 208–216.

Liles, B. Z. (1985). Cohesion in the narratives of normal and language disordered children. *Journal of Speech and Hearing Research, 28,* 123–133.

Liles, B. Z. (1987). Episode organization and cohesive conjunctions in narratives of children with and without language disorders. *Journal of Speech and Hearing Research, 30,* 185–196.

Lindamood, C., & Lindamood, P. (1975). *Auditory discrimination in depth* (Rev. ed.). Austin, TX: Pro-Ed.

Lloyd, J. (1980). Academic instruction and cognitive behavior modification: The need for attack strategy training. *Exceptional Education Quarterly, 1,* 53–64.

Lodico, M. G., Ghatala, E. S., Levin, J. R., Pressley, M., & Bell, J. A. (1983). The effects of strategy-monitoring training on children's selection of effective memory strategies. *Journal of Experimental Child Psychology, 35,* 263–277.

Loftus, G. F., & Loftus, E. F. (1976). *Human memory: The processing of information.* Hillsdale, NJ: Lawrence Erlbaum.

Lopez, O., Becker, J., Wahed, A., Saxton, J., Sweet, R., Wolk, D., . . . Dekosky, S. (2009). Long-term effects of the concomitant use of memantine with cholinesterase inhibition in Alzheimer disease. *Journal of Neurology, Neurosurgery, and Psychiatry, 80,* 600–607.

Lopez-Aranda, M. F., Lopez-Tellez, J. F., Navarro-Lobato, I., Masmudi-Martin, M., Gutierrez, A., & Khan, Z. U. (2009). Role of layer 6 of v2 visual cortex in object-recognition. *Memory, 325,* 87–89.

Maag, J. W., & Reid, R. (1996).Treatment of attention deficit hyperactivity disorder: A multi-modal model for schools. *Seminars in Speech and Language, 17,* 37–58.

MacInnis, D., & Price, L. (1987). The role of imagery in information processing: Review and extensions. *Journal of Consumer Research, 13,* 473–491.

Manjunath, N., & Telles, S. (2001). Improved performance in Tower of London test. *Indian Journal of Physiology and Pharmacology, 45,* 351–354.

Mann, V. (1991). Language problems: A key to early reading problems. In B. Y. L. Wong (Ed.), *Learning about learning disabilities* (pp. 130-162). San Diego, CA: Academic Press.

Margulies, N. (1991*). Mapping inner space.* Tucson, AZ: Zephyr Press.

Marler, J. A., Champlin, C. A., & Gillam, R. B. (2002). Auditory memory for backward masking signals in children with language impairment. *Psychophysiology, 39,* 767–780.

Marslen-Wilson, W. D., & Tyler, L. K. (1980). The temporal structure of spoken language understanding. *Cognition, 8,* 1–71.

Martin, J., Jerger, J., & Mehta, J. (2007). Divided-attention and directed-attention listening modes in children with dichotic deficits: An event-related potential study. *Journal of the American Academy of Audiology, 18,* 34–53.

Martinkauppi, S., Rama, P., Aronen, H. J., Korvenoja, A., & Carolson, S. (2002). Working memory of auditory localization. *Cerebral Cortex, 10,* 889–898.

Massaro, D. W. (1975a). Language and information processing. In D. W. Massaro (Ed.), *Understanding language: An information-processing analysis of speech perception, reading, and psycholinguistics* (pp. 3–28). New York, NY: Academic Press.

Massaro, D. W. (1975b). *Understanding language: An information-processing analysis of speech perception, reading, and psycholinguistics.* New York, NY: Academic Press.

Massaro, D. W. (1976). Auditory information processing. In W. K. W. Estes (Ed.), *Handbook of learning and cognitive processes: Vol. 4: Attention and memory* (pp. 275–320). Hillsdale, NJ: Lawrence Erlbaum.

Massaro, D. W. (1987). *Speech perception by ear and eye: A paradigm for psychological inquiry.* Hillsdale, NJ: Lawrence Erlbaum.

Masterton, R. B. (1992). Role of the central auditory system in hearing: The new direction. *Trends in Neuroscience, 15,* 280–285.

Matkin, N., & Hook, P. (1983). A multidisciplinary approach to central auditory evaluations. In E. Lasky & J. Katz (Eds.), *Central auditory processing disorders* (pp. 223–342). Baltimore, MD: University Park Press.

Mattingly, I. G. (1972). Reading, the linguistic process, and linguistic awareness. In J. F. Kavanaugh & I. G. Mattingly (Eds.), *Language by ear and by eye: The relationship between speech and reading* (pp. 133–148). Cambridge, MA: MIT Press.

McCoy, S. L., Tun, P. A., Cox, L. C., Colangelo, M., Stewart, R. A., & Wingfield, A. (2005). Hearing loss and perceptual effort: Downstream effects on older adults' memory for speech. *Journal of Experimental Psychology, 58,* 22–33.

McKay, K. E., Halperin, J. M., Schwartz, S. T., & Sharma, V. (1994). Developmental analysis of three aspects of information processing: Sustained attention, selective attention and response organization. *Developmental Neuropsychology, 10,* 121–132.

McKenzie, G. G., Neilson, A. R., & Braun, C. (1981). The effects of linguistic connectives and prior knowledge on comprehension of good and poor readers. In M. Kamil (Ed.), *Directions in reading: Research and instruction* (pp. 215–218). Washington, DC: National Reading Conference.

McReynolds, L. V. (1989). Generalization issues in the treatment of communication disorders. In L. V. McReynolds & J. E. Spradlin (Eds.), *Generalization strategies in the treatment of communication disorders* (pp. 1–12). Philadephia, PA: B. C. Decker.

Medway, F. J., & Venino, G. R. (1982). The effects of effort feedback and performance patterns on children's attributions and task persistence. *Contemporary Educational Psychology, 7,* 26–34.

Meichenbaum, D. (1986). Cognitive-behavior management. In F. H. Kanfer & A. P. Goldstein (Eds.), *Helping people change: A textbook of methods* (3rd ed., pp. 346–380). New York, NY: Pergamon Press.

Meichenbaum, D., & Goodman, J. (1971). Training impulsive children to talk to themselves: A means of developing self-control. *Journal of Abnormal Psychology, 77,* 115–126.

Merzenich, M., Grajski, K., Jenkins, W., Recanzone, G., & Peterson, B. (1991). Functional cortical plasticity: Cortical network origins of representations changes. *Cold Spring Harbor Symposium on Quantum Biology, 55,* 873–887.

Merzenich, M., & Jenkins, W. (1995). Cortical plasticity, learning and learning dysfunction. In B. Julesz & I. Kovacs (Eds.) *Maturational windows and adult cortical plasticity: SFI Studies in the sciences of complexity, Vol. XXIII* (pp. 247–272). Reading, PA: Addison-Wesley.

Merzenich, M., Jenkins, W., Johnston, P., Schreiner, C., Miller, S. L., & Tallal, P. (1996). Temporal processing deficits of language-learning impaired children ameliorated by training. *Science, 271,* 77–80.

Merzenich, M., Schreiner, C., Jenkins, W., & Wang, X. (1993). Neural mechanisms underlying temporal integration, segmentation, and input sequence representations: Some implications for the origin of learning disabilities. *Annals New York Academy of Science, 682,* 1–22.

Miller, G. A. (1956). The magical number seven, plus or minus two: Some limits on our capacity for processing information. *Psychological Review, 63,* 81–97.

Miller, G. A., & Gildea, P. M. (1987). How children learn words. *Scientific American, 257,* 94–99.

Miller, G. L., & Knudsen, E. I. (2003, February). Adaptive plasticity in the auditory thalamus of juvenile barn owls. *Journal of Neuroscience, 23,* 1059–1065.

Miller, R. L., Brickman, P., & Bolen, D. (1975). Attribution versus persuasion as a means for modifying behavior. *Journal of Personality and Social Psychology, 31,* 430–441.

Millward, K., Hall, R., Ferguson, M., & Moore, D. (2011). Training speech-in-noise perception in mainstream school children. *International Journal of Pediatric Otorhinolaryngology, 75,* 1408–1417.

Mody, M., Schwartz, Gravel, J. S., & Ruben, R. J. (1999). Speech perception and verbal memory in children with and without histories of otitis media. *Journal of Speech, Language, and Hearing Research, 42,* 1069–1079.

Moncrieff, D., Jerger, J., Wambacq, I., Greenwald, R., & Black, J. (2004). ERP evidence of a dichotic left-ear deficit in some dyslexic children. *Journal of the American Academy of Audiology, 15,* 518–534.

Moncrieff, D., & Musiek, F. (2002). Interaural asymmetries revealed by dichotic listening tests in normal and dyslexic children. *Journal of the American Academy of Audiology, 13,* 428–437.

Moncrieff, D., & Wertz, D. (2008). Auditory rehabilitation for interaural asymmetry: Preliminary evidence of improved dichotic listening performance following intensive training. *International Journal of Audiology, 47,* 484–497.

Moore, D. R. (1993). Plasticity of binaural hearing and some possible mechanisms following late-onset deprivation. *Journal of the American Academy of Audiology, 4,* 227–283.

Moore, D. R., Halliday, L. F., & Amitay, S. (2009). Use of auditory learning to manage listening problems in children. *Philosophical Transactions of the Royal Society, 364,* 409–420.

Morley, B. J., & Happe, H. K. (2000). Cholinergic receptors: Dual roles in transduction and plasticity. *Hearing Research, 147,* 104–112.

Moynahan, E. D. (1978). Assessment and selection of paired associate strategies: A developmental study. *Journal of Experimental Child Psychology, 26,* 257–266.

Murdock, J. Y., Garcia, E. E., & Hardman, M. L. (1977). Generalizing articulation training with trainable mentally retarded subjects. *Journal of Applied Behavior Analysis, 10,* 717–733.

Murphy, C., & Schochat, E. (2011). Effect of nonlinguistic auditory training on phonological and reading skills. *Folia Phoniatrica Logopaedica, 63,* 147–153.

Musiek, F. E. (1999). Habilitation and management of auditory processing disorders: Overview of selected procedures. *Journal of the American Academy of Audiology, 10,* 329–342.

Musiek, F. E., Baran, J. A., & Pinheiro, M. L. (1992). P300 results in patients with lesions of the auditory areas of the cerebrum. *Journal of the American Academy of Audiology, 3,* 5–15.

Musiek, F. E., Baran, J. A., & Shinn, J. (2004). Assessment and remediation of an auditory processing disorder associated with head trauma. *Journal of the American Academy of Audiology, 15,* 117–132.

Musiek, F. E., Bellis, T. J., & Chermak, G. D. (2005). Nonmodularity of the CANS: Implications for (central) auditory processing disorder: A critique of Cacace and McFarland's "The Importance of Modality Specificity in Diagnosing Central Auditory Processing Disorder (CAPD)." *American Journal of Audiology, 14,* 128–138.

Musiek, F. E., & Chermak, G. D. (1995). Three commonly asked questions about central auditory processing disorders: Management. *American Journal of Audiology, 4,* 15–18.

Musiek, F. E., & Gollegly, K. (1988). Maturational considerations in the neuroauditory evaluation of children. In F. Bess (Ed.), *Hearing impairment in children* (pp. 231–252). Parkton, MD: York Press.

Musiek, F. E., Gollegly, K., Lamb, L., & Lamb, P. (1990). Selected issues in screening for central auditory processing of dysfunction. *Seminars in Hearing, 11,* 372–384.

Musiek, F. E., & Hoffman, D. W. (1990). An introduction to the functional neurochemistry of the auditory system. *Ear and Hearing, 11,* 395–402.

Musiek, F. E., & Oxholm, V. (2003). Central auditory anatomy and function. In L. M. Luxon, J. M Furman, A. Martini, & D. C. Stephens (Eds.), *Textbook of audiological medicine* (pp. 517–572). London, UK: Taylor and Francis Group.

Neisser, U. (1976). *Cognition and reality.* San Francisco, CA: W. H. Freeman.

Nickerson, R. S. (1986*).Reflections on reasoning.* Hillsdale, NJ: Lawrence Erlbaum

Ninio, A. (1980). Picture-book reading in mother-infant dyads belonging to two sub-groups in Israel. *Child Development, 51,* 587–590.

Nippold, M. A. (1988). The literate lexicon. In M. Nippold (Ed.), *Later language development* (pp. 29–47). Boston, MA: College-Hill Press.

Nippold, M. A. (1991). Evaluating and enhancing idiom comprehension in language-disordered students. *Language, Speech, and Hearing Services in Schools, 22,* 100–106.

Nippold, M. A., & Fey, S. H. (1983). Metaphoric understanding in preadolescents having history of language acquisition difficulties. *Language, Speech, and Hearing Services in Schools, 14,* 171–180.

Norris, J. A., & Damico, J. S. (1990). Whole language in theory and practice: Implications for language intervention. *Language, Speech, and Hearing Services in Schools, 21,* 212–220.

Ohl, F. W., & Scheich, H. (2005). Learning-induced plasticity in animal and human auditory cortex. *Current Opinion in Neurobiology, 15,* 470–477.

Olswang, L. B., & Bain, B. (1994). Data collection: Monitoring children's treatment progress. *American Journal of Speech-Language Pathology, 3,* 55–66.

Palincsar, A. S., & Brown, A. L. (1984). Reciprocal teaching of comprehension fostering and comprehension monitoring activities. *Cognition and Instruction, 1,* 117–175.

Palincsar, A. S., & Brown, A. L. (1987). Enhancing instructional time through attention to metacognition. *Journal of Learning Disabilities, 20,* 66–75.

Palincsar, A. S., & Klenk, L. (1992). Fostering literacy learning in supportive contexts. *Journal of Learning Disabilities, 25,* 211–225.

Pan, Y., Zhang, J., Cai, R., Zhou, X., & Sun, X. (2011). Developmentally degraded directional selectivity of the auditory cortex can be restored by auditory discrimination training. *Behavioral Brain Research, 225,* 596–602.

Paris, S. G., & Myers, M. (1981). Comprehension monitoring, memory, and study strategies of good and poor readers. *Journal of Reading Behavior, 13,* 5–22.

Paris, S. G., Newman, R. S., & McVey, K. A. (1982). Learning the functional significance of mnemonic actions: A microgenetic study of strategy acquisition. *Journal of Experimental Child Psychology, 34,* 490–509.

Paris, S. G., Wixson, K. K., & Palincsar, A. S. (1986). Instructional approaches to reading comprehension. In E. Z. Rothkopf (Ed.), *Review of research on education* (Vol. 13, pp. 91–218). Washington, DC: American Educational Research Association.

Pearl, R. A. (1982). LD children's attributions for success and failure: A replication with a labeled LD sample. *Learning Disability Quarterly, 5*, 173–176.

Pearson, P. D., & Fielding, L. (1982). Research update: Listening comprehension. *Language Arts, 59*(9), 617–629.

Peele, J., Troiani, V., Grossman, M., & Wingfield, A. (2011). Hearing loss in older adults affects neural systems supporting speech comprehension. *Journal of Neuroscience, 31*, 12638–12643.

Perfetti, C. A. (1985). *Reading ability.* New York, NY: Oxford University Press.

Perfetti, C. A., & McCutchen, D. (1982). Speech processes in reading. *Speech and Language Advances in Basic Research and Practice, 7*, 237–269.

Petacchi, A., Kaernbach, C., Ratnam, R., & Bower, J. (2011). Increased activation of the human cerebellum during pitch discrimination: A positron emission tomography (PET) study. *Hearing Research, 282*, 35–48.

Phillips, D., Hall, S., Harrington, I., & Taylor, T. (1998). "Central" auditory gap detection: A spatial case. *Journal of the Acoustical Society of America, 103*, 2064–2068.

Phillips, D., Taylor, T., Hall, S., Carr, M., & Mossop, J. (1997). Detection of silent intervals between noises activating different perceptual channels: Some properties of "central" auditory gap detection. *Journal of the Acoustical Society of America, 101*, 3694–3705.

Pichora-Fuller, M. K., Schneider, B. A., & Daneman, M. (1995). How young and old adults listen to and remember speech in noise. *Journal of the Acoustical Society of America, 97*, 593–608.

Pichora-Fuller, M., & Souza, P. (2003). Effects of age and age-related hearing loss on the neural representation of speech cues. *Clinical Neurophysiology, 114*, 1332–1343.

Pickles, J. O. (2008). *An introduction to the physiology of hearing* (3rd ed.). London, UK: Emerald.

Pienkowski, M., & Eggermont, J. J. (2011). Cortical tonotopic map plasticity and behavior. *Neuroscience and Biobehavioral Reviews, 35*, 2117–2128.

Pillsbury, H. C., Grose, J. H., Coleman, W. L., Conners, C. K., & Hall, J. W. (1995). Binaural function in children with attention-deficit hyperactivity disorder. *Archives of Otolaryngology-Head and Neck Surgery, 121*, 1345–1350.

Pinheiro, F., & Capellini, S. (2010). Auditory training in students with learning disabilities. *Pro Fono, 22*, 49–54.

Pinheiro, M., & Musiek, F. (1985). *Assessment of central auditory dysfunction: Foundations and clinical correlates.* Baltimore, MD: Williams & Wilkins.

Piquado, T., Cousins, K., Wingfield, A., & Miller, P. (2010). Effects of degraded sensory input on memory for speech: Behavioral data and a test of biologically constrained computational models. *Brain Research, 1365*, 48–65

Poldrack, R., Temple, E., Protopapas, A., Nagarajan, S., Tallal, P., Mezenich, M., & Gabrieli, J. (2001). Relations between neural bases of dynamic auditory processing and phonological processing: Evidence from fMRI. *Journal of Cognitive Neuroscience, 13*, 687–697.

Poplin, M. S. (1988a). Holistic/constructivist principles of the teaching/learning process: Implications for the field of learning disabilities. *Journal of Learning Disabilities, 21*, 401–416.

Poplin, M. S. (1988b). The reductionist fallacy in learning disabilities: Replicating the past by reducing the present. *Journal of Learning Disabilities, 21*, 389–400.

Poremba, A., Saunders, R. C., Crane, A. M., Cook, M., Sokoloff, L., & Mishkin, M. (2003). Functional mapping of the primate auditory system. *Science, 299*, 568–571.

Pratt, M., & Bates, K. (1982). Young editors: Preschoolers' evaluation and production of ambiguous messages. *Developmental Psychology, 18*, 30–42.

Pressley, M. (1982). Elaboration and memory development. *Child Development, 53*, 296–309.

Pressley, M., Borkowski, J. G., & O'Sullivan, J. T. (1984). Memory strategy instruction is made of this: Metamemory and durable strategy use. *Educational Psychologist, 19,* 94–107.

Pressley, M., Johnson, C. J., & Symons, S. (1987). Elaborating to learn and learning to elaborate. *Journal of Learning Disabilities, 20,* 76–91.

Pressley, M., & Levin, J. R. (1987). Elaborative learning strategies for the inefficient learner. In S. J. Ceci (Ed.), *Handbook of cognitive, social and neuropsychological aspects of learning disabilities* (Vol. 2, pp. 175–212). Hillsdale, NJ: Lawrence Erlbaum.

Purdy, S., Kelly, A., & Davies, M. (2002). Auditory brainstem response, middle latency response, and late cortical evoked potentials in children with learning disabilities. *Journal of the American Academy of Audiology, 13,* 367–382.

Rauscher, F., Shaw, G., Levine, L., Wright, E., Dennis, W., & Mewcomb, R. (1997). Music training causes long-term enhancement of children's spatial-temporal reasoning skills. *Journal of Neurology Research, 19,* 2–8.

Recanzone, G. H., Schreiner, C. E., & Merzenich, M. M. (1993). Plasticity in the frequency representation of primary auditory cortex following discrimination training in adult owl monkeys. *Journal of Neuroscience, 13,* 87–103.

Rehm, L. P., Fuchs, C. Z., Roth, D. M., Kornblith, S. J., & Romano, J. M. (1979). A comparison of self-control and assertion skills treatments of depression. *Behavior Therapy, 10,* 429–442.

Reid, L. (1992). Improving young children's listening by verbal self-regulation: The effect of mode of rule presentation. *Journal of Genetic Psychology, 153,* 447–461.

Reid, M. K., & Borkowski, J. G. (1987). Causal attributions of hyperactive children: Implications for training strategies and self-control. *Journal of Educational Psychology, 76,* 225–235.

Riccio, C. A., Hynd, G. W., Cohen, M. J., Hall, J., & Molt, L. (1994). Comorbidity of central auditory processing disorder and attention-deficit hyperactivity disorder. *Journal of the American Academy of Child and Adolescent Psychiatry, 33,* 849–857.

Riccio, C. A., Reynolds, C. R., & Lowe, P. A. (2001). *Clinical applications of continuous performance tests.* New York, NY: John Wiley & Sons.

Ries, P. W. (1994). *Prevalence and characteristics of persons with hearing trouble: United States.* National Center for Health Statistics, *Vital Stat, 24,* 188.

Ringel, B. A., & Springer, C. J. (1980). On knowing how well one is remembering: The persistence of strategy use during transfer. *Journal of Experimental Child Psychology, 29,* 322–333.

Robertson, D., & Irvine, D. R. F. (1989). Plasticity of frequency organization in auditory cortex of guinea pigs with partial unilateral deafness. *Journal of Comparative Neurology, 282,* 456–471.

Ronnberg, J. (2003). Cognition in the hearing impaired and deaf as a bridge between signal and dialogue: A framework and a model. *International Journal of Audiology, 42,* S68–S76.

Rumbaugh, D. M., & Washburn, D. A. (1996). Attention and memory in relation to learning: A comparative adaptation perspective. In G. R. Lyon & N. A. Krasnegor (Eds.), *Attention, memory, and executive function* (pp. 199–220). Baltimore, MD: Paul H. Brookes.

Rumelhart, D. E. (1980). Schemata: The basic building blocks of cognition. In R. Spiro, B. Bruce, & W. Brewer (Eds.), *Theoretical issues in reading comprehension* (pp. 33–58). Hillsdale, NJ: Lawrence Erlbaum.

Rumelhart, D. E. (1984). Understanding understanding. In J. Flood (Ed.), *Understanding reading comprehension* (pp. 1–20). Newark, DE: International Reading Association.

Russo, N., Nicol, T., Zecker, S., Hayes, E., & Kraus, N. (2005). Auditory training improves neural timing in the human brainstem. *Behavioural Brain Research*, *156*, 95–103.

Sahley, T. L., Musiek, F. E., & Nodar, R. H. (1996). Naloxone blockage of (−) pentazocine-induced changes in auditory function. *Ear and Hearing, 17*, 341–353.

Sahley, T. L., & Nodar, R. H. (1994). Improvement in auditory function following pentazocine suggests a role for dynorphins in auditory sensitivity. *Ear and Hearing, 15*, 422–431.

Salvi, R. J., Lockwood, A. H., Frisina, R. D., Coad, M. L., Wack, D. S., & Frisina, D. R. (2002). PET imaging of the normal human auditory system: Responses to speech in quiet and in background noise. *Hearing Research, 170*, 96–106.

Samuels, S. J. (1987). Factors that influence listening and reading comprehension. In R. Horowitz & S. J. Samuels (Eds.), *Comprehending oral and written language* (pp. 295–325). San Diego, CA: Academic Press.

Sarampalis, A., Edwards, B., Kalluri, S., & Hafter, E. (2009). Objective measures of listening effort: Effects of background noise and noise reduction. *Journal of Speech, Language, and Hearing Research, 52*, 1230–1240.

Schacter, D. L., & Tulving, E. (1994). *Memory systems.* Cambridge, MA: MIT Press.

Schochat, E., Musiek, F. E., Alonso, R., & Ogata, J. (2010). Effect of auditory training on the middle latency response in children with (central) auditory processing disorder. *Brazilian Journal of Medical and Biological Research, 43*, 777–785.

Schon, D., Magne, C., & Besson, M. (2004). The music of speech: Music training facilitates pitch processing in both music and language. *Psychophysiology, 41*, 341–349.

Schunk, D. H. (1982). Effects of effort attributional feedback on children's perceived self-efficacy and achievement. *Journal of Educational Psychology, 74*, 548–556.

Sergeant, J. (1996). A theory of attention: An information processing perspective. In G. R. Lyon, & N. A. Krasnegor (Eds.), *Atten-tion, memory, and executive function* (pp. 57–70). Baltimore, MD: Paul Brookes.

Shallice, T., & Vallar, G. (1990). The impairment of auditory-verbal short-term storage. In G. Vallar & T. Shallice (Eds.), *Neuropsychological impairments of short-term memory* (pp. 11–53). New York, NY: Cambridge University Press.

Sharma, M., Purdy, S., & Kelly, A. (2009). Comorbidity of auditory processing, language, and reading disorders. *Journal of Speech, Language, and Hearing Research, 52*, 706–722.

Sharma, M., Purdy, S., Newall, P., Wheldall, K., Beaman, R., & Dillon, H. (2006). Electrophysiological and behavioral evidence of auditory processing deficits in children with reading disorder. *Clinical Neurophysiology, 117*, 1130–1144.

Singly, K., & Anderson, J. (1989). *The transfer of cognitive skill.* Cambridge, MA: Harvard University Press.

Sloan, C. (1986). *Treating auditory processing difficulties in children.* San Diego, CA: College-Hill Press.

Snider, V. E. (1989). Reading comprehension performance of adolescents with learning disabilities. *Learning Disability Quarterly, 12*, 87–96.

Snyder, R. L., Bonham, B. H., & Sinex, D. G. (2008). Acute changes in frequency responses of inferior colliculus central nucleus (ICC) neurons following progressively enlarged restricted spiral ganglion lesions. *Hearing Research, 246*, 59–78.

Solan, H. A., Shelley-Tremblay, J., Silverman, M., & Larson, S. (2003). Effect of attention therapy on reading comprehension. *Journal of Learning Disabilities, 36*(6), 556–563.

Song, J. H., Skoe, E., Wong, P. C., & Kraus, N. (2008). Plasticity in the adult human auditory brainstem following short-term linguistic training. *Journal of Cognitive Neuroscience, 20*, 1892–1902.

Sorqvist, P., Stenfelt, S., & Ronnberg, J. (2012). Working memory capacity and visual-verbal cognitive load modulate auditory-sensory gating in the brainstem: Toward a unified view of attention. *Journal Cognitive Neuroscience, 24,* 2147–2154.

Speece, D., McKinney, J., & Appelbaum, M. (1985). Classification and validation of behavioral subtypes of learning disabled children. *Journal of Educational Psychology, 77,* 67–77.

Stach, B., Loiselle, L., Jerger, J., Mintz, S., & Taylor, C. (1987). Clinical experience with personal FM assistive listening devices. *Hearing Journal, 10,* 24–30.

Stach, B., Spretnjak, M., & Jerger, J. (1990). The prevalence of central presbycusis in a clinical population. *Journal of the American Academy of Audiology, 1,* 109–115.

Stanovich, K. E. (1993). The construct validity of discrepancy definitions of reading disability. In G. R. Lyon, D. B. Gray, J. F. Kavanaugh, & N. A. Krasnegor (Eds.), *Better understanding learning disabilities* (pp. 273–307). Baltimore, MD: Paul H. Brookes.

Sticht, T. G., & James, J. H. (1984). Listening and reading. In P. D. Pearson (Ed.), *Handbook of reading research* (pp. 293–317). New York, NY: Longman.

Stokes, T. F., & Baer, D. M. (1977). An implicit technology of generalization. *Journal of Applied Behavior Analysis, 10,* 349–367.

Stone, C. A., & Wertsch, J. V. (1984). A social interactional analysis of learning disabilities remediation. *Journal of Learning Disabilities, 17,* 194–199.

Strait, D., & Kraus, N. (2011). Can you hear me now? Musical training shapes functional brain networks for selective auditory attention and hearing speech in noise. *Frontiers in Psychology, 2,* 113.

Strouse Carter, A., Noe, C., & Wilson, R. (2001). Listeners who prefer monaural to binaural hearing aids. *Journal of the American Academy of Audiology, 12,* 261–271.

Studdert-Kennedy, M. (1980). Speech perception. *Language and Speech, 23,* 45–66.

Suiter, M. L., & Potter, R. E. (1978). The effects of paradigmatic organization on recall. *Journal of Learning Disabilities, 11,* 247–250.

Swanson, H. L. (1987). Information processing theory and learning disabilities: A commentary and future perspective. *Journal of Learning Disabilities, 20,* 155–166.

Swanson, H. L. (1989). Strategy instruction: Overview of principles and procedures for effective use. *Learning Disability Quarterly, 12,* 3–15.

Swanson, H. L. (1993). Learning disabilities from the perspective of cognitive psychology. In G. R. Lyon, D. B. Gray, J. F. Kavanagh, & N. A. Krasnegor (Eds.), *Better understanding learning disabilities* (pp. 199–228). Baltimore, MD: Paul H. Brookes.

Swanson, H. L., & Cooney, J. B. (1991). Learning disabilities and memory. In B. Y. L. Wong (Ed.), *Learning about learning disabilities* (pp. 104–127). San Diego, CA: Academic Press.

Swanson, T. J., Hodson, B. W., & Schommer-Aikins, M. (2005). An examination of phonological awareness treatment outcomes for seventh-grade poor readers from a bilingual community. *Language, Speech, and Hearing Services in Schools, 36,* 336–345.

Sweetow, R. W. (1986). Cognitive aspects of tinnitus patient management. *Ear and Hearing, 7,* 390–396.

Sweetow, R. W., & Henderson-Sabes, J. H. (2004). The case for LACE, individualized listening and auditory communication enhancement training. *Hearing Journal, 57,* 32–40.

Syka, J. (2002). Plastic changes in the central auditory system after hearing loss, restoration of function, and during learning. *Physiological Reviews, 82,* 601–636.

Tallal, P., Miller, S., Bedi, G., Byma, G., Wang, X., Nagarajan, S. S., . . . Merzenich, M. M. (1996). Language comprehension in language-learning impaired children improved with acoustically modified speech. *Science, 271,* 81–84

Tamm, L., Nakonezny, P., & Hughes, C. (2012). An open trial of a metacognitive executive function training for young children with ADHD. *Journal of Attention Disorders* [Epub ahead of print].

Teale, W. H. (1984). Reading to young children: Its significance for literacy development. In H. Goelman, A. A. Oberg, & F. Smith (Eds.), *Awakening to literacy* (pp. 110–121). London, UK: Heinemann Educational Books.

Thiebaut de Shotten, M., Urbanski, M., Duffau, H., Volle, E., Ley, R., Dubois, B., & Bartolomeo, P. (2005). Direct evidence for a parietal-frontal pathway subserving spatial awareness in humans. *Science, 309,* 2226–2228.

Thomas, A., & Pashley, B. (1982). Effects of classroom training on LD students' task persistence and attributions. *Learning Disability Quarterly, 5,* 133–144.

Thorell, L., Lindqvist, S., Bergman, S., Bohlin, G., & Klingberg, T. (2009). Training and transfer effects of executive functions in preschool children. *Developmental Science, 12,* 106–113.

Tillery, K. L., Katz, J., & Keller, W. D. (2000). Effects of methylphenidate (Ritalin) on auditory performance in children with attention and auditory processing disorders. *Journal of Speech, Language, and Hearing Research, 43,* 893–901.

Torgesen, J. K. (1979). Factors related to poor performance on rote memory tasks in reading-disabled children. *Learning Disability Quarterly, 2,* 17–23.

Torgesen, J. K. (1980). Conceptual and educational implications of the use of efficient task strategies by learning disabled children. *Journal of Learning Disabilities, 13,* 364–371.

Torgesen, J. K., & Houck, G. (1980). Processing deficiencies in learning disabled children who perform poorly on the digit span task. *Journal of Educational Psychology, 72,* 141–160.

Treat, N. J., Poon, L. W., Fozard, J. L., & Popkin, S. J. (1977, August). *Toward applying cognitive skill training to memory problems.* Paper presented at the meeting of the American Psychological Association, San Francisco, CA.

Tremblay, K., & Kraus, N. (2002). Auditory training induces asymmetrical changes in cortical neural activity. *Journal of Speech, Language, and Hearing Research, 45,* 564–572.

Tremblay, K., Kraus, N., Carrell, T., & McGee, T. (1997). Central auditory system plasticity: Generalization to novel stimulation following listening training. *Journal of the Acoustical Society of America, 102,* 3762–3773.

Tremblay, K., Kraus, N., & McGee, T. (1998). The time course of auditory perceptual learning: Neurophysiological changes during speech-sound training. *NeuroReport, 9,* 3557–3560.

Tremblay, K., Kraus, N., McGee, T., Ponton, C., & Otis, B. (2001). Central auditory plasticity: Changes in the N1-P2 complex after speech-sound training. *Ear and Hearing, 22,* 79–90.

Tremblay, K., Piskosz, M., & Sousa, P. (2003). Effects of age and age-related hearing loss on the neural representation of speech cues. *Clinical Neurophysiology, 114,* 1332–1343.

Truesdale, S. (1990). Whole-body listening: Developing active auditory skills. *Language, Speech, and Hearing Services in Schools, 21,* 183–184.

Tun, P., Williams, V., Small, B., & Hafter, E. (2012). The effects of aging on auditory processing and cognition. *American Journal of Audiology, 21,* 344–350.

Uhrich, A., & Swalm, R. (2007). A pilot study of a possible effect from a motor task on reading performance. *Perceptual and Motor Skills, 104,* 1035–1041.

Ungerleider, L. G. (1995). Functional brain imaging studies of cortical mechanisms for memory. *Science, 270,* 769–775.

Van Dijk, T. A. (1985). Semantic discourse analysis. In T. A. Van Dijk (Ed.), *Handbook of discourse analysis. Dimensions of discourse* (Vol. 2, pp. 103–136). London, UK: Academic Press.

Van Kleeck, A. (1994). Metalinguistic development. In G. P. Wallach & K. G. Butler (Eds.), *Language learning disabilities in school-age children and adolescents* (pp. 53–98). New York, NY: Charles E. Merrill.

Wagner, R. K., & Torgesen, J. K. (1987). The nature of phonological processing and its causal role in the acquisition of reading skills. *Psychological Bulletin, 101,* 192–212.

Warren, R. M., & Warren, R. P. (1970). Auditory illusions and confusions. *Scientific American, 223,* 30–36.

Warrier, C. M., Johnson, K. L., Hayes, E. A., Nicol, T., & Kraus, N. (2004). Learning impaired children exhibit timing deficits and training-related improvements in auditory cortical responses to speech in noise. *Experimental Brain Research, 157,* 431–441.

Wartenberg, T. (2009). *Big ideas for little kids: teaching philosophy through children's literature.* Lanham, MD: Rowman & Littlefield.

Watson, C. S., & Foyle, D. C. (1985). Central factors in the discrimination and identification of complex sounds. *Journal of the Acoustical Society of America, 78,* 375–380.

Weaver, C. (1985). Parallels between new paradigms in science and in reading and literary theories: An essay review. *Research in the Teaching of English, 19,* 298–316.

Weaver, C. (1993). Understanding and educating students with attention deficit hyperactivity disorder: Toward a system theory and whole language perspective. *American Journal of Speech-Language Pathology, 2,* 78–89.

Weinberger, N. M., & Diamond, D. M. (1987). Physiological plasticity in auditory cortex: Rapid induction by learning. *Progress in Neurobiology, 29,* 1–55.

Wells, G. (1985). Preschool literacy-related activities and success in school. In D. R. Olson, N. Torrance, & A. Hildyard (Eds.), *Literacy, language, and learning* (pp. 229–255). Cambridge, UK: Cambridge University Press.

Whitman, T. L., Burgio, L., & Johnson, M. B. (1984). Cognitive behavioral interventions with mentally retarded children. In A. Meyers & W. E. Craighead (Eds.), *Cognitive behavior therapy with children* (pp. 193–227). New York, NY: Plenum Press.

Wible, B., Nicol, T., & Kraus, N. (2002). Abnormal neural encoding of repeated speech stimuli in noise in children with learning problems. *Clinical Neurophysiology, 113,* 485–494.

Wible, B., Nicol, T., & Kraus, N. (2005). Correlation between brainstem and cortical auditory processes in normal and language-impaired children. *Brain, 128,* 417–423.

Wiens, J. W. (1983). Metacognition and the adolescent passive learner. *Journal of Learning Disabilities, 16,* 144–149.

Wiig, E. H., Semel, E. M., & Crouse, M. A. B. (1973). The use of morphology by high risk and learning disabled children. *Journal of Learning Disabilities, 6,* 457–465.

Willeford, J. A. (1985). Assessment of central auditory disorders in children. In M. L. Pinheiro & F. E. Musiek (Eds.), *Assessment of central auditory dysfunction* (pp. 239–257). Baltimore, MD: Williams & Wilkins.

Willeford, J. A., & Burleigh, J. M. (1985). *Handbook of central auditory processing disorders in children.* Orlando, FL: Grune & Stratton.

Willott, J. F. (1999). *Neurogerontology: Aging and the nervous system.* New York, NY: Springer.

Willott, J. F., Aitken, L. M., & McFadden, S. L. (1993). Plasticity of auditory cortex associated with sensorineural hearing loss in adult mice. *Journal of Comparative Neurology, 329,* 402–411.

Wilson, C. C., Lanza, J. R., & Barton, J. S. (1988). Developing higher level thinking skills through questioning techniques in the speech and language setting. *Language, Speech, and Hearing Services in Schools, 19,* 428–431.

Wittrock, M. C. (1974). Learning as a generative process. *Educational Psychology, 11,* 87–95.

Wittrock, M. C. (1977). *The human brain.* Englewood Cliffs, NJ: Prentice-Hall.

Wong, B. Y. L. (1987). How do the effects of metacognitive research impact on the learning disabled individual? *Learning Disability Quarterly, 10,* 189–195.

Wong, B. Y. L. (1991). The relevance of meta-cognition to learning disabilities. In B. Y. L. Wong (Ed.), *Learning about learning disabilities* (pp. 232–261). San Diego, CA: Academic Press.

Wong, B. Y. L., & Jones, W. (1982). Increasing metacomprehension in learning-disabled and normally-achieving students through self-questioning training. *Learning Disability Quarterly, 5*, 228–240.

Wong, C., Jin, J., Gunasekera, G., Abel, R., Lee, E., & Dhar, S. (2009). Aging and cortical mechanisms of speech perception in noise. *Neuropsychologia, 47*, 693–703.

Wong, G. (1993). Comparing two modes of teaching a question-answering strategy for enhancing reading comprehension: Didactic and self-instruction. *Journal of Learning Disabilities, 26*, 270–279.

Wong, P., Ettlinger, M., Sheppard, J., Gunasekera, G., & Dhar, S. (2010). Neuroanatomical characteristics and speech perception in noise in older adults. *Ear and Hearing, 31*, 471–479.

Woods, D. L., & Clayworth, C. C. (1986). Age-related changes in human middle latency auditory evoked potentials. *Electroencephalography and Clinical Neurophysiology, 65*, 297–303.

Wren, C. T. (1983). *Language and learning disabilities: Diagnosis and remediation.* Rockville, MD: Aspen.

Wright, B. A., Lombardino, L. J., King, W. N., Puranik, C. S., Leonard, C. M., & Merzenich, M. M. (1997). Deficits in auditory temporal and spectral resolution in language-impaired children. *Nature, 387*, 176–178.

Wu, S. H., & Kelly, J. B. (1992). Synaptic pharmacology of the superior olivary complex studied in mouse brain slice. *Journal of Neuroscience, 12*, 3084–3097.

Zatorre, R. J. (2001). Neural specialization for tonal processing. *Annals of the New York Academy of Sciences, 930*, 193–210.

Zatorre, R. J., Belin, B., & Benhune, V. B. (2002). Structure and function of auditory cortex: Music and speech. *Trends in Cognitive Sciences, 6*, 37–46.

CHAPTER 11

COMPUTER-BASED AUDITORY TRAINING (CBAT) FOR CENTRAL AUDITORY PROCESSING DISORDER

LINDA M. THIBODEAU

Introduction

Auditory training techniques have been advocated for a variety of communication difficulties. Over the years, many techniques have been developed for use with persons with hearing loss (Carhart, 1960; Goldstein, 1939; Sweetow & Palmer, 2005; Wedenberg, 1951). Efforts have also been devoted to development of auditory-based computerized programs for children with language disorders (Merzenich et al., 1996; Tallal et al., 1996; Zwolan, McDonald Connor, & Kileny, 2000). Strong support for performance changes made possible through computer-based auditory training (CBAT) stems from investigations of neural plasticity in animals (Galvan & Weinberger, 2002; Kilgard & Merzenich, 1998b; Recan-

zone, Schreiner, & Merzenich, 1993). With the accumulating evidence documenting improved neurophysiologic representation of acoustic stimuli, as well as improved listening and related functions in children and adults following targeted auditory training, several CBAT programs have been developed for individuals with auditory, language, and learning disorders (e.g., Hayes, Warrier, Nicol, Zecker, & Kraus, 2003; Jirsa, 1992; Kraus, McGee, Carrell, King, Tremblay, & Nicol, 1995; Merzenich et al., 1996; Musiek, Baran, & Shinn, 2004; Russo, Nicol, Zecker, Hayes, & Kraus, 2005; Schopmeyer, Mellon, Dobaj, Grant, & Niparko, 1998; Tallal et al., 1996; Tremblay & Kraus, 2002; Tremblay, Kraus, Carrell, & McGee, 1997; Tremblay, Kraus, & McGee, 1998; Tremblay, Kraus, McGee, Ponton, & Otis, 2001; Warrier et al., 2004). Like other training protocols,

CBAT should be evaluated according to the principles of evidence-based practice (EBP), as explained in Chapter 2.

The primary purpose of this chapter is to provide a framework for the evaluation of CBAT so that researchers and practitioners may address the important variables that may impact outcomes and influence EBP studies. There have been few, randomized, controlled clinical trials with relatively large subject pools ($N > 50$) including comparison groups that have been conducted to determine the effectiveness of various types of computer-based training programs designed for children with language impairments and/or reading difficulty (Gillam et al., 2008; Rouse & Krueger, 2004). Loo, Bamiou, Campbell, and Luxon (2010) conducted a systematic review of CBAT research with two commercially available programs published between 2000 and 2008. They concluded that CBAT may improve auditory processing and phonological awareness, but had minimal effect on the language, spelling, and reading skills of children with deficits in those areas. Therefore, the information presented in this chapter should be viewed only as a guide for the evaluation of available programs, and not as an endorsement of any particular program.

Critical evaluation of CBAT requires consideration of the reason for training, the process of training, and how the participants react to the training. First, there must be some rationale for the type of training and what is being trained. For example, is the training designed to address increased attention or to refine temporal processing? Consistent with a specific rationale, several training factors such as type of stimuli, schedule of training, and method of delivery may gain importance relative to others. Once the training factors have been prioritized,

then the appropriate CBAT program may be selected. Even though all the optimal features may be in place, there may still be other factors as to how the training is conducted that will influence success, such as reinforcement and motivation.

The second purpose of this chapter is to provide a review of some of the currently available CBAT methods. Typically, a speech-language pathologist or audiologist selects the CBAT program and determines the treatment plan, including frequency of treatment and duration of sessions. In some cases, CBAT programs are selected by educational administrative personnel who are responsible for curriculum decisions. This review of currently available CBAT programs may be used as a guide to compare important features that may impact success. All currently available CBAT programs involve some degree of linguistic processing and, therefore, actually may be considered computer-based *auditory-language* training. However, the broader term CBAT is used to represent all the levels possible for training, which may include verbal and nonverbal stimuli.

The final purpose of the chapter is to review research that supports the effectiveness of CBAT and to provide suggestions for future studies. This is an exciting time for the application of CBAT as computers, smartphones, and tablets continue to become more readily available in schools, the home, and even in vehicles, which, in turn, allows greater access to effective training techniques.

Parameters of CBAT

Most are in agreement that auditory training can be an effective intervention for children with central auditory processing disorder (CAPD) (Chermak & Musiek, 2002). As the term implies, such training requires some form of auditory input that could be naturally or electronically produced. In order to propose a model to support the use of CBAT, there are three areas to consider: meaningfulness of the stimuli, active versus passive interaction, and frequency of training. Animal and human research underlying auditory training principles and CBAT discussed in this chapter are elaborated in Chapter 7.

Meaningfulness of the Stimuli

Stimuli for auditory training vary along two dimensions: natural versus synthetic, and speech versus nonspeech. The easiest stimuli to produce quickly, of course, are natural speech and these stimuli are likely the most meaningful to most individuals, particularly children. Synthetic speech, however, allows for more accurate control of parameters such as duration and intensity. Natural, nonspeech sounds (e.g., environmental sounds) are used less frequently, perhaps because of the lack of or reduced cognitive association evoked to maintain interest. The final category, synthetically produced, nonspeech signals such as tones or noise bursts, would be least interesting. However, these nonspeech signals can be easily manipulated for targeted training of basic perceptual features and auditory processes that correspond to speech and language processes. An example of training with such nonspeech stimuli would be the use of frequency sweeps that are analogous to second-formant transitions. Historically, the stimuli for auditory training have evolved from primarily natural speech to synthetically generated stimuli that have become increasingly acces-

sible with improvements in technology and easier access to the Internet. The application of these four types of auditory stimuli is reviewed with respect to their use in auditory training programs.

Natural Speech Stimuli

Human speech is the typical input for naturally produced auditory stimuli. Perhaps the earliest formal auditory training programs that involved natural speech were those designed to enhance communication skills of persons with hearing loss (Carhart, 1960; Wedenberg, 1951). These programs generally involved a hierarchy of skills moving from awareness, to discrimination, to identification, and finally to comprehension. Depending on the age of the child and residual hearing, the parent or teacher would provide activities involving vocabulary that was meaningful to the child at that time. For example, a child would be more inclined to focus on a same/different auditory discrimination task involving animal names following a trip to the zoo. Although natural speech stimuli have been widely used in auditory training, there are no studies documenting the benefits of a particular non-CBAT program with children with hearing loss. Walden and colleagues have demonstrated the benefits of auditory training, however, using natural speech with adults with hearing loss (Montgomery, Walden, Schwartz, & Prosek, 1984; Walden, Erdman, Montgomery, Schwartz, & Prosek, 1981). Another program that has shown promise is LACE, or Listening and Communication Enhancement (Sweetow, 2004).

Synthetic Speech Stimuli

Auditory training specifically designed for adults and children with CAPD often involves a dimension of speech processing requiring central integration, such as dichotic listening, phonemic synthesis, and/or temporal processing. Training in these areas requires more precise stimulus control, which is enabled through the use of synthetic speech or nonspeech signals. By controlling acoustic aspects of the stimuli, graduated difficulty may be introduced; however, this may be offered at the expense of using less interesting and less meaningful stimuli for the client.

Tallal and colleagues explored auditory training with synthetic speech based on the theory that children with language disorders are unable to process the rapid fluctuations of frequency information in speech and, therefore, miss important cues for perception (Merzenich et al., 1996; Tallal et al., 1996). They created CBAT programs in which children were presented synthetic speech with modified acoustic cues to aid recognition. For example, recognition training might begin using speech tokens with second-formant transitions with durations twice that found in normal speech. As the child responds correctly, the transitions can be shortened gradually to normal values.

Natural Nonspeech Stimuli

Environmental sounds are the most common natural, nonspeech stimuli that have been used in auditory training. In the early stages of training, programs for children with hearing loss often include discrimination and identification of common environmental sounds such as those produced by phones, car horns, dogs, alarm clocks, and so forth.

Although not specifically designed for remediation of communication disorders, the Suzuki method of learning music, which involves training with naturally produced, nonspeech stimuli, has implications for the rationale to use CBAT. This intensive auditory-based program designed for music instruction involves daily listening to recordings of songs played on the instrument that is being learned (Suzuki, 1981, 1983). Suzuki reasoned that just as children did not learn to read printed letters before they learned to speak, children can learn to play music prior to learning how to read printed musical notation. Similarly, he recognized that children learn to communicate by hearing the speech of their parents on a daily basis and proposed that it is logical, therefore, to expect that children could learn to play an instrument through repetitive listening to a hierarchy of songs with guided instruction. See discussion of music in auditory training in Chapters 4 and 7.

Synthetic Nonspeech Stimuli

The use of nonspeech stimuli allows for more precise training in discrete frequency, intensity, or temporal domains. These alterations of the stimulus characteristics are easily accomplished in CBAT. Because of the lack of inherent meaningfulness, such stimuli are typically accompanied by attractive pictures that relate to some aspect of the training. For example, Tallal and colleagues (1996) include synthetic, nonspeech stimuli in the Fast ForWord training in a game presented in a circus setting. It includes specific training exercises on frequency sweeps that are analogous to rapid formant transitions in speech. Although results of some studies have been interpreted as support for this type of training for children with language impairments (Rouse & Krueger, 2004; Temple et al., 2003; Troia & Whitney, 2003), evidence suggests that the improvements may not be the result of the characteristics of the nonspeech, synthetic stimuli but rather related to other features of the auditory training program (Gillam et al., 2008), as discussed below.

Nonspeech, synthetic stimuli also have been used to specifically retrain cortical processing of frequency-specific stimuli following reorganization resulting from hearing loss. Research with animals who have noise-induced hearing loss has shown that regions of the cortex that responded to specific frequency stimuli are reorganized to respond to other frequencies when there is no input at the former frequencies as a result of hearing loss (Eggermont & Komiya, 2000; Robertson & Irvine, 1989). In fact, frequency-specific response regions on the cortex actually expand over time such that areas that are no longer stimulated become responsive to sounds in frequency regions where there is no hearing loss (Irvine, 2000; Robertson & Irvine, 1989). It has been proposed that with intensive training with frequencies reintroduced in the hearing loss region, cortical reorganization can return toward the pre-hearing loss state (Willott, 1996). See discussions of plasticity in Chapters 1 and 7 of this volume and in Chapters 1, 3, and 5 of Volume 1 of the Handbook.)

Based on the findings with animals, Scott and Thibodeau examined the possibility that training with frequency-specific stimuli might result in speech recognition benefits for adults with hearing loss (Scott & Thibodeau, 2006). Adults with high-frequency hearing loss were provided amplification that restored high-frequency audibility. They then participated in two weeks (one hour daily) of discrimination training with frequency-sweep stimuli modeled after second-formant transitions. Although there was no change in consonant-vowel-consonant (CVC) identification following training, there was a significant improvement in sentence recognition in noise and self-report of benefit. It is possible that despite the audibility of the signal, the damaged cochlea continued to pass on to the central auditory nervous system a distorted signal, thereby limiting improvements possible in CVC identification. Another likely explanation for lack of improvement in CVC identification may be the result of tonotopic reorganization in the auditory cortex that left particular areas without neural connections (Recanzone, Schreiner, & Merzenich, 1993). It is important to note that this training involved nonspeech, nonmeaningful stimuli with very limited graphic feedback.

Focused (Active) Versus Unfocused (Passive) Experience

The rationale for CBAT must also include consideration of the role of attention in training. Much acoustic information is processed without attention seemingly focused on particular stimuli. For example, one may recall hearing a radio commercial when asked about it even though there was no specific task to record information or respond to that information. Throughout a typical day, there are numerous unfocused (i.e., passive) auditory events that are processed by the auditory system, but not necessarily acknowledged unless circumstances require specific recall of that information. Research with guinea pigs, rats, and monkeys has shown that for measurable cognitive reorganization to occur following training with tones, some form of focused or active attention through pairing electrical stimulation with acoustic stimuli or through conditioned discrimination training is required (Galvan & Weinberger, 2002; Kilgard & Merzenich, 1998a; Recanzone et al., 1993).

Perhaps the most common example of unfocused or passive auditory training in humans is the process of learning language by a normally developing infant. By 12 months of age, the infant shows discrimination patterns specific to the language to which they have been exposed auditorily (Kuhl & Meltzoff, 1996). Another common, unfocused, passive auditory training experience is that which occurs when listeners with hearing impairment receive hearing aids or cochlear implants. Adjustment to the new sound provided by the assistive technology occurs over time as the individual continually acquires more auditory experience. This is referred to as acclimatization and can occur over 6 weeks to 2 years (Cox & Alexander, 1992; Gatehouse, 1992, 1993; Horwitz & Turner, 1997; Tyler & Summerfield, 1996).

Unlike this passive (unfocused) auditory stimulation, auditory training with focused attention employs various techniques that require the listener to actively direct attention to specific information in the stimuli. For example, pairing a visual stimulus with an auditory stimulus that is made progressively more difficult in a discrimination task, or providing a reward for attending increases the likelihood of active, focused attention. Typically, focused auditory attention involves selection of specific stimuli for training (e.g., nonspeech gap detection or speech comprehension of stories). Stemming from findings with animals, research with humans has shown that as a result of brain plasticity, auditory processes, as well as the cognitive processes that support perception can be trained. Improvements in perception following focused auditory attention have been shown for adults with hearing aids (Walden et al., 1981), children with cochlear implants (Zwolan et al., 2000), and children with language impairments (Tallal et al., 1996). Unfortunately, although these studies show improvements, the specific acoustic ability that was trained is unknown, in part because of the lack of carefully defined control groups.

Although a program may be designed for focused attention training, if the tasks are not engaging because of excessive difficulty level or lack of redundancy, attention to the task may be lost. What may have been intended as a focused attention task may become an unfocused attention task. Unlike traditional therapy, where a clinician immediately recognizes the need to redirect a child's attention by changing tasks or reinforcement, a child may progress through CBAT with only the minimal attention needed to press the response key to advance the game, unbeknownst to the clinician or parent. In this situation, the child is probably not truly focusing auditory attention to the task. In experiments with animals, training with unfocused attention has been shown to be less effective (Kilgard & Merzenich, 1998b); therefore, allowing a child to progress through CBAT in the absence of true, focused auditory attention could result in an undesirable attention pattern that could affect performance on other training tasks, as was suggested by Friel-Patti et al. (2001) after reviewing performance of a child with language impairment.

Friel-Patti et al. (2001) described a subject who participated in the CBAT program Fast ForWord for 31 days, yet he did not meet the criterion of 90% completion on five of the seven exercises. In fact, his performance increased over the first ten days on all tasks except one, a nonspeech, frequency-sweep discrimination task. His performance on that task never rose above 5% completion over the 31 training days. Performance on three of the six remaining tasks either reached a plateau (30% and 70% performance level) or declined during the final 10 days of training. In the same way, two other children showed declines in performance near the end of training. It was concluded that the temporal processing system was bombarded with stimuli that could not be discriminated by the children and therefore they were operating at an unsuccessful level, which may have created interference. In other words, the tasks might have interfered with each other as the children responded "with limited and increasingly stressful resources" (Friel-Patti, DesBarres, & Thibodeau, 2001). See Chapter 7 for discussion of passive listening studies with animals in enriched as well as ambient, everyday acoustic environments.

Frequency of Training

Although electrophysical changes to training with acoustic stimuli may be seen with as little as one training session (Atienza, 2002; Gottselig, Brandeis, Hofer-Tinguely, Borbély, & Achermann, 2004), the typical treatment model for children with communication disorders is therapy two or three times per week (Gillam, 1999). This is somewhat constrained by the service delivery model in the public schools where caseloads are so large that students cannot be seen every day. Research by Tremblay and

colleagues have demonstrated, however, that intensiveness of training is crucial to successful outcomes. They reported that nine 20-minute training sessions over five days resulted in significantly improved discrimination of voice onset time cues in synthetic speech in adults with normal communication (Tremblay, Kraus, Carrell, & McGee, 1997). Interestingly, changes in the mismatched negativity potential (MMN) occurred after only four consecutive days of training in all ten subjects, whereas significant behavioral changes in speech discrimination occurred in 9 of the 10 listeners (with additional training) on day ten (Tremblay, Kraus, & McGee, 1998).

Also demonstrating the importance of frequency of training, Russo, Nicol, Zecker, Hayes, and Kraus (2005) found that children who had difficulties encoding the acoustic features of speech showed improvements following intensive training with Earobics relative to control subjects who received no training. Specifically, measures were made of neural timing in the brainstem in response to the presentation of the syllable "da." Children in the training group showed improved stimulus encoding precision relative to the controls. The authors concluded that the training resulted in improvements in neural synchrony concomitant with improvements in perceptual, academic, and cognitive measures. This research suggests that with frequent auditory training, the ability to code information into auditory patterns that may facilitate perception may be enhanced.

In summary, research suggests that the impact of auditory training for language processing can be enhanced through the use of meaningful stimuli. Moreover, employing tasks that direct one's attention to specific aspects of the stimulus and that are presented frequently over a concentrated time period are more likely to result in improved outcomes.

Processing Models of CBAT

A number of theories and models continue to evolve to account for the complex processes involved in auditory perception, speech perception, and spoken language processing. Among these models are those that focus on bottom-up versus top-down processing; interactive and parallel processes versus autonomous and serial processes; passive, nonmediated single factor theories versus active, mediated dual factor theories; and reliance on either feature detection, template matching, filtering, or other means of analyzing relevant dimensions of auditory stimuli (Borden, Harris, & Raphael, 2003; Jusczyk & Luce, 2002; Kent & Read, 2002). Commonly accepted is that auditory-language processing involves multiple sources of information and interactive and parallel networks broadly activated across the brain (ASHA, 1996; Chermak & Musiek, 1997; Musiek, Bellis, & Chermak, 2005).

While no specific model completely explains the benefits derived from auditory training, several comments are in order relative to the individual with CAPD, who, typically, experiences difficulty in the actual coding and organization of the auditory stimulus. Regardless of whether feature detection, template matching, or filtering is used to analyze relevant dimensions of stimuli, individuals with CAPD, and particularly children with CAPD, are likely to have less extensive experience and *data sets* (e.g., stores of acoustic templates with associated meaning) and are more likely to experience difficulty attending to acoustic events, which results in the coding of fewer acoustic features. All of this reduces the probability that acoustic matches will be made and meaning subsequently extracted from the signal. An individual with CAPD may compensate for these limitations in quiet but have considerable difficulty under challenging conditions of noise, reverberation, rapid speech, and so forth. Interfering noise compromises one's ability to store the acoustic trace accurately. It is as if the sharp edges on a complex geometric design become fuzzy. Anything that reduces the distinctiveness of the signal will reduce the accuracy with which the acoustic information is stored and consequently the probability that meaning can be derived. What is unique to CBAT is that the stimuli can be manipulated to strengthen the acoustic templates deciphered at the periphery as well as the neural networks required for cognitive processing. This occurs through the repetitive presentations of acoustic information in a focused-listening task that is experienced frequently (i.e., several times a week) by children who are motivated to attend due to the interesting and rewarding graphics of the CBAT.

Benefits of CBAT

Although the three principles described above (i.e., meaningfulness of the stimuli, focused training, and intensity of treatment) can be accomplished via traditional therapy, CBAT offers several advantages relative to these principles and thereby facilitates training. These advantages include stimulus control, hierarchy of activities, and the inherently interesting vehicle that computers offer to engage children in intensive training.

Precise Stimulus Control

Regardless of the training paradigm, it is crucial that the acoustic accuracy be maintained through the transducer (speaker or headphone), which should be monitored regularly. Through the use of synthetic speech and nonspeech stimuli, precise acoustic features can be manipulated and presented in a graduated sequence of difficulty. For example, if the child's *template* for the word "hotdog" did not include a brief silent interval between the stop consonants /t/ and /d/, then training to recognize small gaps would be productive so that when "hotdog" or other similar two-syllable words are presented, the templates may be refined to include this brief silence between syllables. Training may begin with noise bursts with easily perceptible gaps and through precise digital manipulation the gap duration could be altered in a sequential manner. This is known as an adaptively controlled paradigm where the difficulty level is based on the response to the previous stimulus. For example, if a gap is correctly detected, then the next trial would have a smaller duration gap. If the response to that trial is incorrect, the next gap would be longer in duration to facilitate perception. A typical adaptive gap detection paradigm involves stimulus manipulation so that the participant can correctly detect the gap with 70% accuracy. This type of graduated training could not be accomplished via natural speech, despite repeated presentations of the stimulus word. If the participant is not able to detect that silence, then no amount of repetition of that same interval would facilitate perception.

An example of manipulating the stimulus in the frequency domain that is possible in CBAT involves the perception of second-formant transitions. If the participant is unable to hear the difference between "bad" and "dad," it is likely that he or she is not discriminating differences between second formant transitions that cue the difference between the bilabial and alveolar placement. Repeatedly presenting stimuli that the participant cannot discriminate will not strengthen the accuracy of internal auditory representations. Training should begin with stimuli incorporating large changes in frequency that are greater than that which occur in real speech (Thibodeau, Britt, & Friel-Patti, 2001). Initially, the participant should be able to discriminate these large changes with about 70% accuracy. This 70% level allows for a balance between challenging and successful performance. Once accuracy rate improves beyond 70%, the change in frequency should be slightly reduced and training continued toward the 70% accuracy rate. As has been accomplished by Tallal and colleagues, the use of CBAT allows precise manipulation of the signal in an adaptive manner so that the acoustic differences are increased until 70% performance is reached. Subsequently, frequency differences are decreased gradually until participants are able to discriminate frequency differences characteristic of normal speech (Merzenich et al., 1996).

Access to Levels and Games

Another advantage of CBAT is the easy access to an appropriate training level that the digital format provides. Because the selection of the stimulus to be presented can be chosen based on the previous response (i.e., adaptive training), training becomes more efficient as the participant does not have to sit through either multiple trials where there is no success or where trials are too easy and the participant achieves 100% success. Furthermore, to maintain interest CBAT also easily allows the clinician to hold the training objective constant while changing the game scene. For example, rather than continue selecting a balloon that corresponds to a change in frequency, the scene may change after three minutes so that the child is listening for the monkey that made a different sound. Variety helps to maintain the child's attention and continue practicing to strengthen the auditory representation.

Youth's Interest In Computers

Children are surrounded by electronic images today more than ever. It may not be surprising that a third of children under 6 years of age (36%) have a television in their bedroom (Rideout, Vandewater, & Wartella, 2003). More than 25% of these children have a video recorder/player or digital video disc (DVD) player, while 10% have a video game player, and 7% have a computer in their bedroom. The latest trend is large screen televisions luring youth to the couch to view action-filled reality shows. The scenes may range from youth programs with a potpourri of 3-minute scenes to adult programs with scenes of adventure and survival. In addition, these images can be taken almost anywhere through portable DVD players or downloaded as apps on tablets or mobile phones. Children enjoy electronic entertainment while riding in the car, sitting at siblings' sporting events, or even while waiting for a haircut. Such frequent visual input potentially conditions children to expect entertaining electronic input regularly. In fact, much of their communication with friends occurs without auditory input, as they exchange information electronically through text messaging on mobile phones or instant messaging on computers.

With the increase in access to computers in the schools, home, doctors' offices, coffee shops, movie theaters, and so forth, children are increasingly comfortable with electronic communication and some may chose it as a form of recreation rather than physical activity. Children are also accessing their favorite music via the computer because there is convenient access to downloading songs for a nominal price. Computers are used then to exchange favorite music among friends through software that allows burning of compact discs. With the advent of networking software for local area networks (LAN) and associated interactive games, students are even planning weekend social events around their computers by having LAN parties. Teens gather with their laptops or personal computers and compete with one another through interactive, challenging games.

With the increased exposure, availability, and utility of computers, it is logical to consider their application for remediation of communication disorders. It is doubtful that this will be a passing trend, as computers continue to expand in capability while costs decline. The challenge will be to develop training software compatible with technology, with its fast-paced upgrades, that can be conveniently accessed. For example, complex interactive software may exceed the storage and memory capabilities of the typical home or clinic computer and therefore require Internet resources to function completely. Moreover, within a few years, CBAT software, hardware, or both can become obsolete and require totally different digital signal access, storage, and encoding.

Convenience of Training

Computers are available not only in educational settings, but in most homes. According to a U.S. survey (Rideout et al., 2003), 73% of homes with young children have a computer. More than a third (39%) of 4 to 6 year olds use a computer several times a week. With regard to computer games, one in four (25%) play several times a week or more (Rideout et al., 2003). Children are even accessing media while riding in cars. It is conceivable that some form of auditory training could even take place while on a daily commute or while traveling. Furthermore, hotels are often equipped with Internet access that might also facilitate intensive training regardless of a family's schedule.

Standardization of Training

The use of CBAT allows for consistency in training because the stimuli and activities are controlled by the computer. In some instances, this could be a disadvantage because the child's attention may wander with less human interaction. However, to facilitate comparison across clinics and training protocols, the consistent format

is attractive. Another argument to support the standardization of training is the benefits for training large groups. If a standardized set of activities can be helpful for a large number of children, then administration can be streamlined and cost effectiveness maximized. However, as discussed below under Treatment Outcomes, Efficacy, and Effectiveness, a review of the research shows that gains are made often by only some children on only a subset of the outcome measures. It will continue to be important, therefore, to assess the needs of an individual child throughout training to ensure that he or she is engaged in the process and continuing to make progress.

Design of CBAT

Training Areas

One of the first decisions that must be made, of course, is the purpose of the training. Table 11–1 provides a list of auditory skills or processes that have been suggested for training children with CAPD. There is no single CBAT program that addresses all of these areas; therefore, a combination of programs may be necessary to comprehensively address the processing deficits. Although a global auditory training program may be attractive, most software developers have based the training tasks on the perceived needs of a particular population, such as children with hearing impairment (Oticon's Otto's World of Sounds), language impairments (Fast ForWord), and attention deficit hyperactivity disorder (Brain Train). There has been much crossover, however, in the application of available training programs. This may result in

Table 11-1. Areas of Training for Children with CAPD

Training Area	Possible Stimuli	Software
Awareness	Nonspeech or Speech	Otto's World Earobics Brain Train
Memory	Nonspeech or Speech	Brain Train Earobics Fast ForWord® Learning Fundamentals
Temporal processing, including sequencing, temporal resolution (gap detection)	Nonspeech or Speech	Fast ForWord® Earobics Sound Auditory Training™
Localization	Nonspeech or Speech	LiSN and Learn
Auditory Discrimination	Nonspeech or Speech	Fast ForWord® Otto's World Sound Auditory Training™
Auditory Pattern Perception	Nonspeech or Speech	Brain Train Earobics Fast ForWord® Learning Fundamentals Sound Auditory Training™
Phonological Awareness	Speech	Conversation Made Easy Earobics Fast ForWord® Learning Fundamentals
Auditory Synthesis	Speech	Learning Fundamentals Earobics
Dichotic Processing (Binaural Integration)	Nonspeech or Speech	Sound Auditory Training™ Constraint-Induced Auditory Therapy (CIAT)
Identification in Quiet	Nonspeech or Speech	Brain Train Earobics Fast ForWord® Sound and Way Beyond Sound Auditory Training™

Table 11–1. *continued*

Training Area	Possible Stimuli	Software
Degraded Speech Recognition (Filtered Speech, Compressed Speech, Speech-In-Competition/Noise, Auditory Closure)	Speech	Conversation Made Easy Earobics Learning Fundamentals Sound Auditory Training™
Binaural interaction	Nonspeech or Speech	Sound Auditory Training™
Binaural separation	Nonspeech or Speech	Sound Auditory Training™
Comprehension	Speech	Brain Train Conversation Made Easy Earobics Fast ForWord® Learning Fundamentals
Auditory Vigilance	Nonspeech or Speech	Brain Train Learning Fundamentals

significant problems if the training tasks designed for one group are too difficult for another, which may be counterproductive and lead to frustration. Moreover, overgeneralized use of software with populations not originally intended to be trained with that software can lead to inefficient and ineffective treatment. For example, children with hearing impairment may not have the frequency resolution capabilities to successfully complete the easiest level of the frequency-sweep discrimination task of the program Fast ForWord, which was designed for children with language impairments who have normal hearing sensitivity. It is crucial, therefore, to know the intended audience, and if synthetic stimuli are used, to review the acoustic characteristics of the stimuli at the easiest and most difficult levels. Tasks that are either too difficult or too easy can lead to lack of attention and consequently less training benefit (Prensky, 2001). Similarly, cognitive, visual, and verbal skills required for use of particular CBAT must be considered.

Type of Training Stimuli

The next consideration in designing CBAT might be the choice of stimuli. The four possibilities, including speech versus nonspeech and natural versus synthetic, were described above under Meaningfulness of Stimuli. All of the areas listed in Table 11–1 could be trained using speech stimuli, either natural or synthetic. Depending on the hierarchy of training, discussed in the next section, synthetic stimuli may be necessary to precisely control the difficulty of the task. Interestingly, most of the skill areas listed in Table 11–1 could also be trained with nonspeech stimuli, either natural or synthetic. Although many programs use primarily natural speech, there is no research with children to support the benefits of training with natural speech versus synthetic nonspeech. One study with adults has shown that training with nonspeech stimuli may be generalized to increase discrimination of speech stimuli (Lakshminarayanan & Tallal, 2007).

Table 11–1 lists sample software for school-aged children using each of the stimulus types for each training area.

The choices are more limited, of course, to train comprehension with nonspeech, natural stimuli. For such a task, natural environmental sounds (e.g., fire truck, violin music, alarm clock) could be presented. Recognition could be trained by requiring the client to choose a picture that corresponds to the source. To train comprehension of these sounds, the client would be asked to associate the sound with the meaning the sound conveys by choosing a picture that corresponds to an associated event (e.g., people running from a house with flames, people walking into a concert hall, someone lying in bed with stretched out arms, respectively). Research by Gillam and colleagues (2008) suggests that children with language impairments experience equal gains in expressive and receptive language regardless of whether natural speech, synthesized speech, or nonspeech tokens are used as training stimuli. Given Gillam's findings, the clinician might prefer to use nonspeech stimuli in CBAT to more precisely target the underlying auditory skills without introducing potential confounding variables of speech and language.

Regardless of the type of stimulus used, the clinician must assess the fidelity of the signal presented to the participant. The fidelity of the acoustic representation of stimuli, whether they are brief stimuli or intentionally distorted (e.g., filtered, time compressed, presented in noise) stimuli, is essential to train efficiently and effectively toward the treatment goals. Poor fidelity can result from poor transducers (i.e., earphones and speakers) or poor signal processing itself.

Training Hierarchy

By definition, training implies a hierarchy of tasks. The challenge in CBAT is to determine the optimal starting and difficulty levels within a program. Naturally, the age of the listener is a determining factor, but even within an age group, there can be a wide range of abilities. Diagnostic test findings should provide some guidance in this determination. Ideally, the CBAT would include a "pre-training" assessment to determine the optimal starting levels so that the participant can begin training with relatively high success and gradually move toward more challenging activities. Without this feature, it becomes the responsibility of the audiologist or speech-language pathologist administering the CBAT to determine if the starting level chosen is appropriate to provide initial success required to maintain interest and motivation. As mentioned in the section on Frequency of Training, there is some evidence to suggest that if children are asked to perform tasks that are too difficult, overall attention may decline and result in reduced outcomes.

Irrespective of any particular software, an overall training hierarchy is proposed stemming from Garstecki's work with adults with hearing loss (Garstecki, 1982). In his scheme of auditory-visual training, he proposed starting at the easiest level to be successful and moving through the hierarchy of increasingly more difficult tasks until a plateau in performance is reached (i.e., when no further increases in performance are made despite continued training). Garstecki's hierarchy included four variables: (1) message type—related sentences to unrelated sentences; (2) competing noise type—quiet, single noise, babble, multispeaker; (3) competing noise level—positive to negative ratio; and (4) use of situational cues—relevant background cues, no visual background cues. Table 11–2 illustrates the hierarchy matrix as applied to variables in auditory processing. One might start training with no noise, natural speech, and many picture cues relating to the stimuli. The most difficult task would be training with synthetic, nonspeech stimuli, with multitalker babble at −10 signal-to-noise ratio (SNR) with no picture cues. Generally, one progresses through the matrix one cell at a time, rather than increasing difficulty on several dimensions concurrently.

Adaptive Difficulty Levels

Another significant decision that must be made in designing CBAT is whether the activities will be presented at fixed difficulty level or whether the software will adapt based on the participant's response. As mentioned above, programs that operate at a fixed level might be too easy. This is not as detrimental, however, as starting an activity that might have 20 presentations that are too difficult, thereby discouraging the participant and jeopardizing motivation and persistence on task. Nonetheless, the benefit of having an adaptive program is that the task can continually adjust to more difficult levels as the participant answers correctly. Typically, if the participant answers incorrectly, the next presentation is at an easier level; if the child answers correctly, the next presentation could be at a more difficult level. That is known as *one-up, one-down* or *simple up/down* and allows the participant to perform at an accuracy rate of about

Table 11–2. Hierarchy of Training

	Very Easy	Easy	Difficult	Very Difficult
Stimuli	Natural Speech	Synthetic Speech	Natural Nonspeech	Nonspeech Synthetic
Competing Noise	No Noise	Single Noise	Two Talker Babble	Multi Talker Babble
Noise Level	N/A	+10 SNR	0 SNR	−10 SNR
Situation Cues	Pictures present	Pictures precede task	Single word cue	No Cue

50%. This may actually be frustrating for some children and it might be better to train with a *two-down, one-up* adaptive procedure that results in performance with 70% accuracy (Levitt, 1978). With this tracking rule, a child must respond correctly to two consecutive trials before the difficulty level of the next trial is increased. After every incorrect response, the difficulty level is lowered so the next trial will likely be completed successfully. This *two-down, one-up* procedure allows greater accuracy (70% vs. 50%) and may be considered more enjoyable by some children. Chermak and Musiek (2002) advocate a 30% to 70% training range to achieve a balanced success-failure rate, maintain motivation, and work on the threshold of challenge. See Chapter 2 in Volume 1 of the Handbook for discussion of adaptive methods.

Reinforcement

To increase accuracy of performance, feedback must be provided regarding performance accuracy. In the absence of feedback, the participant is less likely to focus on a particular aspect of the signal that would foster continued accurate performance. Indeed, feedback can be reinforcing and reinforcement has been used successfully to increase learning in children with learning disabilities and mental retardation (Dawson, Hallahan, Reeve, & Ball, 1980; De Csipkes, Smouse, & Hudson, 1975). The reinforcement provided in CBAT typically includes some type of animation that occurs following a certain number of correct responses. The more interesting and novel the animation, the more likely the child will maintain motivation to perform successfully. As the task difficulty increases, reinforce-

ment becomes even more important to maintain attention.

A distinction should be made between reinforcement and feedback. When participants receive some information regarding their performance, they are receiving feedback. Such information is critical to any learning experience. Depending on the form of the information, the feedback also may be considered positive reinforcement, which will likely increase the desired behavior. In CBAT, the goal is to provide positive reinforcement that will encourage the child to persist on task despite increasing difficulty.

Feedback in the form of positive reinforcement may be one of the major factors that maintains participants' engagement in a computer game, an engaged state that facilitates learning. Digital, game-based learning engages the participant through a hierarchy of experiences that cause enjoyment (Prensky, 2001). Prensky proposed that there are a series of relationships that occur through game-based learning that result in motivation to continue. He stated that because games are a form of *fun,* they give the participant enjoyment and pleasure. Games are also a form of *play* that may result in intense and passionate involvement. With rules that provide structure, games have goals that motivate the participant to continue. As the activities move toward the goals, there are outcomes and feedback that cause motivation and learning. When games are adaptive, the participant is allowed to perform at the optimum level and achieve a sense of *winning,* which adds to ego gratification. Games that present competition or challenge may spark creativity and problem solving. Finally, games convey events in a story-like format that can evoke positive emotions (e.g., enjoyment) that perpetuates the cycle of relationships. For participants with CAPD who are offered this series of experiences through CBAT, one would expect their interest to persist and learning to increase relative to non-computer-based strategies where the relationships between reinforcement, goals, and *winning* are less apparent. See Chapter 10 for further discussion of the role of feedback and reinforcement for effective intervention.

Operating Format

When designing software, it is necessary to consider how the program will run on the computer. The choices are to run from a CD, from an installed version stored on the computer's hard drive, from a web-based application, or from some combination of these two approaches. The Web-based applications require an internet connection and often store the response data through the internet rather than locally on the computer. Most programs are designed to be installed and run independently of the CD. When the CD is required during training, less data are stored on the hard drive, but loading the software is required each time it is used, which may be time consuming. This would also be inconvenient if the software were to be used in multiple locations.

Factors That May Influence Success

Treatment Schedule

The scheduling of training includes the time of day training is offered, the length of each training session, and the dura-

tion and frequency of training. As with any intervention program, it is optimal to offer training at a time of day when the participant is most alert. As mentioned previously, the frequency and duration of training are important factors. It is optimal to conduct the CBAT at approximately the same time each day as this helps to facilitate relatively equivalent attention across days and reduce variability in performance (Gillam, 1999). Depending on the time of day and the duration of training that is offered, it may be necessary to have snacks available to help maintain attention.

Several programs recommend a 30- to 90-minute training session three to five times per week, a training regimen in sharp contrast to the typical quantity and frequency with which children receive speech-language and hearing services in schools (Gillam, 1999). This type of schedule may be unrealistic for most families and educational settings due to time conflicts and limited attention span. In contrast, some studies show improvements with as little as 15 minutes of training two times per week (Segers & Verhoeven, 2003). Gillam (1999) reported significantly greater gains achieved by children with specific language impairments when the therapy was provided daily for 90 minutes compared with the gains achieved by children who were served in traditional models. Most CBAT is recommended for a period of at least 4 to 6 weeks (e.g., Earobics and Fast ForWord). When the training is frequent, the child becomes more accustomed to a routine of attending for a certain time period. The experience of attending becomes more familiar and requires less effort with training. It has been shown that frequent auditory training results in increased attention span and ability to complete a complex task (e.g., perseverance) (Scott, 1992).

Auditory Environment

Given the nature of auditory training, it is critical that the child be able to concentrate on the training signals and not be distracted by ambient signals. The use of headphones is often recommended to reduce ambient sounds, particularly when there is more than one training station in a room. In the group situation, there also should be a system for asking a question by raising an indicator to alert the clinician, parent or other monitor to come to that station. Although some may argue that presence of ambient noise during auditory training may improve users' ability to discriminate between important and unimportant sounds, this variable should be systematically varied from quiet to increasing noise levels, an option included in some training programs.

An FM system is another tool to help participants focus attention on the CBAT signal. The FM system may be useful in CBAT to enhance the signal from the computer relative to the surrounding classroom noise. By connecting the signal from the sound output jack of the computer to the audio input on the FM transmitter, the child may hear the auditory signal more readily, yet still be able hear some sounds in the classroom, unlike with headphones that would block most of the environmental sounds. As mentioned above in the section on hierarchy of training, moving from an ideal SNR to less favorable conditions during training will facilitate carryover into the real world where optimal acoustic conditions are rare. See Chapter 12 for discussion of FM technology and signal enhancement. Users who do not have an FM system may benefit from use of headphones to increase the SNR by blocking some of the ambient sound. The computer's volume control settings should be set to a level that provides intelligible stimuli and is comfortable for the user.

Motivation

Motivation may be internal or external. Internal motivation is based on a desire from within oneself to accomplish a task because it is interesting, arouses pleasure, or enhances self-esteem. For example, when a child receives an animated scene to indicate completion of a training level, the child feels a sense of accomplishment that may lead to feelings of greater self-worth. A sense of pleasure may also result from knowing that accomplishing a level means the end of training is near. Hence, motivation may be facilitated by advising the participants at the beginning of training about the number of training levels or games to be accomplished during that session.

Although CBAT typically is designed with interesting graphics and visual reinforcement, maintaining a child's attention during lengthy training periods may require external motivators. Reinforcers may be needed not only for the individual session but also to motivate the child to return week after week. These external motivators may be as simple as some recognition for completion of the training sequence each day to more elaborate rewards after completing each five-minute segment. Tangible, nonsticky, reinforcers may be given at frequent intervals to maintain motivation, particularly when tasks are more difficult. Many programs use progress bars or interesting animations such as a monkey climbing a tree to demonstrate the user's success in training. Small prizes also may be offered for reaching criterion performance each day of the week. Having children share their progress with an interested adult (besides the clinician) on a daily basis also may contribute to their motivation to perform well. Whatever the schedule of reinforcement, reinforcers will be more effective when the participant understands in advance the critical steps needed to obtain them. See Chapters 7 and 10 for further discussion of the role of motivation for effective intervention.

Factors to Consider in Selecting CBAT

Differentiating Software for Training

As a teacher, parent, or clinician considers offering CBAT, there are many factors to examine prior to selecting software. First, the purpose of the training should be determined. If there are specific language concepts to be trained, software that includes activities that focus on these language concepts should be considered. If phonemic processing skills are of concern, for example, software that includes discrimination training of phonemic differences is desirable. Memory and attention skills are indirectly exercised in all CBAT programs. Some programs increase focus on attention and memory by requiring an additional task to be performed before responding, or by adding noise to the task to compete for attention.

Table 11–1 provides some guidance as to the specific areas of central auditory processing particular software is designed to train.

Option to Train With a Home Computer

To increase the frequency of training, it may be desirable to have the option for CBAT in the home. The price of computers has dropped such that many families have systems that meet the minimum requirements of the most sophisticated programs. The challenge for training at home is to control distractions and provide time for focused training without interruptions. When training is conducted in a clinic or school, the child is usually there for the sole purpose for training. When CBAT is conducted in the home, a regular time should be set aside to minimize interruptions caused by carpools, television, or visits from friends. For the older child, it will be paramount to restrict Instant Messaging or chat room access during training because so many teens are accustomed to multitasking by typing messages to several people while ostensibly doing homework on the computer. Such attempts at multitasking would likely detract from the older child's attention to the CBAT and therefore diminish benefit derived.

Because home computers are often shared by multiple users for multiple reasons, the designated training time must be communicated to all members who can plan their computer use accordingly. Furthermore, during home training, there must be a system for accountability to the monitoring professional. If a certain program is recommended for training so many minutes each day, a record keeping log should be provided that can be monitored weekly.

System Requirements

Most software comes with a description of the computer hardware requirements for effective operation. These should always be consulted prior to installation to avoid lengthy and/or unnecessary troubleshooting. An overview of computer requirements for Fast ForWord serves as an example (Table 11–3).

Manufacturers will list the minimal requirements because, typically, the

software is *backward* compatible for a few years. If a program was written to function with the most recent, common operating system, it will typically also work with the previous one or two versions. However, newer operating systems that are developed after the generation of CBAT software may not be compatible. After checking the operating system requirements, one must consider processor and memory requirements. Typically, if the operating system requirements are met, processing and memory requirements for video and sound cards also are acceptable. Programs may require quite different amounts of hard drive space, however, depending on the graphics

Table 11–3. Hardware Requirements For Operating Fast ForWord® Training Programs (http://www.scilearn.com)

Operating System
- Windows® XP Home or Professional Service Pack 2
- Windows® Vista Service Pack 1 Home, Business, Ultimate or Enterprise
- Windows® 7

Memory
- 512 MB of RAM for Windows XP Service Pack 2
- 2 GB of RAM for Vista Service Pack 1 or Windows 7

Sound Card
- Creative Labs SoundBlaster or 100% compatible with DirectSound support

Hard Drive Space
- Scientific Learning Gateway: 500 MB for application, 100 MB per student Multimedia installation: 6 GB

Optical Drive
- DVD ROM Required for installation

Video Card/Monitor
- Minimum supported resolution of 1024 × 768 resolution, 16-bit color

Internet Connection
- Required for Gateway license registration and Progress Tracker

involved. The hard drive storage requirements for Fast ForWord programs range from 140 megabytes for a single program to approximately 3 gigabytes for the entire set of programs (see Table 11–3). One should also consider whether the program requires a CD inserted in the drive to operate program or if all the games are stored on the hard drive. CBAT developers often require CD dependent operation to minimize licensing abuse and to reduce memory requirements during operation.

Some programs require an additional hard disk space for each participant or provide the option to assign an external memory option for storage of individual performance. This may be a significant negative factor if the program is to be used with a large group of students because the initial assignment of data storage media and the daily access to individual disks may be quite time consuming. Some CBAT programs require an Internet connection so that participant performance may be compiled into training reports that store data and show progress across sessions. Requiring Internet access may be a limiting factor in selecting a CBAT program, particularly when the primary concern is individual training rather than planning for a large group of users (e.g., students).

Considerations for CBAT in Schools

The use of CBAT in the schools has been addressed in previous sections regarding interfacing with FM systems, avoiding distracting ambient noise, and group training arrangements. There are three other important considerations, however, that involve the actual installation of the

software, licensing, and interfacing with the current service delivery options.

An important consideration for CBAT in schools is knowing how many students will use the software. Multiple site licenses will be more cost-effective for large group applications. Prior to adding software to school-based computers that may be part of a network, technical support for the network should be consulted regarding installation requirements. In many cases, there are designated personnel to manage software installations to be sure that compatibility requirements are met. As mentioned above, CD-dependent software may be more difficult to manage as young children or busy teachers have to organize data disks or software CDs for training sessions.

Schools must also consider how CBAT will be implemented in relation to the regular curriculum and special services. Will the use of the CBAT be a supplement to the traditional therapy? If FM systems are provided, will the training be offered at a time when the transmitter can be interfaced with the computer for a given student? Finally, as discussed above, can CBAT be made available in schools consistent with an intensive therapy schedule as required for maximum effectiveness?

CBAT Software Comparison

In general, CBAT programs have all been designed to strengthen some aspect of auditory processing or auditory-language processing, whether it is discrimination of nonspeech sounds or comprehension of directions through interesting graphics paired with auditory stimuli. The programs differ in the levels of instruction, the specific training areas, response reinforcement, and how they operate relative to the computer hardware. They range in price from $99 for a single CD for one type of program to over $3000 for a site license for a set of training programs. The more expensive programs typically have more complex adaptive training reflecting more sophisticated algorithms (e.g., Fast ForWord). Such complexity often requires considerable consumer support for troubleshooting and interpretation, which is a factor that adds to the program costs.

CBAT programs also vary in their hardware requirements. Table 11–4 provides basic information for 10 auditory-language training software programs that are currently available. The random access memory (RAM) requirements for the programs listed in Table 11–4 are typically 32 MB, but they range from requiring 8 MB for Foundations of Speech Perception to 256 MB for Sound and Way Beyond. The required hard drive storage space ranges from 10 MB for Earobics to 500 MB for Sound and Way Beyond. CD drive speed could be as low as 2× to run Earobics or as high as 8× to run Otto's World of Sound. One consideration mentioned previously is whether or not the program will operate independently of a CD. This provides greater flexibility for the user to not be dependent on having the CD in place during training. The final column in Table 11–4 indicates whether the program is CD dependent, meaning that a program CD must be in the computer's CD drive to run the program.

As noted in Table 11–4, software has been developed for a variety of audiences. The primary groups that have been targeted for training include those with language impairments and those with hearing loss. Much software also has been developed to treat children with reading difficulties. Many programs include some activities directed at phonemic awareness including discrimination of speech sounds and sound symbol association (see Table 11–1). A new Web-based set of auditory training exercises (Sound Auditory Training, described below) focuses training on fundamental auditory processes using predominantly nonverbal stimuli. As suggested by Gillam et al. (2008), the critical factors contributing to success through auditory training may not be the specific program content, but rather the intensiveness of training.

With the possibility for significant overlap in applications of these programs, the selection of an appropriate program may be difficult. For example, there are several programs designed to enhance language skills. It could be very time consuming to review all these programs to select one for a particular child; therefore, it is suggested that age be the first criterion for program selection. Within that age category, one may determine from a more limited set of programs which ones have appropriate levels for training. For example, for a 10-year old child with auditory processing difficulties with no associated language delays, CBAT software that includes activities focused on memory, attention, and speech recognition in degraded acoustic conditions, such as Captain's Log of Brain Train, may be more useful than software focusing on language concepts, such as MicroLads of Laureate programs. Although a complete analysis of all the components of each of these programs is beyond the scope of this chapter, a brief synopsis of the software listed in Table 11–4 is provided to guide one to appropriate exploration in greater detail.

Table 11–4. Basic Information for 13 Auditory-Language Training Software Programs

Software	Author	Publisher	Date	Web Address	Age	Intended Audience	CD
Brain Train®	Joseph A. Sanford, Ann Turner	Brain Train, Inc.	1989	http://www.braintrain.com/soundsmart/soundsmart_home.htm	Preschool to Adult	Cognitive Impaired	Yes
Conversation Made Easy	Nancy Tye-Murray	Central Institute for the Deaf	2002	http://www.cid.wustl.edu/deafhome/PUBLICATIONS/books.htm	Upper Elementary to Adult	Hearing Impaired	Yes
Earobics®	Jan Wasowicz	Cognitive Concepts	1996	http://www.earobics.com/	Preschool to Adult	Language Impaired, Dyslexic, Auditory Processing	Yes
Fast ForWord®	Paula Tallal, Michael Merzenich	Scientific Learning	1997	http://www.scilearn.com/	Preschool to Adult	Language Impaired, Dyslexic, Pervasive Developmental Disorder	No
Foundations in Speech Perception	Cochlear Corp.	Cochlear Corp.	2000	No Longer Marketed	Elementary	Hearing Impaired	Yes
Laureate Learning Systems®	Mary Sweig Wilson, Bernard J. Fox, Marion Blank, Eleanor Semel, Barbara Couse Adams	Laureate Learning Systems	1982	http://www.llsys.com/professionals602/products/descriptions/mldesc.html	Elementary to Adults	Language Impaired, Developmental disabilities, Physical impairments, Visual impairments, Hearing impairments, Autism, ESL students	Yes

continues

333

Table 11-4. *continued*

Software	Author	Publisher	Date	Web Address	Age	Intended Audience	CD
Learning Fundamentals®	Marna Scarry-Larkin	LocuTour Multimedia	1994	http://www.locutour.com/products/product.php?id=40	Preschool to Teens	Language Impaired, Dyslexic, Attention Problems	No
Listening and Communication Enhancement (LACE)	Robert Sweetow	NeuroTone, Inc.	2004	http://www.neurotone.com/index.html	Adult	Hearing Impaired	No
Otto's World of Sounds	Oticon Corporation	Oticon Corporation	2005	http://www.oticon.com/children/parents-and-relatives/resources/ottos-world-of-sounds.aspx	Elementary	Hearing Impaired	Yes
Sound And Way Beyond	Cochlear Corp.	Cochlear Corp.	2005	http://hope.cochlearamericas.com/sound-way-beyond	Adult	Hearing Impaired	No
LiSN and Learn	Sharon Cameron, Harvey Dillon	National Acoustic Laboratories	2011	http://capd.nal.gov.au/lisn-learn-about.shtml	Elementary	Spatial Processing Disorder	Yes
Constraint-Induced Auditory Therapy (CIAT)	Annette Hurley, Ph.D, D. Bradley Davis, AuD	AUDiTEC	2011	http://www.auditec.com/cgi/Auditec201205PrepressedCompactDiscs.pdf	Children and Adults	Dyslexia, Aphasia, Hearing Impaired	Yes
Brain Fitness	Posit Science Corporation	Posit Science Corporation	2011	http://www.positscience.com/brain-training-products/brain-fitness-program	Adult	Hearing Impaired	Yes

Brain Train

Brain Train is a series of programs using natural speech designed to improve attention, memory, self-control, problem-solving, and listening skills designed for those with brain injury, learning disabilities, attention deficit hyperactivity disorder (ADHD), or other cognitive impairments. Unlike other CBAT, Brain Train includes activities to develop mental math skills and help reduce impulsivity. The software uses natural speech to encourage, praise, and challenge users to perform.

Conversation Made Easy

This series of programs is designed for persons with hearing loss to learn skills to improve conversation skills and therefore increase self-confidence. There are three instruction modules: (1) speech-reading enhancement, (2) repair strategies, and (3) facilitative strategies to optimize the environment. Separate programs are available for adults and teenagers, children with low-level language skill, and children with advanced language skills. For each age, there are three CD -based programs covering sounds, sentences and everyday situations. The actual movies and photos of real-world scenes help to maintain attention. Because of these graphic requirements, however, some computers require changes to the display settings to allow the scenes to be seen.

Earobics

Earobics is a comprehensive, phonological awareness and auditory-language processing training software designed for those with difficulties in reading and language processing. Programs are grouped for application in the school, clinic, or home. The school version consists of a package of games designed to strengthen language development, phonemic awareness, alphabetic knowledge, decoding and spelling, beginning reading, and beginning writing. The clinic version has three levels (i.e., steps) for pre-kindergarten, school-age, and adolescents/adults. The activities focus on the following: Step 1: sound awareness, discrimination of sound in noise and quiet, sequencing sound and associating sound with letters; Step 2: complex directions with and without background noise, memory for sounds and words; Step 3: activities to strengthen reading, spelling and comprehension. The first level targets the fundamentals of auditory processing while the next levels build upon these skills. The home version is similar to the three steps, but designed to be used by only two participants and a guest. Earobics is known for its reasonable cost and access for home use. The graphics are entertaining and activities maintain interest for the respective age level.

Fast ForWord

Fast ForWord training is based on the premise that language and reading difficulties stem from poor temporal processing (Merzenich et al., 1996). Activities are designed to increase temporal resolution and stimuli may be nonspeech tones or acoustically modified speech with lengthened features (i.e., formant transitions) compared with natural speech. Based on the user's success, the stimuli progress from longer to shorter, toward the acoustics of formant transitions found in natural speech. Fast ForWord has many levels for all age levels. In general, programs are designed for young children to develop basic skills necessary for language and reading development; for school-age children to strengthen fundamental cognitive skills of memory, attention, processing and sequencing with a focus on phonological awareness and language structures; and for older students to focus on processing skills similar to the previous level and strengthen reading through sound-letter comprehension, phonological awareness, beginning word recognition and English language conventions.

Foundations in Speech Perception

This program is designed to teach listening skills to children, ages 3 to 12 years, with moderate to severe hearing loss, including those with cochlear implants. Lessons start at the basic level of matching words to pictures and progress to complex tasks such as identifying words or phrases without visual cues. Using recorded natural speech, the activities are adaptive to the child's performance level. Each activity begins with a training task to familiarize the participant with the lesson prior to being scored. There is a hierarchy of training, ranging from basic (matching words with pictures) to advanced (distinguishing between similar sounding words) to complex (identifying words or phrases without visual cues). When a skill is achieved, the program automatically moves the user to the next level. The child can also record their speech and replay it to compare to the computer model. Reinforcement is provided by a computer painting activity at the conclusion of a lesson. The screen layout may be confusing at first because there are blocks to correspond to speech segments that

are discovered through frequent exploration with the computer mouse.

Laureate Learning Systems

Laureate Learning Systems includes over 80 programs that address a wide array of auditory-language processing skills. The programs are designed for those functioning at preverbal level up to adult language levels. They are conveniently organized by category and by linguistic level. The categories include games that are designed for early instructional, early vocabulary, expressive language, early categorization training, syntax training, auditory discrimination, vocabulary and concept development, functional language training, advanced categorization training, and finally reading and spelling. The software also may be selected based on linguistic stages that include interpreted communication, intentional communication, single words, word combinations, early syntax, syntax mastery, and complete generative grammar. The Laureate website includes descriptions of these stages along with training goals and the recommended software. The recommended software for auditory training are "Nouns and Sounds," which includes 100 environmental sounds, and "Following Directions," a program that focuses on discrimination of directions.

Learning Fundamentals

This set of programs is designed for use by parents, clinicians, and teachers and includes four main areas: speech, language, literacy, and attention. Each area has several programs with skill levels that vary from beginning to advanced. For example, in the area of memory the tasks begin with simple sustained attention and move to alternating and divided attention with response delays and auditory distractors. The programs include bright photographs on simple screens designed to allow those with attention difficulties to focus on the concept with minimal distractions. In addition to listening to quality audio recordings of natural speech, speech also may be recorded and compared with the speaker's productions. Four programs also are offered that train phonology, vocabulary, and syntax in Spanish.

Listening and Communication Enhancement (LACE)

The purpose of LACE is to provide interactive, computerized training to improve listening and communication. It is designed for adult hearing aid users to train at home. It is recommended that training be done for 30 minutes a day, 5 days a week, for 4 weeks. The interactive and adaptive tasks are divided into three main categories: degraded speech, cognitive skills, and communication strategies. These activities also train auditory memory, speed of processing, and auditory-verbal closure, which are believed to be important skills for understanding language in noisy or otherwise challenging environments. The results of the training session are plotted for the adult as well as sent to a website so that the audiologist can monitor progress. Although the opportunity to train at home is attractive, the vocabulary may be challenging for some clients with limited urban experience. The response accuracy is based on the honor system because the program will provide the correct answer in print and listeners are to respond yes or no to indicate whether they had perceived the stimulus correctly.

Otto's World of Sounds

Otto's World of Sounds, designed for children with hearing loss, focuses on basic auditory skills of sound detection, discrimination and identification. It is intended for home use and as a supplement to a traditional auditory training program. Through the use of 10 different auditory environments, the child encounters sounds analogous to those in their daily listening experiences. The activities within each environment increase in complexity as more sounds are added as the basis for training discovery, memory, and recognition. This program is based on Otto, a prairie dog, which may be most attractive to younger children. The program is distributed free of charge.

Sound and Way Beyond

Sound and Way Beyond is designed for adults with cochlear implants or those with hearing aids who have severe to profound hearing loss. The eight modules include auditory discrimination of pure tones, discrimination and identification of environmental sounds, male/female voice identification, vowel recognition, consonant recognition, word recognition, everyday sentences, and music appreciation. The modules can be completed at home with no specific recommended schedule.

Sound Auditory Training™

Sound Auditory Training is designed for individuals of all ages diagnosed with CAPD. This Web-based software provides several graphic interfaces (games), as well as a basic response mode for adult users, each of which can be applied to exercise any of the multiple exercises targeting fundamental auditory skills, including frequency discrimination, intensity discrimination, frequency and duration pattern recognition, temporal resolution (gap detection), dichotic processing, and consonant-vowel discrimination and identification in quiet and in competition. The exercises can be completed at home, in clinic, or at school.

In summary, given the numerous options for CBAT programs, various selection criteria may be employed. Obviously age level will be a primary factor in selecting a program. In addition, the selection of programs that use nonspeech stimuli (e.g., Sound Auditory Training, Sound and Way Beyond) may be considered when the goal is primarily "auditory training," whereas other programs that use speech and language stimuli may be considered when the focus is more on "auditory-language" training.

Treatment Outcomes, Efficacy, and Effectiveness

In general, there has been considerable evidence on the effectiveness of auditory training with humans and nonhumans (Bao, Chang, Woods, & Merzenich, 2004; Pan, Zhang, Cai, Zhou, & Sun, 2011), electrophysiological and behavioral measures (Alonso & Schochat, 2009; Cameron & Dillon, 2011; Murphy & Schochat, 2011; Pantev & Herholz, 2011; Tremblay, 2007), and natural speech and computer-generated stimuli (Millward, Hall, Ferguson, & Moore, 2011; Moncrieff & Wertz, 2008; Moore, Rosenberg, & Coleman, 2005; Pinheiro & Capellini, 2010). The focus here is on the evidence for the benefits of auditory training conducted through the use of computer presentations. The tech-

nical report issued by experts in the field of CAPD and published by the American Speech-Language-Hearing Association (ASHA) recognized the potential benefits of CBAT (American-Speech-Language-Hearing-Association, 2005). They reported that intervention for CAPD consists of three concurrent approaches, including direct skills remediation, compensatory strategies, and environmental modifications. Despite their recognition that computer-mediated software has several advantages of "multisensory stimulation in an engaging format that provides generous feedback and reinforcement and facilitates intensive training" (p. 11), they admonish that "additional data are needed to demonstrate the effectiveness and efficacy of these approaches" (p. 11).

Table 11–5 includes a summary of auditory training research that specifically included computer-based techniques. Many of the studies evaluating CBAT methods reported positive treatment outcomes (Gillam, 1999; Merzenich et al., 1996; Sullivan et al., in press; Tallal et al., 1996). However, demonstrating efficacy and effectiveness is more involved, because of the need for control groups, counterbalanced designs, and real-world conditions. On average, most studies show improved scores on some outcome measure following auditory training in children with language impairments (Friel-Patti et al., 2001; Loeb, Stoke, & Fey, 2001; Merzenich et al., 1996; Tallal et al., 1996), hearing loss (Schopmeyer, Mellon, Dobaj, Grant, & Niparko, 1998; Sullivan et al., 2013; Zwolan et al., 2000), and reading difficulties (Rouse & Krueger, 2004; Tallal et al., 1996; Troia & Whitney, 2003). Only one of the studies summarized in Table 11–5 involved a randomly assigned control group that received no CBAT (Rouse & Krueger, 2004).

Table 11–5. Summary of CBAT Research

STUDY				SUBJECTS				PROCEDURES	RESULTS
Author	Year	Title	Journal	Exper N =	Control N =	Ages	Diagnosis	CBAT	Effect
Merzenich, Jenkins, Johnston, Schreiner, Miller, & Tallal	1996	Temporal Processing Deficits of Language-learning Impaired Children Ameliorated by Training	*Science*	11	11	5;4 to 10;0	Language Impaired	Group 1: Modified Speech in FFW games Group 2: Video Games and training with natural speech	Positive Treatment for both groups, Greater gains on Receptive Tasks for Group 1
Tallal, Miller, Bedi, Byma, Wang, Nagarajan, Schreiner, Jenkins, & Merzenich	1996	Language Comprehension in Language-Learning Impaired Children improved with Acoustically Modified Speech	*Science*	7	None	5:0 to 9;0	Language Impaired and Poor Readers	Portions of FFW	Positive Treatment Effect
Schopmeyer, Mellon, Dobaj, Grant, & Niparko	1998	Use of Fast ForWord to Enhance Language Development in Children With Cochlear Implants	7th Symposium on Cochlear Implants in Children	11	None	4;10 to 11;5	Hearing Impaired using Cochlear Implant	FFW	Positive Treatment Effect

continues

Table 11–5. *continued*

STUDY				SUBJECTS				PROCEDURES		RESULTS
Author	Year	Title	Journal	Exper N =	Control N =	Ages	Diagnosis	CBAT		Effect
Zwolan, Connor, & Kileny	2000	Evaluation of the Foundations in Speech Perception Software as a Hearing Rehabilitation Tool for Use at Home	*Journal of the American Academy of Rehabilatative Audiology*	7	7	5;0 to 12;0	Hearing Impaired using Cochlear Implant	Group 1: FSP Group 2: No Treatment		Positive Treatment Effect
Friel-Patti, DesBarres, & Thibodeau	2001	Case Studies of Children Using Fast ForWord	*American Journal of Speech-Language Pathology*	5	None	5;10 to 9;2	Language Learning Disability	FFW		Positive Treatment Effect for some Students
Loeb, Stoke, & Fey	2001	Language Changes Associated with Fast ForWord	*American Journal of Speech-Language Pathology*	4	None	5;6 to 8;1	Language Impaired	FFW in Homes		Positive Treatment Effect for some Students

	STUDY			SUBJECTS				PROCEDURES	RESULTS
Author	Year	Title	Journal	Exper $N=$	Control $N=$	Ages	Diagnosis	CBAT	Effect
Gillam, Crofford, Gale, & Hoffman	2001	Language Change Following Computer-Assisted Language Instruction with Fast ForWord or Laureate Learning Systems Software	*American Journal of Speech-Language Pathology*	2	2	6;11 to 7;5	Language Impaired	Group 1: FFW Group 2: CBAT-Tones	Positive Treatment Effect for some Students
Marler, Champlin, & Gillam	2001	Backward and Simultaneous Masking Measured in Children with Language-Learning Impairments Who Received Intervention With Fast ForWord or Laureate Learning Systems Software	*American Journal of Speech-Language Pathology*	2	2	6;10 to 9;3	Language Impaired	Group 1: FFW Group 2: CBAT-Lang	No Treatment Effect
Thibodeau, Friel-Patti, & Britt	2001	Psychoacoustic Performance in Children Completing Fast ForWord Training	*American Journal of Speech-Language Pathology*	5	5	5;10 to 9;1	Language Impaired and Normal Language	Group 1: CBAT-Tones Group 2: CBAT-Tones	No Treatment Effect

continues

341

Table 11–5. *continued*

| STUDY | | | SUBJECTS | | | | PROCEDURES | | RESULTS |
Author	Year	Title	Journal	Exper N=	Control N=	Ages	Diagnosis	CBAT	Effect
Troia & Whitney	2003	A Close Look at the Efficacy of Fast ForWord Language for Children with Academic Weaknesses	*Contemporary Educational Psychology*	25	12	Grades 1 to 6	Academic Weakness	Group 1: FFW Group 2: No Treatment	Limited Treatment Effect
Hayes, Warrier, Nicol, Zecker, & Kraus	2003	Neural Plasticity following Auditory Training in Children with Learning Problems	*Clinical Neurophysiology*	27	15	8;0 to 12;0	Learning Impaired	Group 1: Earobics Group 2: No Treatment	Positive Treatment Effect on some measures
Segers & Verhoeven	2003	Effects of Vocabulary Training by Computer in Kindergarten	*Journal of Computer Assisted Learning*	67	97	4;0 to 6;0	Normal Language	Group 1: CBAT-Lang Group 2: No Treatment	Positive Treatment Effect
Temple, Deutsch, Poldrack, Miller, Tallal, Merzenich, & Gabrieli	2003	Neural Deficits in Children with Dyslexia Ameliorated by Behavioral Remediation: Evidence from Functional MRI	*Proceedings of the National Academy of Sciences*	20	None	8;0 to 12;0	Poor Readers	FFW	Positive Treatment Effect

continues

STUDY				SUBJECTS				PROCEDURES	RESULTS
Author	Year	Title	Journal	Exper N =	Control N =	Ages	Diagnosis	CBAT	Effect
Pokorni, Worthington, & Jamison	2004	Phonological Awareness Intervention: Comparison of Fast ForWord, Earobics, and LiPS	*Journal of Educational Research*	36	16	7;6 to 9;0	Poor Readers	Group 1: FFW Group 2: Earobics Group 3: Non CBAT	No Treatment Effect
Rouse & Krueger	2004	Putting Computerized Instruction to the Test: a Randomized Evaluation of a "Scientifically Based" Reading Program	*Economics of Education Review*	272	240	5;0 to 7;9	Poor Readers	Group 1: FFW Group 2: No Treatment	Limited Treatment Effect
Troia	2004	Migrant Students with Limited English Proficiency Can Fast ForWord Language Make a Difference in Their Language Skills and Academic Achievement?	*Remedial and Special Education*	99	92	Grades 1 to 6	Normal Verbal IQ, Native Spanish Speaker	Group 1: FFW Group 2: Trad Tx	Limited Treatment Effect

Table 11–5. *continued*

| | STUDY | | | SUBJECTS | | | | PROCEDURES | RESULTS |
| | | | | Exper N= | Control N= | Ages | Diagnosis | | |
Author	Year	Title	Journal					CBAT	Effect
Warrier, Johnson, Hayes, Nicol, & Kraus	2004	Learning Impaired Children Exhibit Timing Deficits and Training-Related Improvements in Auditory Cortical Responses to Speech in Noise	*Experimental Brain Research*	13	11	8;0 to 13;0	Learning Problems	Group 1: Earobics Group 2: No Treatment	Positive Treatment Effect
Segers & Verhoeven	2004	Computer-supported Phonological Awareness Intervention for Kindergarten Children with Specific Language Impairment	*Language, Speech, and Hearing Services in the Schools*	24	12		Language Impaired	Group 1: CBAT-Phon Awareness Group 2: CBAT-Syn Sp Group 3: CBAT-Vocab	Positive Treatment Effect but not for Synthetic Speech

continues

	STUDY				SUBJECTS				PROCEDURES	RESULTS
Author	Year	Title	Journal	Exper N=	Control N=	Ages	Diagnosis	CBAT	Effect
Cohen, Hodson, O'Hare, Boyle, Durani, McCartney, et al.	2005	Computer-Based Intervention Through Acoustically Modified Speech (Fast ForWord) in Severe Mixed Receptive-Expressive Language Impairment: Outcomes from a Randomized Controlled Trial	Journal of Speech, Language, and Hearing Research	50	27	6;0 to 10;0	Receptive Specific Language Impairment	Group 1: FFW Group 2: CBAT-Lang Group 3: No Treatment	No Treatment Effect
Russo, Nicol, Zecker, Hayes, & Kraus	2005	Auditory Training Improves Neural Timing in the Human Brainstem	Behavioural Brain Research	9	10	8;0 to 12;0	Learning Impaired	Group 1: Earobics Group 2: No Treatment	Positive Treatment Effect on some measures
Gillam et al.	2008	The Efficacy of Fast ForWord Language Intervention in School-Age Children With Language Impairment: A Randomized Controlled Trial.	Journal of Speech, Language, and Hearing Research	216	N/A	6;0 to 8;11	Language Impaired	Group 1: FFW Group 2: CBAT-Lang Group 3: Trad Tx Group 4: CBAE	No Treatment Effect

Table 11-5. *continued*

| STUDY | | | | SUBJECTS | | | | PROCEDURES | | RESULTS |
Author	Year	Title	Journal	Exper N=	Control N=	Ages	Diagnosis	CBAT		Effect
Cameron & Dillon	2011	Development and Evaluation of the LiSN & Learn Auditory Training Software for Deficit-Specific Remediation of Binaural Processing Deficits in Children: Preliminary Findings	*Journal of the American Academy of Audiology*	9	Self	6:9 to 11:4	Spatial Process-ing Deficit	LiSN & Learn		Positive Treatment Effect for Speech Reception Thresholds, Memory, and Attention
Sullivan, Thibodeau, & Assmann	in press	Auditory Training of Speech Recognition with Interrupted and Continuous Noise Maskers by Children with Hearing Impairment	*Journal of the Acoustical Society of America*	16	8	8;0 to 12;0	Hearing Impaired	Group 1: Continuous Noise Group 2: Interrupted Noise		Greater Positive Treatment Effect for Interrupted Noise vs Continuous

Note: *Exper* = Experimental, *CBAT* = Computer-Based Auditory Training, *FFW* = Fast ForWord®, *CBAT-Lang* = Computer-Based Auditory Training with Language Focus, *CBAT-Tones* = Computer-Based Auditory Training with Tone Stimuli, *CBAT-Vocab* = Computer-Based Auditory Training with focus on Vocabulary training, *CBAT-Syn Sp* = Computer-Based Auditory Training with Synthetic Speech Stimuli, *Trad Tx* = Traditional Therapy, *FSP* = Foundations of Speech Perception, *Non CBAT* = Auditory Training that was not computer based, *CBAE* = Computer-Based Academic Enrichment.

Efficacy is demonstrated when results show that the treatment is capable of working in the best-case scenario, that is, when appropriate listeners participate and the treatment protocol is followed (Robey & Schultz, 1998). Effectiveness, however, is demonstrated when the program is shown to be effective in real life situations where there may be fewer controls (Robey & Schultz, 1998). In the few studies properly designed to demonstrate efficacy of CBAT (e.g., included control groups that did not receive CBAT), support was not seen for a specific CBAT; however, these studies did reveal gains derived from intensive treatment with CBAT (Chen, Corwell, Yaseen, Hallett, & Cohen, 1998; Gillam, 1999; Pokorni, Worthington, & Jamison, 2004; Rouse & Krueger, 2004; Troia & Whitney, 2003). One study conducted by Gillam et al. (2008) designed to separate intensiveness of treatment from treatment mode found that the improvements in language skills by children who received intensive intervention from a speech-language pathologist were equivalent to those achieved by children who received intervention for the same time period via CBAT.

Sweetow and Palmer (2005) reviewed the limited published research regarding the efficacy of auditory training with individuals with hearing loss. They provided many insights into the quality of research needed for CBAT with children with CAPD. Of the 213 articles they reviewed concerning adults with hearing loss, 42 were identified as studies with potential results related to effectiveness of auditory training. Of these, only 6 met inclusion criteria that required sufficient detail to allow evaluation of the quality of the research and a study design that involved a randomized controlled trial. These 6 studies did support, in fact, the efficacy of auditory training, particularly for the treatments that involved training with meaningful, sentence materials (synthetic approach), rather than noncontextual speech syllable drills (analytic approach). Sweetow and Palmer (2005) provide a framework for evaluation of research with CBAT.

Table 11–6, adapted from Sweetow and Palmer (2005), includes the criteria upon which CBAT research can be evaluated. The lack of a control group is perhaps the most important variable limiting many CBAT studies. Interestingly, several studies have demonstrated that the benefits of Fast ForWord or Earobics are no greater than the gains seen following the same intense computer experience but with academic enrichment games (Chen et al., 1998; Gillam, 1999; Pokorni et al., 2004). This finding suggests that the gains that were made were not the result of specific training activities in the software, but perhaps the result of more generalized training of attending to auditory patterns and the strengthening of possible auditory representation used in perception.

In addition to comparing different types of CBAT, it is also interesting to compare a single CBAT treatment with a no-treatment control group. At least three studies have examined the benefits of Earobics compared with a control group that received no treatment (Hayes, Warrier, Nicol, Zecker, & Kraus, 2003; Russo et al., 2005; Warrier, Johnson, Hayes, Nicol, & Kraus, 2004). Results of each study confirmed significant benefits received by the experimental (treatment) group relative to the control group. These studies demonstrate the benefits of CBAT, and when considered in conjunction with the studies reviewed above that demonstrated absence of significant differences

Table 11–6. Criteria For Evaluation of CBAT Research (Adapted From Sweetow & Palmer, 2005)

1. Randomized assignment to treatment groups

2. Inclusion of a control group

3. Power analysis supports the number of subjects included

4. Experimenters and/or subjects blinded to the treatment

5. Psychometrically sound outcome measures related to communication disorders and/or treatment

6. Feedback employed in the training paradigms

7. Assessment of long-term benefits following dismissal from treatment

8. Generalization to other treatment settings

in treatment outcomes across different types of CBAT, it seems apparent that the intensity and frequency of treatment are perhaps the most important variables influencing treatment outcome.

Summary

CBAT can be an effective training tool for children with CAPD and associated disorders. Three important elements influence the benefit derived from training: meaningfulness of stimuli, engagement of active or focused attention, and intensive training. Although research has supported the use of CBAT for children with language impairments (many of whose clinical profiles included reference to auditory or listening difficulties), there have been few studies specifically designed to determine the efficacy of CBAT for children diagnosed with CAPD. (It is important to note, however, that many of these same studies measured abnormal auditory evoked potential activity in their subjects with language

impairment and learning impairment prior to treatment, suggesting the presence of central auditory deficits in these subjects [Jirsa, 1992; Russo et al., 2005; Tremblay, Kraus, McGee, Ponton, & Otis, 2001; Warrier et al., 2004].) CBAT seems ideally suited to strengthen auditory perception skills through repetitive tasks that can be presented in an engaging format with reinforcement that allows intensive training necessary for maximum benefit.

Currently there are several programs available that range in price, sophistication, and ease of use. Selection of software is expedited by first selecting the age category followed by training area. Additional research involving individuals diagnosed with CAPD in well-designed studies incorporating randomly assigned control groups are needed to determine the efficacy of CBAT, including the most important program features underlying treatment success. Further research is needed to determine the most appropriate stimuli, hierarchy of tasks, and training format (home vs. school vs. clinic) to use with children with CAPD.

References

Alonso, R., & Schochat, E. (2009). The efficacy of formal auditory training in children with central auditory processing disorder: behavioral and electrophysiological evaluation. *Brazillian Journal of Otorhinolaryngology*, *75*, 726–732.

ASHA (American Speech-Language-Hearing Association). (1996). Central auditory processing: Current status of research and implications for clinical practice. *American Journal of Audiology*, *5(2)*, 41–54.

ASHA. (2005). *(Central) auditory processing disorders*. Retrieved from http://www.asha.org/members/deskref-journals/deskref/default

Atienza M., Cantero, J. L., & Dominguez-Marin, E. (2002). The time course of neural changes underlying auditory perceptual learning. *Learning and Memory*, *9*, 138–150.

Bao, S., Chang, E. F., Woods, J., & Merzenich, M. M. (2004). Temporal plasticity in the primary auditory cortex induced by operant perceptual learning. *Nature Neuroscience*, *7*, 974–981.

Borden, G. J., Harris, K. S., & Raphael, L. J. (2003). *Speech science primer* (4th ed.). Baltimore, MD: Lippincott Williams & Wilkins.

Cameron, S., & Dillon, H. (2011). Development and evaluation of the LiSN & Learn auditory training software for deficit-specific remediation of binaural processing deficits in children: Preliminary findings. *Journal of the American Academy of Audiology*, *22*, 678–696.

Carhart, R. (1960). Auditory training. In S. R. S. Hallowell Davis (Ed.), *Hearing and deafness* (pp. 368–386). New York, NY: Holt, Rinehart and Winston.

Chen, R., Corwell, B., Yaseen, Z., Hallett, M., & Cohen, L. G. (1998). Mechanisms of cortical reorganization in lower-limb amputees. *Journal of Neuroscience*, *18*, 3443–3450.

Chermak, G., & Musiek, F. (1997). *Central auditory processing disorders: New perspectives*. San Diego, CA: Singular.

Chermak, G., & Musiek, F. (2002). Auditory training: Principles and approaches for remediating and managing auditory processing disorders. *Seminars in Hearing*, *23*, 297–308.

Cohen, W., Hodson, A., O'Hare, A., Boyle, J., Durrani, T., McCartney, E., . . . Watson, J. (2005). Effects of computer-based intervention through acoustically modified speech (Fast ForWord) in severe mixed receptive-expressive language impairment: Outcomes from a randomized controlled trial. *Journal of Speech, Language, and Hearing Research*, *48*, 715–729.

Cox, R. M., & Alexander, G. C. (1992). Maturation of hearing aid benefit: Objective and subjective measurements. *Ear and Hearing*, *13*, 131–141.

Dawson, M. M., Hallahan, D. P., Reeve, R. E., & Ball, D. W. (1980). The effect of reinforcement and verbal rehearsal on selective attention in learning-disabled children. *Journal of Abnormal Child Psychology*, *8*, 133–144.

De Csipkes, R. A., Smouse, A. D., & Hudson, B. A. (1975). Influence of reinforcement on the paired-associate learning of retarded and nonretarded children. *American Journal of Mental Deficiency*, *80*, 357–359.

Eggermont, J. J., & Komiya, H. (2000). Moderate noise trauma in juvenile cats results in profound cortical topographic map changes in adulthood. *Hearing Research*, *142*, 89–101.

Friel-Patti, S., DesBarres, K., & Thibodeau, L. (2001). Case studies of children using Fast ForWord. *American Journal of Speech-Language Pathology*, *10*, 203–215.

Galvan, V. V., & Weinberger, N. M. (2002). Long-term consolidation and retention of learning-induced tuning plasticity in the auditory cortex of the guinea pig. *Neurobiology of Learning and Memory*, *77*, 78–108.

Garstecki, D. C. (1982). Rehabilitation of hearing-handicapped elderly adults. *Ear and Hearing*, *3*, 167–172.

Gatehouse, S. (1992). The time course and magnitude of perceptual acclimatization to frequency responses: Evidence from monaural fitting of hearing aids. *Journal of the Acoustical Society of America, 92,* 1258–1268.

Gatehouse, S. (1993). Role of perceptual acclimatization in the selection of frequency responses for hearing aids. *Journal of the American Academy of Audiology, 4,* 296–306.

Gillam, R. (1999). Computer-assisted language intervention using Fast ForWord: Theoretical and empirical considerations for clinical decision-making. *Language, Speech, and Hearing Services in Schools, 30,* 363–370.

Gillam, R., Crofford, J., Gale, M., & Hoffman, L. (2001). Language change following computer-assisted language instruction with Fast ForWord or Laureate Learning Systems software. *American Journal of Speech-Language Pathology 10,* 231–247.

Gillam, R., Loeb, D., Hoffman, L., Bohman, T., Champlin, C., Thibodeau, L., . . . Friel-Patti, S. (2008). The efficacy of Fast ForWord language intervention in school-age children with language impairment: A randomized controlled trial. *Journal of Speech, Language, and Hearing Research, 51,* 97–119.

Goldstein, M. A. (1939). *The acoustic method for the training of the deaf and hard-of-hearing child.* St. Louis, MO: Laryngoscope Press.

Gottselig, J. M., Brandeis, D., Hofer-Tinguely, G., Borbély, A., & Achermann, P. (2004). Human central auditory plasticity associated with tone sequence learning. *Learning and Memory 11,* 162–171.

Hayes, E. A., Warrier, C. M., Nicol, T. G., Zecker, S. G., & Kraus, N. (2003). Neural plasticity following auditory training in children with learning problems. *Clinical Neurophysiology, 114,* 673–684.

Horwitz, A. R., & Turner, C. W. (1997). The time course of hearing aid benefit. *Ear and Hearing, 18,* 1–11.

Irvine, D. R. (2000). Injury- and use-related plasticity in the adult auditory system. *Journal of Communication Disorders, 33,* 293–311.

Jirsa, R. E. (1992). The clinical utility of the P3 AERP in children with auditory processing disorders. *Journal of Speech and Hearing Research, 35,* 903–912.

Jusczyk, P. W., & Luce, P. A. (2002). Speech perception and spoken word recognition: Past and present. *Ear and Hearing, 23,* 2–40.

Kent, R. D., & Read, C. (2002). *The acoustic analysis of speech* (2nd ed.). New York, NY: Delmar.

Kilgard, M. P., & Merzenich, M. M. (1998a). Cortical map reorganization enabled by nucleus basalis activity. *Science, 279,* 1714–1718.

Kilgard, M. P., & Merzenich, M. M. (1998b). Plasticity of temporal information processing in the primary auditory cortex. *Nature Neuroscience, 1,* 727–731.

Kraus, N., McGee, T., Carrell, T., King, C., Tremblay, K., & Nicol, T. (1995). Central auditory system plasticity associated with speech discrimination training. *Journal of Cognitive Neuroscience, 7,* 25–32.

Kuhl, P. K., & Meltzoff, A. N. (1996). Infant vocalizations in response to speech: Vocal imitation and developmental change. *Journal of the Acoustical Society of America, 100*(4 Pt 1), 2425–2438.

Lakshminarayanan, K., & Tallal, P. (2007). Generalization of non-linguistic auditory perceptual training to syllable discrimination. *Restorative Neurology and Neuroscience, 25,* 263–272.

Levitt, H. (1978). Adaptive testing in audiology. *Scandinavian Audiology Supplementum, 6,* 241–291.

Loeb, D., Stoke, C., & Fey, M. (2001). Language changes associated with Fast ForWord-Language: Evidence from case studies. *American Journal of Speech-Language Pathology, 10,* 216–230.

Loo, J., Bamiou, D., Campbell, N., & Luxon, L. (2010). Computer-based auditory training (CBAT): Benefits for children with language- and reading-related learning difficulties. *Developmental Medicine and Child Neurology, 52,* 708–717.

Marler, J. A., Champlin, C. A., & Gillam, R. B., (2001). Backward and simultaneous masking measured in children with language-learning impairments who received intervention with Fast ForWord or Laureate Learning System software. *American Journal of Speech-Language Pathology, 10,* 258–268.

Merzenich, M. M., Jenkins, W. M., Johnston, P., Schreiner, C., Miller, S. L., & Tallal, P. (1996). Temporal processing deficits of language-learning impaired children ameliorated by training. *Science, 271,* 77–81.

Millward, K., Hall, R., Ferguson, M., & Moore, D. (2011). Training speech-in-noise perception in mainstream school children. *International Journal of Pediatric Otorhinolaryngology, 75,* 1408–1417.

Moncrieff, D., & Wertz, D. (2008). Auditory rehabilitation for interaural asymmetry: Preliminary evidence of improved dichotic listening performance following intensive training. *International Journal of Audiology,* 484–497.

Montgomery, A. A., Walden, B. E., Schwartz, D. M., & Prosek, R. A. (1984). Training auditory-visual speech reception in adults with moderate sensorineural hearing loss. *Ear and Hearing, 5,* 30–36.

Moore, D., Rosenberg, J., & Coleman, J. (2005). Discrimination training of phonemic contrasts enhances phonological processing mainstream school children. *Brain and Language, 94,* 72–85.

Murphy, C. D., & Schochat, E. (2011). Effect of nonlinguistic auditory training on phonological and reading skills. *Folia Phoniatrica Logopaed, 63,* 147–153.

Musiek, F. E., Baran, J. A., & Shinn, J. (2004). Assessment and remediation of an auditory processing disorder associated with head trauma. *Journal of the American Academy of Audiology, 15,* 117–132.

Musiek, F. E., Bellis, T. J., & Chermak, G. D. (2005). Nonmodularity of the CANS: Implications for (central) auditory processing disorder. *American Journal of Audiology, 14,* 128–138.

Pan, Y., Zhang, J., Cai, R., Zhou, X., & Sun, X. (2011). Developmentally degraded directional selectivity of the auditory cortex can be restored by auditory discrim training. *Behavioural Brain Research 225,* 596–602.

Pantev, C., & Herholz S. C. (2011). Plasticity of the human auditory cortex related to musical training. *Neuroscience and Biobehavioral Reviews, 35,* 2140–2154.

Pinheiro, F., & Capellini, S. (2010) .Auditory training in students with learning disabilities. *Pro Fono, 22,* 49–54.

Pinker, S. (1990). *Language acquisition.* Cambridge, MA: MIT Press.

Pokorni, J., Worthington, C., & Jamison, P. (2004). Phonological awareness intervention: Comparison of Fast ForWord, Earobics, and LiPS. *Journal of Educational Research, 97,* 147–157.

Prensky, M. (2001). *Digital game-based learning.* New York, NY: McGraw-Hill.

Recanzone, G. H., Schreiner, C. E., & Merzenich, M. M. (1993). Plasticity in the frequency representation of primary auditory cortex following discrimination training in adult owl monkeys. *Journal of Neuroscience, 13,* 87–103.

Rideout, V., Vandewater, E., & Wartella, E. (2003). *Zero to six: Electronic media in the lives of infants, toddlers, and preschoolers* (No. 3378): Henry J. Kaiser Family Foundation.

Robertson, D., & Irvine, D. R. (1989). Plasticity of frequency organization in auditory cortex of guinea pigs with partial unilateral deafness. *Journal of Comparative Neurology, 282,* 456–471.

Robey, R., & Schultz, M. (1998). A model for conducting clinical/outcome research: An adaptation of the standard protocol for use is aphasiology. *Aphasiology, 12,* 787–810.

Rouse, C., & Krueger, A. (2004). Putting computerized instruction to the test: A randomized evaluation of a "scientifically based" reading program. *Economics of Education Review, 23,* 323–338.

Russo, N. M., Nicol, T. G., Zecker, S. G., Hayes, E. A., & Kraus, N. (2005). Auditory training improves neural timing in the human brainstem. *Behavioral Brain Research, 156,* 95–103.

Schochat, E., Musiek, F. E., Alonso, R., & Ogata, J. (2010). Effect of auditory training on the middle latency response in children with (central) auditory processing disorder. *Brazilian Journal of Medical and Biological Research, 43,* 777–785.

Schopmeyer, B., Mellon, N., Dobaj, H., Grant, G., & Niparko, J. (1998). *Use of Fast ForWord™ to enhance language development in children with cochlear implants.* Paper presented at the Seventh Symposium on Cochlear Implants in Children, Iowa City, IA.

Scott, J., & Thibodeau, L. (2006, April). *The effects of auditory training on hearing aid acclimatization.* Paper presented at the annual convention of the American Academy of Audiology. Minneapolis, MN.

Scott, L. (1992). Attention and perseverance behaviors of preschool children enrolled in Suzuki violin lessons and other activities. *Journal of Research in Music Education, 40,* 225–235.

Segers, E., & Verhoeven, L. (2003). Effects of vocabulary training by computer in kindergarten. *Journal of Computer Assisted Learning 19,* 557–566.

Segers, E., & Verhoeven, L. (2004). Computer-supported phonological awareness intervention for kindergarten children with specific language impairment. *Language, Speech, and Hearing Services in Schools, 35,* 229–239.

Sullivan, J., Thibodeau, L, & Assmann, P. (in press). Auditory training of speech recognition with interrupted and continuous noise maskers by children with hearing impairment. *Journal of the Acoustical Society of America.*

Suzuki, S. (1981). *Ability development from age zero.* Miami, FL: Warner Brothers.

Suzuki, S. (1983). *Nurtured by love: The classic approach to talent education.* Miami, FL: Warner Brothers.

Sweetow, R., & Palmer, C. V. (2005). Efficacy of individual auditory training in adults: A systematic review of the evidence. *Journal of the American Academy of Audiology, 16,* 494–504.

Tallal, P., Miller, S. L., Bedi, G., Byma, G., Wang, X., Nagarajan, S. S., . . . Merzenich, M. M.(1996). Language comprehension in language-learning impaired children improved with acoustically modified speech. *Science, 271,* 81–84.

Temple, E., Deutsch, G. K., Poldrack, R. A., Miller, S. L., Tallal, P., Merzenich, M. M., & Gabrieli, J.D. (2003). Neural deficits in children with dyslexia ameliorated by behavioral remediation: Evidence from functional MRI. *Proceedings of the National Academy of Sciences of the USA, 100,* 2860–2865.

Thibodeau, L., Friel-Patti, S., & Britt, L. (2001). Psychoacoustic performance in children completing Fast ForWord™ training. *American Journal of Speech-Language Pathology, 10,* 248–257.

Tremblay, K. (2007). Training-related changes in the brain: Evidence from human auditory evoked potentials. *Seminars in Hearing, 28,* 120–132.

Tremblay, K., & Kraus, N. (2002). Auditory training induces asymmetrical changes in cortical neural activity. *Journal of Speech, Language, and Hearing Research, 45,* 564–572.

Tremblay, K., Kraus, N., Carrell, T. D., & McGee, T. (1997). Central auditory system plasticity: Generalization to novel stimuli following listening training. *Journal of the Acoustical Society of America, 102,* 3762–3773.

Tremblay, K., Kraus, N., & McGee, T. (1998). The time course of auditory perceptual learning: Neurophysiological changes during speech-sound training. *NeuroReport, 9,* 3557–3560.

Tremblay, K., Kraus, N., McGee, T., Ponton, C., & Otis, B. (2001). Central auditory plasticity: Changes in the N1-P2 complex after speech-sound training. *Ear and Hearing, 22,* 79–90.

Troia, G., & Whitney, S. (2003). A close look at the efficacy of Fast ForWord language for children with academic weaknesses. *Contemporary Educational Psychology, 28,* 465–494.

Tyler, R. S., & Summerfield, A. Q. (1996). Cochlear implantation: Relationships with research on auditory deprivation and acclimatization. *Ear and Hearing, 17*(3 Suppl.), 38S–50S.

Walden, B. E., Erdman, S. A., Montgomery, A. A., Schwartz, D. M., & Prosek, R. A. (1981). Some effects of training on speech recognition by hearing-impaired adults. *Journal of Speech and Hearing Research, 24,* 207–216.

Warrier, C. M., Johnson, K. L., Hayes, E. A., Nicol, T., & Kraus, N. (2004). Learning impaired children exhibit timing deficits and training-related improvements in auditory cortical responses to speech in noise. *Experimental Brain Research, 157,* 431–441.

Wedenberg, E. (1951). Auditory training of deaf and hard of hearing children. *Acta Oto-laryngologica, 94*(Suppl.), 1–129.

Willott, J. F. (1996). Physiological plasticity in the auditory system and its possible relevance to hearing aid use, deprivation effects, and acclimatization. *Ear and Hearing, 17*(3 Suppl.), 66S–77S.

Zwolan, T., McDonald Connor, C. M., & Kileny, P. (2000). Evaluation of the foundations in speech perception software as a hearing rehabilitation tool for use at home. *Journal of the Academy of Rehabilitative Audiology, 33,* 39–51.

CHAPTER 12

SIGNAL ENHANCEMENT: PERSONAL FM AND SOUND-FIELD TECHNOLOGY

CAROL FLEXER

Management for children with central auditory processing disorder (CAPD) typically includes three events: direct therapeutic remediation, compensatory strategies, and environmental modifications. This chapter focuses on the environmental modifications piece by exploring the functional use of personal FM and sound-field FM and IR (infrared) technology as a partial treatment for CAPD. While functioning to improve the signal-to-noise ratio (SNR), this technology may not solve all of a child's CAPD issues; other treatments discussed in this Handbook may be necessary. Nevertheless, current studies demonstrate the potential of SNR-enhancing technologies to positively influence academic behavior and perhaps even cause changes in consistency of neural responses to sound

for children with CAPD (Hall, 2011; Hornickel, Zecker, Bradlow, & Kraus 2012).

The classroom is one of the most challenging learning domains for all children, and especially those with CAPD. Youngsters spend much of their time in noisy classroom environments where teachers demand constant, detailed listening to critical, often fast-paced instruction that is spoken at a distance from them. The major factors that affect auditory learning in the classroom include the hearing and attention capabilities of the child and the actual classroom environment (e.g., noise, reverberation and distance from the speaker). Additional variables include the speech of the teacher and of pupils, and their relative positions in the room.

A child with CAPD has the same neurological, linguistic, and psychosocial limitations experienced by all children, plus extra auditory *baggage*. Children with CAPD, as well as those with attention deficit hyperactivity disorder (ADHD) typically have normal hearing sensitivity at the time of diagnosis (note: they may have had otitis media–caused fluctuating hearing loss during infancy or preschool years) but have difficulty processing auditory stimuli due to deficits or dysfunction of the central nervous system, or in the case of ADHD, attention deficits and distractibility issues (Chermak, Hall, & Musiek, 1999). They often are annoyed, confused, and even agitated by typical classroom noise levels, with subsequent difficulty focusing on their teacher's voice.

Let us begin by exploring the listening limitations common to all children, including those with CAPD.

How Children Hear

We "hear" with the brain. The ears are just a way in. The problem with hearing loss and with poor auditory environments is that accurate sound representation does not reach the brain. The purpose of having favorable listening environments and amplification technologies is to enhance acoustic saliency by channeling complete words efficiently and effectively to the brain (Cole & Flexer, 2011).

To begin at the beginning, studies in brain development show that stimulation of the auditory centers of the brain is critical (Berlin & Weyand, 2003; Boothroyd, 1997; Chermak, & Musiek, 2007; Sharma, Dorman, & Spahr, 2002). Sensory stimulation influences the actual growth and organization of auditory brain pathways (Bhatnagar, 2002; Diamond & Lee, 2011; Merzenich 2010; Sharma, Dorman, & Spahr, 2002; Tallal, 2005). If complete acoustic events are received, then that is how the brain will be organized. Conversely, if hearing loss or poor listening environments filter some or all speech sounds from reaching auditory centers of the brain, then the brain will be organized differently. "When we want to remember (or learn) something we have heard, we must hear it clearly because memory can be only as clear as its original signal . . . muddy in, muddy out" (Doidge, 2007, p. 68). Therefore, anything that can be done to access, grow, and *program* those important and powerful auditory centers of the brain with acoustic detail expands children's opportunities for enhancement of life function. Poor acoustic environments or a child's hearing loss, no matter how minimal, can be roadblocks to sufficient sounds getting to the brain unless amplification technologies are used. Signal enhancement, such as that provided by personal or sound-field technology, is really about brain stimulation and the positive impact on the development of auditory-neural pathways.

It is important to recognize that children are not small adults. They are not able to listen like adults listen. Indeed, children bring different listening capabilities to a communicative and learning situation than do adults in two main ways. First, the central auditory nervous system is not fully myelinated until or perhaps even past the teenage years; thus a child does not bring a complete neurological system to a listening situation (Bhatnagar, 2002; Boothroyd, 1997; Merzenich, 2010). Second, children do not have the years of language and life experience that enable adults to fill in the gaps of missed or inferred information (such filling in of gaps is called auditory/cognitive closure). Leibold and Neff (2011) explained that children require years of listening experience to learn to focus on the most informative aspects of complex speech sounds in the presence of interfering noise. Therefore, because children require more complete, detailed auditory information than adults, all children need a quieter room and a louder signal (Anderson, 2004; Valente et al., 2012). Unlike adults, who receive sound into *developed* brains, the brains of children are still developing.

Typical mainstream classrooms are auditory-verbal environments; instruction is presented through the teacher's spoken communication (Smaldino & Flexer, 2012). The underlying assumption is that children can hear clearly, and attend to and focus on the teacher's speech. Thus, children in a mainstream classroom, whether or not they have hearing problems, must be able to hear the teacher in order for learning to occur. If children cannot consistently and clearly hear and focus on the teacher, the major premise of the educational system is undermined. The point is, all children and especially those with CAPD, require a favorable SNR (Valente, Pievinsky, Franco, Heinrichs-Graham, & Lewis, 2012).

Signal-to-Noise Ratio

The major factors that affect auditory learning in the classroom include the hearing and attention capabilities of the child and the actual classroom environment. Additional variables include the speech of the teacher and pupils, and their relative positions in the room. Because the speech of talkers is filtered through the physical environment of a room and the auditory/attentional system of the listener, these variables are of primary consideration (Boothroyd, 2004; Rubin, Flagg-Williams, Aquino-Russell, & Lushinaton, 2011).

The SNR is the intensity relationship between a primary signal, such as the teacher's speech, and background noise. Noise is anything and everything that conflicts with the auditory signal of choice and may include other talkers, heating or cooling systems, classroom or hall noise, playground sounds, computer noise, and wind, among others (Nelson & Blaeser, 2010). The quieter the room and the more favorable the SNR, the clearer the auditory signal will be for the brain. The further the listener is from the desired sound source and the noisier the environment, the poorer the SNR and the more garbled the signal will be for the brain. The dominant source of masking noise in a room is the children in the room and the number of acoustic events that are co-occurring. This masking effect is especially true for the consonants that carry most of the intelligibility of speech necessary for accurate perception (Wroblewski et al., 2012). Background noise in a room tends to mask the less intense consonant phonemes significantly more than the more intense vowel phonemes. As mentioned earlier, all children—especially those with CAPD—need a quieter environment and a louder signal than do adults in order to learn (Anderson, 2004; Anderson & Arnoldi, 2011).

Adults with normal hearing and intact listening skills require a consistent SNR of approximately +6 dB for the reception of intelligible speech (Bess & Humes, 2003). Children need a much more favorable SNR because their neurological immaturity and lack of life and language experiences reduce their ability to perform auditory/cognitive closure. It has long been known that all children require the signal to be about 10 times louder than competing sounds (Nabelek & Nabelek, 1985). Due to noise, reverberation, and variations in teacher position, the SNR in a typical classroom is unstable and averages out to only about +4 dB and may be 0 dB—often less than ideal even for adults with normal hearing and normal auditory processing capabilities (Smaldino & Flexer, 2012). Interestingly, children with sensorineural hearing loss have a spatial processing disorder, a particular type of auditory processing disorder that makes them less able to attend to target sounds coming from one direction by suppressing sounds coming from other directions (Ching, van Wanrooy, Dillon, & Carter, 2011).

A key concept regarding the value of enhancing the SNR is acoustic saliency. Many children with CAPD also present comorbid language deficits (Chermak & Musiek, 2007). Tallal (2005) found that children with language impairment make more errors on acoustically nonsalient as compared with acoustically salient grammatical morphemes. In a sentence context, acoustically nonsalient morphemes are shorter in duration and softer than louder phonemes in adjacent portions of the utterance (Anderson & Arnoldi, 2011; Tallal, 2005); Therefore, the environmental management of enhancing the SNR of spoken instruction for children with CAPD has the added benefit of increasing acoustic saliency of more difficult to hear speech sounds (Valente et al., 2012; Wroblewski, Lewis, & Stelmachowicz, 2012).

A critical factor in acoustic accessibility is the room's reverberation time (RT). Reverberation time refers to the amount of time it takes for a steady-state sound to decrease 60 dB SPL from its peak amplitude. In a reverberant room, speech is reflected from various hard room surfaces, causing some speech elements to be delayed in reaching the ear of the listener (Valente et al., 2012; Wroblewski et al., 2012). The reflected speech overlaps with the direct speech signal (the signal not reflected before reaching the listener's ear) and covers up or masks certain acoustic speech components. Because vowels are more intense than consonants, a long RT tends to produce a prolongation of the spectral energy of vowels, which then covers up less intense consonant components (Smaldino & Flexer, 2012). A reduction of consonant information can have a significant effect on speech recognition because the vast majority of the acoustic information that is important for speech recognition is provided by consonants (Smaldino, 2011). Speech recognition, therefore, tends to decrease with increases in reverberation time. Speech recognition in adults with normal hearing is not significantly degraded until the RT exceeds approximately 1 second. Listeners with hearing problems, however, need considerably shorter RT (0.4 to 0.5 seconds) for optimal communication (Crandell, Smaldino, & Flexer, 2005). Because of this increased difficulty, acoustical guidelines for populations who experience hearing loss suggest that RT should not exceed 0.4 to 0.5 seconds in communication environments used by these individuals (ASHA, 2005).

All children benefit from learning in a classroom with low reverberation levels (Valente et al., 2012). Although there are some acoustic conditions that cannot be controlled, it is essential that we control the conditions we can in order to provide children with an appropriate listening and learning environment.

Signal-to-Noise Ratio Enhancing Technologies

It has long been recognized that a remote microphone improves the SNR for a listener. That is, a microphone worn by a talker who uses radio (FM) or light waves (IR) to send the talker's voice to the listener who wears a receiver makes the desired signal louder and more clear by overcoming distance, background noise, and to some extent excessive reverberation, especially in the personal FM configuration (Mendel, Roberts, & Walton, 2003; Smaldino & Flexer, 2012). Numerous studies show that academics, literacy, attention, and behavior improve when children have better access to the desired signal (Crandell, Smaldino, & Flexer, 2005; Smaldino & Flexer, 2012.). The question remains: Will children with CAPD show similar benefits of FM use? That is, can personal and/or sound-field technology be considered a viable treatment for children with CAPD? Given that children in general benefit from an enhanced SNR (Rubin, Flagg-Williams, Aquino-Russell, & Lushinaton, 2011), will children with CAPD benefit more? Will the use of such technology reduce the necessity of additional treatments for some children? How can we determine if SNR enhancing technology is effective for a particular student? The following sections explore these issues.

Necessary Versus Sufficient Distinctions

A discussion of environmental modifications must be preceded by a discussion of "necessary versus sufficient" benefit.

There is general agreement that acoustic accessibility is a necessary prerequisite for academic success. However, acoustic accessibility and enhanced signal saliency in the absence of additional treatments may not be sufficient for some children with CAPD (Chermak & Musiek, 2007).

An analogy in the visual realm might involve a child who has difficulty drawing geometric figures. A necessary first step in addressing this problem would be ensuring clear lighting that enhances visual saliency of the drawing field. The lighting alone might be insufficient to correct a child's drawing of geometric designs; additional treatments may be necessary. One does not remove the lights if they did not solve the entire problem. One keeps the lighting as a necessary first step and then adds additional instruction and accommodations. In a similar vein, one does not remove SNR-enhancing technologies if they do not solve the entire problem. One adds other treatments discussed in this Handbook to achieve sufficiency.

Personal FM Technology

Personal FM systems are like individual, private radio stations where the talker (typically the teacher) wears the wireless microphone transmitter, and the children wear the receiver coupled to their ears via headphones, ear buds, or through personal hearing aids. The purpose of a personal FM system is to improve the SNR by effectively overcoming the typical classroom acoustic problems of distance and noise (Crandell, Kreisman, Smaldino, & Kreisman, 2004; Dillon, 2012).

Traditional personal FM systems, typically designed for children with hearing loss, have been too powerful for children with normal hearing sensitivity. Since children with CAPD tend to have normal hearing sensitivity at the time of diagnosis, typical FM systems may result in over-amplification that could cause distortion of the speech signal and even hearing loss through noise exposure. In addition, personal FM styles may be perceived as undesirable by parents and pupils with CAPD. If personal FM systems are selected as an environmental treatment option, they must have low-power output and minimum gain to avoid over-amplification.

The iSense by Phonak (Figure 12–1) was designed specifically for listeners with normal hearing sensitivity. The iSense is a miniaturized FM receiver that can be used with a variety of FM transmitters. The discreet, ear-level receiver is easily fit by an audiologist. Its primary purpose is to improve listening and attention skills and perhaps the academic abilities of children with CAPD and ADHD by improving the SNR and enhancing signal saliency.

A study by Updike (2005) asked if personal FM systems, specifically the Edu-Link (the prior version of the iSense), actually improved the attention and achievement of children with ADHD and CAPD. Specifically, Updike wanted to know if the EduLink could be used as a tool to enhance the speech discrimination skills, classroom behavior, and academic performance of children with ADHD and CAPD. Updike studied 12 children 8 to 10 years old: 6 with diagnosed CAPD and 6 with diagnosed ADHD. All were given the following tests: hearing screening, tympanometry, acoustic reflex thresholds (screening), word recognition

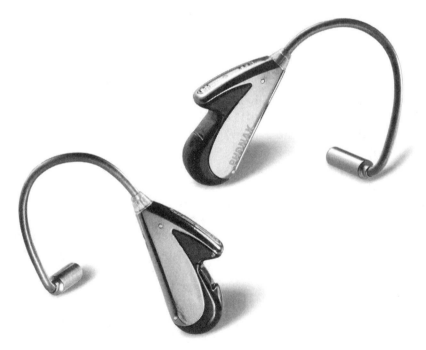

Figure 12–1. The iSense, a miniaturized FM receiver, was designed for listeners with normal hearing sensitivity and can be used with a variety of FM transmitters. Photo Courtesy of Phonak.

testing, and the SCAN Subtest 3–Competing Words (Keith, 1986). The results of the study clearly illustrated that with the use of the personal FM system, the word recognition of students with CAPD and ADHD for phonetically balanced kindergarten word lists (PBK) performance improved significantly in quiet and in noisy classrooms using a +5 dB SNR for both student groups; attending and classroom behaviors improved significantly as measured by attention surveys and classroom observations for both student groups; academic scores improved significantly in all subject areas in both fall and spring semesters for students with CAPD; academic scores improved significantly in some subject areas for students with ADHD; and both teachers and students highly approved of the EduLink personal FM system. An appropriately fit personal FM system can improve the SNR by +15 to +20 dB (Hawkins & Yacullo, 1984).

Johnston and colleagues (2009) evaluated 10 children with a positive diagnosis of CAPD who were fitted with Phonak EduLink FM devices for home and classroom use. Prior to FM use, baseline measures showed significantly lower speech-perception scores and decreased academic performance and psychosocial problems for children with CAPD when compared with an age-and gender-matched control group. During the school year, repeated measures demonstrated speech perception improvement in noisy classroom environments as well as significant academic and psychosocial benefits for children with CAPD when compared with matched groups. Compared with the control group, the children with CAPD showed greater speech perception advantage with FM technology. Importantly, after prolonged FM use, even when not wearing the EduLink, speech perception abilities were improved in the children with CAPD, suggesting the possibility of enhanced auditory system function.

Hall (2011) conducted case studies on triplet adolescent males (age 13 years) who were having academic difficulties in middle school; two of the brothers (subjects B and C) were diagnosed with CAPD following testing. A personal FM system was recommended for subjects B and C for classroom use. Follow-up monitoring revealed child B was resistant to FM use and did not follow recommendations, but child C did. Child C, who followed recommendations for FM use demonstrated marked improvement in auditory processing and in school performance as evidenced by grades, over the course of an academic year. Furthermore, at the end of the period of intervention, the same central auditory test battery showed no evidence of CAPD for child C. On the other hand, child B who did not comply with daily use of a personal FM system in middle school, showed no progress in auditory processing and continued to experience academic problems.

Friederichs and Friederichs (2005) investigated whether changes in electrophysiological late event potential patterns could be used to reflect clinical changes in children with CAPD resulting from using the EduLink personal FM system. They found that auditory event related potentials are in fact sensitive to performance changes in children with CAPD who used an EduLink personal FM system. Specifically, they found that in the case of infrequent tone responses, development of the classical P2/P3 distribution pattern with an increase in P2 amplitude was observed in the experimental group after both 6 months and 1 year of FM use; this maturation was not observed in the control group. The

EduLink did not replace, but rather augmented other intervention measures such as speech-language therapy.

A recent study by Hornickel et al. (2012) evaluated the use of the EduLink personal FM system (prior version of the iSense personal FM system) on auditory neurophysiology and reading skills in children with dyslexia and CAPD and compared their auditory neurophysiology to typically developing children. Specifically, 38 children who attended private schools with rich academic environments for children with severe reading and learning impairments were monitored and tested over the course of one year; 19 used the EduLink and all received the same curriculum. An age- and sex-matched group of 26 typically developing children was included in the study. Reading ability, phonological awareness and auditory brainstem function response to speech were tested. Children who used the EduLink improved on phonological awareness and reading. The matched control group of 19 children with dyslexia who attended the same schools but did not use the EduLink did not improve on these measures. An exciting finding revealed that children with dyslexia who used the EduLink had more consistent auditory brainstem responses to speech after one year. This change was not observed for children with dyslexia in the same classrooms who did not use the FM system, nor in the age- and sex-matched group of 26 typically developing children. The absence of changes in both control groups suggest that without the FM intervention, neural response consistency is not expected to change in either typically developing or dyslexic children. Children with the greatest improvement in phonological awareness showed the greatest improvement in neural response consistency. These decreases in auditory variability as seen electrophysiologically, suggested a fundamental change in how the auditory system represents and accesses speech. Hornickel et al. (2012) posited that inconsistent neural processing of sound underlies and reflects the variability in auditory processing that is common in children with dyslexia. The authors further suggest that the personal FM system resulted in neural and behavioral changes due to improved clarity of the acoustic signal and a subsequent enhancement of auditory attention as a result of improved SNR. FM systems enhance the SNR of the teacher's voice, which may contribute to the arousal, orientation, and attention by the students, thereby lessening a portion of the cognitive burden required for learning.

To summarize, studies conducted to date support the effectiveness of personal FM systems for children with CAPD in obtaining short-term and long-term objectives, including measurable changes in brain function. Certainly additional research is needed; however, these initial studies strongly suggest that personal FM systems could be considered as a viable treatment option, with or without additional accommodations.

Sound-Field Systems— FM or Infrared

This section provides general information about sound-field technology and its use in the classroom for all children, and particularly for those with CAPD. Sound-field technology, now referred to as CADS (classroom audio distribution systems) is an effective educational tool that allows control of the acoustic environment in a classroom thereby facilitating acoustic accessibility of teacher instruction for all children in the room (Crandell, Smaldino, & Flexer 2005). A sound-field system looks like a wireless public address system, but it is designed specifically to ensure that the entire speech signal, including the weak high frequency consonants, reaches every child in the room. By using this technology, an entire classroom can be amplified through the use of one, two, three, or four portable or wall- or ceiling-mounted loudspeakers.

The teacher wears a wireless microphone transmitter, just like the one worn for a personal FM unit, with the teacher's voice sent via radio waves (FM) or light waves (IR) to an amplifier that is connected to the loudspeakers (Figure 12–2A). There are no wires connecting the teacher with the equipment. The radio or light wave link allows the teacher to move about freely, unrestricted by wires (Figure 12–2B).

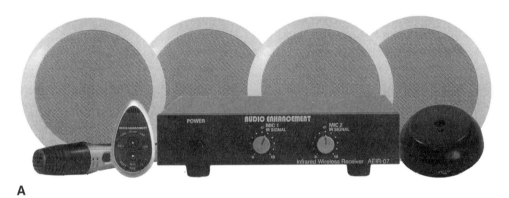

A

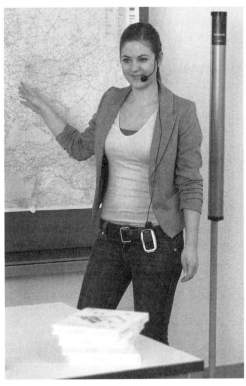

Figure 12–2. Classroom Audio Distribution Systems (CADS) function by having the teacher wear a wireless microphone transmitter, which transmits the teacher's speech via light waves— infrared (**A**), or radio waves—FM (**B**) (Digital Modulation) to an amplifier and loudspeakers. **A** is IR-2007 Dual Channel Infrared Receiver System by Audio Enhancement shown with student handheld pass-around microphone, an all-in-one teacher "pendant-style" microphone, four speakers, and ceiling-mounted dome sensor, provided courtesy of Audio Enhancement. **B** is the DigiMaster 5000 portable loudspeaker with teacher-worn Inspiro wireless dynamic FM transmitter. Photos courtesy of Phonak.

B

Classroom Audio Distribution Systems: A More Descriptive Term

The term CADS is more descriptive of sound-field function. Some teachers, parents, and acoustical engineers interpret the labels "sound-field amplification" and "classroom amplification" to mean that all sounds in the classroom are made louder. This misunderstanding may give the impression that sound is blasted into a room, causing rising noise levels, interfering with instruction in adjacent rooms, and provoking anxiety in pupils. In actuality, when the equipment is installed and used appropriately, the reverse is true. The amplified teacher's voice can sound soothing, as it is evenly distributed throughout the room easily reaching every child. The room quiets as students attend to spoken instruction. In fact, the listener is aware of the sound distribution and ease of listening only when the equipment is turned off. The overall purpose of the equipment is to improve *acoustic saliency* by having the details of spoken instruction continually reach the brains of all pupils. In addition, other audio sources (e.g., computer, iPod, DVD, SmartPhone) can be channeled through the CADS. Hence, the term CADS more accurately describes how sound-field systems function and is the preferred terminology.

Children Who Might Benefit From CADS

It could be argued that virtually all children could benefit from CADS because the improved SNR creates a more favorable learning environment. If children can hear better, clearer, and more consistently, they should have an opportunity to learn more efficiently (Rosenberg et al., 1999). Indeed, some school systems have established the use of CADS in every classroom as a district goal (Knittel, Myott, & McClain, 2002).

No one disputes the necessity of creating a favorable visual field in a classroom. A school building never would be constructed without lights in every classroom. However, because hearing is invisible and more difficult to understand, the necessity of creating a favorable auditory field may be questioned by school personnel. Nevertheless, studies continue to show that CADS facilitate opportunities for improved academic performance (Crandell, Smaldino, & Flexer, 2005; Flexer, 2004).

Millett and Purcell (2010) evaluated the benefit of IR CADS in 12 first-grade classrooms compared with 12 classrooms without CADS in Canada. They identified a greater change in the percentage of students reading at grade level over one year in the CADS-equipped classrooms, as well as trends toward improved reading outcomes for students at risk for reading difficulty (though changes were not statistically significant).

In addition to children with CAPD, populations that seem to be especially in need of SNR-enhancing technology to focus attention and overcome hearing problems include children with fluctuating conductive hearing impairments, unilateral hearing impairments, minimal permanent hearing impairments, cochlear implants, cognitive disorders, learning disabilities, attention problems, articulation disorders, and behavior problems (Anderson & Arnoldi, 2011; Rosenberg et al., 1999; Smaldino & Flexer, 2012). Children with CAPD are in particular need of this equipment as a first line of treatment because by definition their auditory neural brain centers are impaired (Friederichs & Friederichs, 2005; Hornickel et al., 2012).

Maag and Anderson (2007) evaluated the effects of CADS on the speed at which three elementary-school students with ADHD responded to teacher commands. Following introduction of the amplification system, improvements were seen for all tasks evaluated, including difficult tasks such as multiple instructions given simultaneously. Teachers who use CADS report that they also benefit (Rosenberg et al., 1999). Many state they need to use less energy projecting their voices; they have less vocal abuse, and are less tired by the end of the school day. Teachers also report the system increases their efficiency as teachers, requiring fewer repetitions, thus allowing for more actual teaching time. Morrow and Connor (2011) used ambulatory phonation monitoring and analysis to evaluate elementary school music teachers' vocal load. Analysis revealed significant decreases in vocal intensity and phonation time when amplification was in use, evidence of reduced overall vocal load. These results support previous findings of significantly decreased strain on teachers' voices when CADS are in use (e.g., Blair, 2006).

With an increasing number of schools incorporating principles of inclusion (as stipulated in Public Law 94-142—now referred to as IDEA) where children who would have been in self-contained placements are in the mainstream classroom, CADS offer a way of enhancing the classroom learning environment for the benefit of all children. It is a win-win situation.

Selection, Installation, and Monitoring of CADS

Not all classroom acoustic environments are improved by use of CADS. For exam-

ple, Wilson, Marinac, Pittv, and Burrows (2011) reported that IR CADS installation resulted in small but significant improvements in listening and auditory analysis for children aged 7 to 9 in some, but not all, Australian classrooms included in their study. Classrooms in schools with lower background noise and reverberation times tended to show more benefit from CADS, leading the authors to suggest that CADS may not be beneficial in acoustically unsuitable rooms such those with open classroom plans. Lubman (2008) argued that installation of CADS should not be regarded as a substitute for appropriate noise control in classrooms. Shield, Greenland, and Dockrell (2010) offered information about appropriate noise control and strategies to maximize intelligibility in open-plan classroom environments.

Multiple issues need to be considered for the effective selection and installation of CADS. Perhaps the primary issue is the number and positioning of loudspeakers (Boothroyd, 2004; Dillon, 2012). How many loudspeakers and where to place them are probably the most frequently asked questions when considering CADS. More data-based studies are needed to investigate these questions because there are many geometric and acoustic variables present in each individual classroom environment, as demonstrated by Wilson et al. (2011). Classroom variables include size, shape, construction materials, and seating arrangements. Learning styles also vary considerably: whole group instruction, individual learning, small group interactive learning, learning centers, independent learning, self-contained classes, and open-concept classrooms. Teaching style is another important variable and includes single-teacher lecture, team teaching, or multiple teaching occurring simultaneously at several learning centers throughout the room. The students themselves add yet additional variables as a function of their ages, numbers in a class and the presence of comorbid disabling conditions. Therefore, a pragmatic approach is useful for ordering and installing CADS. This pragmatic approach considers the individual classroom, the individual teacher and teaching style(s) used in the classroom, and the nature of the pupils who learn in that particular classroom. Boothroyd (2004) noted that a simulation approach is another strategy that holds great promise for resolving many of the unknowns in loudspeaker placement.

A typical CADS design goal is to increase the signal intensity of the talker's voice uniformly by about 10 dB throughout the classroom (Crandell, Kreisman, Smaldino, & Kreisman, 2004; Dillon, 2012). In order to accomplish this goal, one must know something about the room and also about the loudspeakers used in the CADS. Interestingly, in some cases, reverberation can actually benefit speech perception when students are seated close to the class loudspeakers. Although late room reflections interfere with the speech signal and are considered noise (Crandell et al., 2004), earlier reflections add to the original speech signal and actually increase the intensity of the original signal in a positive way (Boothroyd, 2004). By seating the student close to a loudspeaker, two goals are accomplished: The intensity of the signal is increased by amplification, and the addition of noise by late reverberation is avoided because the student receives only early reflections (Dillon, 2012; Smaldino & Flexer, 2012; Wroblewski et al., 2012).

Desktop or totable sound-field systems have been introduced to provide improved sound-field conditions for individual students. Figure 12–3 depicts a small loudspeaker placed on a student's desk. Usually, students with exceptional listening needs (e.g., students with cochlear implants or students with more severe central auditory processing problems) use this form of sound-field amplification. Obviously, other students in the classroom do not benefit from this kind of system because the sound improvements are localized to the student's immediate area, not broadcast uniformly throughout the classroom.

Adequate acoustic dispersion of the teacher's voice throughout the classroom is a function of many factors, including the wattage of the sound-field amplifier, the directionality of the loudspeakers, and the location and number of the loudspeakers in the room. It has been common practice to use multiple loudspeakers in order to accomplish adequate dispersion, although there is little research to base this decision on other than intuition and what sounds good to the installer. It is well recognized that carelessly installed, multiple loudspeakers can alter the acoustic spectrum of the talker's signal and increase the negative effects of reverberation (Siebein, 2004). On the other hand, single, point loudspeakers may not allow for an even distribution of sound throughout the room (Boothroyd, 2004).

There is some evidence that four or more loudspeakers installed and distributed in the ceiling provide the best dispersion of sound to all students in the room (Dillon, 2012). Several different loudspeaker designs, such as bending wave flat panel and high directivity loudspeakers, may provide more placement options (Prendergast, 2001). Ongoing research is needed in this area to ascertain the best

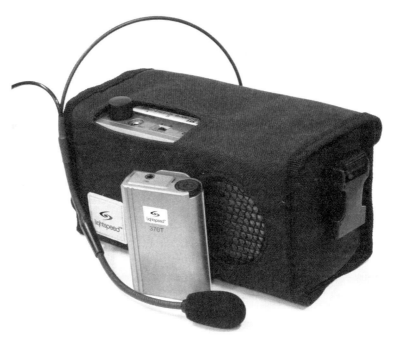

Figure 12–3. A small loudspeaker (desk-top system) placed on a pupil's desk can increase the loudness of the teacher's speech thereby improving the SNR for a particular student. (LES-391 desk-top speaker, courtesy of LightSPEED Technologies).

way to accomplish adequate dispersion of speech energy in classrooms.

Obviously, the goal is for all students in the learning field to have access to an even, consistent, and favorable SNR at a 10 dB improvement over unamplified speech (Crandell et al., 2004). Thus, if group learning is the mode of teaching, the entire classroom needs to be amplified evenly; all the pupils need to be able to hear the teacher at all times. The larger the classroom, typically the greater number of loudspeakers (three or four) needed so that each child is closer to a loudspeaker than he or she could be to the teacher (Dillon, 2012). Close proximity avoids loss of critical speech elements as the sound signal is transmitted across a physical space.

If the classroom has learning centers, a loudspeaker can be positioned close to each for maximum effective amplification at the critical locations (Crandell, Smaldino, & Flexer, 2005). If only one learning center is used at a time, then the other loudspeakers should be turned off. If a small resource classroom is used, one or two loudspeakers should provide an even and consistent SNR throughout the area.

If the classroom and class size is small, with only one teacher-instructed learning center in use at any given time, the teacher could carry a single battery-powered loudspeaker to each teaching location to amplify that specific environment. This single, portable loudspeaker arrangement has worked very effectively in some preschool settings.

Understanding CADS From a Universal Design Rather Than From a Treatment Perspective

Historically, amplification technologies such as hearing aids, personal FM systems, and now cochlear implants have been recommended as treatments for hearing loss. Because there certainly are populations for whom an enhanced SNR can mean the difference between passing and failing in school, CADS came to be recommended as treatments for hearing problems. If viewed as a treatment, CADS is recommended for a particular child and managed through the special education system. When recommended for a specific child with CAPD, CADS fits in the treatment category. However, with the recognition that all children require an enhanced SNR, comes the necessity of moving beyond thinking of CADS as a treatment. CADS need to be integrated into the general education arena. The concept of universal design can be useful in this regard.

The concept of universal design originated in the architectural domain, with the common examples of curb cuts, ramps, and automatic doors. After years of use, it was found that the modifications that were originally believed to be relevant for only a few people turned out to be useful and beneficial for a large percentage of the population (Gargiulo & Metcalf, 2013). In terms of learning, universal design means that the assistive technology is not specially designed for an individual student but rather for a wide range of students. Universally designed approaches are implemented by general education teachers rather than by special education teachers (Gargiulo & Metcalf, 2013). It is critical to note that implementation of CADS is shift-ing from the special education to the general education arena (Smaldino & Flexer, 2012). Universal design is good news for children with CAPD because it means they will be going into classrooms that are automatically equipped with the SNR-enhancing equipment necessary to address their limitations.

Teacher Inservices: A Necessity for Effective Equipment Use

Difficulties with CADS arise primarily from lack of teacher and administrator information about the rationale and use of the technology, and inappropriate setup and function of the equipment itself (Boothroyd, 2002; Smaldino & Flexer, 2012).

Initial inservices to teachers and administrators need to emphasize the "brain development" purpose of acoustic accessibility (Cole & Flexer, 2011). The relationship of hearing to literacy needs to be targeted, as does the fact that children listen differently than adults (as discussed earlier). Moreover, the concept of SNR needs to be explained. Microphone techniques need to be demonstrated to teachers so they can learn how to use the equipment to teach incidental listening strategies. It should be emphasized that teachers can use a much softer and more interesting voice because CADS provides the vocal projection. Problems can result when teachers place limitations on their teaching, or when they teach the same way with the technology as without it. A second microphone in the classroom—a pass-around microphone for the students—can greatly enhance teacher effectiveness. The pass-around microphone also allows children to hear each other, thereby increasing incidental learning and creating an auditory feedback loop through enhanced auditory self-monitoring of speech.

When advocating for SNR-enhancing technology for all children, and especially for a child with CAPD, one should emphasize that acoustic accessibility is not a luxury—it is a necessity—and one guaranteed by Section 504 of the Rehabilitation Act of 1973. Hearing is a first-order event for children in mainstreamed classrooms. If children cannot clearly and consistently hear classroom instruction, the entire premise of the educational system is undermined. Few families or schools have money for devices that are perceived as frills. However, when hearing takes its proper place at the head of the line relative to academic opportunities, then recommendations for SNR-enhancing technologies are taken seriously.

Legal Issues

Section 504 of the Rehabilitation Act of 1973

In most states, children with CAPD does not qualify for special education services through the Individuals with Disabilities Education Act or IDEA—unless they also have other documented/covered disabilities. Unlike special education legislation, Section 504 is not based on failure; rather it is predicated on accessibility (Rehabilitation Act of 1973). The law is a civil rights act that prohibits recipients (such as agencies and organizations) of federal funds from discriminating against "qualified individuals with disabilities in the United States." Specifically, a recipient of federal funds that operates a public elementary or secondary education program

shall provide a free appropriate public education (FAPE) to each qualified person with a disability who is in the recipient's jurisdiction, regardless of the nature or severity of the person's disability. The emphasis in Section 504 is equal opportunity or equal access. Section 504 does not link the child's disability to his or her need for special education services, but rather to the existence of limitations on a major life activity (Rehabilitation Act Amendments of 1992). Therefore, Section 504 is financed by general education and not by special education funds. On the other hand, IDEA requires that a child's disability be linked directly to the need for special education services in order to benefit from the educational process (IDEA, 2004).

The 504 plan can outline access support with accommodations. However, 504's regulations are not as clearly defined or as financially supported as IDEA's. Any student who qualifies for an individualized educational plan automatically qualifies for a 504 Plan, but the reverse is not true. In order to qualify for a 504 Plan, some documentation must be provided showing that equal access cannot be obtained without it. See Chapter 5 for school policies, processes and services for children with CAPD.

Show the Need for Technology

The key to securing technology from the school system is to obtain data documenting need (Ackerhalt & Wright, 2003; Anderson & Smaldino, 2012). A multifactored evaluation (MFE), which is a thorough evaluation by a multidisciplinary team, is necessary to document the need for a child to receive special services. The last category on most MFE forms is "assistive technology needs." In order for assistive technology to be recommended within any legislative framework, some type of evaluation must be conducted. We must document that the child's failure in the regular education system is linked to hearing difficulties in the classroom and that the child with CAPD cannot obtain an appropriate education unless personal FM or CADS are utilized.

Hearing Assistance Technology Guidelines From the American Academy of Audiology

The American Academy of Audiology's *Clinical Practice Guidelines for Remote Microphone Hearing Assistance Technologies for Children and Youth Birth–21 Years* (AAA, 2008) provides a rationale and comprehensive protocol for devices that use remote microphones, such as personal FMs and CADS. These guidelines apply not only to children with all degrees of hearing loss, but also to children with normal hearing who have special listening requirements, which includes children with CAPD. The protocol contains a core statement that addresses the complex process of hearing assistance technology selection, fitting, and management, plus supplements that outline procedures for fitting and verification of ear level FM (Supplement A) and classroom audio distribution systems (CADS) (Supplement B). The guidelines discuss regulatory considerations and qualifications of personnel as well as candidacy, fitting, and verification protocols. Monitoring and managing equipment is discussed in detail, including procedures for checking systems to be sure they are working. Strategies for implementing guidelines in the schools

are offered. For access to the full document, please refer to http://www.audiology.org/resources/documentlibrary/Documents/HATGuideline.pdf.

Efficacy Measures for SNR Enhancing Technology

Efficacy can be defined as the extrinsic and intrinsic value of a treatment (Crandell, Smaldino, & Flexer, 2005). Even though an environmental modification might have general value, some measurement needs to be made to show that the individual student in question is obtaining some benefit (Anderson & Smaldino, 2012). Benefit may be measured through educational performance, behavioral speech perception tests, direct measures of changes in brain development, or through functional assessments. Functional assessments are the most common and easily administered efficacy measure.

Functional Assessments as a Measure of Efficacy for a Child With CAPD

Functional assessments as a measure of efficacy are typically accomplished by having the teacher, student, or parent complete a questionnaire before and after use of the personal FM or CADS. Several functional assessment measures are available commercially and described below, including the SIFTER, LIFE-R, CHAPS, and the Fisher's Auditory Problems Checklist.

SIFTER: Screening Instrument for Targeting Educational Risk

The SIFTER is a one-page form that is easily filled out by the teacher or teachers at multiple intervals during a school year (Anderson, 1989). The form allows the teacher to observe and rate the student's performance as compared with typical students in the class relative to five content areas of academics, attention, communication, class participation, and school behavior. The total score in each area is recorded as pass, marginal, or fail. Even though the SIFTER was originally developed to identify students at risk for listening problems, it has proven to be useful in establishing efficacy of intervention in the classroom. When used in a pretest/posttest paradigm, any change in the child's classroom performance as a result of the FM intervention can be noted and documented.

LIFE-R: Listening Inventories for Education–Revised

Using the LIFE-R (Anderson, Smaldino & Spangler, 2011), the student self-rates his or her ability to hear and understand in each of 15 listening situations. A separate form allows the teacher to evaluate the student's listening difficulty. Sections include classroom listening situations and situations outside the classroom. The addition of student input about their personal classroom listening difficulties improves the overall validity of this subjective approach to efficacy. See the following website to obtain the LIFE-R: http://successforkidswithhearingloss.com/wp-content/uploads/2011/08/Teacher-LIFE-R.pdf.

CHAPS: Children's Auditory Performance Scale

This questionnaire, appropriate for children age 7 and older, consists of six subsections that were selected to represent the most often reported auditory difficulties experienced by children diagnosed as having CAPD (Smoski, Brunt, & Tannahill, 1998). The 36-item scale concerns six listening conditions: quiet, ideal, multiple inputs, noise, auditory memory/sequencing, and auditory attention span. Parents or teachers are asked to judge the amount of listening difficulty experienced by the child in question as compared with the listening difficulty of a typical child of similar background and age.

Fisher's Auditory Problems Checklist

This checklist (Fisher, 1985; modified by Johnson & Seaton, 2012), completed by a parent and/or teacher, provides a screening/rating of the child's attention, comprehension, discrimination, speech in noise, localization, sensitivity, long- and short-term memory, and speech and language problems.

Summary

The key issue explored in this chapter concerns the role of SNR-enhancing technology in the overall intervention program for children with CAPD. To summarize, this first issue or perhaps question is: What outcome/results are we expecting the technology to provide? There are both short- and long-term positive results demonstrated by studies summarized in this chapter. Short-term results include better auditory focus, increased attention span, longer time on task, and fewer disruptive behaviors. Of course, measuring these results can be tricky and may involve videotaping, or at the least, multiple pre-FM use and post-FM classroom observations and functional assessments. In addition, the child with CAPD may have spent many years "practicing" his diffuse focus and disruptive behaviors, so these unwanted behaviors may not disappear overnight. Long-term results are based on learning and practicing new skills and strategies and may include measurable changes in auditory neurophysiology. Since children are growing new neural connections in the brain and creating expanded "data files" of life and language experience, new skills could take many months to show up as improved learning and performance. Measurement of new skills could include improved grades, accurate class participation, and higher marks on standardized tests. In addition, improvement documented on functional tools, such as the SIFTER, LIFE-R, and CHAPS also could be useful.

The second issue explored in this chapter concerns expectations. Are we expecting the equipment to solve all of the student's problems, to be the "magic bullet"? Or, have we targeted a few, critical behaviors we are expecting the equipment to address. That is, extensive research has demonstrated that SNR-enhancing technology is a *necessary* first step toward create a viable classroom learning environment for students. However, that technology may not be *sufficient* to address all of the challenges experienced by a particular child with CAPD; additional accommodations and therapies may, and often are required as well.

An evaluation strategy could begin by identifying short- and long-term desired outcomes of FM use and the tools needed to measure those outcomes. Next, one ought to identify if the desired outcomes are expected to occur with or without additional accommodations or treatments, or prior to providing additional accommodations or treatments. What is realistic?

In summary, environmental modifications in the form of personal FM systems or CADS likely are viable first steps toward enhancing signal saliency and auditory focus for the child with CAPD. Numerous studies suggest that every classroom ought to have acoustic accessibility; including acoustic treatments to reduce noise and reverberation and well-installed and -used CADS as a *necessary* learning condition for all children. The universal use of CADS reduces the need for special education referrals; the technology may preclude many potential problems, including classroom listening difficulties experienced by children with CAPD (Flexer & Long, 2004).

References

AAA (American Academy of Audiology). (2008). *Clinical practice guidelines for remote microphone hearing assistance technologies for children and youth birth–21 years*. Retrieved from http://www.audiology.org/resources/documentlibrary/Documents/HATGuideline.pdf

Ackerhalt, A. H., & Wright, E. R. (2003). Do you know your child's special education rights? *Volta Voices, 10,* 4–6.

Anderson, K. (1989). *Screening instrument for targeting educational risk (SIFTER)*. Tampa, FL: Educational Audiology Association.

Anderson, K. (2004). The problem of classroom acoustics: The typical classroom soundscape is a barrier to learning. *Seminars in Hearing, 25,* 117–129.

Anderson, K., & Arnoldi, K. A. (2011). *Building skills for success in the fast-paced classroom*. Hillsboro, OR: Butte.

Anderson, K. L., & Smaldino J.J. (2012). Providing audiology services to school children: More than just preferential seating. (2012). *Hearing Journal, 65*, 50–54.

Anderson, K., Smaldino, J., & Spangler, C. (2011). *Listening Inventory for Education-Revised (LIFE-R)*. Retrieved from http://successforkidswithhearingloss.com/wp-content/uploads/2011/08/Teacher-LIFE-R.pdf

ASHA (American Speech-Language-Hearing Association). (2005). *Acoustics in educational settings: Position statement*. Retrieved from http://www.asha.org/policy/PS2005-00028.htm

Berlin, C. I., & Weyand, T. G. (2003). *The brain and sensory plasticity: Language acquisition and hearing*. Clifton Park, NY: Thomson Delmar Learning.

Bess, F. H., & Humes, L. E. (2003). *Audiology the fundamentals* (3rd ed.). Philadelphia, PA: Lippincott Williams & Wilkins.

Bhatnagar, S. C. (2002). *Neuroscience for the study of communicative disorders* (2nd ed.). Philadelphia, PA: Lippincott Williams & Wilkins.

Blair, J. C. (2006). Teachers' impressions of classroom amplification. *Educational Audiology Review, 23*, 12–13.

Boothroyd, A. (1997). Auditory development of the hearing child. *Scandinavia Audiology, 26*(Suppl. 46), 9–16.

Boothroyd, A. (2004). Room acoustics and speech perception. *Seminars in Hearing, 25*, 155–166.

Chermak, G. D., & Musiek, F. E. (2007). *Handbook of central auditory processing disorder*. San Diego, CA: Plural.

Ching, T. Y., van Wanrooy, E., Dillon, H., & Carter L. (2011). Spatial release from masking in normal-hearing children and children who use hearing aids. *Journal of the Acoustical Society of America, 129*, 368–375.

Cole, E., & Flexer, C. (2011). *Children with hearing loss: Developing, listening, and talking, birth to six* (2nd ed.). San Diego, CA: Plural.

Crandell, C. C., Kreisman, B. M., Smaldino, J. J., & Kreisman, N. V. (2004). Room acoustics intervention efficacy measures. *Seminars in Hearing, 25*, 201–206.

Crandell, C. C., Smaldino, J. J., & Flexer, C. (2005). *Sound-field amplification: applications to speech perception and classroom acoustics* (2nd ed.). New York, NY: Thomson Delmar Learning.

Diamond, A., & Lee, K. (2011). Interventions shown to aid executive function development in children 4 to 12 years old. *Science, 333*, 959–964.

Dillon. H. (2012). *Hearing aids* (2nd ed.). New York, NY: Thieme Medical.

Doidge, N. (2007). *The BRAIN that changes itself*. London, UK: Penguin Books.

Fisher, L. I. (1985) Learning disabilities and auditory processing. In R. J. Van Hattum (Ed.), *Administration of speech-language services in the schools* (pp. 231–292). Houston, TX: College-Hill Press.

Flexer, C. (2004). The impact of classroom acoustics: Listening, learning, and literacy. *Seminars in Hearing, 25*, 131–140.

Flexer, C., & Long, S. (2003). Sound-field amplification: Preliminary information regarding special education referrals. *Communication Disorders Quarterly, 25*, 29–34.

Friederichs, E., & Friederichs, P. (2005). Electrophysiologic and psycho-acoustic findings following one-year application of a personal ear-level FM device in children with attention deficit and suspected central auditory processing disorder. *Journal of Educational Audiology, 12*, 29–34.

Gargiulo, R. M., & Metcalf, D. (2013). *Teaching in today's inclusive classrooms: A universal design for learning approach* (2nd ed.). Belmont, CA: Cengage Learning.

Hall, J. W. (2011). Auditory processing disorder: Application of FM technology. In J. R. Madell, & C. Flexer (Eds.), *Pediatric audiology casebook* (pp. 32–36). New York, NY: Thieme Medical.

Hawkins, D. B., & Yacullo, W. (1984). Signal-to-noise ratio advantage of binaural hearing aids and directional microphones under different levels of reverberation. *Journal of Speech and Hearing Disorders, 49,* 278–286.

Hornickel, J., Zecker, S., , Bradlow, A., & Kraus, N. (2012). Assistive listening devices drive neuroplasticity in children with dyslexia. *Proceedings of the National Academy of Sciences, 109(41),* 16731–16736.

IDEA. (2004). *Individuals with Disabilities Education Improvement Act of 2004,* PL 108–446, 20 U.S.C. &1400 et seq.

Johnson, C. D., & Seaton. J. (2012). *Educational audiology handbook* (2nd ed.). Clifton Park, NY: Delmar-Cengage Learning.

Johnston, K. N., John, A. B., Kreisman, N. V., Hall, J. W., & Crandell, C. C. (2009). Multiple benefits of personal FM system use by children with auditory processing disorder (APD). *International Journal of Audiology, 48,* 371–383.

Keith, R. W. (1986). *SCAN: A screening test for auditory processing disorders.* San Antonio, TX: Psychological Corporation.

Knittel, M. A. L., Myott, B., & McClain, H. (2002). Update from Oakland schools sound-field team: IR vs. FM. *Educational Audiology Review, 19,* 10–11.

Leibold, L. J., & Neff, D. (2011). Masking by remote-frequency noise band in children and adults. *Ear and Hearing, 32,* 663–666.

Lubman, D. (2008). *Sound field amplification competes with noise control.* Paper presented at the 156th meeting of the Acoustical Society of America, Miami, FL.

Maag, J. W., & Anderson, J. M. (2007). Sound-field amplification to increase compliance to directions in students with ADHD. *Behavioral Disorders, 32,* 238–253.

Mendel, L. L., Roberts, R. A., & Walton, J. H. (2003). Speech perception benefits from sound field fm amplification. *American Journal of Audiology, 12,* 114–124.

Merzenich, M. M. (2010, April). *Brain plasticity-based therapeutics in an audiology practice.* Learning Lab presented at the American Academy of Audiology National Conference, San Diego, CA.

Millett, P., & Purcell, N. (2010). Effect of sound field amplification on grade 1 reading outcomes. *Canadian Journal of Speech-Language-Pathology and Audiology, 31,* 17–24.

Morrow, S. L., & Connor, N. P. (2011). Voice amplification as a means of reducing vocal load for elementary school teachers. *Journal of Voice, 25,* 441–446.

Nabelek, A., & Nabelek, I. (1985). Room acoustics and speech perception. In J. Katz (Ed.), *Handbook of clinical audiology* (3rd ed.). Baltimore, MD: Williams & Wilkins.

Nelson, P. B., & Blaeser, S. B. (2010). Classroom acoustics: What possibly could be new? *ASHA Leader, 15,* 16–19.

Prendergast, S. (2001). A comparison of the performance of classroom amplification with traditional and bending wave speakers. *Journal of Educational Audiology,* 2001 annual issue.

Rehabilitation Act Amendments of 1992, P.L. 102-569. (1992, October 29). *United States Statutes at Large, 106,* 4344–4488.

Rehabilitation Act of 1973, P.L. 93-112. (1973, September 26). *United States Statutes at Large, 87,* 355–394.

Rosenberg, G. G., Blake-Rahter, P., Heavner, J., Allen, L., Redmond, B. M., Phillips, J., & Stigers, K. (1999). Improving classroom acoustics (ICA): A three-year FM sound field classroom amplification study. *Journal of Educational Audiology, 7,* 8–28.

Rubin, R. L., Flagg-Williams, J. B., Aquino-Russell, C. E., & Lushinaton, T. P. (2011). The classroom listening environment in the early grades. *Canadian Journal of Speech-Language Pathology and Audiology, 35,* 344–359.

Sharma, A., Dorman, M. F., & Spahr, A. J. (2002). A sensitive period for the development of the central auditory system in children with cochlear implants: Implications for age of implantation. *Ear and Hearing, 23,* 532–539.

Shield, B., Greenland, E., & Dockrell, J. (2010). Noise in open plan classrooms in primary schools: A review. *Noise and Health, 12,* 225–234.

Siebein, G. W. (2004). Understanding classroom acoustic solutions. *Seminars in Hearing, 25*, 141–154.

Smaldino, J. (2011). New developments in classroom acoustics and amplification. *Audiology Today, 23*, 30–36.

Smaldino, J., & Flexer, C. (2012). *Handbook of acoustic accessibility: Best practices for listening, learning and literacy in the classroom*. New York, NY: Thieme Medical.

Smoski, W. J., Brunt, M. A., & Tannahill, J. C. (1998*). Children's Auditory Performance Scale (CHAPS)*. Tampa, FL: Educational Audiology Association.

Tallal, P. (2005). *Improving language and literacy is a matter of* Time. Paper presented at Speech, Language and Learning Center Beth Israel Medical Center, New York City.

Updike, C. (2005, July). *Children with ADD and APD: Do personal FM systems improve their attention and achievement?* Presented at the Educational Audiology Association Conference.

Valente, D. L., Plevinsky, H. M., Franco, J. M., Heinrichs-Graham, E. C., & Lewis, D. E. (2012). Experimental investigation of the effects of the acoustical conditions in a simulated classroom on speech recognition and learning in children. *Journal of the Acoustical Society of America, 131*, 232–246.

Wilson, W. J., Marinac, J., Pittv, K., & Burrows, C. (2011). The use of sound-field amplification devices in different types of classrooms. *Language, Speech and Hearing Services in Schools, 42*, 395–407.

Wroblewski, M., Lewis, D. E., & Stelmachowicz, P. G. (2012). Effects of reverberation on speech recognition in stationary and modulated noise by school-aged children and young adults. *Ear and Hearing, 33*, 731–744.

CHAPTER 13

CLASSROOM MANAGEMENT
Collaboration With Families, Teachers, and Other Professionals

JEANANE M. FERRE

Central auditory processing disorder (CAPD) refers to a deficit in the perceptual processing of auditory stimuli and the neurobiological activity underlying that processing (ASHA, 2005a). Central auditory processing disorder is not the result of higher order language, cognitive, or related disorders, but may be associated with difficulties in higher order language, learning, and communication function. That is to say, CAPD may coexist with, but is not the result of, dysfunction in other modalities (ASHA, 2005a). In the diagnostic process, the audiologist administers well-controlled tests designed to determine the presence or absence of the disorder and to identify the specific perceptual processes that are impaired. In assessment, related professionals use formal and informal procedures to obtain evidence of the extent to which there exist difficulties in other sensory processing or higher order cognitive, language, or learning skills, as well as evidence of the functional strengths and weaknesses of the listener (ASHA, 2005a). This evaluation process leads to the differential diagnosis of central auditory processing disorder from neurocognitive and other related disorders and to the determination of the impact the disorder is likely to have on a listener's academic success, communication skills, and psychosocial well-being. The evaluation process is followed logically by intervention; the comprehensive, therapeutic treatment and management of the disorder designed to reduce or resolve specific impairments and to minimize the adverse impact of the disorder on the listener's life functions.

Intervention— A Balancing Act

For intervention to be effective, it is necessary to "balance" treatment and management components (Figure 13–1). In remediation or treatment, deficit-specific procedures designed to improve deficient skills are implemented. In management, efforts are directed toward minimizing the impact of the disorder in the listener's everyday life settings. The reader will find detailed discussions of issues related to treatment and specific treatment approaches in Chapters 7 through 11 of this volume. Chapters 12, 14, and 15 include discussions of CAPD management using technology and issues associated with management among adolescents and adults. In this chapter, environmental modifications and compensatory strategies commonly employed to minimize the adverse effects of CAPD on school-age children are described. Case studies are used to illustrate the importance and role of collaboration among professionals, students and their families in the management of CAPD among school-age children.

The Management Team

While most would agree that the audiologist's role in the diagnostic process is both essential and obvious, there is less agreement when it comes to intervention. Too often, the refrain is heard, "Audiologists *diagnose*, speech-language pathologists or others *treat*." Emanuel, Ficca, and Korczak (2011) found that while most audiologists (81%) believed that audiologists should provide recommendations for treatment, only 40% believed the audiolo-

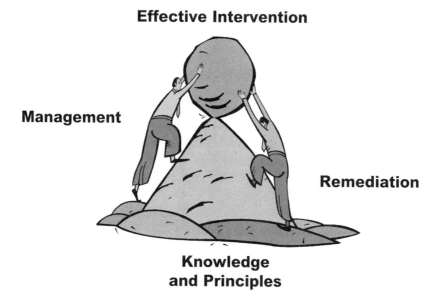

Effective Intervention

Management

Remediation

Knowledge and Principles

Figure 13–1. Intervention—the balanced efforts in management and remediation based on sound principles and accumulated neuroscientific knowledge.

gist should be responsible for provision of treatment of CAPD. Furthermore, presence of a CAPD can exacerbate and be exacerbated by other sensory and neurocognitive disorders, and CAPD manifests with a variety of clinical profiles. For these reasons, it is essential that case management, like the assessment process, be multidisciplinary in nature (Figure 13–2). Results from a comprehensive evaluation of auditory and language function should be included when discussing the overall academic, communicative, and psychosocial needs of the listener.

As a member of the assessment and intervention team, the audiologist offers insight regarding possible impact of central auditory processing disorder as it relates to other life skills. The audiologist works with other team members to develop and, as needed, to implement specific, meaningful, and realistic treatment and management strategies designed to improve auditory and related skills, as well as to minimize the day-to-day impact of the disorder on the listener's academic success, communication abilities, and/or sense of self. The audiologist applies scientific principles in developing and implementing deficit-specific treatment and management goals and strategies, to gauge the success of those strategies, and to extend intervention principles to all environments in order to maximize benefit.

In most cases, input from related professional disciplines, including, but not limited to, neuropsychology/psychology, special education, speech-language pathology, occupational therapy (OT), and physical therapy (PT)—is incorporated in the intervention process. This input may include diagnoses of comorbid conditions and identification of specific communication or academic difficulties to which the CAPD is a contributing or exacerbating factor. Parents, families, and other caregivers can offer important information regarding the disorder's impact on the student's day-to-day listening and psychosocial well-being and, therefore, parents and family members

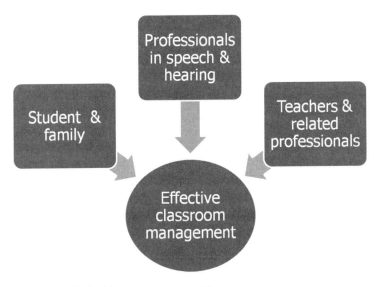

Figure 13–2. The management team.

also should be considered integral to the intervention team. In addition to understanding treatment goals, parents, teachers, and others need to know how to manage the central auditory processing disorder on a daily basis. This aspect of intervention extends beyond individualized *pull-out/push-in* sessions (i.e., therapy provided outside the classroom/ therapy provided within the classroom) with the speech-language pathologist or educational specialist, by complementing the efforts of specialists throughout the day, at school, and at home. These additional strategies encourage parents and teachers to modify the way they talk to and with children with central auditory processing disorder, help them choose activities to enhance listening skills, and modify the classroom and home environment to enable all children to meet their potential.

Interactive Intervention Approach

The goal of intervention for central auditory processing disorder should be to maximize the listener's access to and use of incoming auditory information. To that end, one must identify the components of a communication event. Ferre's (1998) M^3 intervention program characterizes any communication event—between parent and child, teacher and student, or student-to-student, as the interplay of three key components. These key components are the listening environment (the *medium*), the information/signal being communicated (the *message*), and the integrity of the listener (the *me*) (Figure 13–3). Compromises in any of these three components (e.g., poor room acoustics, sig-

nals having poor acoustic or linguistic quality, impaired auditory processing or active listening skills) adversely affect communication outcomes. Conversely, creating positive change in any of the key components (e.g., reducing classroom noise, speaking clearly, *looking and listening* while communicating) will enhance communication and the likelihood of success.

Focus on the Environment

It is estimated that up to 60% of classroom activities involve students listening to and participating in spoken communication with teachers or other students (ANSI, 2002). Thus, it is essential that classrooms be free of acoustical barriers. When assessing the listening environment, consideration should be given to both acoustic and nonacoustic variables that can affect speech perception. Acoustic variables include presence, nature, and level of background noise, signal strength relative to background noise, reverberation time, and distance between speaker and listener (Crandell & Smaldino, 2002). Nonacoustic factors include lighting, access to visual cues, and presence of visual and/or physical distractions (Ferre, 1997, 2007). (See Chapter 2 for discussion of these acoustic variables.)

Background Noise

Background noise refers to any auditory disturbance in a room that interferes with listening (Crandell & Smaldino, 2002). Noise within a room can come from internal sources (in the building, but outside the room), external sources (outside the building) and in-room sources. Background noise can adversely affect

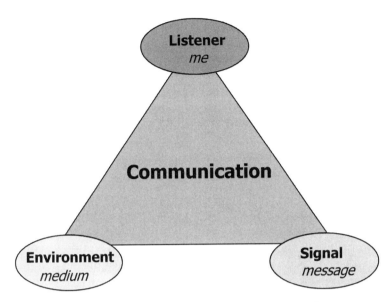

Figure 13–3. The communication triangle. What we hear—*message*; where we hear—environment or *medium*; and how we hear —*me* as the key elements in communication.

speech perception by masking the acoustic and linguistic cues of a message and by distracting the listener from the communication event (Bradley & Sato, 2008; Crandell & Smaldino, 2002).

The audiologist can use a sound level meter to measure the intensity of noise, as well as its spectral and temporal aspects that also contribute to the degree to which the noise interferes with listening (Nabalek & Nabalek, 1994). Speech spectrum noise, multitalker babble, and real-life in-room noise appear to affect more adversely the speech recognition skills of young children, college-age students and adults with academic difficulties than does pink or nonspeech-like noise (Chermak, Vonhof, & Bendel, 1989; Jamieson, Kranjc, Yu, & Hodgett, 2004; Papso & Blood, 1989).

Signal-to-noise ratio (SNR) refers to the intensity of the signal relative to the background noise. Holding other factors constant, as the SNR becomes less favorable, speech recognition becomes poorer for all listeners (Cooper & Cutts, 1972). For listeners with normal hearing, speech recognition is not severely reduced until the SNR reaches 0 dB (Crandell & Smaldino, 2002). SNRs that are at least 2 to 15 dB more favorable than those needed by normal hearing listeners are required by very young listeners and those with hearing impairment, speech-language disorders, limited English proficiency, academic disabilities, or central auditory processing disorder (Bronzaft, 1982; Crandell & Smaldino, 1996, 2002; Evans & Maxwell, 1997; Finitzo-Heiber & Tillman, 1978; Maxwell & Evans, 2000; Plomp & Mimpen, 1979).

Reverberation

Reverberation, or echo, refers to the persistence of a sound in an enclosed space due to the multiple reflections of sound waves off hard surfaces. A room's reverberation may be expressed in terms of its reverberation time (RT), or the amount of time required for the sound to significantly decay (i.e., decrease by 60 dB) after the signal source has stopped. As noted above, the audiologist measures a room's RT using a sound level meter. However, new technologies have made it possible to estimate a room's RT using computer software (e.g., RevMeter Pro app for iPhone).[1] Reverberation affects speech recognition by masking direct sound (Nabalek & Nabalek, 1994). While all rooms have some reverberation, large and irregularly shaped rooms tend to have longer RTs than smaller rooms or those with greater amounts of absorptive material. For normal hearing adults, recognition is not adversely affected until the RT exceeds 1.0 second (Finitzo-Hieber & Tillman, 1978); however, for children with impaired hearing, language, or processing skills, speech perception may be compromised at RTs as low as 0.4 seconds (Crandell, Smaldino, & Flexer, 1995).

Classroom Noise Abatement

Classroom noise abatement programs should seek to maintain an SNR of at least +15 with reverberation time of 0.4 seconds or less (ASHA, 1995, 2005b). Reverberation times can be somewhat longer (i.e., 0.6 seconds) in small and mid-size classrooms, and up to 0.7 seconds in larger classrooms, without degrading speech intelligibility for normal hearing listeners, provided an SNR of +15 or better is maintained (ANSI, 2002).

Classroom noise abatement techniques ranging from relatively simple to rather extensive, can be implemented to achieve these SNR and RT goals. Extensive, and often expensive, solutions for improving classroom acoustics include reduction or elimination of open classrooms; relocation of teaching spaces away from playgrounds, gymnasiums, or cafeterias; building infrastructure changes such as double-paned windows, noise control devices on heating, air conditioning, and ventilation systems; use of smaller and less irregularly shaped classrooms; changes in lighting fixture type (i.e., from fluorescent to incandescent) and location; and lowered ceiling levels. Simpler and less expensive classroom noise abatement can be accomplished by closing windows, carpeting rooms, using curtains, drapes, and/or acoustic ceiling tiles, placing baffles within the listening space, and damping highly reflective surfaces. Placing bookcases perpendicular to each other or creating a 6- to 8-inch space between side-by-side bookcases can create baffles and minimize noise. Cork bulletin boards and the use of fabric to cover hard surfaces increases sound absorption and dampens reflective surfaces. Felt pads or rubber caps on the bottoms of chair and table legs minimize furniture-to-floor noise. For more detailed information on specific acoustical modifications in the classroom the reader is referred to Sillman (2000), Cran-

---

[1]iPhone is a registered trademark of Apple Corporation. The RevMeter Pro application is available from Apple's "App Store." Due to limitations in the dynamic range of the iPhone microphone, the software measures decays of only 20 or 30 dB (i.e., RT20, RT30) with the software makers suggesting that these values be multiplied by 3 or 2, respectively, to estimate RT60 values. The app is not recommended for use in obtaining exact measurements of RT.

dell and Smaldino (2001), and Crandell and Smaldino (2004).

In the home, parents and caregivers should be reminded about simple ways to reduce noise and minimize acoustic barriers to listening such as closing doors and windows; reducing radio, stereo, and television volume; using carpet and drapes; rearranging furniture and changing lighting; and minimizing the number of speakers talking at the same time.

Distance From Source

Distance between the speaker and listener can affect speech recognition. Generally, sound intensity decreases with increasing distance from the source (Ostergaard, 2000). Sound in a room may be direct or reverberant. Direct sound is the sound reaching the listener without obstruction. Reverberant sound is sound energy comprising reflected waves within the space. As distance from the speaker increases, the amount of reverberant sound tends to increase and dominate the signal. Boothroyd (2004) noted that for students seated near the back of a classroom, the signal was composed almost entirely of reverberant sound while listeners near the front of the room received almost all-direct sound. He suggested that a distance of 3 to 6 feet from the source would create optimal audibility, with speech recognition decreasing beyond that critical distance.

Nonacoustic Factors

When assessing the physical space, attention also should be given to nonacoustic factors such as lighting, presence of visual cues, and presence of visual and physical distractions. Room lighting can affect ability to use visual cues and main-tain attention on task. Replacing fluorescent lighting with incandescent lighting not only eliminates the hum often produced by these lights, it also improves access to visual cues by reducing harshness and glare. Speakers should avoid being *backlit*, that is, standing with the light coming from behind the speaker rather than on the speaker's face. Teachers should be reminded to speak *after* looking down at their notes or writing on a board rather than *while* writing or reading. The importance of maintaining eye contact and using visual cueing to assist and gauge understanding should be discussed with teachers, specialists, and parents.

Preferential classroom seating can be used to counteract the adverse effects of distance and poor lighting and enhance the listener's ability to use available relevant visual cues. In preferential seating, an effort is made to maximize both the acoustic and visual aspects of the signal based on the summative benefits of bimodal processing (Erber, 1969; Sanders & Goodrich, 1971). The listener's speech perception is enhanced when seated nearer the speaker. Most students with central auditory processing disorder benefit from use of visual cues and should be encouraged to *look and listen* to maximize speechreading opportunities. Schow and Nerbonne (1996) noted that speechreading is optimal at a distance of 5 feet from the speaker, decreasing significantly as distance from the speaker increases. Teachers can be encouraged to use the *Arc of the Arms Rule* (Ferre, 1997) that places the listener near and facing the speaker at no more than a 45-degree angle. This seating arrangement, especially when the "listening arc" is situated away from distracting noise, enhances both signal audibility and accessibility of speechreading cues (Ferre, 1997). Depending on the type of auditory processing deficit that has been identified, it may be necessary to move students to a different listening, study or testing environment. Study/work carrels can be used to minimize visual distractions at school and in the home. Consultation with the OT/PT may result in changes in seating ergonomics (e.g., chair type or design) to minimize physical distractions that can interfere with listening or studying.

Summary

It has been established that by improving classroom acoustics, the listening and learning skills of all children can be enhanced (ANSI, 2002; Crandell & Smaldino, 2002). Before implementing environmental modifications, the audiologist should verify with other team members the specific needs of the student with CAPD in the classroom and at home. In addition, the specific profile of processing deficits should be identified clearly and modifications appropriately customized to that profile, as not all modifications outlined above may be beneficial for all profiles of central auditory processing disorder, as illustrated in the case histories at the end of this chapter. Considerations when assessing the listening environment are included in Appendix 13–A.

Focus on the Message

In addition to enhancing the environment, attention should be given to management strategies that enhance the acoustic, linguistic and related instructional aspects of the signal or message. Acoustic signal enhancement can be accomplished through assistive listening technology and by using clear speech techniques. Linguistic modifications include rephrasing information and adding nonauditory sensory cues. Instructional modifications include using preview material, adjusting length and type of message, and modifying response time and response mode.

Assistive Listening Technology

Technology (i.e., assistive listening devices [ALDs]) may be recommended to enhance the signal. The ALD is designed to improve the SNR reaching the listener's ear. Unlike traditional amplification where both the speech signal and the ambient noise are both amplified, the physical configuration of the personal ALD selectively amplifies the signal and has the effect of pulling the target signal away from the noise via mild gain amplification, thereby pushing the noise further into the perceptual background. This results in a significantly more favorable SNR and, in turn, improved speech reception. Sound-field FM (i.e., frequency modulated) systems enhance the target signal for groups of listeners. When used with proper diagnosis and monitoring, assistive listening technology can lead to improved auditory attention, short-term memory, auditory discrimination, and speech perception (Blake, Field, Foster, Plott, & Wertz, 1991; Crandell & Smaldino, 2002; Flexer, 2007; Rosenberg, 1998; Shapiro & Mistal, 1985; 1986; Stach, Loiselle, Jerger, Mintz, & Taylor, 1987). Direct signal enhancement via personal and sound-field technology is discussed in detail in Chapter 12.

Clear Speech

In direct signal enhancement discussed above, the listener's speech recognition is enhanced. In clear speech, the focus is on improving speech recognition by modifying the speaker's speech. Schum (1997) noted that in typical conversational speech it is not uncommon for speakers to articulate quickly, fail to project the voice, omit unnecessary or redundant sounds, and to run words and sounds together. These behaviors can adversely affect speech recognition not only for normal hearing listeners (Helfer, 1997), but also for those with hearing loss and auditory-based learning disabilities (Bradlow, Kraus, & Hayes, 2003; Payton, Uchanski, & Braida, 1994; Schum, 1996). A common complaint among students with central auditory processing disorder is mishearing parts or all of a message. In clear speech, the speaker is trained to speak at a slightly reduced rate and to use a slightly increased volume (Picheny, Durlach & Braida, 1985, 1986). In so doing, spectral boundaries and characteristics are enhanced, signal timing and prosody improves, and relative consonant-to-vowel intensities increase (Bradlow et al., 2003; Ferguson & Kewley-Port, 2003; Krause & Braida, 2004; Picheny et al., 1986). With a minimal amount of instruction and practice, most talkers can be trained to produce clear speech (Caissie, Campbell, Frenette, Scott, Howell, & Roy, 2005; Schum, 1996). With additional training, clear speech can even be achieved without necessarily reducing overall speaking rate (Krause & Braida, 2002, 2004). By coupling clear speech with an auditory-visual presentation, speech recognition is enhanced further (Helfer, 1997). Both the audiologist and the speech-language pathologist are in unique positions to assist classroom teachers, related professionals and parents in learning to use clear speech to improve day-to-day communication. A useful resource for teaching clear speech activities is the *Communication Is a Two-Way Street* pamphlet available from Oticon Corporation (http://www.oticonus.com).

Linguistic Modifications

Other beneficial changes to the message involve alterations to the nonacoustic and nonverbal aspects of the signal. By rephrasing a misheard signal, the speaker presents the listener with a more linguistically familiar and less ambiguous target, thereby fostering improved comprehension. For example, the ambiguous "Stop that!" can be replaced with the more explicit, "Stop tapping your pencil (feet, desk)." To gauge a listener's comprehension, use, "Tell me what you think I said" or "Tell me what you heard" rather than, "Do you understand?" That is, ask the listener to paraphrase the message to assess reception and understanding. Encourage students to repeat or restate whatever portions of the message they received, for example, "I heard you ask me 'where are you going', is that right?" or "I heard two things to do, but not three." Positively reinforce the effort and then *fill-in* the missing or misheard information. Adding complementary visual cues, examples, demonstrations, and manipulatives (e.g., using three-dimensional shapes during a geometry lesson, using colored beads to explain sorting or math concepts) can improve understanding, particularly for unfamiliar or abstract information. Limiting the overall amount of information given at one time, breaking long messages down into shorter (5- to 6-word) sequences, and adding or emphasizing *tag* words (e.g., *first, last, before, after, if, then*) enhances message salience and understanding (Ellis, 1989). When listening in class, some students with CAPD will require a recording device (e.g., smart pen) or a note-taker or scribe to assist note taking and improve the ability to *get the message* (Ferre, 2006).

Instructional Modifications

Preteaching or previewing material is designed to enhance familiarity, and thereby scaffold the listener's overall comprehension challenge. In general, the more familiar one is with the target, the easier the processing becomes. Books on tape, copies of teachers' notes/texts, Cliffs Notes™[2], seeing movies, and reading aloud to children can enhance familiarity with the subject, task demands, main ideas, key elements, and vocabulary. The increasing use of computer technology in the classroom enhances access to information for all students. Teachers are able to post syllabi, notes, entire lectures/class presentations, and curricular resources to a school's website or electronic blackboard and/or directly to a student's personal storage device (e.g., tablets, cell phones), enabling all students, including those with central auditory processing disorder and related learning issues to access information and increase familiarity.

For children with central auditory processing disorder, knowledge of the rules, structure, and task demands *up front* can minimize overload. It is important to note that for many of these children this knowledge is not acquired through mere exposure, but through explicit instruction, repeated practice and review and usage across a variety of contexts and settings (Ferre, 2006). When the message is in the form of a test, closed-set questions (i.e., multiple choice or fill-in) rather than more open-ended questions (e.g., essays) are preferred for students

with CAPD. In addition to test taking in quiet, separate environments, some students may need extended time for test taking or need test questions read to them to ensure understanding.

Many children with CAPD report experiencing excessive auditory fatigue. Scheduling *listening breaks* throughout the day, in which auditory message demands are limited, can minimize auditory overload. For example, do not schedule a spelling lesson right after a reading class. Intersperse lecture classes with activities that are more hands-on or less academically challenging (e.g., physical education). Do not schedule homework or therapy immediately after school. Instead, schedule some minutes of *down time* or physical activity after the school day ends and before therapy or homework sessions (Ferre, 2002). For homework, break tasks down and provide work breaks between activities. The student should do homework for an amount equal to no more than 1.5 times the time spent on homework by typically achieving same-age peers (e.g., if typical students spend 60 minutes on all homework, student in question should spend no more than 90 minutes). Encourage students to assist in structuring their homework. For example, have the student choose the order in which the assignments will be completed, number of minutes spent on each task, and/or the number of items to be accomplished in specified amount of time. Gradually increase the amount of time or number of items to be completed in that amount of time.

Sometimes the listening challenge simply exceeds the capability of the student with CAPD such that course substi-

---

[2]Cliffs Notes™ is a registered trademark of Hungry Minds, Inc.

tutions or waivers may be required. For example, consideration may be given to a nonverbal alternative to meet foreign language requirements. Many states not only recognize American Sign Language as a foreign language, but also accept it for credit at the high school and collegiate levels (LCNDEC, 2004). Some students may require a waiver or substitution (e.g., a culture course) for a foreign language requirement based on the nature and severity of their auditory processing difficulties. A highly structured and well-ordered language such as Hebrew or Latin may meet the second language needs of some children with CAPD.

Finally, how students are asked to respond to the message may require modification. For some students with central auditory processing disorder, it may be necessary to provide extended time, allow dictated responses on written exams, reduce use of oral exams, or allow answers to be written in a test booklet rather than transferred to a score sheet, especially for standardized testing. As with modifications to the environment, any modification to the type, quality, or length of the message or comparable adjustments to the required response to the message should be made only after clearly defining the specific profile of the central auditory processing disorder and establishing the specific needs of the individual student. Appendix 13–B provides a checklist of aspects of the message that may be modified to enhance instructional success.

Focus on the Listener

As illustrated in Figure 13–3, the listener plays an important role in the communication event. As noted previously,

direct treatment in CAPD intervention is designed to reduce not only the specific auditory deficit but also its adverse impact (Bellis, 2003; Chermak, 2007; Musiek, Chermak, & Weihing, 2007). Students with central auditory processing disorder need to understand the nature of their deficit and how it affects their lives (Ferre, 1997, 1998) and be able to respond to the question, "How can *I* change the environment, the message, or myself to improve the listening situation?" Students can be taught and encouraged to use (or ask others for) many of the modifications discussed in this chapter.

One way to encourage this self-reflection, proactivity, and assertiveness is by encouraging students to use *rules for good communication* (Ferre, 1997). Ten simple *rules* can help students learn to monitor the listening environment, message quality, and their own listening behavior to manage the impact of their CAPD. Top-down compensatory strategies or central resource training can teach the student to use specific compensatory strategies in order to improve access to and understanding of auditorily presented information, including metacognitive and metalinguistic strategies, active listening strategies, and problem-solving strategies (Chermak, 1998, 2007; Kelly, 1995). Compensatory strategies or central resource training is discussed in-depth in Chapter 10.

Computer-assisted games, including apps, increasingly are being used as part of many students' individualized intervention to extend rehabilitation beyond the therapy environment so as to maximize mastery and ensure generalization of skills (ASHA, 2005a). At school, teachers can engage whole classrooms in *low-tech* games and activities that enhance both bottom-up auditory perceptual and top-down cognitive-linguistic and listening skills. By including a few minutes in each school day of group game play designed to improve use of visual cues (e.g., Charades, Pictionary®), enhance auditory vigilance (e.g., musical chairs, Simon Says), build active listening and/or problem-solving skills (e.g., *ending sound game* in which each player says a word beginning with the final sound of the previous player's word—*caT-TaP-PiG-GoaT* Clue®, Battleship®), or expand vocabulary and working memory (Twenty Questions, Catch-Phrase®, Taboo®, Tribond®), all students are able to strengthen the *me* referred to previously as a vital component of the *communication equation*.[3]

As a member of the management team, the audiologist can facilitate the student's use of compensatory strategies. Both the student and team members need a clear understanding of the student's specific listening needs. Audiologists should work with parents and teachers to understand instructional styles and curricular demands in order to ensure that appropriate modifications are implemented. As the expert in central auditory processing disorder, the audiologist provides resources for materials, products, and activities that can be used, often informally, at home and school to enhance auditory, listening, and related skills, improve understanding of the disorder, enhance use of compensatory strategies and develop students' self-advocacy skills. Finally, the audiologist can facilitate access to appropriate related professionals and support groups as needed.

A checklist of self-advocacy tips that can be shared with students, teachers, and families is presented in Appendix 13–C.

Communicating Central Auditory Processing Test Results to the Team

As a member of the intervention team, the audiologist should convey diagnostic test results, impressions, and recommendations both in writing and through participation at the student's case conference or team meeting. Both formats provide the opportunity to educate the student, parents, teachers, and related professionals about central auditory processing disorder, in general, as well as the specific auditory processing and related listening/learning needs of the particular student.

A clearly written diagnostic report is essential to this communication. The statement of problem, reason for referral, and relevant case history information should be included, followed by a reporting of test results in which vocabulary, professional terms, and acronyms have been clarified. Although results from individual tests are important, a summary of the cumulative audiologic test battery findings may be more appreciated by parents and related professionals with whom the student works. The audiologic characteristics and nature of the specific profile (i.e., deficient skill areas) should be explained clearly and concisely, followed by a discussion of the possible impact on communication, academics, day-to-day listening, and psychosocial skills. Recom-

---

[3]Catch-Phrase® and Taboo® are registered trademarks of Hasbro, Inc.; Battleship® and Clue® are registered trademarks of Milton Bradley, Inc.; Pictionary® is a registered trademark of Pictionary, Inc. and Parker Brothers, Tribond® is a registered trademark of Mattel, Inc.

mendations should be based on sound principles of intervention, including deficit-specific rationale, taking into account recognized educational philosophies and practices, and including descriptions of desired changes and prognosis. Audiologists should be familiar with educational options in their geographic area, as well as state and local service eligibility criteria. Chapter 5 reviews educational policies and services relevant to intervention for students with CAPD.

Finally, both oral and written reports should include recommendations and timelines for measuring outcomes, both subjectively and objectively. Effectiveness of classroom management strategies may be reflected, formally, in improved grades and improved function as reflected on listening performance checklists such as the CHAPS (Children's Auditory Performance Scale) (Smoski, Brunt, & Tannahill, 1998). Less formal evidence may include observation of increased use of self-advocacy techniques by the student, decreased fatigue, reports of less frequent need for repetition and reinstruction, and students' self-reports of improved *hearing* at home or in the classroom.

Case Studies of Students With Central Auditory Processing Disorder

To summarize and conclude this chapter, cases studies illustrating the application of an interactive, collaborative approach to CAPD intervention in an educational setting are presented. Central auditory test results of the students described in the following case studies were interpreted using the Bellis-Ferre model (1999) for characterizing specific pro-

files. It is well established that students with CAPD represent a heterogeneous population with respect to the functional impact of their processing deficit(s) as well as their performance across tests of central auditory function (ASHA, 2005a; Bellis, 2007; Ferre & Wilber, 1986; Jerger, Martin, & Jerger, 1987). As noted previously, differential diagnosis is used to differentiate among disorders having similar symptoms and/or manifestations. The Bellis-Ferre model is a theoretical framework in which individual test scores as well as inter- and intratest patterns of performance are examined in order to relate central auditory test findings to both their presumed underlying neurophysiological bases and functional sequelae (ASHA 2005a; Bellis, 1996, 1999, 2006; Bellis & Ferre, 1999; Ferre, 1997, 2006). The model delineates five profiles of CAPD based on key central auditory test findings, and describes typical behavioral manifestations associated with each deficit. The reader will note similarities in manifestations and test results among the profiles as well as findings considered unique to that profile.

The model consists of three primary profiles of CAPD, characterized by presumed underlying site of central nervous system dysfunction, and two secondary profiles that, while yielding unique patterns of results on central auditory tests, may be described more appropriately as manifestations of supramodal or cognitive-linguistic disorders and not true central auditory disorder. It is important to note that any central auditory processing profiling system should not be used as a terminal classification system into which a student's test scores or behaviors must be fit; but rather as a starting point for conceptualizing and clarifying those findings. The students described herein represent prototypical cases using the Bellis-Ferre model; their central auditory test results could be described using other conceptualizations of models. Regardless of the model one chooses to interpret assessment findings, it is imperative that a multidisciplinary approach be used in the assessment process, test scores across disciplines be related to functional needs, and management and treatment be collaborative in order to be effective (ASHA, 2005a; Bellis, 2006, 2007; Chermak, 2007; Ferre, 2006). For a detailed discussion of these profiles, the reader is referred to Bellis (2003). Brief descriptions of these profiles precede the case illustrations. Table 13–1 summarizes key management strategies appropriate for each deficit profile. See Chapter 8 in Volume I of the Handbook for discussion of the use and limitations of CAPD profiles.

Auditory Decoding Profile

The auditory decoding profile is characterized by poor discrimination of fine acoustic differences in speech with behavioral characteristics similar to those observed among children with peripheral hearing loss. This profile is presumed to reflect left hemisphere dysfunction. Weak discrimination means that the auditory system is working harder than it should be to extract the fine acoustic changes within the speech spectrum. Difficulty extracting and/or discriminating the fine acoustic differences in the speech spectra places the student at risk for listening difficulties when noise is present, in highly reverberant environments (e.g., gym, cafeteria), when visual and/or contextual cues are not available, or when listening to a soft-spoken speaker or one

with an accent or dialect different than the listener's. Even under optimal listening conditions, the auditory system of the individual with CAPD is working harder than the system of the normal listener to analyze incoming acoustic information. As the acoustic or linguistic conditions deteriorate and/or linguistic-cognitive demands increase, the student will expend more energy just to process the acoustic information, leaving less energy for higher order processing. As auditory overload occurs, fatigue sets in and listening comprehension deteriorates. Students with poor decoding require management strategies that improve access to and use of an acoustically clear signal.

When considering the environment, classroom management will focus on improving signal clarity through noise abatement, use of preferential seating, and trial use of an ALD. Auditory decoding deficit can create secondary difficulties in communication (e.g., vocabulary, syntax, semantics, second language acquisition) and academic skills (e.g., reading decoding, spelling, notetaking, direction following). To mitigate these potential effects, the student needs message modifications that include use of clear speech, repetition or rephrasing, the addition of visual cues that clarify/complement auditory target, technology to aid message access (e.g., digital recorder/smart pen), and curricular changes (e.g., nonverbal second language, course taken *pass-fail*).

Integration Profile

The integration deficit profile likely is due to inefficient interhemispheric communication and is characterized by deficiencies in the ability to perform tasks that

Table 13–1. Summary of Management Strategies for Central Auditory Processing Disorders

CAP Deficit Profile	Improving Access to Signal	Accommodations
DECODING DEFICIT—acoustic analysis issues – Focus on signal quality—acoustic	Preferential seating near/facing speaker Classroom noise abatement Trial use FM System Speakers use Clear Speech Repeat information as needed	ASL for second language requirement Preteaching/previewing Adjust schedule to minimize overload Multisensory learning environment Supplement verbal with visual/tactile cues
INTEGRATION DEFICIT—synthesis issues – Focus on quantity and structure	Look OR Listen Repeat with demonstration, DO NOT rephrase Limit overall amount of information given Present information sequentially Recording device, scribe as needed	Extended time on tests, assignments Music while studying Movement/listening breaks Books on tape, study guides Test answers in booklet, not computer sheet
PROSODIC DEFICIT—poor analysis/synthesis – Focus on quality & structure	Repeat with emphasis on key words Use Clear Speech Preferential seating Classroom noise abatement Placement with highly animated teacher	Explicit multisensory learning environment Preteaching/previewing Movement/listening breaks Extended time, test type adjustments Adjust schedule to minimize overload
ASSOCIATIVE DEFICIT—difficulty with "rules" – Focus on signal quality—linguistic	Rephrasing, not repetition Clarify message as needed Use Clear Language- Say what you mean Speak the "same" language Use visuals & manipulatives	Preteaching rules and vocabulary Waive second language requirement Enhance familiarity Assess IQ using non language-biased tests Change test format—ask the "right" questions
OUTPUT-ORGANIZATION—poor execution – Focus on quantity/structure of response	Minimize distractions—auditory, visual, tactile Break tasks down Consider FM system Recording device or scribe	Preteaching Outlines, checklists Closed set tests Increased computer use Test answers in booklet, not computer sheet

require intersensory and/or multisensory communication. A student with this profile may complain that there is too much information, and has difficulty intuiting task demands, starting complex tasks, transitioning from task to task, or completing tasks in a timely fashion. Ability to function in noise depends less on the acoustic aspects of the noise and more on task demands. For example, this student, while completing a highly familiar task may be unaffected by environmental noise. However, while studying or taking a test, each having greater task demands, this student may be bothered by noise at levels that typical peers would consider inconsequential. Impact on communication is variable, and academic difficulties in reading, spelling, writing, and other integrative tasks typically are observed. For the student with impaired integration, management focuses on modifications, accommodations, and compensations that adjust the quantity and structure of the signal.

Environmental modifications include use of noise reducing earplugs or noise canceling earphones while studying or taking tests, seating designed to minimize simultaneous multisensory input (e.g., *look or listen*), an experiential learning environment, and listening and movement breaks during the day. Message or curricular adjustments include repetition with related cues, use of manipulatives, use of examples and demonstrations, shortened and/or simplified instructions, *preteaching*, extended time, closed set tests, and highly structured second language learning.

Prosodic Profile

The prosodic deficit profile is characterized by deficits using prosodic features of a speech signal, a predominantly right hemisphere function. The student displays difficulty in auditory pattern recognition, important for perceiving running speech, and may have difficulty recognizing and using patterns in other sensory systems (e.g., visual, tactile). Difficulties are observed in pragmatic language (e.g., reading facial expressions, body language, and gestures; recognizing or using sarcasm or heteronyms), rhythm perception, music, and nonverbal learning. Children with prosodic deficits have difficulty recognizing and attaching meaning to auditory patterns. Like the student with poor discrimination, this student needs modifications that improve the acoustic and linguistic clarity of the signal (e.g., repetition with clear speech, classroom noise abatement). Like the student with poor integration, they also need adjustments to the structure of the signal (e.g., reduced overall length of message, use of tag words, knowledge of demands or expectations).

In the classroom, the student with prosodic deficit benefits from an explicit, experiential, well-structured hands-on learning environment. A teacher with a melodic voice, who uses an animated teaching style and ample demonstration and examples is a good match for the student with the prosodic deficit profile, as such a teaching style maximizes access to prosodic features of speech and providing the how-to instruction and practice that the student needs (Bellis, 2003; Bellis & Ferre, 1999; Ferre, 2006). Teachers should repeat information using clear speech and with emphasis (stress) on key words, altering message pacing (e.g., "Look out the window" vs. "Look, out the window"), and/or using associated visual cues, examples, and demonstrations. These techniques would allow the student to know task demands up front in order not to be overwhelmed. Management includes noise abatement, untimed activities, provision of listening breaks, highly structured second language learning, adjustment to workload, and note-taking assistance (e.g., scribe, digital recording device).

Associative Deficit Profile

Associative deficit is a secondary central auditory test profile characterized by significant auditory-language processing difficulties, believed to be related to dysfunction in the communication between the primary (Heschl's gyrus) and secondary or auditory association (Wernicke's area) cortices of the dominant (usually left) hemisphere (i.e., intrahemispheric integration). On central auditory tests, performance on degraded speech and temporal discrimination tasks are normal, with poor scores for verbal mediation (i.e., labeling) response on pattern tasks and marked difficulty, typically bilateral or right-ear deficits, on dichotic listening tasks that tax binaural integration and separation skills. Deficiency in these skills impacts language processing, as the listener has difficulty attaching linguistic meaning to incoming acoustic signals quickly and efficiently. As such, the listener has difficulty extracting the key information from a spoken message. In general, listeners with this auditory-language association deficit don't speak the same language as their peers and do not glean linguistic meaning as easily as non-impaired listeners. The listener with this deficit profile tends to take most statements literally and often sees ambiguity even in seemingly straightforward messages (Bellis, 2003, 2006; Bellis & Ferre, 1999; Ferre, 2006). Functional listening and learning difficulties include issues in verbal and/or written comprehension, especially for unfamiliar or linguistically ambiguous targets; poor functional spelling, note-taking, direction following, and/or receptive/expressive language skills (Bellis, 2003, 2006; Bellis & Ferre, 1999; Ferre, 2006).

Management of associative deficits focuses on maximizing the ability to *use the rules*. The most significant environmental modification for this student is placement in an educational environment that uses a systematic, logical, multisensory, rule-based approach to language/learning. *Whole language* environments are not appropriate for the child with associative deficit.[4] Because auditory-language association deficit can adversely affect language processing skills, language-based IQ tests (e.g., Stanford-Binet, WISC) will underestimate true intellectual potential. Evaluation using a non language-biased measure (e.g. Universal Nonverbal Intelligence Test) tends to provide a more reliable estimate of intellectual potential. Message-related strategies include rephrasing using simpler language; using clear, concise, and explicit language; limiting use of ambiguous messages; use of multiple choice or closed set fill-in-the-blank tests (i.e., no open-ended test questions); preteaching of new material; imposition of external organization (e.g., always telling the

---

[4]Whole language environments are those that teach language arts, specifically reading and writing, by emphasizing the learning of whole words and phrases through context rather than through phonics or sound-symbol exercises. Whole language learning presumes that the learner will assimilate information according to known rules, expectations, and experiences without the need for explicit, stimulus-driven, instruction.

student before beginning the specific task parameters); and waiver of foreign language requirement (Bellis, 2003; Ferre, 2006).

Output-Organization Deficit Profile

Output-organization deficit is a secondary central auditory test profile characterized by poor scores on central auditory tests requiring the reporting of multiple or precisely sequenced targets, with normal performance seen on single target and/or free recall tasks. Atypical crossed reflexes or abnormalities in otoacoustic emission results may be seen (Bellis, 2003). Behaviorally, the student exhibits difficulties in planning, applied problem-solving, listening comprehension, direction following, spelling, writing, expressive speech and language skills, including articulation and word finding and retrieval, and the ability to complete assignments in a timely fashion and/or to *get started* on long assignments. This deficit profile may reflect dysfunction in the frontal and prefrontal cortices responsible for executive functioning or disordered efferent (i.e., motor) pathway function (Bellis, 2003; Bellis & Ferre, 1999; Fahy & Richard, 2005; Ferre, 1997; Richard, 2001). Management for poor output-organization skills includes training in the rules of information organization and practice in how to do this organization. Repetition or rephrasing works only if information is broken down into smaller linguistic units. Use of tag words (e.g., *first, last, before, after, now*) is helpful, as are outlines, checklists, and assignment notebooks. Finally, the student with impaired output–organization requires production-related adjustments

such as a digital recorder/smart pen or a scribe for note-taking, changes in writing demands and workload, and extended time on tests.

Case Profiles

Diana, age 9 years, 8 months, was referred for evaluation by the school speech-language pathologist as part of a multidisciplinary case study. Speech-language evaluation indicated poor sound blending, vocabulary, and word memory skills. Parents reported that Diana had an embolism in the left hemisphere that was reportedly stable; however, MRI data were not available at the time of testing. Diana was enrolled in a dual curriculum (English-Hebrew) regular education environment. Academic achievement was at expected levels for English-language curriculum, but significantly below grade level in Hebrew-language classes. Results of central auditory evaluation revealed normal peripheral auditory function and impaired auditory closure and related discrimination skills as evidenced by abnormal performance on low redundancy speech tasks (e.g., low-pass filtered speech, time compressed speech, with and without reverberation, listening in noise). Performance on tasks of binaural integration, binaural separation, and temporal patterning were within normal limits for age, suggesting no specific deficits in these areas. Overall pattern of performance provided evidence of *auditory decoding* profile, suggesting dysfunction in the primary auditory cortex and consistent with reported presence of left hemisphere embolism. At the student's case conference, additional pull-out therapy time was added to allow the speech-language pathologist to include auditory rehabilitation (e.g., discrimination training, speechreading, compensatory strategies training, self-advocacy training). Recommended management strategies for this student included the following:

- Preferential classroom seating
- Additional noise abatement at school and home with draperies added to the classroom
- Direct signal enhancement via personal FM system and use of a recording device in Hebrew classes only
- Repetition of information as needed
- Use of clear speech by parents and teachers
- Adjusted class schedule to minimize auditory fatigue (e.g., Hebrew classes moved to mornings)
- Preteaching new information, especially vocabulary
- Multisensory instruction (e.g., verbal information supplemented with written and graphic materials)
- Informal checklist developed collaboratively by the speech-language pathologist and the audiologist to gauge strategy effectiveness.

Robbie, age 10 years, 6 months, is in a self-contained classroom for students with learning disabilities with reports of limited improvement. He was referred for testing as part of a triennial evaluation to clarify auditory needs. Central auditory evaluation indicated normal peripheral auditory function and evidence of specific deficit in auditory pattern recognition skills, characterized by excessive left ear suppression on dichotic listening tests and inability to mimic or label temporal patterns. Overall test results indicated a prosodic profile, suggesting right hemisphere dysfunction.

In addition to speech-language therapy currently in place to improve social and pragmatic language skills, therapy was recommended to improve temporal patterning skills, recognition and use of prosody, self-advocacy and compensatory skills, and speech-reading ability. The small classroom size and nature of Robbie's learning environment precluded the need for specific recommendations for noise abatement, preferential seating, or a multisensory learning environment that would be offered for other children with this profile. The following management strategies were recommended:

- Repetition of targets emphasizing key items and components of the message
- Use of clear speech by teacher and classroom aide
- Use of more animated instructional style by teacher
- Preteaching and use of concrete manipulatives for instruction of abstract concepts
- Digital recording of lectures, provision of copies of teachers' notes
- Extended time for tests and assignments
- Classroom aide to track improvement/progress via observation checklist.

Claire, age 8 years, 9 months, was seen for testing at the parents' request. Claire received private OT for reported sensory integration disorder and special education services in reading and written language. Parents reported that Claire had two febrile seizures during early childhood. Annual electroencephalography (EEG) testing to monitor brain activity reportedly indicated generally immature responses but no specific abnormalities.

Central auditory evaluation indicated normal peripheral auditory function, normal performance on degraded speech tests, good ability to mimic tonal patterns but poor ability to label patterns, and excessive left ear suppression on dichotic listening tests. Evaluation results indicated an integration profile, suggesting deficient interhemispheric communication, consistent with report of generalized neurologic immaturity. Activities to improve auditory-visual integration skills were recommended for inclusion in Claire's therapy plan, to be implemented by both the OT and the special education resource teacher. In addition, the following management strategies were recommended:

- Use of manipulatives for instruction of abstract concepts
- Use of sequential, rather than simultaneous, presentation of directions (e.g., students told to look at and copy written instructions from the board first, then teacher presented instructions verbally)
- Presentation of information with demonstration and modeling
- Repetition rather than rephrasing of instructions
- Increased opportunities for previewing of new, unfamiliar material
- Provision of books on tape
- Extended time for tests
- For computer-scored tests, Claire be allowed to write answers in test booklet rather than transfer to computer-scored answer sheet
- Integration skills to be tracked at three month intervals by OT and audiologist.

Maggie, age 12 years, 6 months, was seen for assessment upon referral of her neuropsychologist. Medical history was positive for recurrent middle ear effusion. MRI and EEG reports noted "atypical activation over left temporal-parietal region compared with right hemisphere activity." Maggie's individualized education plan (IEP) included educational and speech-language support. Central auditory testing revealed age appropriate performance on temporal patterning and degraded speech tests, with bilateral suppression across all dichotic listening tasks, including dichotic digits, dichotic rhyme, and competing sentences, resulting in a diagnosis of associative type auditory (language) processing deficit. In addition to recommendations for additional assessment of language processing and related memory skills, the following educational accommodations and compensations were implemented:

- Placement in a multisensory, experiential learning environment, not a whole language educational environment
- Knowledge of task parameters up front with explanations of any changes in demands
- Classroom buddy to assist, as needed, with clarification of instructions
- Change in math curriculum from whole-language program (Everyday Mathematics®) to explicit multisensory program (e.g., Touch Math®, Math-U-See®)[5]
- Use of clear speech and clear language (i.e., speaking at slightly slower rate with slightly increased loudness and minimizing ambigu-

---

[5]Everyday Mathematics® is a registered trademark of McGraw-Hill Education. TouchMath® is a registered trademark of Innovative Learning Concepts, Inc. Math-U-See® is a registered trademark of Math-U-See, Inc.

ous statements, jargon, and nonspecific references)

- For instructions, all students to be alerted regarding total number of steps to be given (e.g., "I want you to do three things") with tag words used such as *first, last, before, after,* and so forth, with insertion of brief (1- to 2-second) pause between items
- Provision of *thinking time* before requiring a response
- Preteaching new vocabulary and abstract concepts
- Extended time for all examinations, with tests taken in separate, quiet room, and questions read to her to ensure understanding
- Time spent on homework not to exceed 50% more than time spent by typical sixth grader
- Middle school foreign language requirement waived
- School psychologist to administer nonverbal, non language-biased IQ test (e.g., Universal Nonverbal Intelligence Test [UNIT™]) to gain more reliable estimate of intellectual potential.[6]

Stephanie, age 16 years, 9 months, was seen for reevaluation per the school district's request. Stephanie's history includes diagnoses of attention deficit disorder, for which numerous medication trials had been initiated with no positive outcomes reported, and speech-language impairment for which she had received ongoing therapy since early childhood. Initial central auditory processing evaluation at age 13 years indicated auditory decoding deficit for which Stephanie subsequently received computer-assisted auditory training. Re-evaluation revealed no significant change in performance compared with results at age 13 years despite auditory training. At the multidisciplinary case conference that included Stephanie and her parents, the decision was reached to discontinue bottom-up auditory training with continuation of short-term therapy provided by the speech-language pathologist to include aural rehabilitation with focus on compensatory strategy training, including use of visual cues (e.g., speech-reading). In addition, the following environmental modifications and educational accommodations were agreed upon by all team members:

- Provision of teachers' notes, presentations, and handouts via electronic blackboard
- Advanced exposure to/preteaching of science class vocabulary
- Elimination of oral exams in foreign language class, with course to be taken on a pass-fail basis as Stephanie did not want a course waiver or alternative language
- Extended time on all tests with district-supported request for extended time on the ACT®[7]
- Schedule adjustment—English, originally following Spanish as penultimate period of the day, swapped with first period physical education class to minimize fatigue and provide end-of-day opportunity for movement
- Parents purchased Phonak ISense™ FM system for Stephanie's use through remainder of high school and during college.[8]

---

[6]UNIT™ is a registered trademark of Riverside Publishing
[7]ACT® is a registered trademark of ACT, Inc.
[8]ISense™ is a registered trademark of Phonak, Inc.

Drew, age 12 years, 9 months, was seen upon referral of his speech-language pathologist. This seventh grader presented with mood regulation issues, dyspraxic speech, issues in written and verbal expression, and poor handwriting. Central auditory testing revealed evidence of an output-organization deficit profile with excessive ordering errors on patterning tasks in which target labels were given backward (e.g., high-low-high for low-high low, short-short-long for long-long-short), fair-poor listening in noise, and marked difficulty recognizing multiple dichotic targets, with no difficulty for single targets. At Drew's IEP meeting, the team agreed to the following additions to his educational plan:

- Assessment and treatment as needed, of executive functions and word finding skills
- Extended time on all tests, including standardized measures and class projects
- Written assignments completed on computer (e.g., word processing program)
- Provision of digital recording pen (e.g., smartpen purchased by parents) with laptop interface for note-taking
- Test-taking in a separate quiet room with scribe to record test answers.

As the preceding cases illustrate, while several management strategies may be appropriate for many types of CAPD profiles, it is important that the team resist a "one size fits all approach" and customize each plan based upon a particular student's communicative and educational needs as well as their individual strengths. There is overlap across management strategies for various types of CAPD because each represents impairment in auditory skills, perceptual and/or functional. Regardless of deficit type, all share a need for an optimized listening/learning environment (the *medium*), acoustically and/or linguistically clear signal (the *message*), and support to maximize self-advocacy and residual skill sets (the *me*). While sharing diagnostic and intervention characteristics, each CAPD type presents unique diagnostic indicators and each student presents with unique educational, communicative, and daily listening and learning challenges. As Myklebust (1954) pointed out nearly 60 years ago, even students with similar problems vary in their functional needs and must be served individually in order to maximize potential. The cases described here illustrate the importance of, and success in, collaboration and teaming to develop individualized intervention programs for students with central auditory processing disorder. This shared responsibility among professionals, families, and students utilizes resources efficiently and is most likely to achieve intervention goals and lead to positive treatment outcomes.

References

American National Standards Institute. (2002). *ANSI S12.60-2002. Acoustical performance criteria, design requirements and guidelines for schools.* Melville, NY: Author.

ASHA (American Speech Language Hearing Association). (1995). *Guidelines for acoustics in educational settings.* Rockville, MD: Author.

ASHA. (2005a). *Technical report: (Central) auditory processing disorders.* Rockville, MD: Author.

ASHA. (2005b). *Guidelines for addressing acoustics in educational settings.* Rockville, MD: Author.

Bellis, T. (2003). *Assessment and management of central auditory processing disorders in the educational setting* (2nd ed.). Clifton Park, NY: Thomson Delmar Learning.

Bellis, T. (2007). Historical foundations and the nature of (central) auditory processing disorder. In F. Musiek & G. Chermak (Eds.), *Handbook of (central) auditory processing disorder: Auditory neuroscience and diagnosis* (Vol. I, pp. 119–136). San Diego, CA: Plural.

Bellis, T., & Ferre, J. (1999). Multidimensional approach to differential diagnosis of central auditory processing disorders in children. *Journal of the American Academy of Audiology, 10,* 319–328.

Blake, R., Field, B., Foster, C., Plott, F., & Wertz, P. (1991). Effect of FM auditory trainers on attending behaviors of learning-disabled children. *Language-Speech-Hearing Services in the Schools, 22,* 111–114.

Boothroyd, A. (2004). Room acoustics and speech perception. *Seminars in Hearing, 25,* 155–166.

Bradley, J., & Sato, H. (2008) The intelligibility of speech in elementary school classrooms. *Journal of the Acoustical Society of America, 123,* 2078–2086.

Bradlow, A., Kraus, N., & Hayes, E. (2003). Speaking clearly for children with learning disabilities, sentence perception in noise. *Journal of Speech, Language, and Hearing Research, 46,* 80–97.

Bronzaft, A. L. (1982). The effect of a noise abatement program on reading ability. *Journal of Environmental Psychology, 1,* 215–222.

Caissie, R., Campbell, M., Frenette, W., Scott, L., Howell, I., & Roy, A. (2005). Clear speech for adults with a hearing loss. Does intervention with communication partners make a difference? *Journal of the American Academy of Audiology, 15,* 157–171.

Chermak, G. (1998). Managing central auditory processing disorders, Metalinguistic and metacognitive approaches. *Seminars in Hearing, 19,* 379–392.

Chermak, G. (2007). Central resource training, cognitive, metacognitive and metalinguistic skills and strategies. In G. Chermak & F. Musiek (Eds.), *Handbook of (central) auditory processing disorder: Comprehensive intervention* (Vol. II, pp. 107–166). San Diego, CA: Plural.

Chermak, G. D., Vonhof, M. R., & Bendel, R. B. (1989). Word identification performance in the presence of competing speech and noise in learning disabled adults. *Ear and Hearing, 10,* 90–93.

Cooper, J., & Cutts, B. (1971). Speech discrimination in noise. *Journal of Speech and Hearing Research, 14,* 332–337.

Crandell, C., & Smaldino, J. (1996). Speech perception in noise by children for whom English is a second language. *American Journal of Audiology, 5,* 47–51.

Crandell, C., & Smaldino, J. (Eds). (2001). Classroom acoustics, understanding barriers to learning. *Volta Review, 101,* 1–73.

Crandell, C., & Smaldino J. (2002). Room acoustics and auditory rehabilitation technology. In J. Katz (Ed.), *Handbook of clinical audiology* (5th ed., pp. 607–630). Philadelphia, PA: Lippincott Williams & Wilkins.

Crandell, C., & Smaldino, J. (Eds.). (2004). Classroom acoustics. *Seminars in Hearing, 25*(2).

Crandell, C., Smaldino, J., & Flexer, C. (1995). *Soundfield FM amplification, theory and practical applications.* San Diego, CA: Singular.

Ellis, E. (1989). A metacognitive intervention for increasing class participation. *Learning Disabilities Focus, 5,* 36–46.

Emanuel, D., Ficca, K., & Korczak, P. (2011). Survey of the diagnosis and management of auditory processing disorder. *American Journal of Audiology, 20,* 48–60.

Erber, N. (1969). An interaction of audition and vision in recognition of oral speech stimuli. *Journal of Speech and Hearing Research, 12,* 423–425.

Evans, G. W., & Maxwell, L. (1997). Chronic noise exposure and reading deficits. The mediating effects of language acquisition. *Environment and Behavior, 29*, 638–656.

Fahy, J., & Richard, G. (2005). *The source for development of executive functions.* East Moline, IL: Linguisystems.

Ferguson, S., & Kewley-Port, D. (2002). Vowel intelligibility in clear and conversational speech for normal-hearing and hearing-impaired listeners. *Journal of the Acoustical Society of America, 112*, 259–271.

Ferre, J. (1997). *Processing power: A guide to CAPD assessment and management.* San Antonio, TX: Pearson Assessments.

Ferre, J. (1998). The M^3 model for treating central auditory processing disorders. In M. G. Masters, N. A. Stecker, & J. Katz (Eds.), *Central auditory processing disorders, mostly management* (pp. 103–115). Boston, MA: Allyn & Bacon.

Ferre, J. (2002). Managing children's auditory processing deficits in the real world. What teachers and parents want to know. *Seminars in Hearing, 23*, 319–326.

Ferre, J. (2006). Management strategies for APD. In T. K. Parthasarathy (Ed.), *An introduction to auditory processing disorders in children* (pp. 161–185). Mahwah, NJ: Lawrence Erlbaum Associates.

Ferre, J. (2007). The ABCs of CAP: Practical strategies for enhancing central auditory processing skills. In D. Geffner & D. R. Swain (Eds.), *Auditory processing disorders* (pp. 187–205). San Diego, CA: Plural.

Ferre, J., & Wilber, L. (1986). Central auditory processing skills of normal and LD children: An experimental test battery. *Ear and Hearing, 7*, 336–343.

Finitzo-Heiber, T., & Tillman, T. (1978). Room acoustical effects on monosyllabic word discrimination ability for normal and hearing impaired children. *Journal of Speech and Hearing Research, 21*, 440–448.

Flexer, C. (2007). Signal enhancement, personal FM and sound field technology. In G. Chermak & F. Musiek (Eds.), *Handbook of (central) auditory processing disorder: Comprehensive intervention* (Vol. II, pp. 207–224). San Diego, CA: Plural.

Helfer, K. (1997). Auditory and auditory-visual perception of clear and conversational speech. *Journal of Speech, Language, and Hearing Research, 40*, 432–443.

Jamieson, D. G., Kranjc, G., Yu, K., & Hodgett, W. E. (2004). Speech intelligibility of young school-aged children in the presence of real-life classroom noise. *Journal of the American Academy of Audiology, 15*, 508–517.

Jerger, S., Martin, R., & Jerger, J. (1987). Specific auditory perceptual dysfunction in a learning disabled child. *Ear and Hearing, 8*, 78–86.

Kelly, D. (1995). *Central auditory processing disorders: Strategies for use with children and adolescents.* San Antonio, TX: Pearson Assessments.

Krause, J., & Braida, L. (2002). Investigating alternative forms of clear speech, the effects of speaking rate and speaking mode on intelligibility. *Journal of the Acoustical Society of America, 112*, 2165–2172.

Krause, J., & Braida, L. (2004). Acoustic properties of naturally produced clear speech at normal speaking rates. *Journal of the Acoustical Society of America, 115*, 362–378.

LCNDEC (Laurent Clerc National Deaf Education Center). (2004). *States that recognize American Sign Language as a foreign language.* Washington, DC: Gallaudet University: Author.

Maxwell, L., & Evans, G. (2000). The effects of noise on pre-school children's pre-reading skills. *Environmental Psychology, 20*, 91–98.

Musiek, F., Chermak, G., & Weihing, J. (2007). Auditory training. In G. Chermak & F. Musiek (Eds.), *Handbook of (central) auditory processing disorder: Comprehensive intervention* (Vol. II, pp. 77–106). San Diego, CA: Plural.

Myklebust, H. (1954). *Auditory disorders in children: A manual for differential diagnosis.* New York, NY: Grune & Stratton.

Nabalek, A., & Nabalek, I. (1994). Room acoustics and speech perception. In J. Katz (Ed.), *Handbook of clinical audiology* (4th ed., pp. 624–637). Baltimore, MD: Williams & Wilkins.

Ostergaard. P. (2000). Physics of sound and vibration. In E. Berger, L. Royster, J. Royster, D. Driscoll, & M. Layne (Eds.), *The noise manual* (pp. 19–39). Fairfax, VA: American Industrial Hygiene Association.

Papso, C. F., & Blood, I. M. (1989). Word recognition skills of children and adults in background noise. *Ear and Hearing, 10,* 235–236.

Payton, K., Uchanski, R., & Braida, L. (1994). Intelligibility of conversational and clear speech in noise and reverberation for listeners with normal and impaired hearing. *Journal of the Acoustical Society of America, 95,* 1581–1592.

Picheny, M., Durlach, N., & Braida, L. (1985). Speaking clearly for the hard of hearing I: Intelligibility differences between clear and conversational speech. *Journal of Speech and Hearing Research, 28,* 96–103.

Picheny, M., Durlach, N., & Braida, L. (1986). Speaking clearly for the hard of hearing II, Acoustic characteristics of clear and conversational speech. *Journal of Speech and Hearing Research, 29,* 434–446.

Plomp, R., & Mimpen, A. (1979). Speech-reception threshold for sentences as a function of age and noise level. *Journal of the Acoustical Society of America, 66,* 1333–1342.

Richard, G. (2001). *The source for processing disorders.* East Moline, IL: LinguiSystems.

Rosenberg, G. G. (1998). FM sound-field research identifies benefits for students and teachers. *Educational Audiology Review, 15,* 6–8.

Sanders, D., & Goodrich, S. (1971). Relative contribution of visual and auditory components of speech intelligibility as a function of three conditions of frequency distortion. *Journal of Speech and Hearing Research, 14,* 154–159.

Schow, R., & Nerbonne, M. (1996). *Introduction to audiologic rehabilitation* (3rd ed.). Boston, MA: Allyn & Bacon.

Schum, D. (1996). Intelligibility of clear and conversational speech of young and elderly talkers. *Journal of the American Academy of Audiology, 7,* 212–218.

Schum, D. (1997). Beyond hearing aids, clear speech training as an intervention strategy. *Hearing Journal, 50,* 36–39.

Smoski, W., Brunt, M., & Tannahill, C. (1998). *Children's Auditory Performance Scale.* Tampa, FL: Educational Audiology Association.

Shapiro, A., & Mistal, G. (1985). ITE-aid auditory training for reading and spelling-disabled children: Clinical case studies. *Hearing Journal, 38,* 14–16.

Shapiro, A., & Mistal, G. (1986). ITE-aid auditory training for reading and spelling-disabled children: A longitudinal study of matched groups. *Hearing Journal, 39,* 14–16.

Sillman, E. (Ed). (2000). Improving acoustics in American schools. *Language-Speech-Hearing Services in Schools, 31,* 4.

Stach, B., Loiselle, L., Jerger, J., Mintz, S., & Taylor, C. (1987). Clinical experience with personal FM assistive listening devices. *Hearing Journal, 40,* 24–30.

Appendix 13–A. Checklist for Assessing the Listening Environment

*E*ducate the listener, family and teachers about environmental impact on listening

*N*oise—check noise levels at school and home

*V*erify suspected adverse effects with management team

*I*ndividualize the plan—choose modifications that are deficit specific

*R*everberation—minimize echo in classroom or at home

*O*ptimize access to visual and related cues

*N*ew technology—investigate assistive listening device options

*M*inimize distance between speaker and listener

*E*liminate acoustic barriers whenever possible

*N*ote impact, both positive and negative, that environmental changes have on the listener

*T*ell parents and teachers how to enhance school and home using least restrictive means

Appendix 13–B. Checklist for Message Modifications That Enhance Listening Comprehension

*M*ake sure you have the listener's attention

*E*ye contact and visual cues help

*S*peak clearly

*S*ay what you mean

*A*void ambiguity

*G*ive listening breaks to minimize fatigue

*E*xtend response time for both verbal and written messages

Appendix 13–C. Checklist for Self-Advocacy and Good Communication Rules

*S*it still—we keep or bodies still while listening.

*E*veryone makes mistakes—don't give up on yourself.

*L*isten to the message not just the words—listen for the meaning.

*F*igure it out—use all the clues and guess when you can.

*A*llow yourself time to put your thoughts together before answering.

*D*o ask your buddy, peer, or teacher for help.

*V*oice concerns or questions if you don't understand.

*O*kay to get ahead in your reading and learn new vocabulary words ahead of time.

*C*hoose a quiet place to study or try to move away from noise.

*A*sk for repetition, clarification, or an example if you didn't hear or understand information.

*C*hange your environment when you can to help you hear well.

*Y*ou can use your eyes to hear better—use visual cues.

CHAPTER 14

INTERVENTION APPROACHES FOR ADOLESCENTS AND ADULTS WITH CENTRAL AUDITORY PROCESSING DISORDER

JANE A. BARAN

Introduction

The preceding chapters in Section II of this text have provided detailed information on many of the intervention approaches that can be used to remediate or alleviate the functional deficits experienced by individuals with central auditory processing disorder (CAPD). Although much of the focus in these chapters was on the application of these procedures with children, each of the approaches discussed can be incorporated into an efficacious intervention plan for the adolescent or adult with CAPD. As is the case with children, intervention programs developed for adolescents or adults with CAPD should be individualized to address the specific deficit areas that were uncovered during the diagnos-

tic process (AAA, 2010; ASHA, 2005a; Baran, 1998, 2002, 2007; Chermak & Musiek, 1997). In addition, it is important that the presence of any comorbid conditions be considered as the behavioral manifestations associated with many comorbid conditions (e.g., peripheral hearing loss, attention deficit disorder, behavioral disorder, etc.) can impact the utility of a given management plan or approach for the child or the adult with CAPD (AAA, 2010; ASHA, 2005a; Baran, 1998, 2002, 2007; Chermak & Musiek, 1997).

Older individuals with CAPD often present unique challenges and circumstances that will impact the design and effectiveness of their rehabilitative programs as is also discussed in Chapter 15. Brain plasticity, which is optimal during early childhood, slows as one ages (Musiek & Berge, 1998; Whitelaw & Yuskow,

2008). As a result of this recognized change in brain plasticity with advancing age, there may be less emphasis on auditory training approaches in the intervention programs used with adults and greater reliance on intervention approaches that are designed to improve the quality of the signal or enhance the individual's cognitive and linguistic resources; however, as discussed later in this chapter, auditory training approaches should be given serious consideration as a component of an intervention plan for the adult with CAPD as even the older, more mature brain is capable of changing in response to auditory training activities (Baran, 2002, 2007; Musiek, Shinn, & Hare, 2002). Also, as children mature into adolescents and adults, their lives are reconfigured in different and complex ways and they are called upon to function in many different contexts. Children are commonly viewed as existing or functioning in one context at a time (i.e., as learners in school or as family members outside of school). Adults, on the other hand, are not configured primarily within the context of a single setting, but rather within and across the context of a number of settings—many of which often overlap (e.g., home, family, work, community, recreational activities) (Baran, 2002, 2007; Kleinman & Bashir, 1996). Therefore, distinctively different behaviors and performance are expected of the adult. Children with CAPD and other related disabilities are provided educational support services that focus on the specific disability; however, there are few support services available for adults with CAPD, and the focus is typically not on the individual's disability, but rather on such things as job performance, community involvement, family relationships, and parental effectiveness—all of which can be negatively impacted by

the disorder. Moreover, the effects of the disorder often are not consistent across contexts or even within a single context. An individual may experience little or no difficulty functioning in a given context, but then begin to experience difficulty at another time in the same setting or environment. Fatigue or changes in the listening environment (e.g., an air conditioner being turned on) may be sufficient to create a situation where the individual's compensatory strategies or cognitive resources are taxed, and problems arise. Different contexts will present different listening demands due to such variables as room acoustics, degree of familiarity with the topic(s) of conversation, the number of participants in the conversation, and so forth. Finally, cultural and personal values, motivation, and the availability of support from family or friends can all impact the development and success of a management program designed for the adolescent or adult with CAPD.

It is essential, therefore, that each of these factors and influences (specific auditory deficits, comorbid disorders or disabilities, age, motivation, communication contexts, communication styles, personal roles and responsibilities, and cultural values) be taken into consideration when designing an intervention program for the adolescent or adult patient with CAPD. Failure to do so is likely to result in the development of a rehabilitative program that will not meet with optimal success.

Nature of CAPD in Adolescents and Adults

Patient Characteristics

Adolescents and adults with CAPD present with a variety of etiologic bases and behavioral symptoms. Professionals who provides rehabilitative or intervention services for adolescents and adults with CAPD are likely to encounter four distinct groups of patients in their clinical practices. These groups include: (1) individuals with central auditory deficits associated with confirmed compromise of the central auditory nervous system (CANS), such as in cases of head injuries, cerebrovascular accidents, and degenerative neurologic or neurodegenerative diseases (e.g., multiple sclerosis, Alzheimer's disease), (2) individuals who are experiencing degenerative processes within the CANS that are related to "normal" aging processes, (3) individuals who were initially identified with CAPD at an earlier age and who were likely to have received one or more of the interventions discussed in the previous chapters, and (4) individuals who present for the first time as adults with a diagnosis of CAPD, often in the absence of other significant findings (Baran, 2002, 2007; Musiek, Baran, & Pinheiro, 1994). Many of the individuals who fall into this latter group were likely to have experienced auditory difficulties in the past that went undiagnosed. In these cases, the individuals either identified and adopted strategies on their own that helped them compensate for their auditory problems, or they received individualized attention from teachers and/or parents who helped them deal effectively with their auditory difficulties in the absence of a specific diagnosis and any type of formalized intervention program (Baran, 2002).

The preceding comments focused on individuals with auditory problems that are related to some type of compromise of the CANS; however, there are other patients who will present with auditory difficulties that will not be directly related to involvement of the CANS. Generally these patients (like many of the patients with CAPD) will present with significant hearing difficulties in the absence of a peripheral hearing loss. In many of these patients, the functional deficits may initially appear to be auditory in nature (i.e., related to CANS dysfunction), but when more comprehensive testing is undertaken, it may be determined the deficits are related to some other type of underlying etiology or cause (Jerger & Musiek, 2000). Common etiologic bases for the auditory deficits in these individuals include psychological or emotional difficulties, language differences (e.g., communication contexts where one of the conversational partners is an individual for whom English is a second language and the other is a native speaker of English), or significant changes in the acoustic environment (Baran, 1996; Baran & Musiek, 1994; Saunders & Haggard, 1989). In other patients, the deficits reported may be related to some type of subclinical compromise of the auditory system that is not detected by routine peripheral hearing assessment (Baran, 1996; Baran & Musiek, 1994). For many of these individuals (e.g., those with psychological or emotional problems), referral to another professional for intervention is critical as the types of services that will be required are clearly outside the scopes of practice of either audiologists or speech-language pathologists.

Although it is possible to categorize patients with CAPD into one of the four groups identified above, it is not possible to associate "specific" and "unique" auditory deficits with each of these four groups. CAPD represents a complex and heterogeneous group of deficits and there is considerable overlap in the deficits experienced by individuals who fall into these four categories of patients. Table 14–1 presents a list of some of the

Table 14–1. Common Presenting Symptomatology Associated With Auditory Processing Disorders and Related Disorders in Adolescents and Adults

Inordinate difficulty hearing in noisy or reverberant environments
Lack of music appreciation
Difficulty following conversations on the telephone
Difficulty following multistep directions/instructions
Difficulty taking notes during lectures
Difficulty following long conversations
Difficulty learning a foreign language
Difficulty learning technical or discipline-specific vocabulary where the language is largely unfamiliar or novel
Difficulty in directing, sustaining, or dividing attention
Auditory memory deficits
Spelling difficulties
Reading difficulties
Organizational problems
Behavioral, psychological and/or social problems
Academic or vocational difficulties

Source: From Masters, M. Gay; Stecker, Nancy A.; Katz, Jack, *Central Auditory Processing Disorders: Mostly Management, 1st Edition*, © 1998, p. 199. Reprinted by permission of Pearson Education, Inc., Upper Saddle River, NJ.

commonly reported symptoms noted by individuals being seen for central auditory processing diagnostic evaluations. As can readily be seen as one considers this table, this is a rather extensive list of deficits; however, it should be noted that many, if not most, of the patients seen for CAPD evaluations will not experience all of these deficits. Therefore, it is important when developing an intervention plan for a given patient that the professional takes into consideration any functional deficits that were reported by the patient during intake procedures and the specific auditory deficits that were identified during the diagnostic process,

as well as any additional information that may have been uncovered during the diagnostic process (e.g., the existence of comorbid conditions).

Comorbid Conditions

Many patients with CAPD will also present with one or more comorbid conditions that can impact the intervention program that is being developed to address the individual's auditory deficits. These comorbid conditions can include speech and language disorders, learning disabilities, attention deficit disorders with or without hyperactivity, frank neurologic involvement of the CANS, peripheral hearing loss, psychological disorders, and emotional disorders (Baran & Musiek, 1999; Chermak & Musiek, 1997). There has been much interest in establishing potential cause and effect relationships between each of these disorders and CAPD; however, these causal relationships have been difficult to establish, and they remain elusive for the most part at this time (Baran, 2002). (See Musiek, Bellis, & Chermak, 2005 for discussion of the relationship between brain organization and comorbidity.) What is generally appreciated by the professional and research community is that these relationships are complex, interconnected, and most likely not unidirectional. Also, it is important to understand that it is possible that in some individuals the two conditions (or in some cases more than two conditions) simply coexist and are not directly linked to one underlying cause or etiology. Take for example, the case of a person who has a peripheral hearing loss and then acquires a CAPD as a result of a neurologic insult. In this patient the two conditions are clearly not related to the same etiology and therefore they exist as separate conditions. Regardless of the precise nature of these relationships (i.e., causal, related, or simply coexisting), it will be critical for the professional to take all presenting conditions into consideration when developing a management or intervention program for the patient with CAPD and other comorbid conditions, as these other conditions can (and often will) impact the individual's ability to benefit from interventions that are specifically designed to address the auditory deficits.

The behavioral symptoms (see Table 14–1) often noted in adolescents and adults with CAPD are not unique to CAPD, with many, if not most, of these behavioral symptoms being associated with more than one of the other disorders mentioned above. It is important, therefore, that a comprehensive, and preferably multidisciplinary, assessment of the individual's auditory, linguistic, cognitive, academic, and vocational functioning be undertaken before a CAPD intervention plan is developed, especially if deficits or problems are anticipated in any of these other areas.

Overview of Intervention Approaches

Intervention approaches used to remediate or alleviate the auditory deficits associated with CAPD can be categorized into three major categories based upon their goals and objectives. These goals and objectives are as follows: (1) to improve signal quality, (2) to improve the individual's auditory perceptual skills, and (3) to enhance the individual's language and cognitive skills (AAA, 2010; ASHA, 1996, 2005a). Chermak and Musiek (1997) have proposed an alternative classification system that divides the procedures into two main categories based upon the nature of the mechanisms that underlie the processing requirements involved. In this classification system, the approaches are classified as either bottom-up (i.e., stimulus-driven) or top-down (i.e., concept-driven) (Chermak & Musiek, 1997). Bottom-up procedures involve those approaches specifically used to facilitate the individual's ability to receive and process acoustic signals, whereas top-down approaches encompass those procedures that are specifically designed to facilitate the *interpretation* of auditory information according to linguistic rules and conventions, other available sensory information, and knowledge and experience (Figure 14–1). Although there is not necessarily a one-to-one conversion from one categorization scheme to the other, for the most part approaches that are designed to improve the signal quality or to improve the individual's auditory perceptual skills would be classified as bottom-up or stimulus-driven procedures, whereas approaches that are used to enhance the individual's linguistic and cognitive skills would be classified as top-down or concept-driven procedures.

Many of the intervention options used with children can be used with adolescents and adults; however, as indicated earlier, adolescents and adults with CAPD often present with unique challenges and special needs, and brain plasticity, which is optimal during childhood, is typically reduced in the older individual, with the amount of plasticity decreasing with increasing age (Musiek, Baran, & Schochat, 1999). Therefore, alterations or changes in the neural substrate of the CANS as a result of auditory training may be less likely to occur; they may require more time and training; and they may be less extensive following auditory training than is typically seen in a younger person. However, even more mature brains do maintain some level of plasticity (Musiek et al., 1999). Therefore, auditory training techniques should not be summarily dismissed as an option for inclusion in an intervention plan for the adolescent or adult with CAPD. Given the expectation of reduced brain plasticity for the older patient, it is likely that the intervention plan developed for an adult with CAPD will focus less on formal and

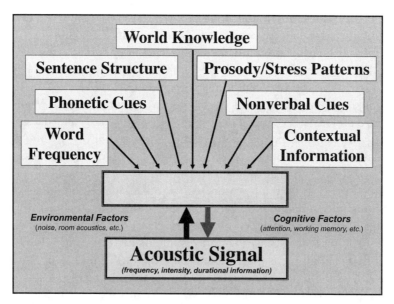

Figure 14–1. A schematic showing the relationship between bottom-up (i.e., stimulus-driven) and top-down (i.e., concept-driven) processes in the processing of verbal stimuli.

informal auditory training approaches that are specifically designed to improve the individual's auditory perceptual skills and more on the types of intervention strategies that are designed to improve the signal quality and/or enhance the individual's compensatory cognitive and linguistic strategies and skills.

As the individual with a CAPD matures from childhood, through adolescence, and then into his or her adult years, new academic, vocational, psychological, and emotional issues often surface and/or preexisting issues become more consequential. Along with increasing age and maturity comes exposure to new and varied listening contexts (e.g., large college classrooms, technical or trade schools with noisy classrooms, civic or religious group meetings)—all of which can place increased demands on the individual's auditory processing skills. Previously successful individuals may now find that the strategies that once served them well fail to provide the assistance they need to face the challenges they experience as adolescents and young adults in these new contexts. As a result, additional management options such as academic or vocational modifications, psychological counseling, career counseling, and transition planning must be considered when an intervention plan is being developed for the adolescent or adult with CAPD. Some of these interventions may be provided most efficiently by the audiologist, whereas other services may be more appropriately provided by other professionals (e.g., speech-language pathologists, psychologists, special educators, vocational rehabilitation counselors). For these reasons, the value of a multidisciplinary approach to management of CAPD cannot be underestimated.

Signal Enhancement Approaches

Signal enhancement procedures typically involve the use of specialized equipment, environmental modifications, and/or speaker training techniques that are specifically designed to improve the quality of the acoustic signal that reaches the auditory system of the individual with CAPD. Commonly used approaches include the provision of either a personal FM (frequency-modulated) system or a classroom/group amplification system, the reduction of extraneous or competing environmental noise through the application of sound attenuating materials in the listening environment (e.g., classroom, workplace), the assignment or personal selection of preferential seating, the enhancement of the acoustic parameters of a spoken message through a variety of means, such as through the use of clear speech procedures (Picheny, Durlach, & Braida, 1985, 1986, 1989), and the use of specialized technology (e.g., telephone amplifiers). Although the use of a personal FM system would often be beneficial for the adolescent or adult student with CAPD, this type of device is frequently rejected by older students, especially those in their teenage years as these students are likely to be concerned about "appearances" and are often subjected to considerable peer pressure in this regard. In these instances, the professional will need to explore alternative methods of enhancing the quality of the acoustic signal (e.g., classroom amplification devices). Finally, it should be noted that all of the approaches listed above can be applied in a variety of contexts (e.g., home, school, or workplace) with appropriate modifications (Baran,

1998; Bellis, 2004; Chermak & Musiek, 1992, 1997; Musiek, 1998; Musiek et al., 1999; Musiek & Schochat, 1999; Masters, Stecker, & Katz, 1998; Ray, Sharff, & Glassford, 1984; Rosenberg, 2002). For additional discussion of personal FM systems, classroom modifications and group amplification systems, and other approaches to maximize the acoustics of the listening environment, the reader is referred to Chapters 4, 12, and 13.

Auditory Training

Auditory training approaches involve those intervention techniques that are specifically directed at improving the individual's auditory perceptual skills. As discussed earlier, these approaches tend to be more effective with younger patients than with older patients as neurophysiologic changes in the CANS are more likely to occur in younger patients due to the higher level of plasticity noted in these individuals. However, even more mature brains maintain some level of plasticity. Therefore, auditory training techniques should not be immediately dismissed as an option for inclusion in an intervention plan for the adolescent or adult with CAPD. As would be the case for children, the selection of the specific type or types of auditory training should be made based on the results of a comprehensive central auditory assessment through which the specific auditory deficit areas can be identified and then targeted for remediation. Musiek and his colleagues have identified a number of auditory processes that can be assessed using specific auditory tests and they have outlined specific intervention procedures that can be used to address each deficit area identified by these tests

(Table 14–2) (Musiek, 1999; Musiek et al., 1999; Musiek & Schochat, 1998). Information on these procedures as well as a discussion of other issues and considerations in the selection of formal and informal auditory training procedures can be found in these resources, as well as in Bellis (2003), Musiek et al. (2002), Chermak and Musiek (1997, 2002) and Chapters 7, 8, and 9 of this Handbook.

Linguistic and Cognitive Interventions

As the individual with CAPD matures into adolescence and then adulthood, the rehabilitative program designed for the individual is less likely to focus on specific skill acquisition (e.g., phonological awareness training, auditory discrimination training) and is more likely to focus on the development of metalinguistic and metacognitive skills and strategies (i.e., central resources training). Many well-conceived strategies have been developed and used with individuals with CAPD. Specific information on these procedures can be found in a number of sources and will not be detailed here (Baran, 1998, 2002; Bellis, 2003, Chermak, 1998; Chermak & Musiek, 1992, 1997; Masters et al., 1998; Musiek, 1998; Musiek et al., 1999; Musiek & Schochat, 1999). The reader is also referred to Chapter 10 for an in-depth discussion of metalinguistic and metacognitive approaches.

Although many of the strategies that have been described in these publications may appear to be obvious, and therefore should require little instructional effort or therapeutic intervention, this may not be the case (Baran, 2002, 2007). If the application of a given strategy was obvious to the individual with

Table 14–2. Examples of Test-Related Auditory Processes and Suggested Auditory Training Procedures

Auditory Process	Tests That Assess Process	Habilitation Techniques
Auditory closure	Distorted speech tests (e.g., filtered speech, compressed speech)	Miller-Gildea vocabulary building
Auditory discrimination	Difference limens for intensity, frequency, duration	Discrimination training, auditory vigilance
Binaural interaction	Dichotic rhyme, localization and lateralization tests	Signal detection in sound-field with changing target positions
Binaural integration	Dichotic speech tests: divided attention	Intensity-altered dichotic listening, temporally altered dichotic listening, auditory vigilance tasks
Binaural separation	Dichotic speech tests: directed attention	Intensity-altered dichotic listening, temporally altered dichotic listening, auditory vigilance tasks
Temporal processing	Two element ordering, pattern perception tests, click fusion	Gap detection, sequencing tasks, prosody training

Source: From Musiek, F. E., Baran, J. A., & Schochat, E. (1999). Selected management approaches to central auditory processing disorders. *Scandinavian Audiology, 28*(Suppl. 51), 63–76. Retrieved from http://www.tandf.co.uk/journals

CAPD, then it is likely that this individual would have adopted the use of the strategy without the need for any type of specific instruction. Moreover, even if an individual "self" identifies a strategy that works well for a given situation or context, if that individual does not learn how to generalize the adopted strategy to new situations or contexts, the individual is likely to continue to experience communicative breakdowns or failures in new contexts. For these reasons, it is advisable that formalized, strategy instruction be considered as a potential component of the management plan that is being developed for adolescents or adults with CAPD (Baran, 2002, 2007).

Although there have been a number of different approaches described for strategy instruction interventions, these procedures usually involve a number of common activities or steps. Most instructional approaches will include: (1) some type of preassessment of current strategy use and commitment to the use of newly acquired strategies, (2) the identification and description of the strategies, (3) the modeling of the strategies, (4) verbal rehearsal of the strategies, (5) controlled practice and feedback on the application of the strategies, and (6) generalization of the strategies to new contexts. The reader interested in additional information on the application of strategy instruction procedures is referred to the following resources (Baran, 1998, 2002; Bender, 2004; Deschler, Alley, Warner, & Schumaker, 1981; Deschler, Shumaker, Lenz, & Ellis, 1984; Hallahan, Lloyd, Kauffman, Weiss, & Martinez, 2005; Harris, Graham, & Pressley, 1991).

Ecological Perspectives

Auditory processing problems are complex and the manner in which they are manifested can vary with different contexts. Often persons with CAPD will experience problems in one context, but they may fail to show evidence of their auditory difficulties in another context, as elaborated below. Even within a given context, it is not uncommon for an auditory deficit to be noted at certain times and not evident at other times. As mentioned earlier, older students and adults need to function in a number of different contexts with varying communicative demands. Children are typically viewed within two relatively distinct and separate contexts. During the day they are viewed as "learners" and function primarily within the context of school. Outside of school, they are viewed primarily as members of a family, even when they are engaged in school-related activities, such as completing homework assignments (Baran, 2002, 2007; Kleinman & Bashir, 1996). However, distinctively different behaviors and roles are expected of the adult. The lives of adolescents and adults are not so neatly compartmental-

ized, as they are expected to function in a number of different and often overlapping contexts (home, work, community and civic organizations, recreational settings) (Baran, 2002, 2007; Kleinman & Bashir, 1996).

At the same time, adults with CAPD (as well as many adolescents, especially those who leave school prior to high school graduation) do not often enjoy the same level of support that is typically provided to the child with such a disability. For the postsecondary student or the adult, there may be no educational team, advocate, or parent to inform others of the difficulties that the individual is experiencing. For the adolescent who is moving into the upper grades (e.g., junior high and high school placements), new challenges are likely to arise—even for those students who may still be on an individualized education plan (IEP). The student in the upper grades is expected to move from classroom to classroom to complete coursework with various teachers who have expertise in particular subject matters. With each different course comes a different teacher with his or her own unique teaching style and philosophy—some of which may be complementary to the individual's learning and communication style/needs, while others may prove to be at odds with the individual's learning style and needs. Not only will the teachers change throughout the course of the school day, but so will the environment within which the student must function. Differences in classroom acoustics, the location of the classrooms relative to noise sources both inside and outside of the school building, and the size and composition of the various classes in which the student is enrolled will all function to provide the student with CAPD with more or less favorable listening environments as he or she changes classes throughout the day.

These issues become even larger when the individual transitions from a secondary educational program to a postsecondary or technical school placement. In these latter contexts, classes are generally much larger, especially for freshman enrolled in large postsecondary institutions, as first year college students are typically enrolled in general education or "core" courses, which tend to be among the largest courses offered at an institution. As a result of the large number of students enrolled in these courses and the large classrooms that are needed to accommodate these large enrollments, classroom noise often becomes more of a problem and instructors often do not have the opportunity to get to know each student's individual learning style and needs (at least not in a timely manner). In addition, the instructors are less likely to be able to monitor students' faces for indications that they have understood or grasped the information being presented. Moreover, the postsecondary student is less likely to have an individual who can serve as an advocate on his or her behalf. Therefore, it is important that the older student with CAPD assume responsibility for his or her own listening and academic success, and he or she will need to document his or her disability and secure an accommodation plan through his or her college or university. In other words, it will be important for the older student with CAPD to acquire the skills and confidence needed to become an effective self-advocate.

The postsecondary student needs not only to become an effective self-advocate, but also needs to become "strategic" to succeed. Strategies that worked well in elementary or high school may not provide the same assistance in the new and more advanced academic context. In order to succeed in a postsecondary program the older student must be able to assess each new listening situation, to identify the strategies that might help compensate for any processing difficulties that are anticipated in the novel listening environment, to select the strategy (or strategies) that appears/appear to be the best alternative(s) given the circumstances, and to find another, alternative strategy if the selected strategy fails to meet the individual's needs in the particular context. In other words, adolescents and adults with CAPD need to not only know how to implement a strategy, but they also need to become *strategic* —knowing when or under which conditions to deploy a strategy (Baran, 1998, 2007; Chermak & Musiek, 1997). What worked in one environment or context may not prove to be useful in another environment or context—or possibly, even within the same environment or context if factors either intrinsic to the individual (e.g., increased fatigue) or extrinsic to the individual (e.g., increases in environmental noise levels) function to negate the usefulness of a "proven" and commonly used strategy.

Although much of the previous discussion has focused on the adolescent or the adult with CAPD who is in a secondary or postsecondary educational placement, much of what has been discussed would be important for the adolescent or adult with CAPD regardless of whether the individual is a student, an employee, a community member, and so forth. Contexts or environments seldom remain constant. In fact, changes in the listening environment are more commonly the rule rather than the exception. It is important, therefore, that individuals with CAPD learn to become *strategic,* as it is likely that the manifestations of their auditory deficits will change both within and across contexts (Baran, 2002, 2007).

Working With Multiculturally and Linguistically Diverse Clients and Families

It is likely that most professionals working with adolescents and adults with CAPD will work with a culturally and linguistically diverse clientele, especially when one considers the changing demographics of the U.S. population. Recent demographic projections suggest that by 2050 the number of Americans racially classified as other than "non-Hispanic White" will exceed the number of Americans who fall into the "non-Hispanic White" classification (Passel & Cohn, 2008; Taylor & Cohn, 2012). These changing demographics underscore the need for professionals to be prepared to work with an increasing number of individuals who may not share the same racial/ethnic backgrounds or cultural values as the professional. To do so, the professional must gain an understanding and appreciation of the cultural differences that may mold an individual's (and his or her family's) needs and expectations and that may also influence or determine the individual's ability to access or benefit from professional services.

In some cultural groups, the parameters defining a communication disorder are influenced by the group's cultural values (Battle, 1997). Behaviors that are considered to be abnormal in one cultural group may well meet the norm for acceptable behavior in another cultural group. So what is perceived to be a disorder by members from the predominant cultural group(s) in the United States, may not be considered a disorder by other cultural groups. Also, in some cultural groups, seeking help for a communication disorder may not be considered as an option, even if the presence of the disorder is recognized. Different cultures assign different meanings to health, wellness, and disability (Battle, 1997). In some cultures, these definitions or meanings may impact access to rehabilitative or intervention services. For example, individuals from a Chinese culture may believe that an individual with a disability or disorder is a curse that has been visited upon the family as a result of the sins or wrongdoings of one's ancestors. In other cultures, an individual with a disability is viewed as a gift from a higher being. In either case, it is unlikely that the individual or the family of the individual with a disorder holding these beliefs will seek counseling and/or intervention services (Battle, 1997).

In Western cultures there is a commonly held assumption that individuals need to change to fit the system, but many cultural groups believe that the system can be altered to fit the individual (Battle, 1997). Also, there is an assumption among persons from Western cultures that individuals with disorders are helped by formal intervention services, whereas in many non-Western cultures there is a commonly held belief that the individual can be helped by the natural support of the family and the community. These differences in cultural values and beliefs will clearly influence an individual's willingness to seek out rehabilitative services (see Battle, 1997, 2002, for additional discussion of these topics).

An understanding of a cultural group's values and traditions can provide a framework for working with an individual from a cultural background that is different from that of the individual providing the services. It is essential, nonetheless, to consider each patient as an individual. Over time, individuals from a different cultural background may take on some of the values of the mainstream group as they are immersed in the Western culture. This process of internalizing some of the values of the new culture to which the individual is exposed is referred to as acculturation (Battle, 2002). As a result of this process, the individual's values may no longer overlap completely with the original culture and it will be important for the professional providing services to understand the individual's new (and often hybrid) values system.

In addition to cultural differences, there may be linguistic differences or communication style differences that may impact the rehabilitative process. Such linguistic differences are obvious when one is working with a non-English-speaking client and his or her family. However, some of these differences may not be as obvious when one is working with an individual for whom English is a second language. In many languages, there are differences in language use that may carry over into the second language, which if not recognized by the professional providing services may be misinterpreted as a language or auditory processing deficit. Take for example the use of silence in conversions. For most Americans, silence in a conversation is interpreted as a hesitancy to speak or an inability to process or respond appropriately. However, in other cultural and linguistic groups, silence can indicate respect for elders (Japanese, Native American), agreement with the previous speaker's message or intent (Russian, Spanish, and French), or disagreement or inability to accept a speaker's attitude, opinions, or beliefs (Chinese) (Battle, 1997). There are many other examples of language use (both form and function) that can be culturally determined. The reader interested in a more in-depth discussion of these topics is referred to Battle (1997).

To summarize, it is essential that the provider who is offering services to individuals from different racial, cultural, or ethnic groups have an appreciation and an understanding of the potential differences in behaviors, values, and/or beliefs that may be represented among the individuals with whom the professional is working. Such an understanding will assist the professional in designing a culturally appropriate intervention for each individual that then should meet with the greatest support and involvement from both the patient and his or her family.

Academic Modifications for Secondary and Postsecondary Students

Secondary and postsecondary programs often present new challenges for the individual with CAPD. As the individual moves from the early grades through middle school, high school, and then onto to college, class sizes often become larger, especially in postsecondary programs. Unfortunately, large classes pose unique challenges for the student with a CAPD. As discussed above, faculty are not likely to get to know each student individually in large classes and there is likely to be more noise present in larger classrooms (e.g., college students often come late to class and some students will leave early, some students will shuffle papers, and others will converse with classmates). In addition, the postsecondary student is less likely to have an advocate or a case manager to help the student gain access to the support services and/or academic modifications that are needed to ensure success.

At the postsecondary level, there is an increased reliance on independent learning and the student is expected to take responsibility for his or her own success or failure. Depending upon the nature of the services received as a student in previous school placements, the individual may enter a postsecondary educational placement ill-equipped to face these new challenges. Many students who have been on IEPs for several years have not had to function independently as there typically has been an individual or a team of professionals within the school assigned the responsibility of ensuring that the goals and the objectives of the individual's IEP are met. Although this type of service delivery may work well for younger students, it does little to prepare students as they transition from secondary to postsecondary placements; that is, unless the IEP specifically addresses some of the new skills that the individual will need to acquire to be successful in college or in an alternative postsecondary placement (e.g., technical or vocational school). As discussed below, if students are to be prepared to meet these new academic demands and expectations they should receive both self-advocacy training and counseling and guidance on how to transition effectively into the new educational program. Both of these services will be most beneficial if they are provided before the time that the student matriculates into the postsecondary placement.

Facing increasing numbers of students requiring individual academic planning and support (e.g., students with learning and/or cognitive disabilities) as well as a number of federal mandates (e.g., Section 504 of the Rehabilitation Act of 1973 and the Americans with Disabilities Act of 1990), universities and colleges have instituted academic support services for their students with disabilities (Baran, 2002, 2007). However, the range of services available across university campuses varies along a continuum from minimal support services to more comprehensive support programs. Even in the institutions with more extensive programs, the services available to students are not likely to be as extensive or as individualized as those that were afforded them as students in elementary or secondary educational programs (Baran, 2002). (See Chapter 5 for discussion of elementary and secondary school policies, processes, and services for students with CAPD.)

Table 14–3 lists some of the more common academic modifications often recommended to assist adult learners with their learning challenges. Some of these recommendations are more appropriate for secondary students, whereas others are more realistic for postsecondary students. For example, it is common practice for faculty in postsecondary institutions to provide a syllabus at the beginning of each course, which outlines course objectives, topics to be covered in class, the sequencing and time of coverage of these topics, as well as specific readings and other assignments that are linked to

Table 14–3. Examples of academic modifications for students in secondary and postsecondary academic placements

Test administration in alternative environments (e.g., less noisy, fewer distractions)
Provision of note-taking services
Provision of tutoring services (may also include peer tutoring)
Reduced course loads
Waiver of a foreign language requirement or approval of a course substitution for a foreign language requirement (e.g., American Sign Language, a culture course)
Creative scheduling of classes to ensure that course requirements and task demands are equally distributed over the course of the academic program
Preferential seating (if seating is assigned)
Tape recordings of lectures and presentations
Video recordings of lectures and presentations
Assignment or selection of course section where instructor's teaching philosophy and style are consistent with student's needs
Provision of outlines, lecture notes, or reading assignments prior to class presentation so that student can review materials in advance
Other accommodations to address comorbid learning difficulties (e.g., untimed tests, alternative test formats)

Source: From Masters, M. Gay; Stecker, Nancy A.; Katz, Jack, *Central Auditory Processing Disorders: Mostly Management, 1st Edition,* © 1998, p. 207. Reprinted by permission of Pearson Education, Inc., Upper Saddle River, NJ.

each topic. Therefore, it is unlikely that a recommended modification/accommodation for the college student would include a request that faculty provide this information prior to each class. In secondary programs, however, it is less likely that students would be provided this type of information for the entire course—most of which are year-long courses. In these instances, a reasonable accommodation would be for the teacher to provide reading assignments prior to the day/time that a topic is to be covered in class. The student with CAPD can then review this information prior to its coverage in the class, thus increasing the likelihood that the information will be processed, understood, and hopefully internalized when it is presented in class.

Preferential seating is a common accommodation that is often recommended for a student with CAPD. In secondary programs where seating is often assigned, it may be reasonable to recommend to the teaching staff that a given individual be provided preferential seating (i.e., seating that provides the greatest auditory and visual access to the primary signal, typically the teacher) when seating assignments are made. Often, such preferential seating involves providing a seat at the front of the classroom for the student with CAPD; however, when classroom discussions are taking place, a more advantageous seating position is likely to be in the center of the classroom. In postsecondary settings, however, seating assignments rarely are made by the instructor. In these cases, although preferential seating would be beneficial, and therefore recommended, it would typically be the student's responsibility for ensuring that he or she has secured such seating. This may mean coming to class early so that the desired seating will still be available.

One of the major challenges for many postsecondary students is fulfilling a university's or college's foreign language requirement—a common requirement for graduation at many colleges and universities. Some universities will waive this requirement for the student with CAPD with sufficient documentation of the disability, whereas others will not waive the requirement, but rather will offer a course substitution (or substitutions) to satisfy this course requirement. The most common modification accepted at many colleges is the substitution of a course that will expose the student to the culture of a different country (Baran, 2002). Another modification of the foreign language requirement accepted by some universities is the substitution of a course in American Sign Language. This modification of the foreign language requirement is particularly attractive for many students with CAPD, since the reliance on auditory skills for acquisition of the language is significantly reduced when compared with the heavy auditory demands of learning a foreign language that is taught primarily through the auditory modality.

The preceding comments highlight the need to consider the unique circumstances that surround each student before recommending any of the accommodations listed in Table 14–3. What works for one student in one context will not necessarily work (or be appropriate) for another student in what may appear on the surface to be the same context.

Vocational Modifications

Although academic modifications recommended for individuals with CAPD are more extensively discussed in the literature, equally important is the need for vocational modifications when young adults graduate from high school and enter the workforce. Unfortunately, this is an area where limited assistance is readily available for young adults with CAPD who may be in need of (and eligible for) this type of support because there are few professionals who provide this type of intervention and support. Consultations with the employer can help the employer understand the deficits that the employee is experiencing as well as how these deficits or difficulties may interact with job demands. In addition, the work environment can be evaluated and recommendations for potential modifications that will improve the listening environment may be offered (e.g., the application of sound attenuating materials, the relocation of a work area away from a significant noise source). Such protections are afforded to employees with disabilities by federal mandates (e.g., the Americans with Disabilities Act of 1990) and should be more readily available to individuals with CAPD and related disabilities. It is therefore essential that more professionals (i.e., audiologists) become involved in the provision of these types of intervention services. When equipped with professional advice and recommendations, employers can implement workplace modifications that will help ensure that employees with disabilities can meet with job success and job satisfaction.

Career Counseling and Transition Planning

Career counseling and transition planning are often overlooked components of an intervention plan for the older student with CAPD. Many adolescents and young adults with CAPD have spent most of their time and energy throughout their educational programs learning how their auditory deficits affect their functioning as "learners." Often these individuals fail to develop an understanding of how these same auditory deficits may affect their performance in the workplace—where the listening demands and performance expectations may be very different from those that were encountered in the educational setting. This lack of understanding as to how their auditory deficits may potentially interact with new listening and performance demands may set the stage for frustration, possible job loss, and loss of self-esteem as these individuals enter the job market. Some of these undesirable outcomes may be avoided, or at least minimized, if students are provided guidance in this area before graduation through the use of appropriate counseling services. Students who can identify their strengths and weaknesses and who are prepared to explore a variety of career options will be more likely to choose a career where they can meet with reasonable success

(Baran, 2002, 2007). In some cases, we have found that students may have chosen realistic career paths, but that parental or societal pressures are pushing these students toward careers for which they are ill-equipped, uninterested, and unmotivated. Counseling may help these students learn how to become more self-assertive in dealing with these parental and societal pressures. Also, career counseling and transition planning can help students who are preparing to enter the workforce learn how to adapt to a new environment (i.e., the workplace) where many of the accommodations that they were previously accustomed to having may not be available. As a result new accommodations may need to be identified and negotiated.

Even when a good "fit" exists between and among the individual's interests, strengths, and career, vocational or educational choices, it is likely that the individual with CAPD will encounter new and unanticipated challenges as he or she moves from one context to another (as discussed above). By working with a counselor, the individual may be able to begin to identify the potential difficulties that may be encountered in the new academic program or job placement. Equipped with this knowledge, the individual can plan how he or she will react to these difficulties if they are encountered. Finally, an essential component of the intervention plan for individuals with CAPD or related disorders is that of self-advocacy training. Although all of these interventions can be incorporated into the management program of a college student or the adult with CAPD, they are likely to be most useful to the individual if they are provided, or at least introduced, during the junior/senior high school years.

Self-Advocacy Training

Young students with disabilities in the educational mainstream typically have an IEP that specifies the various interventions and support services that will be received. They are also likely to have an advocate, case manager, or other professional who ensures that the child's educational needs are being met. As a consequence, many young students do not develop the skills and abilities needed to take on this advocacy role as the need arises and they may struggle in new and challenging situations rather than ask for assistance or accommodations. This is particularly true at the postsecondary level, where it is unlikely that the student will have an individual who advocates for the student. Without specific training in the development of self-advocacy skills, the postsecondary student may not be equipped to access the assistance and/ or accommodations that will be needed in this new educational setting.

Although problems related to poor development of self-advocacy skills often surface in postsecondary environments, they also may be experienced in the workplace. Employees with CAPD who are not able to advocate for their own needs may find themselves at risk for loss of employment or lack of advancement or promotion due to perceived employee ineffectiveness (Baran, 2002, 2007). These individuals also may find that they are not accepted by colleagues in the workplace, as they are perceived by coworkers as being disinterested, aloof, snobby, or antisocial, since they may not readily participate in the conversations that often take place in the workplace because of their auditory deficits (Baran, 2002, 2007).

Management Considerations for Individuals With CAPD and Peripheral Hearing Loss

There are many individuals who will experience both a peripheral hearing loss and a CAPD. This particular comorbidity is more likely to affect adults as they age. In these individuals the CAPD either coexists with, or is secondary to the peripheral hearing loss. In either case, many of the interventions discussed in this chapter can be used to alleviate the auditory problems that these individuals may experience. However, this group of individuals can present unique challenges for the audiologist involved in the selection and fitting of hearing aids. Current preferred practice patterns in the field of audiology outline routine assessment procedures that should be used to evaluate the status of the auditory periphery prior to the fitting of amplification. Unfortunately, the assessment of the integrity and function of the CANS in patients with peripheral loss who are being seen for fitting of amplification is currently not standard practice (ASHA, 2006; Musiek & Baran, 1996). However, recent practice guidelines have recommended that adults presenting with certain types of hearing complaints (e.g., hearing complaints that exceed expectations based upon pure-tone findings, less than anticipated benefit from amplification in individuals who have been fitted with hearing aids) and/or significant case history information (i.e., case history information that suggests possible central nervous system disease/dysfunction, including dementia, cerebrovascular disease, head injury, etc.) be screened for

CAPD (AAA, 2010; ASHA, 2006; see Dillon, 2012 for additional discussion).

Today most patients with hearing loss are considered to be good candidates for amplification given the advances that have occurred in hearing aid technology over the past several years and binaural fittings have become the standard of care for the vast majority of patients with bilateral hearing losses as the benefits of binaural amplification have been well documented (Dillon, 2012; Taylor & Mueller, 2011). In spite of the documented benefits of binaural fittings for most patients with bilateral hearing losses, there appears to be a small subgroup of individuals with bilateral hearing losses for whom binaural amplification may be contraindicated. As clinicians and researchers learn more about the functioning of the CANS and the potential for less-than-optimal binaural processing of auditory information in some patients with CANS disorders, the customary practice of recommending binaural hearing aids for patients with bilateral hearing loss must be questioned.

Jerger and his colleagues (1993) found evidence of binaural interference using aided speech recognition and middle latency response (MLR) measures in four patients with symmetrical hearing losses. Aided speech recognition scores were obtained under three test conditions (aided right ear, aided left ear, and binaural fitting) for three of these subjects, and in all three cases, sizable performance differences were noted between the scores obtained under the two monaural conditions in spite of the finding of symmetrical pure-tone hearing measures. More significant, however, was the observation that the binaural test condition resulted in reduced performance when the score obtained under this condition was compared with the aided speech recognition score of the better ear for each of the three subjects.

These same investigators also obtained MLRs for three of their four subjects under three conditions (monaural right, monaural left, and binaural presentation) and noted a similar pattern of results; that is, the waveforms derived under the binaural presentation condition for all three subjects were noticeably poorer than the waveforms derived from the better ear in each case (Jerger et al., 1993). For these subjects, the presentation of an auditory stimulus to the second or "poorer ear" somehow interfered with the processing of information presented to the "better ear." Although the exact mechanisms underlying this phenomenon have not been definitively established, it is likely that some type of distortion is being introduced by the existing compromise of either the peripheral and/or the central system. Three possible mechanisms include: (1) inefficient transfer of information between the hemispheres, (2) differential aging of the two hemispheres, and (3) asymmetrical cochlear distortions. (See Dillon, 2012, for a more in-depth discussion of these mechanisms.) Regardless of the exact mechanism(s) that may underlie this interference phenomenon, there remains an important implication of these findings; that is, that binaural processes within the auditory system must function appropriately if a patient is to make optimal use of binaural amplification.

Musiek and Baran (1996) outlined four other instances where binaural amplification may be contraindicated for patients with comorbid peripheral hearing loss and CANS dysfunction. They suggested that binaural amplification may be contraindicated under the following conditions: (1) if a symmetrical hearing loss is present, but the central auditory test performance of one ear is markedly poorer than that of the other ear, (2) if an asymmetrical hearing loss is present, and the central auditory test performance of the *better ear* is significantly poorer than that of the poorer ear, (3) if a symmetrical hearing loss is present and abnormal middle and/or late potentials are noted over one hemisphere versus the other (i.e., a significant electrode effect), and (4) if a symmetrical hearing loss is present and an ear effect is noted on electrophysiologic testing (pp. 415–423). Case studies highlighting each of these four conditions or case profiles can be found in the reference cited above. (Also see Chapter 11 in Volume 1 of this Handbook.)

The cases presented by Jerger et al. (1993) and Musiek and Baran (1996) provide evidence of less-than-optimal binaural processing in at least a subgroup of patients with peripheral hearing loss. For an individual to take full advantage of binaural amplification, all of the binaural processes within the CANS must function at their optimum level. As the binaural processes of the CANS are not assessed by routine audiological testing, it is important that the audiologist consider the need to assess CANS function when working with patients with peripheral hearing loss, especially if the patient is considered to be at risk for CAPD. (See Musiek & Baran, 1996, for discussion of alternative methods to incorporate such testing into the evaluation procedures used with patients who are being seen for hearing aid selection and fitting procedures.)

Professional Teaming

The effective intervention program for an adult or adolescent with CAPD is likely to involve contributions from more than one professional. As noted above, it is frequently the case that the individual with CAPD will also experience one or more comorbid conditions (e.g., speech and language disorder, attention deficit disorder with or without hyperactivity, psychological or emotional disorders). The coexistence of one or more of these disorders can significantly impact the effectiveness of any of the intervention programs or strategies that are specifically designed to address the individual's auditory processing deficits. It is therefore important that each of these areas be assessed by the professional with the appropriate training and credentials to conduct such evaluations, and that these professionals then collaborate on the development of an intervention plan for the individual (AAA, 2010; ASHA, 2005b).

Even in those less typical cases where CAPD appears to be the only deficit area, both the audiologist and the speech-language pathologist likely will be involved in the development and delivery of an intervention plan or program. The audiologist will likely take responsibility for interventions designed to improve the quality of the signal (e.g., provision of a personal FM system, consultation with a school system to install a classroom amplification system) and to improve the listening environment (e.g., working with school personnel to improve classroom acoustics). In addition, the audiologist should be involved in the provision of auditory training activities, especially those training activities that can be provided most effectively with the use of sophisticated electronic instrumentation that permits the precise control of the stimulus parameters (e.g., the dichotic interaural intensity difference [DIID] procedure) (Musiek et al., 2004; also see Chapter 9). The speech-language pathologist's role in the management program is to work with the individual to enhance the individual's cognitive and linguistic resources (e.g., working with the individual to identify metacognitive and metalinguistic strategies that can improve the individual's ability to follow conversations, communicate more effectively, etc.). In addition, speech-language pathologists are often involved in the delivery of auditory training programs, especially informal auditory training (e.g., auditory discrimination training) (see Chapter 7) and computerized auditory-language training programs (see Chapter 11), as these are procedures that fall within their scope of practice and for which they are likely to receive reimbursement (ASHA, 2004; Chermak & Musiek, 2002).

When working with adolescents and many young adults with CAPD, it is important to also include teachers, special educators, and guidance counselors in the "professional team." These professionals arc in position to help ensure that interventions designed by the audiologist, speech pathologist and/or other professional carry over to the school setting and that newly acquired skills and/or strategies generalize to other settings. In addition, these individuals can play important roles in career counseling, transition planning, and self-advocacy training.

Role of Paraprofessionals and Family Members

Paraprofessionals can play an important role in the provision of services to individuals with CAPD. Aides in the classroom can assist students by insuring that instructions, course content and homework assignments are received and understood by the individual with CAPD. They can provide additional explanation and clarification of concepts or topics that are not fully understood because the verbal message is not processed efficiently. They also can monitor the student's attention during class time, help the student refocus if lapses in attention occur, and provide other important support services in the classroom.

Speech-language pathology assistants can augment or reinforce the remedial services that are being provided by the school's speech-language pathologists. In many schools, the speech-language pathologist's caseload is quite high, often limiting the amount and frequency of services that can be provided to the child with a disability. Speech-language pathology assistants can provide additional instruction and practice on the activities planned by the speech-language pathologist, which should lead to more timely attainment of therapy goals and objectives. These individuals can also play significant roles in implementing some of the strategy instruction techniques outlined above (e.g., they could be helpful in modeling behaviors for the student, listening to student's description of the strategies).

At the postsecondary level, tutors and note-takers can provide invaluable services to the college student with CAPD. As noted above, postsecondary courses and programs often present new challenges for the student with CAPD. Class sizes are often large, the acoustics of the classroom are frequently less than ideal, and new vocabulary items are likely to be introduced in advanced courses that may not be accurately perceived by the student with CAPD. Each of these variables may hinder the reception and acquisition of course materials that are presented auditorily. Tutors and note-takers can help facilitate the acquisition of information and concepts that may be missed in the classroom due to the presence of CAPD.

Finally, family members and friends can take on important roles in the rehabilitative program for the adolescent or adult with CAPD. They can, and will, play a significant role in the application of some recommended procedures (e.g., clear speech, which requires that the conversational partner with whom the person is communicating take responsibility for modifying his or her own speech according to the parameters specified in the approach). They also can take on the role of facilitator or monitor for many of the informal procedures that may be recommended for implementation at home, as many of these procedures will require a second person to provide feedback about the appropriateness of an individual's responses and/or to present the necessary auditory stimuli. (See Chapter 13 for elaboration of clear speech.)

Documenting Treatment Efficacy

It is important for professionals working with individuals with CAPD to be able to document patient outcomes. As the health care industry works to control rising costs, it is demanding evidence of the effectiveness of treatment procedures. As noted by Musiek et al. (2005), "a solid base of evidence documents improved psychophysical performance, neurophysiologic representation of acoustic stimuli, and listening and related function in children and adults following targeted auditory training" (p. 2); however, additional studies are needed to produce

the level of evidence (e.g., randomized controlled trials; meta-analysis of randomized controlled trials) needed to establish the efficacy of various interventions (Chermak, 2002). An accumulating number of empirical studies have begun to document the efficacy of treatment approaches. (See Chapter 3 for a review.) However, CAPD is a relatively young area of clinical research and the investigative energies in the field of CAPD have followed a natural evolution. Following Bocca and his colleagues' (1954, 1955) finding that individuals with temporal lesions experience auditory deficits in spite of normal peripheral audiological findings, much of the clinical research that followed examined the nature of the auditory deficits in patients with confirmed lesions of the CANS as assessed by a number of auditory tasks/tests (Baran & Musiek, 1999). These investigations served to increase our understanding of normal and abnormal brain function and to link specific auditory processes with an area (or areas) of the brain. What then followed was research on the clinical application of these tests to the assessment of auditory processing abilities in children and the development of clinically feasible tests of central auditory function. More recently, research efforts have focused on the efficacy of CAPD intervention programs. One of the first investigations in this area was a study conducted by Jirsa (1992), which was then followed by additional studies that focused on the effects of intervention for CAPD with children (e.g., Alonso & Schochat, 2009; Hayes, Warrier, Nicol, Zecker, & Kraus, 2003; Schochat, Musiek, Alonso, & Ogata, 2010; Schochat, Musiek, & Baran, 2005; Warrier, Johnson, Hayes, Nicol, & Kraus, 2004).

Although there are no large-scale studies that have examined the efficacy of intervention approaches with adults, there have been some case studies that have shown changes in behavioral and electrophysiologic measures in adults with CAPD following intervention (e.g., Musiek et al., 2004; Weihing & Musiek, 2007). In addition, there have been a number of studies with adults that have used various auditory evoked potential measures to see if neurophysiologic changes could be documented following training on novel auditory perceptual tasks (e.g., Kraus et al., 1995; Song, Skoe, Banai, & Kraus, 2011; Tremblay & Kraus, 2002; Tremblay, Kraus, Carrell, & McGee, 1997; Tremblay, Kraus, & McGee, 1998; Tremblay, Kraus, McGee, Ponton, & Otis, 2001). (See Chapter 7 of Volume 1 of this Handbook.) Each of these studies documented one or more electrophysiologic changes associated with the training, and as such provide some evidence that behavioral interventions can result in physiologic changes in adults. Additional studies with adolescents and adults with CAPD using similar methodologies (i.e., behavioral training approaches and electrophysiologic assessment measures) are likely to demonstrate similar findings—thus supporting the efficacy of these approaches with adults despite the anticipated reduced plasticity of the mature brain.

Although much of the interest recently has been in using an objective measure (e.g., MLR, mismatched negativity) to document changes in neurophysiologic function associated with behavioral changes affected by auditory training, this is by no means the only approach to documenting treatment efficacy. Equally as important are ecological or functional measures that document changes in the individual's performance in a variety of contexts (e.g., school, home, work, and community). For these types of documentation, other measures would be needed. These could include various types of behavioral rating scales, communication effectiveness measures, and other performance measures that probe listening, communication, and academic achievement, and so forth.

Documenting Effectiveness for an Individual

Absent large scale investigations that document treatment efficacy for the various approaches that are being used in remediation and management of CAPD with adolescents and adults, it is important for the professional to document on an individual basis the changes (i.e., the outcome measures) that are occurring, presumably as a result of intervention. Electrophysiologic measures as well as behavioral test measures can be used to document these changes; however, additional quantitative and qualitative measures should be included. Data collected should include measures that would document changes (or lack thereof) in a variety of contexts in which the individual would need to use the newly acquired processing skills and/or strategies. For adolescents in structured environments, these could include teacher questionnaires that probe for changes in auditory behaviors and academic performance. For the adult patient who is not in a structured environment, this could include a journal or a checklist where the individual indicates when a desired strategy or behavior was used. Additionally, the journal could include some type of evaluation or rating of the success of the strategy or behavior. The use of these latter techniques can also encourage self-monitoring and the use of executive processes, which can further enhance the treatment program (Chermak & Musiek, 1997). (See Chapter 2 for further discussion of evidence-based practice and treatment efficacy.)

Case Study

History

This case, which has been reported previously (Musiek, Baran, & Shinn, 2004), involves a 41-year-old female who sustained a traumatic head injury secondary to a horseback riding accident. The patient lost consciousness for a brief period of time at the time of the accident, but then recovered consciousness quickly and demonstrated few abnormal symptoms immediately following the accident. She was able to walk without major difficulty and she showed no signs of amnesia, although she was slightly disoriented. She also experienced some disequilibrium and a tinnitus that was localized in her head following her accident. A neurologic exam conducted within a few days of the incident, however, was essentially normal. Based on these findings and the patient's initial posttrauma symptoms, it was the opinion of the attending physician that this patient had sustained a mild concussion.

A few days after the accident, the patient began to experience some additional and/or worsening symptoms. She began to experience dizziness and her previously experienced disorientation became more of a problem. She also began sleeping excessively. In addition, she began experiencing difficulty understanding conversations and recalling information. The patient's physician indicated that these symptoms were not unusual following a concussion and he felt that these symptoms would resolve with time; however, there was little change in the patient's symptoms after a year had lapsed and other symptoms became apparent over this time frame. Listening became more of a challenge. The patient had difficulty maintaining attention, and she often needed "extended" time to process information. She also reported that the hearing in her left ear was poorer than that in her right ear and that she experienced extreme difficulty with the comprehension of auditory directives, hearing in the presence of background noise or competing messages, and following the speech of speakers who spoke rapidly. Additional problems experienced by the patient included reading comprehension difficulties, memory, planning, and organizational problems (i.e., difficulties in executive function), and mathematical computation difficulties. At the time of her audiological evaluation (13 months posttrauma), the patient noted that her tinnitus had resolved and that she had noted some "slight" improvements in her hearing abilities. Although somewhat improved, the patient's auditory problems continued to have a significant negative impact on her ability to function in normal everyday activities.

Audiological Evaluation

This patient was seen for an audiological evaluation at 13 months postaccident. Results of testing conducted at this time revealed normal peripheral auditory function; however, abnormal results were evident on four of five central auditory tests administered (i.e., dichotic digits, competing sentences, duration patterns, and compressed speech) (Figure 14–2). In addition, subtle electrophysiologic abnormalities were suggested by the MLR tests. These included smaller Na–Pa amplitudes for the right ear relative to the left ear, and poorer waveform morphology for right ear versus left ear recordings (Figure 14–3).

Rehabilitative Program

Because the patient lived some distance from our clinical facility, the decision was made to instruct her on a number of therapy approaches that she could work on daily with the assistance of her family. As the patient was highly motivated, we were confident that she would follow through on our recommendations. The specific therapy procedures recommended for her included clear speech, re-auditorization strategies, a modified dichotic interaural intensity difference (DIID) procedure, a modified auditory memory enhancement procedure, temporal sequence training, auditory discrimination training, and the use of metacognitive strategies. The reader is referred to Musiek et al.

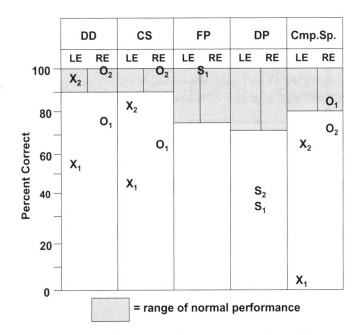

Figure 14–2. Central auditory test results for a 41-year-old female with a history of a mild head injury. Results are displayed for both pre- and postintervention assessments. Key: DD = dichotic digits; CS = competing sentences; FP = frequency patterns; DP = duration patterns; Cmp.Sp. = compressed speech; O_1, X_1, and S_1 = pretherapy test results for the right ear, left ear, and sound field, respectively; O_2, X_2, and S_2 = posttherapy test results for the right ear, left ear, and sound field, respectively (adapted from Musiek et al., 2004, with permission).

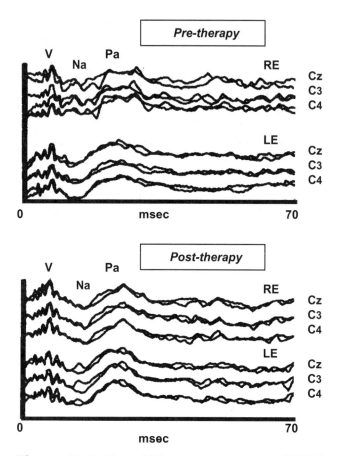

Figure 14–3. The middle latency responses (MLRs) from a 41-year-old female with a history of a mild head injury. Results are displayed for the right and left ears at three electrode sites (Cz, C3, C4) derived pre- and postintervention (adapted from Musiek et al., 2004, with permission).

(2004) for a detailed discussion of each of these procedures and how they were modified for this particular patient.

Postintervention Assessment

Postintervention testing was completed at approximately seven months following our initial assessment of this patient. A screening pure-tone test revealed normal test results. In light of this find-

ing and the previous findings of normal peripheral function, other peripheral tests were not readministered. The four central auditory tests for which performance was found to be abnormal during the earlier testing session were readministered, as was the MLR procedure. As can be seen in Figures 14–2 and 14–3, comparisons of the pre- and postintervention results revealed improvements on a number of the test measures. Test scores improved to within normal limits for both ears on the dichotic digits test and to within normal limits for the right ear and close to normal performance for the left ear on the competing sentences test. Although test performance on the compressed speech test dropped slightly in the right ear, it improved significantly in the left ear. The MLR results showed better waveform morphology across all electrode sites for both ears and increased amplitudes for the Na–Pa wave across three electrode sites when pre- and postintervention comparisons were made.

Postintervention Patient Status

The patient reported that she had noted a number of improvements in her auditory skills and cognitive functioning following her participation in the rehabilitative program. She reported that she could follow and participate in most conversations, although she did acknowledge some continuing difficulty with people who speak rapidly. She also indicated that she could talk on the telephone with the receiver to her left ear and that she was better able to "tune out" auditory distractions and to attend to tasks. She also reported an enhanced ability to recall information and improved short-term and working memory. In addition, concentration skills were reportedly improved, as were organizational skills, and speed of processing. She did, however, continue to experience some auditory and cognitive skills deficits. She reported that processing speed, although improved, had not improved to preaccident levels, that comprehension of some messages remained problematic, and that attending to multiple speakers at the same time and following rapidly

presented speech continued to present some difficulties for her.

Comments

This particular case was chosen for presentation, as it highlights several important considerations and factors that are relevant to the management of the adult with CAPD. These include the following: (1) that patient motivation is an important variable that will affect treatment outcomes, (2) that electrophysiologic measures can be useful in documenting neurophysiological changes associated with improved behavioral measures, (3) that engagement of family members in the rehabilitative program can help facilitate the achievement of program goals and objectives, and (4) that auditory training can be used effectively with adults, even though the brain is known be less plastic as one ages.

Concluding Comments

Central auditory processing disorder represents a complex and heterogeneous group of auditory deficits that can result from a variety of etiologic bases. For many individuals, the disorder will be a developmental disorder that persists from childhood into adulthood. For others, the disorder will be the result of some type of frank neurologic compromise of the CANS (i.e., an acquired disorder), whereas for others the disorder will be the result of normal aging processes. Although there are some clear differences in the etiologic bases of CAPD, these differences do not seem to translate into distinct profiles of auditory deficits. It is important, therefore, that the specific auditory deficits that an individual is experiencing be identified before any management approaches are implemented so that the intervention program can target these specific deficits.

Ecological and context-specific perspectives provide a useful framework for understanding the nature and changing manifestations of CAPD. These perspectives can be used to inform the development of an intervention program. In addition, several other variables are important to consider as one prepares to work with a given individual. Variables such as age, comorbid conditions, communication styles, cultural values, and language differences all can impact an individual's ability to access and benefit from intervention. Therefore, it is essential that each intervention program be individualized to meet the unique needs of each patient. In addition, it is important that each patient's intervention program be continually monitored and systematically evaluated to determine the need for program modifications, which may be indicated if inadequate progress is being made or if the patient's needs change.

References

AAA (American Academy of Audiology). (2010). *Diagnosis, treatment and management of children and adults with auditory processing disorder.* [Clinical practice guidelines]. Retrieved from http://www.audiology.org/resources/documentlibrary/Documents/CAPD%20Guidelines%208-2010.pdf

Alonso, R., & Schochat, E. (2009). The efficacy of formal auditory training in children with (central) auditory processing disorder: Behavioral and electrophysiological evaluation. *Brazilian Journal of Otorhinolaryngology, 75*(5), 726–732.

American with Disabilities Act of 1990, 49 U.S.C. §§ 12101 et seq.

ASHA (American Speech-Language-Hearing Association). (1996). Central auditory processing: Current status of research and implications for practice. *American Journal of Audiology, 5*(2), 41–54.

ASHA. (2004). *Preferred practice patterns for the profession of speech-language pathology* [Preferred practice patterns]. Retrieved from http://www.asha.org/policy/PP2004-00191.htm

ASHA. (2005a). *(Central) auditory processing disorders* [Technical report]. Retrieved from http://www.asha.org/policy/TR2005-00043.htm

ASHA. (2005b). *(Central) auditory processing disorders—the role of the audiologist* [Position statement]. Retrieved from http://www.asha.org/policy/PS2005-00114.htm

ASHA. (2006). *Preferred practice patterns for the profession of audiology.* Retrieved from http://www.asha.org/policy/PP2006-00274.htm

Baran, J. A. (1996). Audiologic evaluation and management of adults with auditory processing disorders. *Seminars in Speech and Language, 17*(3), 233-244.

Baran, J. A. (1998). Management of adolescents and adults with central auditory processing disorders. In G. A. Masters, N. A. Stecker, & J. Katz (Eds.), *Central auditory processing disorders: Mostly management* (pp. 195–214). Boston, MA: Allyn & Bacon.

Baran, J. A. (2002). Managing auditory processing disorders in adolescents and adults. *Seminars in Hearing, 23*(4), 327-335.

Baran, J. A. (2007). Managing (central) auditory processing disorder in adolescents and adults. In G. A. Chermak & F. E. Musiek (Eds.), *Handbook of (central) auditory processing disorder: Comprehensive intervention* (Vol. II, pp. 243–272). San Diego, CA: Plural.

Baran, J. A., & Musiek, F. E. (1994). Evaluation of the adult with hearing complaints and normal audiograms. *Audiology Today, 6*(5), 9–11.

Baran, J. A. & Musiek, F. E. (1999). Behavioral assessment of the central auditory nervous system. In F. E. Musiek & W. F. Rintelmann (Eds.), *Contemporary perspectives in hearing assessment* (pp. 549–602). Boston, MA: Allyn & Bacon.

Baran, J. A., Shinn, J. B., & Musiek, F. E. (2006). New developments in the assessment and management of auditory processing disorders. *Audiological Medicine, 4*(1), 35–45.

Battle, D. E. (1997). Multicultural considerations in counseling communicatively disordered persons and their families. In T. A. Crowe (Ed.), *Applications of counseling in speech-language pathology and audiology* (pp. 118–141). Baltimore, MD: Williams & Wilkins.

Battle, D. E. (2002). Communication disorders in a multicultural society. In D. E. Battle (Ed.), *Communication disorders in multicultural populations* (pp. 3–32). Boston. MA: Butterworth-Heinemann.

Bellis, T. J. (2003). *Assessment and management of central auditory processing disorders in the educational setting: From science to practice* (2nd ed.). Clifton Park, NY: Thomson Learning.

Bender, W. A. (2004). *Learning disabilities: Characteristics, identification, and teaching strategies* (5th ed.). Boston, MA: Allyn & Bacon.

Bocca, E., Calearo, C., & Cassinari, V. (1954). A new method for testing hearing in temporal lobe tumours: Preliminary report. *Acta Otolaryngologica, 44*(3), 219–221.

Bocca, E., Calearo, C., Cassinari, V., & Migliavacca, F. (1955). Testing "cortical" hearing in temporal lobe tumours. *Acta Otolaryngologica, 45*(4), 289–304.

Chermak, G. D. (1998). Metacognitive approaches to managing central auditory processing disorders. In G. A. Masters, N. A. Stecker, & J. Katz (Eds.), *Central auditory processing disorders: Mostly management* (pp. 49–62). Boston, MA: Allyn & Bacon.

Chermak, G. D. (2002). Deciphering auditory processing disorders in children. *Otolaryngology Clinical North America, 35*(4), 733–749.

Chermak, G. D., & Musiek, F. E. (1992). Managing central auditory processing disorders in children and youth. *American Journal of Audiology, 1*, 62–65.

Chermak, G. D., & Musiek, F. E. (1997). *Central auditory processing disorders: New perspectives.* San Diego, CA: Singular.

Chermak, G. D., & Musiek, F. E. (2002). Auditory training: Principles and approaches for remediating and managing auditory processing disorders. *Seminars in Hearing, 23*(4), 297–308.

Deschler, D. D., Alley, G. R., Warner, M. M., & Schumaker, J. B. (1981). Instructional practices for promoting skill acquisition and generalization in severely learning disabled adolescents. *Learning Disability Quarterly, 4*(4), 415–421.

Deschler, D. D., Schumaker, J. B., Lenz, B. K., & Ellis, E. S. (1984). Academic and cognitive interactions for LD adolescents. Part II. *Journal of Learning Disabilities, 17*(3), 170–179.

Dillon, H. (2012). *Hearing aids* (2nd ed.). Turramurra, NSW, Australia: Boomerang Press.

Hallahan, D. P., Lloyd, J. W., Kauffman, J. M., Weiss, M. P., & Martinez, E. A. (2005). *Learning disabilities: Foundations, characteristics, and effective teaching* (3rd ed.). Boston, MA: Allyn & Bacon.

Harris, K. R., Graham, S., & Pressley, M. (1991). Cognitive-behavioral approaches in reading and written language: Developing self-regulated learners. In N. N. Singh & L. L. Beale (Eds.), *Learning disabilities: Nature, theory, and treatment* (pp. 415–541). New York, NY: Springer-Verlag.

Hayes, E. A., Warrier, C. M., Nicol, T. G., Zecker, S. G., & Kraus, N. (2003). Neural plasticity following auditory training in children with learning problems. *Clinical Neurophysiology, 114*(4), 673–684.

Jerger, J., & Musiek, F. E. (2000). Report of the consensus conference on the diagnosis of auditory processing disorders in school-aged children. *Journal of the American Academy of Audiology, 11*(9), 467–474.

Jerger, J., Silman, S., Lew, H. L., & Chmiel, R. (1993). Case studies in binaural interference: Converging evidence from behavioral and electrophysiologic measures. *Journal of the American Academy of Audiology, 4*(2), 122–131.

Jirsa, R. E. (1992). The clinical utility of the P3 AERP in children with auditory processing disorders. *Journal of Speech and Hearing Research, 35*(4), 903–912.

Kleinman, S. N., & Bashir, A. S. (1996). Adults with language-learning disabilities: New challenges and changing perspectives. *Seminars in Speech and Language, 17*(3), 201–216.

Kraus, N., McGee, T., Carrell, T., King, C., Tremblay, K., & Nichol, T. (1995). Central auditory system plasticity associated with speech discrimination training. *Journal of Cognitive Neuroscience, 7*(1), 25–32.

Masters, G. A., Stecker, N. A., & J. Katz (Eds.). (1998). *Central auditory processing disorders: Mostly management*. Boston, MA: Allyn & Bacon.

Moncrieff, D. W., & Wertz, D. (2008). Auditory rehabilitation for interaural asymmetry: Preliminary evidence of improved dichotic listening performance following intensive training. *International Journal of Audiology, 47*(2), 84–97.

Musiek, F. E. (1999). Habilitation and management of auditory processing disorders: Overview of selected procedures. *Journal of the American Academy of Audiology, 10*(6), 329–342.

Musiek, F. E., & Baran, J. A. (1996). Amplification and the central auditory nervous system. In M. Valente (Ed.), *Hearing aids: Standards, options, and limitations* (pp. 407–437). New York, NY: Thieme Medical.

Musiek, F. E., Baran, J. A., & Pinheiro, M. L. (1994). *Neuroaudiology: Case studies*. San Diego, CA: Singular.

Musiek, F. E., Baran, J. A., & Schochat, E. (1999). Selected management approaches to central auditory processing disorders. *Scandinavian Audiology, 28*(Suppl. 51), 63–76.

Musiek, F. E., Baran, J. A., & Shinn, J. (2004). Assessment and remediation of an auditory processing disorder associated with head trauma. *Journal of the American Academy of Audiology, 15*(2), 117-132.

Musiek, F. E., Bellis, T. J., & Chermak, G. D. (2005). Nonmodularity of the CANS: Implications for (central) auditory processing disorder: A critique of Cacace and McFarland's "The importance of modality specificity in diagnosing central auditory processing disorder (CAPD)." *American Journal of Audiology, 14*(2), 128–138.

Musiek, F. E., & Berge, B. E. (1998). A neuroscience view of auditory training/stimulation and central auditory processing disorders. In G. A. Masters, N. A. Stecker, & J. Katz (Eds.). *Central auditory processing disorders: Mostly management* (pp. 15–32). Boston, MA: Allyn & Bacon.

Musiek, F. E., & Schochat, E. (1998). Auditory training and central auditory processing disorders. *Seminars in Hearing, 19*(4), 357–365.

Musiek, F. E., Shinn, J., & Hare, C. (2002). Plasticity, auditory training and auditory processing disorders. *Seminars in Hearing, 23*(4), 263–276.

Passel, J., & Cohn, D. (2008). *U.S. population projections: 2005–2050. Washington, DC: Pew Hispanic Center. February; Census Bureau 2011 population estimates.* Retrieved from http://www.pewsocialtrends.org/2008/02/11/us-population-projections-2005-2050/

Picheny, M. A., Durlach, N. I., & Braida, L. D. (1985). Speaking clearly for the hard of hearing. I. Intelligibility differences between clear and conversational speech. *Journal of Speech and Hearing Research, 28*(1), 96–103.

Picheny, M. A., Durlach, N. I., & Braida, L. D. (1986). Speaking clearly for the hard of hearing. II. Acoustic characteristics of clear and conversational speech. *Journal* of *Speech and Hearing Research*, *29*(4), 434–446.

Picheny, M. A., Durlach, N. I., & Braida, L. D. (1989). Speaking clearly for the hard of hearing. III. An attempt to determine the contribution of speaking rate to differences in intelligibility between clear and conversational speech. *Journal of Speech and Hearing Research*, *32*(3), 600–603.

Ray, H., Sarff, L. S., & Glassford, J. E. (1984, Summer/Fall). Sound field amplification: An innovative educational intervention for mainstreamed learning disabled students. *Directive Teacher*, *4*, 18–20.

Rosenberg, G. G. (2002). Classroom acoustics and personal FM technology in management of auditory processing disorder. *Seminars in Hearing*, *23*(4), 309–318.

Saunders, G. H., & Haggard, M. P. (1989). The clinical assessment of obscure auditory dysfunction—1. Auditory and psychological factors. *Ear and Hearing*, *10*(3), 200–208.

Schochat, E., Musiek, F. E., Alonso, R., & Ogata, J. (2010). Effect of auditory training on the middle latency response in children with (central) auditory processing disorder. *Brazilian Journal of Medical and Biological Research*, *43*(8), 777–785.

Schochat, E., Musiek, F. E., & Baran, J. A. (2005). *Effects of auditory training on the MLR of children with APD.* Paper presented at the annual meeting of the American Academy of Audiology, Washington, DC.

Section 504 of the Rehabilitation Act of 1973, as amended, 29 U.S.C. § 794.

Song, J. H., Skoe, E., Banai, K., & Kraus, N. (2011). Training to improve hearing speech in noise: biological mechanisms. *Cerebral Cortex*, *22*(5), 1180–1190.

Stein, R. (1998). Application of FM technology to management of central auditory processing disorders. In G. A. Masters, N. A. Stecker, & J. Katz (Eds.), *Central auditory processing disorders: Mostly management* (pp. 89–92). Boston, MA: Allyn & Bacon.

Taylor, B., & Mueller, H. G. (2011). *Fitting and dispensing hearing aids.* San Diego, CA: Plural.

Taylor, P., & Cohn, D. (2012). *A milestone on route to a majority minority nation.* Washington, DC: Pew Research Center. Pew Social & Demographic Trends. Retrieved from http://www.pewsocialtrends.org/2012/11/07/a-milestone-en-route-to-a-majority-minority-nation/

Tremblay, K. L., & Kraus, N. (2002). Auditory training induces asymmetrical changes in cortical neural activity. *Journal of Speech, Language, and Hearing Research*, *45*(3), 564–572.

Tremblay, K., Kraus, N., Carrell, T. D., & McGee, T. (1997). Central auditory system plasticity: Generalization to novel stimuli following listening training. *Journal of the Acoustical Society of America*, *102*(6), 3762–3773.

Tremblay, K., Kraus, N., & McGee, T. (1998). The time course of auditory perceptual learning: Neurophysiological changes during speech-sound training. *NeuroReport*, *9*(16), 3357–3560.

Tremblay, K., Kraus, N., McGee, T., Ponton, C., & Otis, B. (2001). Central auditory plasticity: Changes in the N1-P2 complex after speech-sound training. *Ear and Hearing*, *22*(2), 79–90.

Warrier, C. M., Johnson, K. L., Hayes, E. A., Nicol, T., & Kraus, N. (2004). Learning impaired children exhibit timing deficits and training-related improvements in auditory cortical responses to speech in noise. *Experimental Brain Research*, *157*(4), 431–441.

Weihing, J A., & Musiek, F. E. (2007). Dichotic interaural intensity difference (DIID) training. Principles and procedures. In D. Geffner & D. Ross-Swain (Eds.), *Auditory processing disorders: Assessment, management, and treatment* (pp. 281–300). San Diego, CA: Plural.

Whitelaw, G. M., & Yuskow, K. (2008). Neuromaturation and neuroplasticity of the central auditory system. In T. K. Parthasarathy (Ed.), *An introduction to auditory processing disorders in children* (pp. 21–38). Mahwah, NJ: Lawrence Erlbaum Associates.

CHAPTER 15

CONSIDERATIONS FOR THE OLDER ADULT PRESENTING WITH PERIPHERAL (AND CENTRAL) AUDITORY DYSFUNCTION

GABRIELLE SAUNDERS, M. SAMANTHA LEWIS, DAWN KONRAD-MARTIN, and M. PATRICK FEENEY

Introduction

The aging process impacts every system of the body, leading to overall decline in physical, cognitive, and psychological function. Many of these changes affect auditory processing, communication skills, and the ability and motivation to benefit from audiological rehabilitation (AR), either directly or indirectly. Some of these age-related changes and the ways in which they impact communication and AR are discussed below. For each, we describe the age-related changes that occur, the implication of these changes as they pertain to hearing, communication, and AR, and some practical clinical suggestions to minimize their impact. First, however, we provide an overview of age-related changes in the auditory system.

Age-Related Changes in the Auditory System

It is well known that the ability to understand speech deteriorates with age, symptomatic of a plethora of changes within the auditory system collectively termed presbycusis. Aging is often accompanied by a decline in hearing sensitivity, due to sensory changes within the ear. Other changes occur in the auditory nerve and brain, however, making it more difficult for the older individual to make use of important timing cues within the speech signal. General cognitive decline associated with normal aging may also contribute to the difficulty an older listener has understanding speech. Normal hormonal changes and common pathologic conditions among the elderly, such as cardiovascular disease and diabetes can further compromise auditory function. An individual's lifetime exposure to noise or ototoxic drugs, while not considered a part of "normal aging," also contributes to the condition of the auditory system late in life.

This section begins with a discussion of age-related pure-tone threshold loss because, for better or worse, the clinical audiogram is the lynchpin of audiometric testing and treatment today.

Hearing Loss

According to the U.S. Census Bureau, there are now nearly 40 million people over the age of 65 years in the United States. The already large population of older Americans will increase dramatically in the coming years to an estimated 88.5 million people over age 65 by the year 2050 (U.S. Census Bureau, 2008). As the population of older adults increases, so will the prevalence of age-related hearing loss and its personal, societal and economic burdens. Hearing loss is highly prevalent in older adulthood, affecting roughly half of adults between the ages of 60 and 69 years. Figure 15–1 shows hearing loss prevalence as a function of age in decades for nearly 6000 individuals who took part in the National Health and Nutrition Examination Survey (Agrawal, Platz, & Niparko, 2008). The figure shows the percentage of individuals in each age cohort that has hearing loss, defined either as having pure-tone average (PTA) of ≥25 dB HL for frequencies of 0.5, 1 & 2 kHz (light bars) or a PTA ≥25 dB HL for frequencies of 3, 4, and 6 kHz (dark bars). As can be seen in the figure, prevalence increases when higher frequencies are included in the defini-

tion. Using the higher frequency PTA, prevalence reaches over 75% between the ages of 60 and 69 years. A separate study shows that over age 69 years, the prevalence of hearing loss continues to increase such that 59.9% of people aged 73 to 84 years had hearing loss as defined by a PTA ≥25 dB HL for frequencies of 0.5, 1 and 2 kHz, with the prevalence as high as 76.9% when the definition of hearing loss consists of 2, 4, and 8 kHz (Helzner et al., 2005). The prevalence of hearing loss is generally reported to be higher in males. A recent study showed that among right ears of 568 males between the ages of 70 and 79 years, 95% had PTA ≥21 dB HL for frequencies of 1, 2, and 4 kHz (Wilson, Noe, Cruickshanks, Wiley, & Nondahl, 2010). Since 20 dB HL is considered by clinical audiologists to be the limit of normal hearing, these results confirm that hearing loss is a common feature of aging. In fact, it ranks among the top three chronic health conditions for adults over the age of 65 years (Plies & Lethbridge-Cejku, 2007).

Longitudinal studies provide information about the rate at which hearing loss progresses over a lifetime. Figure 15–2 presents results from a large Swedish study on gerontology and geriatrics (Jonsson & Rosenhall, 1998). These results show that high frequencies generally decline more rapidly with age compared with lower frequencies, and the decline in hearing with age is greater among men in the higher frequencies (at least up to age 80 years in this report), consistent with a substantial literature (Brant & Pearson, 1994; Echt, Smith, Backscheider Burridge, & Spiro, 2010; Pearson et al., 1995). Among a group of 188 adults aged 60 years and over, threshold shifts averaged across age and gender, increased with increasing pure-tone frequency from

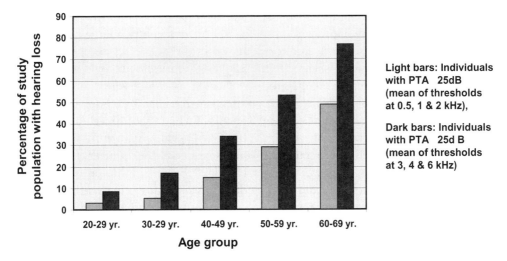

Figure 15–1. Data from: Agrawal, Y., Platz, E., and Niparko, J. (2008). Prevalence of hearing loss and differences by demographic charateristics among U.S. adults. *Archives of Internal Medicine, 168*(14), 1522–1530.

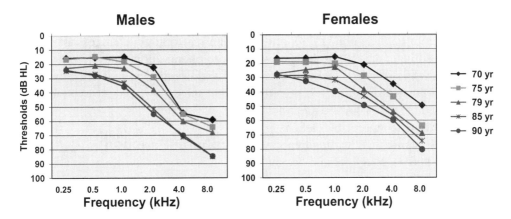

Figure 15–2. Data from the Gerontological and Geriatric Study (1971), Gotteborg, Sweden. Published by Jonsson, R., and Rosenhall, U. (1998). Hearing in advanced age. A study of presbycusis in 85-, 88- and 90-year-old people. *Audiology, 37*(4), 207–218.

0.7 dB per year at 0.25 kHz to 1.2 dB per year at 8 kHz (Lee, Matthews, Dubno, & Mills, 2005). Lower frequency thresholds (0.5-2 kHz) change at a lower rate than do higher frequency thresholds for both sexes (Congdon et al., 2004). Overall, these findings show that hearing loss affects the entire audiometric frequency range in the later decades of life, at which time the need for AR is substantial.

Depending on the older patient, amplification may be necessary, but insufficient to address his or her age-related communicative deficits. Understanding speech involves complex processes that begin in the cochlea with analysis of the acoustic components of the speech signal and proceed through semantic and syntactic analyses involving both auditory and cognitive neural functions. Deficits at any stage of processing may be reflected in altered perception of speech.

A classic study of age-related hearing loss compared three groups of subjects on measures of speech understanding, young normal hearing adults, young hearing-impaired adults, and old hearing-impaired adults (Jerger, 1972). The normal hearing group performed better than the two hearing-impaired groups, as expected. The older hearing-impaired group performed the worst—significantly more poorly than the young adults with the same degree of hearing impairment. This general observation holds for a variety of complex speech understanding conditions, such as for speech in noise (Plomp & Mimpen, 1979), and when using higher level linguistic processing (Wingfield, McCoy, Peelle, Tun, & Cox, 2006). Such results are interpreted as evidence that factors beyond audibility likely contribute to age-related deficits in speech understanding. A leading hypothesis is that there is an age-related decline in central auditory processing involving specific modalities, such as the encoding of temporal cues (Gordon-Salant & Fitzgibbons, 2001), and/or in more global cognitive modalities, such as working memory and processing speed (Craik, 2000; McCoy et al., 2005; Zanto, Toy, & Gazzaley, 2010).

The prevalence of central auditory processing abnormality in older adulthood varies across reports. One study, conducted using data from 1026 older adults aged 64 to 93 years from the Framingham Heart Study cohort, found central auditory processing was abnormal in only 22.6% of the subjects based on results of

a competing speech test (Cooper & Gates, 1991). More recently, a large population-based study of 2015 Australians over the age of 55 years showed evidence of central auditory processing abnormalities affecting roughly 74% adults based on results of a battery of speech understanding tests, primarily competing speech measures (Golding, Carter, Mitchell, & Hood, 2005). The higher prevalence rate of this newer study is in closer agreement with results of numerous clinical studies in which central auditory processing disorder was suspected in more than 50% of older patients (e.g., Jerger, Jerger, Oliver, & Pirozzolo, 1989; Shirinian & Arnst, 1982; Stach, Spretnjak, & Jerger, 1990). Certainly, these results suggest that a more comprehensive understanding of the older hearing-impaired patient requires gaining an appreciation of normal and pathologic changes not just to the peripheral auditory system, but also the central auditory, and cognitive processing stages of the auditory system.

Peripheral Function

Outer and middle ear changes associated with aging are thought to impact auditory function in relatively minor ways. Middle ear changes include a decrease in middle ear stiffness caused by changes in the elasticity of tissues (reviewed by Zafar, 1994). A related clinical finding among older individuals is the presence of an air-bone gap at 4 kHz (Glorig & Davis, 1961; Nondahl, Tweed, Cruickshanks, Wiley & Dalton, 2012). Effects of age are more pronounced using measures of wideband energy reflectance and absorption, which show a decrease in reflectance from 0.8 to 2 kHz as well as a substantial increase near 4 kHz (Feeney

& Sanford, 2004). A common problem related to changes in the elasticity of the outer ear is collapse of the ear canal during audiometric testing when supra-aural headphones are used. This problem can be easily prevented by using appropriately calibrated insert earphones to present air conducted stimuli.

According to the Working Group on Speech Understanding and Aging (1988), there is evidence for at least two major categories of inner ear presbycusis. A flat or gently sloping audiometric configuration indicative of *Metabolic or Strial Presbycusis* is thought to be associated with degeneration of the stria vascularis, a capillary rich lining that covers the lateral wall of the cochlea. The stria vascularis provides the electrochemical driving force for the cochlear receptor cells or hair cells, and is particularly important for outer hair cells to function properly. A steeply sloping audiometric configuration indicative of *Sensory Presbycusis*, is thought to be associated with damaged and missing hair cells within the organ of Corti, with the greatest damage involving the outer hair cells located near the high-frequency coding basal portion of the cochlea. In the healthy cochlea, the outer hair cells act as biomechanical amplifiers in the ear, increasing the sensitivity of the inner hair cells, which transmit sensory information to the auditory nerve. In addition to amplifying soft sounds, the outer hair cells compress the response to loud sounds so that the auditory nerve can encode information for a wide range of stimulus levels. The outer hair cells also receive information from the brain via efferent nerve pathways that descend from the brainstem through the medial olivocochlear bundle. This feedback loop alters the peripheral processing of incoming auditory stimuli.

Animal models are critical for understanding the aging auditory system because environmental and genetic factors can be controlled, lifespan is significantly shorter, and experimental approaches can sometimes be more direct as compared with human research. Hair cell damage and loss appears to play a diminished role in animal models of presbycusis where noise overexposure is not a factor (Tarnowski, Schmiedt, Hellstrom, Lee, & Adams, 1991), suggesting that outer hair cell damage among older humans might not be purely an age effect. Aging alters the efferent feedback loop to the outer hair cells, whether examined in humans or in lower mammals (Jacobson, Kim, & Romney, 2003). Atrophy of the stria vascularis is also a common finding among older animals reared in quiet (Suryadevara, Schulte, Schmiedt, & Slepecky, 2001). Results in animal models confirm another important finding in humans as well. Presbycusis is associated with a substantial reduction in the number and size of spiral ganglion cells of the auditory nerve (Keithley & Feldman, 1979; Schulte, Gratton, & Smythe, 1996). Together, these age-related changes alter peripheral signal processing and limit the excitatory input to the brain with the following impacts, as summarized below.

Age-related changes in the outer hair cells and the stria vascularis reduce the biomechanical amplification of responses to low-level sounds, which causes the well-known loss of sensitivity to sound that is "hearing loss." Outer hair cell changes also make cochlear processing more linear. One effect is that a reduced range of sound levels is able to be encoded by the ear. Soft sounds can be amplified by a hearing aid in order to be heard, but this may come at the expense of compressing the level differences inherent in the speech signal into a small output range, which can obscure speech sounds. Other perceptual consequences of a loss of nonlinearity due to outer hair cell damage include reduced frequency resolving capability, which impairs the ability to discriminate frequencies and hear out signals in noise. Reduced auditory nerve input to central neurons is expected to decrease the precision with which responses across groups of neurons fire synchronously. Over time, the loss of auditory nerve input to the brain destabilizes the tight regulation of excitatory/inhibitory neurotransmission present in the normal adult auditory system, causing permanent changes in brain regions involved in temporal processing (Wang et al., 2009).

Central Auditory Function and Cognition

The effect of age on neural structures and neural processing is not limited to the periphery. The central auditory system also undergoes substantial degenerative changes with age, some of which are secondary to the loss of peripheral input, others which are primary age changes (for an in-depth review see Canlon, Illing, & Walton, 2010). Studies have shown an age-related reduction in the number, size and connectivity of neurons in the brainstem, midbrain, and auditory cortex (Briner & Willott, 1989; Iontov & Shefer, 1984; Kirikae, Sato, & Shitara, 1964; Vaughan, 1977). There is also a marked age-related reduction in inhibitory neurotransmission within the dorsal cochlear nucleus, lateral superior olive, and the inferior colliculus, which likely affects the encoding of the timing cues on which the auditory system heavily relies (Caspary, Milbrandt, & Helfert,

1995; Gleich, 1994; Willott, Milbrandt, Bross, & Caspary, 1997). A recent study in rats tested the hypothesis that age-related inhibitory changes in the brainstem coincide with behavioral temporal processing impairments (Wang et al., 2009). The study showed that aged rats had decreased glycinergic inhibitory neurotransmission within the dorsal cochlear nucleus and weakened temporal sharpening mechanisms of dorsal cochlear nucleus neurons, coupled with impaired gap detection and amplitude modulation sensitivity. Furthermore, the decreased inhibitory neurotransmission found in that study was associated with plastic changes in the brainstem that are a characteristic response to a loss of auditory nerve input to the brain. Recording from single neurons in the inferior colliculus, Walton, Frisina, and O'Neill (1998) used the ability to detect brief silent gaps separating two noise bursts as a measure of temporal processing acuity over the age span. The range of gap durations able to be encoded was similar for neurons in young and older mice. However, compared with young mice, 50% fewer neurons in older mice had gap thresholds of 2 ms or less. Walton also found that most neurons with onset-type response patterns in old mice displayed prolonged recovery from the initial burst, suggesting there is more jitter in the response to rapidly presented sound stimulation among older mice.

The substantial downregulation of inhibitory neurotransmission observed in the brainstem and midbrain extends to the primary auditory cortex where reduced GABAergic transmission has been documented (Ling, Hughes, & Caspary, 2005). In addition, cell bodies of neurons in certain layers of the cortex decrease in size with advanced age in rats (Vaughan & Vincent, 1979), but the most pronounced anatomical change in the auditory cortex is a pruning back of dendrites of cortical pyramidal cells, which results in a decrease in dendritic density (Vaughan, 1977). Certainly, many of the central auditory changes described above are consistent with reports that it is challenging for older individuals to discriminate fluctuations in temporally dynamic sounds, segregate competing sounds, and locate sound sources, which could contribute to the speech understanding difficulties experienced by older individuals.

It is likely that degraded input associated with hearing impairment or central auditory dysfunction places even greater demands on higher level cognitive resources (Shinn-Cunningham & Best, 2008). In fact, functional imaging studies show that when performance is matched between groups of older and younger adult humans on tasks that assess verbal and spatial working memory, there is an apparent "overactivation" in the brains of the older adults, often in prefrontal locations (Grady & Craik, 2000; Reuter-Lorenz, 2002; Reuter-Lorenz et al., 2000). Extra effort expended on the initial stages of speech recognition by listeners with even mild hearing loss may cause measurable failures in the cognitive operations of comprehension and memory for what has been heard (McCoy et al., 2005; Salthouse, 2010). A recent review of the literature from the American Academy of Audiology Task Force on Central Presbycusis confirms that deficits at lower levels of processing can impact cognitive function and, conversely, that deficits involving cognitive processing can impact measures designed to examine comparatively lower levels of processing (Humes et al., 2012). This highlights the difficulty separating peripheral, central auditory and cognitive deficits. (See Chapter 18 in Volume 1 of the Handbook for additional discussion of the aging of the CANS.)

Genetic Predisposition

Presbycusis has a genetic component currently estimated at 35% to 55% from studies of families and twins (Karlsson, Harris, & Svartengren, 1997; Wingfield et al., 2007). Examination of participants in the Framingham Heart Study looking across generations and between siblings indicated a stronger correlation between hearing in mothers and their children than between fathers and their children. This suggests that some forms of presbycusis are due to mitochondrial DNA mutations, since mitochondrial DNA is inherited from the mother's egg (Gates, Couropmitrcc, & Mycrs, 1999). It is likely that multiple genes influence the degree of hearing loss from presbycusis, the age at onset of the hearing loss, and the audiometric configuration.

Age-Related Changes in Mitochondria

Mitochondria are involved in producing adenosine triphosphate (ATP), the main energy source for a variety of cellular metabolic processes, and in other processes such as the formation of reactive oxygen species (free radicals), calcium homeostasis and regulation of programmed cell death or apoptosis (reviewed in Fischel-Ghodsian, 2003). Cellular energy production involves the mitochondrial respiratory chain, which depends on the coordinated action of both nuclear and mitochondrial genes. Free radicals or reactive oxygen and nitrogen species are generated by the mitochondria even in healthy tissue where these highly unstable and reactive molecules are involved in cellular regulatory mechanisms, intercellular signaling or bacteriocidal functions (Evans & Halliwell, 1999). Antioxidant defense mechanisms normally keep levels of free radicals in check; however, even under normal conditions they induce low level oxidative stress which damages cellular lipids, proteins and DNA. Antioxidant defense mechanisms can become overwhelmed, allowing greater damage to ensue. Studies in mice have shown that decreased cellular metabolism, due to respiratory chain dysfunction and increased levels of oxidative stress and accumulated somatic mitochondrial DNA mutations, is an underlying cause of age-related hearing loss (Niu, Trifunovic, Larsson, & Canlon, 2007; Yamasoba et al., 2007)

Age-Related Changes in Hormones

Recent reports suggest that hormonal changes also influence presbycusis. For example, presbycusis develops more slowly among menopausal women undergoing estrogen therapy compared with women who did not receive treatment (Hederstierna, Hultcrantz, Collins, & Rosenhall, 2007). Women undergoing combined estrogen and progestin hormone replacement therapy had poorer hearing compared with women taking only estrogen or no hormone treatment at all (Guimaraes et al., 2006).

Hypertension and Cardiovascular Disease

Cardiovascular disease appears to exacerbate presbycusis, with associations found only among women. A similar association among men may have been obscured by higher rates of noise-induced hearing loss (Gates, Cobb, D'Agostino, & Wolf, 1993; Torre, Cruickshanks, Klein, Klein, & Nondahl, 2005). Similarly, hearing loss in the low and mid frequencies was correlated with high systolic and diastolic blood pressure among women over age 79 years, with no consistent correlations among the men or younger women studied (Rosenhall & Sundh, 2006).

Diabetes

Diabetes mellitus is a metabolic disease with microvascular, macrovascular and neural complications. Evidence is accumulating showing that diabetes is associated with hearing loss. Bainbridge, Hoffman, and Cowie (2008) examined hearing data from 5140 individuals who took part in the National Health and Nutrition Examination Survey (NHANES) between 1999 and 2004. Prevalence of hearing loss was 15% for participants without diabetes, but was double (30%) for participants with diabetes. Those aged 20 to 49 years had the greatest prevalence disparity of high-frequency impairment of mild or greater severity in the better ear, suggesting that diabetes may accelerate the process of peripheral sensory impairment seen most typically in the general population during the fifth decade of life.

Tobacco Use, Noise Exposure, and Exposure to Ototoxic Agents

Smoking has been associated with hearing loss though the risk of hearing loss attributable to smoking is fairly small in most reports (Nomura, Nakao, & Morimoto, 2005). For example, one epidemiological study showed that smokers have a 1.69 times greater chance of having hearing loss than nonsmokers, and that living with a smoker increased the risk of hearing loss among nonsmokers (Cruickshanks et al., 1998).

Noise overexposure causes direct mechanical damage to the hair cells and supporting cells within the cochlea (Pujol & Puel, 1999). Intense metabolic activity caused by noise overexposure increases free radical formation leading to oxidative stress and an upregulation of apoptosis primarily affecting the cochlear outer hair cells (LePrell, Yamashita, Minami, Yamasoba, & Miller, 2007). Other presumably excitotoxic effects of noise include a loss of afferent nerve terminals and a delayed, but substantial degeneration of the cochlear nerve (Kujawa & Liberman, 2009). Gates et al. (2000) examined the rate of change of hearing over 15 years among older men as a function of the presence and depth of an audiometric "notch" (threshold elevation of ≥15 dB in the 3 to 6 kHz region of the audiogram). The age-related change in hearing thresholds varied by noise-notch category. Thresholds in the 3 to 6 kHz range increased less over time and thresholds adjacent to the notch region increased more over time for the men with noise notches considered to be large. These findings suggest that the damage caused from noise continues to progress well after the exposure.

There are hundreds of medications with ototoxic potential for affecting the auditory and/or vestibular end organs (Palomar, Abdulghani, Bodet, Andreu, & Palomar, 2001). Therapeutic drugs such as aminoglycoside antibiotics and the platinum-based chemotherapy agent cisplatin are among the most commonly prescribed ototoxic medications. The ototoxic action of aminoglycoside antibiotics and cisplatin primarily involves damage and loss of outer hair cells beginning at the high-frequency coding cochlear base due to induction of apoptosis associated with increased oxidative stress; however, the stria vascularis and spiral ganglion are also targets of cisplatin ototoxicity (Alam et al., 2000; Hellberg et al., 2009; Rybak, 2007; Schweitzer, 1993). Work in animal models suggests that compared with cisplatin, carboplatin produces a greater mixture of inner and outer hair cell damage, and oxaliplatin produces greater damage to the auditory nerve (Ding, Allman, & Salvi, 2012). Evidence that chemotherapeutics cause oxidative stress within brain tissues has also been found, with documented damage to the inferior colliculus following exposure to cisplatin (Rybak, 2005).

Certain solvents involving mixtures of xylene, toluene, and/or methyl ethyl ketone and heavy metals including lead, mercury, trimethyltin, and arsenic are ototoxic. The specific mechanisms involved in the toxicology of ototoxic industrial chemicals and solvents differ across agents, but all produce cochlear injury that includes outer hair cells loss, as reviewed in detail by Pouyatos and Fechter (2007). These solvents and heavy metals are also neurotoxic, producing injury within the brain including documented changes within the central auditory system (Fuente & McPherson, 2007; Musiek, Baran, Shinn, & Jones, 2011).

Impacts and Recommendations

The myriad of changes that accompany aging suggest that each older patient may have unique perceptual and cognitive limitations as well as rehabilitative needs. A systematic approach to clinical intervention that considers deficits in specific types of processing and at multiple processing levels is important for the therapeutic management of patients with presbycusis. For example, techniques appropriate for addressing a loss in peripheral hearing sensitivity alone are substantially different from those appropriate for also addressing central-auditory deficits or cognitive declines. In fact, based on a review of the literature, Stach, Loiselle, and Jerger (1991), have suggested that individuals presenting with both peripheral and central auditory dysfunction tend to be less satisfied with, obtain worse performance with, and derive less benefit from traditional hearing aids than individuals with peripheral hearing sensitivity loss alone. For these individuals, the authors recommended use of remote-microphone technology, as a means for enhancing the signal-to-noise ratio and thereby helping improve speech understanding in the presence of noise.

The Stach et al. (1991) recommendation of remote-microphone technology for individuals that present with both peripheral and central auditory dysfunction is not surprising given the technical report published by the American Speech-Language-Hearing Association (ASHA Working Group on Auditory Processing Disorders, 2005) and the clinical practice guidelines published by the American Academy of Audiology (2010) on central auditory processing disorders. Both documents indicate that intervention for central auditory processing disorders should involve both bottom-up and top-down approaches. Although any intervention should be patient-specific and done in conjunction with other team member, when appropriate, typical strategies have included: (1) envi-

ronmental modifications, (2) training of auditory skills where the deficits exist, and (3) compensatory communication strategies to build self-reliance and promote generalizability of skills into everyday activities.

Environmental modifications can include both bottom-up and top-down approaches to improving an older adults ability to receive and understand auditory information (ASHA Working Group on Auditory Processing Disorders, 2005). These may be simple changes like recommending that the older adult sit closer to the speaker or more complex like making changes to the acoustics of the rooms for which the listener frequents (see ASHA Working Group on Auditory Processing Disorders, 2005 for additional recommendations). As suggested by Stach et al. (1991), this may also include the provision of remote-microphone technology (e.g., a personal frequency-modulation [FM] system). FM technology, as commonly used, consists of a remote microphone/transmitter and a receiver. The microphone/transmitter can be worn by a speaker (family member, lecturer, and teacher) or coupled directly to an electronic device (TV, radio tuner, telephone). The receiver can be a standalone unit coupled to head/earphones or it can be incorporated into an ear-level device such as a hearing aid. The advantage of an FM system is that it effectively reduces acoustic energy in the environment between the microphone and receiver (i.e. background noise) resulting in a significant improvement in signal-to-noise ratio. Improved speech-in-noise performance associated with FM technology among adults with hearing loss has been well documented (Boothroyd, 2004; Jerger, Chmiel, Florin, Pirozzolo, & Wilson, 1996; Lewis, Crandell, Valente,

& Enrietto, 2004). Perhaps more importantly, assessment of the use of FM systems by adults with hearing loss who had significant complaints of understanding speech in everyday listening environments resulted in numerous improvements in self-report of functional abilities (Chisolm, Noe, McArdle, & Abrams, 2007). See Chapter 12 for greater discussion of FM technology.

Training of auditory skills is generally considered a bottom-up treatment approach designed to reduce or resolve the processing difficulties (ASHA Working Group on Auditory Processing Disorders, 2005). There is an accumulating body of literature documenting that auditory training has the potential to change auditory behaviors (Tremblay & Kraus, 2002; Tremblay, Kraus, McGee, Ponton, & Otis, 2001). However, as discussed below, it is often difficult to show transfer of trained skills to real-world listening situations.

Compensatory training includes provision of information about communication strategies that are aimed at helping the individual focus on the use of central resources (e.g. language, memory, problem solving). It can also consist of training exercises that involve building vocabulary, active listening, problem-solving, auditory closure (filling in missing parts of speech) and attribution training (strengthening the listener's locus of control; Bellis, 2006). Compensatory strategy training is considered a top-down treatment approach designed to minimize the impacts of the processing problems that are not resolved through environmental management and auditory training (ASHA Working Group on Auditory Processing Disorders, 2005). These three forms of intervention combined are the recommended approach to addressing age-related hearing loss.

Age-Related Changes in the Visual System

According to the Centers for Disease Control and Prevention (Desai, Pratt, Lentzner, & Robinson, 2001), at least 1.7 million people report concomitant hearing loss and vision loss (dual sensory impairment [DSI]) and that the prevalence increases with age (Jee et al., 2005; Schneider et al., 2012). Although substantial research has examined the impacts of single sensory impairments, the effect of acquired DSI has been less well studied, nonetheless, it is clear that DSI has psychological, psychosocial, and functional effects, although authors of a recent review concluded that data are inconclusive regarding whether the impacts of DSI are greater than the sum of the impacts of the two single sensory impairments (Schneider et al., 2011). Self-reported DSI is associated with higher rates of depression or depressive symptoms relative to individuals with hearing loss alone or vision loss alone or no sensory impairment (Capella-McDonnall, 2005; Lupsakko, Mantyjarvi, Kautiainen, & Sulkava, 2002), as well as diminished functional independence (Keller, Morton, Thomas, & Potter, 1999) and decreased participation in social activities (Crews & Campbell, 2004).

As with hearing loss, many age-related changes in the visual system are considered to be a part of normal aging. These include presbyopia (changes in accommodative ability of the eye associated with a less flexible lens and weaker ciliary muscles), decreased light transmission of the ocular media and decreased pupil size, losses in contrast sensitivity, greater sensitivity to and delayed recovery from glare, delayed dark adaptation, and reduced visual field and color discrimination (Michael & Bron, 2011; Rubin et al., 1997; Watson & Echt, 2010). Like presbycusis, most age-related changes are not amenable to correction; consequently, environmental, and/or compensatory strategies are required. In addition to normal age-related changes, there are several pathologic conditions associated with aging, the most common ones being macular degeneration, diabetic retinopathy, cataract, and glaucoma. These result in a variety of consequences such as inability to see fine detail or to read fine print, dependence on high luminance, decreased acuity, scattered field loss over the retina, blurred vision and poor contrast sensitivity (see Watson & Echt, 2010 for review).

Impacts and Recommendations

Poor visual acuity can impact communication and AR. In terms of communication, it results in a decreased ability to make use of speechreading cues and nonverbal information, such as facial expressions, gestures, eye gaze and posture. Use of speechreading cues can result in up to 50 to 60% better sentence identification over using auditory or visual cues alone (Walden, Busacco, & Montgomery, 1993). Furthermore, because the cues provided by speechreading are complementary to those provided by amplification (speechreading provides place-of-articulation cues, whereas amplification provides place, manner and voicing cues; Walden, Grant, & Cord, 2001), their absence has an interactive effect on hearing aid effectiveness. In terms of AR, poor vision impacts the ability to follow the hearing aid orientation and the ability to use and maintain hearing aids—specifically, changing settings, cleaning the hearing aids and replacing the batteries.

The data of Parving and Philip (1991) showed that poor vision has measurable impacts on hearing-aid outcome. They reported that 40% of hearing-aid users in their tenth decade (≥90 years) could not use the volume control wheel, 36% could not change the hearing-aid battery, and 34% could not clean the earmold.

There are relatively simple ways to address some of these issues. First, it is the clinician's responsibility to recommend to the patient that they select hearing aids that are larger, more visible, and use bigger batteries. The clinician should also select relevant automatic hearing aid signal processing features so that the need for additional manipulations of the hearing aid is minimized. For instance, adaptive directionality, if appropriate, and an automatic telecoil might be advantageous over manually operated options. Second, it is also the clinician's responsibility to have available assistive technology to help the visually impaired patient. Smith et al. (2001) recommended having a handheld magnifier available. Such magnifiers can provide magnification of between 1.5 and 20 times and can be equipped with battery-operated lights. They are inexpensive and widely available for purchase. A superior solution, although more costly, is a video magnifier (closed-circuit television). A closed-circuit television is superior to a handheld magnifier because it frees up both hands of the user, does not require steady hands during use, and can provide greater magnification than that provided by a handheld magnifier. A closed-circuit television consists of a stand-mounted video camera that projects magnified objects or text onto a video screen. The image can be shown in black and white or color and can be used in conjunction with a personal computer. These are especially useful when demonstrating the use and care of a hearing aid. Third, there are simple environmental adaptations that can easily be implemented, such as ensuring a well-lit clinic space that uses incandescent overhead lighting to avoid creating glare (Kricos, 2007), and making sure the clinician's face is not backlit, to optimize visibility of his or her face for speechreading. Finally, all written materials should be clear and simple, with redundancy to reinforce important points, but they should not include information over and above that directly required by the patient. Forty-four percent of persons older than 65 years read at fifth grade level or below, whereas another 30% read at approximately fifth-grade to eighth-grade levels (Kirsch, Jungeblat, Jenkins, & Kolstad, 1993). Therefore, the materials should be presented at an appropriate reading level, they should be written in the active voice, personal pronouns should be used, and they must be direct, specific, and concrete (Center for Medicare Education, 2006). Research shows that the print should be a minimum of 14-point, it should have wide spaces between the lines, and a sans serif font should be used (Echt, 2002). Multiple columns on a page should be avoided, the text should be justified on the left but unjustified on the right, and the materials should be printed in high-contrast black and white, or in saturated colors to optimize contrast sensitivity on matte paper to prevent difficulties related to glare (Erber, 2003; Kitchel, 2006).

Age-Related Cognitive Decline

The effect of aging on cognition as reported in both cross-sectional and longitudinal studies is mixed. Some functions decline, such as encoding new memories, executive processes (e.g., manipulation of information stored in working memory and selectively attending to specific information in the presence of other information that might compete for attention), and the speed of processing information. Other functions remain relatively unaffected by age, such as short-term memory, autobiographical memory (for one's life events), and emotional processing (Hedden & Gabrieli, 2005; Salthouse, 2011). Short-term memory, as measured by the digit span task in which a series of digits is heard and repeated, shows little decline until after age 70 years, but then declines more quickly with age (Gregoire & Van der Linden, 1997). However, Heinrich and Schneider (2011) showed that for elderly listeners with mild high-frequency hearing loss, performance on a paired-associate memory paradigm that assesses short-term memory declined as the speech presentation level increased. The effect was duplicated in young listeners when distorted speech was presented at a high presentation level, but elderly listeners showed the effect at lower presentation levels. Thus, interpretation of memory effects for speech materials in elderly listeners could be complicated by this presentation-level effect.

The brains of older adults have progressively lower volumes of gray matter than the brains of younger adults (Haug & Eggers, 1991), which in part appears to be related to lower synaptic densities (Terry & Katzman, 2001). A major cortical area affected by healthy aging is the frontostriatal system (prefrontal cortex through connections to and from the basal ganglion) for which function declines with decreases in dopamine and serotonin (Volkow et al., 1996), with a concomitant loss in frontal white-matter tracts (Head et al., 2004). These changes are correlated with age-related declines in memory and executive function (Hedden & Gabrieli, 2005).

Mild cognitive impairment (MCI) refers to a condition involving memory complaints and poor performance on memory tasks without the rapid decline of memory and cognition found in dementia. Individuals with MCI may be in an early more treatable stage of Alzheimer's disease (Hedden & Gabrieli, 2005). In comparison with healthy aging where neurological deficits are found in the prefrontal cortex and basal ganglia affecting executive function and processing speed, MCI and Alzheimer's disease are characterized by neurological changes in the hippocampus and medial temporal lobe that correspond to deficits in long-term memory (Buckner, 2004; Hedden & Gabrieli, 2005).

There appears to be a relationship between cognitive decline and deficits in hearing thresholds and central auditory processing. Lin, Ferrucci, et al. (2011) evaluated the relationship between average hearing thresholds in the better ear and tests of memory and executive function in 347 participants from the Baltimore Longitudinal Study of Aging (BLSA). They found that greater hearing loss was significantly associated with poorer scores on mental status, memory, and executive function tests. The same group (Lin, Metter et al., 2011) evaluated hearing in 639 participants from the BLSA who were dementia-free in 1990–1994 and followed them for 12 years. A total of 58 cases of incident dementia were eventually diagnosed over that time for this group, and the risk of acquiring dementia increased log-linearly with the degree of baseline hearing loss. Similar finding were reported by Uhlmann, Larson, Rees, Koepsell, and Duckert (1989). Lin, Metter, et al. (2011) hypothesized that mecha-

nisms for such a relationship between hearing loss and dementia may be an exhaustion of cognitive reserve (i.e., an individual's capacity to cope with neuropathology), as a result of social isolation, environmental deafferentation (deprivation of input to the auditory cortex), or a combination of these. A study by Gates, Beiser, Rees, D'Agnostino, and Wolf (2002) performed hearing evaluations and the Synthetic Sentence Identification with Ipsilateral Competing Message (SSI-ICM) test on 740 dementia-free members of the Framingham Heart Study cohort. A central auditory processing deficit on the SSI-ICM was defined as a score of 50% or less in at least one ear. Prospective evaluation of these individuals for an average of 8.4 years revealed that 40 of them received a diagnosis of probable Alzheimer's disease. The presence of a central auditory processing deficit on the initial SSI-ICM test had a positive predictive value for subsequent probable Alzheimer's disease of 47% with a sensitivity of only 17%. Gates et al. (2010) compared the results of a battery of tests chosen to evaluate multiple dimensions of executive control function, including behavioral inhibition, concept generation, and verbal and visuospatial working memory, with the results of three central auditory processing tests in 313 elderly participants: 232 cognitively normal, 60 with MCI, and 21 with dementia. Executive function results were significantly associated with all three central auditory processing tests and with the hearing thresholds in the poorer ear even after controlling for effects of MCI and dementia. In further examination of the same cohort, Gates, Anderson, McCurry, Feeney, and Larson (2011) reported that subjects who scored less than 50% correct on the Dichotic Sentence Identification test had a hazard ratio for incident dementia of 9.9 (95% confidence interval, 3.6–26.7), which means they were nearly 10 times more likely to develop dementia than those subjects with scores better than 50%. This prompted Gates et al. (2011) to recommend a test of central auditory processing for older adults reporting hearing difficulty.

Impacts and Recommendations

General recommendations for lifestyle choices in the elderly may be useful in lowering the risk for developing cognitive difficulties. These include staying intellectually engaged, maintaining cardiovascular physical activity, minimizing chronic stress, and maintaining a healthy diet high in poly- and monounsaturated fatty acids (e.g., fish and olive oil) and antioxidants (e.g., fruits and vegetables; Hedden & Gabrieli, 2005). Given the demonstrated relationship between cognitive decline and poor hearing thresholds, even in individuals without pathological cognitive deficits, it is critical that elderly individuals with peripheral hearing loss be provided with amplification devices, hearing assistive technology (HAT), and AR, as appropriate, as soon as possible. This underscores the need for appropriate hearing screening as part of annual physical exams and for community-based hearing screenings.

Knowing that memory deficits may plague many elderly hearing-impaired individuals, it is critical to spend adequate time reviewing recommendations, as well as providing easy-to-follow written instructions and training materials with illustrations to help individuals and family members carry out rehabilitation programs in the home. Follow-up phone conversations with the patient or family member can help resolve issues that would reduce the effectiveness of a successful rehabilitation program.

Palmer, Adams, Bourgeois, Durrant, and Rossi (1999) conducted hearing aid evaluations and hearing aid fittings in the home of patients with Alzheimer dementia. Monaural hearing aid fittings with minimal external controls were used to simplify the fitting process and minimize confusion for the patients. Caregivers reported a reduction in problem behaviors as a result of successful hearing aid use in these individuals. Several psychosocial approaches to cognitive rehabilitation for patients with dementia were proposed by Dröes, van der Roest, van Mierlo, and Meiland (2011) that could be conducted by a psychologist, occupational therapist, physical therapist, or nursing staff in group or individual settings. These could also include computer programs for cognitive training in dementia patients (Tárraga et al., 2006). Irrespective of the type of planned cognitive rehabilitation for an individual, it is critical to evaluate and treat any existing hearing disorder to allow the individual to maximally benefit from cognitive rehabilitation. This emphasizes the importance of a team approach to rehabilitation for patients with cognitive disorders, and the need for an audiologist to be on the team to manage the patient's AR.

Independent of cognitive decline, there is mounting evidence that home-based computer training using auditory, visual and cognitive exercises can improve memory (Berry et al., 2010; Zelinski et al., 2011), as well as self-rated health assessment (Wolinsky et al., 2010). In addition, such programs may also prolong the individual's ability to continue independent driving (Edwards, Delahunt, & Mahncke, 2009), and improve driving safety over time among elderly individuals (Edwards, Myers, et al., 2009).

Such programs should be considered as supplements to AR, especially those that focus on auditory training, the general goal of which is to compensate for any degradation in the auditory signal due to internal (hearing loss) or external (noise) factors (Sweetow & Palmer, 2005). Auditory training makes use of the fact that neurons in the brain can reorganize and restructure following, for example, training or changes in sensory input (Kraus et al., 1995; Ramachandran, 2005; Reuter-Lorenz & Lustig, 2005).

Auditory training as a rehabilitation tool is based on the rationale that hearing aids do not restore the auditory system to normal, hearing-aid processed signals differ acoustically from unprocessed signals, and that the auditory cortex of most patients acquiring hearing aids has been deprived of normal auditory input for many years. Following the widespread availability of personal computers and internet access, computer-based auditory training programs have been developed. Some are available commercially, such as the Listening and Communication Enhancement program (Sweetow & Sabes, 2006) or Fast ForWord (Merzenich et al., 1996), and Brain HQ (Mahncke, Connor, Appelman, et al., 2006), while others to date have only been used in laboratory studies (e.g., the Speech Perception Assessment and Training System [SPATS]; Miller et al., 2007; CasperSent [Boothroyd, 2008] and the Frequent-Word auditory training protocol [Humes, Burk, Strauser, & Kinney, 2009]). While these programs differ in the specific skills trained, there are similarities across programs regarding the underlying training principles that are applied. Such principles include the use of adaptive algorithms that adjust training difficulty as the user's skills progress in order to maintain

a difficulty level at the upper limits of the user's ability, the provision of feedback to promote learning and rewards to increase motivation, and the expectation that the user will train almost daily over several weeks. In a review of the auditory training literature, Chisolm and Arnold (2012) conclude that most studies showed statistically significant improvements as a function of training when assessed immediately post-intervention. However, a fundamental assumption of any auditory training program is that the skills learned within the program will "generalize" or "transfer" to untrained stimuli. Data on this are somewhat mixed. Some studies with hearing-impaired individuals show good generalization from a training program to other stimuli (Miller et al., 2007; Stecker et al., 2006; Sweetow & Sabes, 2006), whereas others show little or no generalization (Agnew, Dorn, & Eden, 2004; Burk & Humes, 2008; Burk, Humes, Amos, & Strauser, 2006; Saunders, McArdle, Chisolm, Smith, & Wilson, 2011). Thus, although auditory training might be a good solution for some patients with peripheral hearing loss, its effectiveness has not been conclusively demonstrated. The reader is referred to Chapter 3 for a review of the efficacy of auditory training with patients presenting with central auditory processing disorder, and to Chapter 7 for review of auditory training principles and procedures.

Age-Related Changes in Manual Dexterity

With advancing age comes diminished manual dexterity (Carmeli, Partish, & Coleman, 2003). As with vision, there are normal age-related changes in manual dexterity which include decreased grip strength, limitations in wrist movement, loss of fine motor control, unsteady movements and decreased sensitivity, as well as pathologic conditions, such as arthritis and Parkinson's disease,- which exacerbate these difficulties (Carmeli et al., 2003; Proud & Morris, 2010). Arthritis is one of the most common chronic conditions afflicting the elderly, diagnosed in approximately 50% of adults over the age of 65 years (Morbidity and Mortality Weekly Report, 2010). Parkinson's disease is a common neurodegenerative disease with a typical age of onset of 65 years. Its prevalence increases with age, from about 553.52/100,000 among those 65 to 69 years of age, to 2,948.93/100,000 individuals among those 85 years and older. It is most common among caucasian males, and is more common in urban then rural populations (Wright Willis, Evanoff, Lian, Criswell, & Racette, 2010).

Impacts and Recommendations

Diminished manual dexterity has direct effects on several aspects of AR, with the most obvious being hearing aid insertion, manipulation of the hearing aid controls, and handling of the battery. Research has shown strong associations between manual dexterity, ability to handle hearing aids, and hearing aid outcomes (Humes, Wilson, & Humes, 2003; Kumar, Hickey, & Shaw, 2000; Singh Pichora-Fuller, Hayes, von Schroeder, & Carahan, 2012; Tomita, Mann, & Welch, 2001). Furthermore, Meister, Lausberg, Kiessling, von Wedel, and Walger (2002) found that ease of handling becomes significantly more important with age. Singh et al. (2012) note that there is considerable individual variability in the capacity of older individuals to manipulate and handle hearing aids, and thus clinicians should assess manual dexterity, rather than assume all older individuals will have handling difficulties. Dexterity can be assessed using the 3-item "Manual Dexterity and Vision" scale from the *Attitudes Towards Loss of Hearing Questionnaire* (Saunders, Cienkowski, Forsline, & Fausti, 2005) or one or more of the measures described by Singh et al. (2012).

Data are somewhat mixed about which hearing aid style is easiest to handle. Johnson, Danhauer, and Krishnamurti (2000) and Upfold, May, and Battaglia (1991) reported that in-the-ear (ITE) hearing aids were the easiest to insert and remove, whereas the participants in the study of Stephens and Meredith (1990) found that BTE hearing aids were most easily handled. The changing of hearing-aid batteries poses similar handing problems, and although in general larger hearing aids use larger batteries, even the largest batteries are only a few millimeters in diameter and thus are problematic for many older individuals. At least two manufacturers of hearing-aid batteries have developed tools that negate the need to hold the battery itself through the use of long battery tabs and magnets and, while not available yet in the United States, there are recent developments, such as solar powered hearing aids, that may entirely obviate the need for hearing aid batteries. In the mean time, the audiologist can consider having the patient practice manipulating dummy aids before a hearing aid style is selected. By carefully selecting hearing aid signal processing features, the need for changing hearing aid settings can be minimized. Indeed many of today's hearing aids do not have volume controls, use adaptive directionality, automatically adjust noise reduction settings, and have switchless telecoils that are activated when in the presence of a stationary magnetic field. The pros and cons of these automated options should be discussed with any patient who exhibits manual dexterity issues.

For individuals who simply cannot handle hearing aids, there is at least one extended wear hearing aid commercially available that is inserted deeply in the ear canal by a professional and remains there until the batteries need to be replaced between 8 and 12 weeks later. This type of device overcomes many manual dexterity issues, as all hearing aid manipulation is done by a hearing care professional. Hearing aids, however, may not be the ideal solution for all patients. For some, provision of HAT, such as a telephone amplifier and an FM or infrared television access system, may be more appropriate. It is therefore recommended that the first step in AR be to establish the patient's listening needs and priorities. This can be achieved using a questionnaire such as the Client Oriented Scale of Improvement (COSI; Dillon, James, & Ginis, 1997) or the Glasgow Hearing Aid Benefit Profile (GHABP; Gatehouse, 1999). The COSI has the patient specify the listening situations in which he or she specifically wants to improve his or her ability to hear. The GHABP has the patient specify the communication situations in which he or she considers it important to hear as well as possible. Depending on the patient's needs and priorities, the clinician can select the most appropriate forms of AR.

As mentioned earlier, it should be noted that there is some evidence that older adults that present with both peripheral and central auditory dysfunction may not be as successful as individuals that present with peripheral hearing loss alone when it comes to using traditional amplification (see Stach, Loiselle, & Jerger, 1991). These individuals may require amplification that has the capability of improving the signal-to-noise ratio like hearing aids equipped with directional microphone technology and/or the use of remote-microphone technology. (See Chapter 12 for discussion of FM technology.) There is also evidence that some of these individuals, despite having symmetrical pure-tone hearing thresholds, may prefer using only one hearing aid as compared to two (e.g., Cox, Schwartz, Noe, & Alexander, 2011). To illustrate, Cox et al. (2011) found that almost half of the subjects (43 out of 94 subjects) in their study reported preferring the use of one hearing aid over the use of two. These same authors also evaluated a variety of potential variables (selected from the literature) to determine which, if any, accurately predicted which subject would prefer using one hearing aid. Although there were some variables that were associated with this preference, like dichotic listening, binaural loudness summation, and a greater number of reported hearing problems unaided (Abbreviated Profile of Hearing Aid Benefit; Cox & Alexander, 1995), the predictive accuracy of these tests was not 100% accurate. There are some promising tests and electrophysiological procedures that have been evaluated (e.g., binaural interference); however, there is no test or battery of tests which accurately predicts which individuals will prefer using one hearing aid (e.g. Cox, et al., 2011; Jerger, 2011; Jerger, Silman, Lew, & Chmiel, 1993). Clinicians, however, should be aware of this possibility and recognize that these patients may require additional clinical time. The clinician also needs to be aware that the desired form of AR may change over time as the patient ages; highlighting the need to maintain regular contact with this patient population.

Loss of Independence With Age

Hearing loss has been associated with an increased use of community support services and informal support (i.e., help from friends/nonspouse family; Schneider et al., 2010). Individuals providing that support are often considered to be caregivers, individuals who assume responsibility for the physical and emotional needs of another. Ongoing provision of care or "caregiving" often has a negative impact on the caregiver, especially when he or she is older. Indeed, caregivers are at an increased risk for depression, illness and, even death (Schulz & Beach, 1999). Specific to hearing, it has been shown that caregivers of individuals with greater levels of hearing disability and handicap reported more symptoms of distress via the Malaise Inventory (Rutter, Tizard, & Whitmore, 1970) than when hearing disability and handicap were less significant (Tolson, Swan, & Knussen, 2002). This distress was significantly related to the patient's symptoms of depression and the caregivers' perception of hearing-related hassles (e.g., having to repeat oneself).

The use of hearing aids when needed is helpful in alleviating the care burden. For instance, in a study of hearing loss and depressive mood, the utilization of hearing aids not only improved depressive symptoms and quality of life for the patients, but caregiver burden also was reduced (Boi et al., 2012). Likewise, in the Tolson et al. (2002) study, although

patient depression scores and caregiver ratings of global distress did not change, hearing aid use reduced the caregiver's perception of hearing-related "hassles." Finally, both the hearing-impaired individual and his or her family reported positive benefits to themselves in many aspects of quality of life, including relationships at home and with the family, feelings about self, life overall, social life, and emotional health, following use of hearing aids (Kochkin & Rogin, 2000).

Data from the 2010 National Survey of Residential Care Facilities show that each day in 2010, 733,300 persons were residents of some form of residential care facility (Caffrey et al., 2012), of whom 11% were under age 65 years, 9% were aged between 65 to 74 years, 27% were 75 to 84 years and 54% were over 85 years. The prevalence of hearing impairment in this population is typically higher than that among those living independently in the community. For instance, Mahoney (1992) reported that 96% of the nursing home residents that she tested had a mild degree of hearing loss or greater, with 55% having a moderate to profound degree of hearing loss. Likewise, Garahan, Waller, Houghton, Tisdale, and Runge (1992) reported that over three-quarters of the residents (without dementia) had at least a mild degree of hearing loss and over half of these same residents had at least a moderate or severe hearing loss in their better hearing ear.

Unfortunately, and problematically, only 14% to 30% of nursing home residents use hearing aids (Cohen-Mansfield, & Taylor, 2004a), and use is little better even when the facility has an AR program in place (Schow, 1982). This low utilization might be because many older individuals are unaware of their hearing loss. This is well illustrated by the data of Mahoney (1992) who reported that only 41% of nursing home residents reported hearing difficulties and 86% of residents were somewhat to very satisfied with their ability to hear, even though 96% had a mild loss or greater. Another factor that may explain the low use of hearing aids in assisted care facilities is the lack of awareness of hearing loss on the part of nursing home staff, even though the residents rely on them for support. For example, Garahan et al. (1992) reported that there was no record made in the patient's chart of hearing impairments by either the physician or the nurse in almost half of the residents with hearing loss, and Cohen-Mansfield and Taylor (2004a) noted that hearing screening in residential facilities is almost absent.

Caffrey et al. (2012) reported that almost four out of ten residents in residential care facilities required assistance with three or more activities of daily live, specifically 73% needed help bathing, 53% with dressing, 36% with toileting, 25% with transferring (mobility limitation) and 22% with eating. Thus, as pointed out by Caffrey et al. (2012) and Gough and McKim (1986), most also likely rely on staff to maintain their hearing aids, select the appropriate setting, insert the aids and to contact the hearing aid supplier to make any necessary adjustments. Unfortunately, it cannot be assumed that medical professionals from other fields have been trained to work with individuals with hearing loss. Kato, Hickson, and Worrall (1996) noted that staff with less formal nursing training were less educated about the potential communication problems of patients than those with more formalized nursing education, whereas a survey of dietitians, half of whom worked in a nursing home,

showed that 78% had not been trained to work with special populations (Wright, Smifiklas-Wright, Blood, & Wright, 1997). Likewise, Cohen-Mansfield and Taylor (2004b) reported that almost half of their certified nursing assistants stated that they had not received training on the use and care of hearing aids. Most members of staff, however, were able to conduct basic hearing aid checks, change the batteries and turn the hearing aids on and off.

Knowledge of how to handle hearing aids, however, does not necessarily mean better hearing aid function among nursing home residents. Anand and Court (1989) found that over half (25/49) of the hearing aids belonging to nursing home residents were not working either because of a dead battery or earwax obstruction. It is important to note, however, that the majority of staff who participated in the study of Kato et al. (1996) expressed an interest in learning more about the communication problems of their residents. Rather encouragingly, a communication training program developed by the Action for Dysphasic Adults for nursing home staff resulted in improved self-perception of knowledge and competence regarding communication impairments, and they scored more highly on a test assessing their knowledge of communication strategies (Brayn, Axelrod, Maxim, Bell, & Jordan, 2002).

Impacts and Recommendations

It is important to include caregivers in the AR process and when appropriate, to tailor instructional materials to the caregiver as well (e.g., when the caregiver takes primary responsibility for AR). Caregivers can include the patient's partner, other family members, close friends, and health care workers. It should not be assumed that any of these individuals have had prior training in the use and care of hearing aids, HAT, and/or good communication strategies for individuals with hearing loss. If possible, caregivers should be invited to attend the clinical appointments so that this information can be shared with them directly. Written educational materials also should be provided. If the patient resides in an assisted care facility, the audiologist should offer to provide in-service training to the staff. Tools for such training can be obtained from the VA RR&D National Center for Rehabilitative Auditory Research by contacting the first author.

Unfortunately, it seems likely that much hearing loss in assisted living facilities goes unrecognized by staff. Audiologists should consider partnering with these facilities to provide audiology services (including, but not limited to, hearing screenings), staff education, and recommendations about ways to modify room acoustics to enhance communication in order that older frail individuals receive audiological care, which has the potential to improve their quality of life and well-being.

Age-Related Changes in Mobility

Mobility is critical to maintaining independence. Mobility decreases with age, both as a result of chronic conditions that detrimentally impact the ability to move, such as obesity and musculoskeletal pain, as well as age-related declines in muscle strength and balance (Rantakokko, Mänty, & Rantanen, 2012). As a result, walking speed declines, capacity to walk far decreases (Rantanen, Guralnik, & Ferrucci, 2001), and the frequency of falls and associated injuries increases. For example, between 20% and 40% of community-dwelling individuals over age 65 years fall every year, and about half of those who fall, do so repeatedly (Peel, 2011). Falls are associated with ongoing decline in mobility over time (Rantakokko et al., 2012), and a lack of mobility has been associated with decline in social engagement (Thomas, 2011) which, in turn, is associated with decreased quality of life (Hudakova & Hornakova, 2011; Oxley & Whelan, 2008), loneliness (Smith, 2012), and constriction in life space (Shah et al., 2012).

Driving can be a way to compensate for physical mobility limitations. However, also associated with aging are changes that lead to unsafe driving and thus the need to cease doing so. Indeed, the rate of traffic accidents has been shown to increase dramatically with age. Preusser, Williams, Ferguson, Ulmer, and Weinstein (1998) reported that compared to drivers aged 40 to 49 years, those aged 65 to 69 years were 1.29 times more at risk of being involved in a fatal crash, while those aged 85 years and older were 3.74 times more at risk. Yee, Cameron, and Bailey (2006) found that the total fatality rate of individuals over age 65 years was almost double that of those younger than 65 years. Elderly victims had a higher rate of chest injuries and longer intensive care unit stays compared with the younger group.

Impacts and Recommendations

Decreased mobility, whether due to physical limitations or the need to stop driving due to safety concerns, presumably makes access to healthcare services more difficult. Although there are no published data we are aware of that document the relationship between mobility and hearing aid acquisition and use, there are data showing that when deciding whether to seek help for hearing loss, individuals weigh the pros and cons of doing so. This includes comparing the impact hearing loss has relative to the impact(s) of co-occurring health conditions (Carson, 2005). This, in combination with MarkeTrak VII data showing that 52% of nonadopters of hearing aids stated they had more serious priorities than acquiring a hearing aid (Kochkin, 2007), suggests that an individual with mobility limitations is unlikely to take an active role in AR.

The increased availability of teleaudiology, or remote audiological care, should open new doors for individuals with limited mobility. In recent years there have been numerous technological innovations, such as the advent of low-cost webcams, affordable and reliable broadband Internet connectivity, and computerized audiological equipment for diagnostics, as well as hearing aid and cochlear implant programming. Indeed, remote video-otoscopy (Birkmire-Peters, Peters, & Whitaker, 1999; Sullivan, 1997), remote hearing aid fittings (Fabry, 1996; Swanepoel, Eikelboom, Ferrari, & Rumkumar, 2012), and applications for testing of hearing remotely (Krumm, Hogarth, & Martin, 2001; Smits, Kapteyn, & Houtgast, 2004) are becoming widespread. There is a system now available that permits remote monitoring of ototoxic changes resulting from chemotherapy, with which patients can test high-frequency hearing from home and then transmit the infor-

mation to a hearing healthcare professional (Jacobs et al., 2012). Also, under development, is a self-fitting hearing aid. The plan is for this wearable device to incorporate a tone generator to enable user-controlled, automated, in situ audiometry, a formula for selecting hearing aid settings, and a trainable algorithm through which the users could fine tune the hearing aid output (Convery, Keidser, Dillon, & Hartley, 2011). Furthermore, several hearing aid manufacturers have online or downloadable applications (i.e., apps) for remote AR that train speechreading skills, understanding of speech in noise, and communication strategies. Remote audiological and AR tools such as these should permit greater access to hearing healthcare for those with limited mobility, as well as those in rural or underserved communities (Nemes, 2010) in the United States, as they already are in remote parts of Australia, Brazil, and India (Swanepoel et al., 2012). While some available applications are as yet not approved by the U.S. Food and Drug Administration (FDA), audiologists should become familiar with the options teleaudiology offers and consider its use for patients with limited mobility, and should also be aware that studies indicate that patients benefit from and are willing to participate in remote AR (Thoren, Oberg, Wanstrom, Anderson, & Lunner, 2012).

Age-Related Changes in Lifestyle

Successful aging is associated with participation in more leisure activities, physical activity and engagement in life (Chaves, Camozzato, Eizirik, & Kaye,

2009; Garfein & Herzog, 1995; Li et al., 2006; Menec, 2003) and thus the lifestyles of older individuals are at least as diverse as those of younger individuals (Lähteenmäki & Kaikkonen, 2004). Despite this, some audiological literature suggests older adults place less importance on communicating in noise (Meister et al., 2002) and report less need for doing so (Erdman & Demorest, 1998; Garstecki & Erler, 1996). To elaborate, Meister et al. (2002) asked people aged 20 to 91 years to rank the importance of eight hearing aid attributes (e.g., hearing for speech in quiet, hearing for speech in noise, hearing aid sound quality, ease of handling, how much feedback the user would experience, and how well the user could localize sounds while using the hearing aid). They found that up to age 73 years, understanding of speech in noise was the most important attribute, followed by understanding of speech in quiet, with the other attributes holding similar or lower importance. People who were aged 73 years and over, however, said that hearing speech in quiet was the most important attribute, followed by hearing speech in noise. Similarly, Garstecki and Erler (1996) found that older individuals reported fewer needs to communicate in difficult listening situations than younger individuals, and Erdman and Demorest (1998) reported that among their participants communication needs decreased with age. A recent study (Wu & Bentler, 2012), however, provides conflicting evidence for changes in communication needs. In that study adults with mild to moderate sensorineural hearing loss kept a journal of listening situations encountered over a week, while simultaneously using a wearable dosimeter to measure the sound levels to which they were exposed over that week. Half of the participants were younger than 65 years of age, and half were aged between 65 and 90 years. According to the journal entries, there were no differences in the types of listening environments encountered or in the time spent in each. Similarly, although there was a significant difference in overall sound levels to which the participants were exposed, with younger individuals experiencing higher levels than older ones, that difference was only 2.8 dB across all environments for the whole week. Thus, on balance, these data suggest that the difference in communication needs of older and younger individuals is less varied than the difference across individuals in a single age group.

Impacts and Recommendations

In terms of AR, and in particular selection and programming hearing aids, one cannot assume that older individuals have vastly different communication needs than those of younger individuals. Thus, when planning AR for an older individual, it is critical to tailor it to the individual's communication priorities and lifestyle. This could be done simply through an interview, or as mentioned above, by having patients complete the COSI or the GHABP. Once this information has been obtained, the clinician can then focus AR towards a successful outcome for those particular listening situations important to the patient. For individuals whose primary need is to communicate one-on-one in a quiet setting, the best approach might be a hearing aid with minimal, optional features. For someone who encounters complex communication situations with background noise, a personal FM system with a wireless microphone might prove most effective. For others, whose communication needs are primarily limited to their home, one or more HAT devices (such as a telephone amplifier and an infrared television access system) might prove easier to use and be most effective.

Acceptance and Awareness of Hearing Loss

There is evidence that older individuals are more accepting of hearing impairment than younger individuals. That is, for the same degree of impairment, older individuals report fewer difficulties than younger individuals (Gordon-Salant, Lantz, & Fitzgibbons, 1994; Lutman, Brown, & Coles, 1987; Uchida, Nakashima, Ando, Nino, & Shimokata, 2003), and the level of impairment at which older individuals report hearing difficulties is greater than the level of impairment at which younger individuals report difficulties (Merluzzi & Hinchcliffe, 1973). There are several possible explanations for this. First, it may be that older individuals expect a degree of hearing impairment as they age and accept it. Second, older individuals judge their hearing ability in relation to that of others in their age group and tend to underestimate their hearing impairment (Maurer & Schow, 1995). Third, some older individuals may be simply unaware that their hearing has deteriorated because the onset was so gradual (Pacala & Yueh, 2012). Regardless of the underlying explanation, misperception of hearing impairment probably manifests as a reluctance to acquire hearing aids or to participate in other types of AR.

Impacts and Recommendations

The first step in working with an older patient's misperception of hearing impairment is for the family to understand this, and to realize that the probability of a successful hearing aid outcome will increase if the hearing-impaired individual accepts their need for hearing aids (Brooks & Hallam, 1998; Jerram & Purdy, 2001). This is especially important because as many as 50% of hearing-aid users are prompted by family members to seek help and acquire hearing aids (Kochkin, 2009; Wilson & Stephens, 2002). The Performance-Perceptual Test (PPT) of Saunders, Forsline, and Fausti (2004) might help some individuals become aware of their hearing impairment. In the PPT, actual and perceived ability to understand speech in noise is measured using the same test materials, test procedure and unit of measurement. By comparing the two, the extent to which individuals either underestimate or overestimate their hearing ability is obtained. It has been shown that individuals who overestimate their hearing report fewer difficulties than expected. By explaining this to hearing-impaired individuals it can help them become more aware of their limitations and be more open to using hearing aids (Saunders & Forsline, 2012).

When programming hearing aids for the older, first-time hearing aid user, it is also important for the clinician to remember that it is likely that the individual has had some degree of hearing impairment for many years and thus provision of amplification may lead to a negative reaction. Preparing patients through counseling about realistic expectations and advising them to avoid large groups and noise when first using their hearing aids is important. Furthermore, most hearing aid manufacturers now incorporate features that automatically increase gain over time until the target output is reached, so the users can adjust gradually to the incoming sound.

Bereavement

With age comes increased likelihood of bereavement, especially of spouses, siblings and friends. Loss of a spouse has been associated with reductions in functional health (d'Epinay, Cavalli, & Guillet, 2009-2010; van den Berg, Lindenboom, & Portrait, 2011), reduced emotional well being (d'Epinay et al., 2009-2010; Norris & Murrell, 1990), increased risk of institutionalization (Nihtilä & Martikainen, 2008), and mortality (Elwert & Christakis, 2008; Hart, Hole, Lawlor, Smith, & Lever, 2007; Jagger & Sutton, 1991; van den Berg et al., 2011). These negative consequences are highest in the period immediately after the death, and tend to lessen as time passes (Bowling, 2009; Murrell, Himmelfarb, & Phifer, 1988; Nihtilä & Martikainen, 2008; van den Berg et al., 2011). There are, of course, many different reactions to bereavement, and recovery time varies (Ott, Lueger, Kelber, & Prigerson, 2007), as does the complexity of the grief reaction (Newson, Beolen, Hek, Hofman, & Tiemeir, 2011). It is interesting to note, however, that other forms of loss, such as divorce or separation, and loss of a job or a home can actually have greater effects on health than bereavement (Murrell et al., 1988). An individual's susceptibility to the negative effects of bereavement is influenced by many factors, including preexisting mental and physical health conditions, social support, suddenness of death, and other life events (Norris & Murrell, 1990). Likewise, there are factors that seem to protect or buffer the individual from the negative effects of bereavement. For instance, Norris and Murrell (1990) reported that social embeddedness (i.e., the degree to which a person is entrenched in a social network) and involvement in new activities reduced the effects of bereavement on depression and physical health, respectively. Aber (1992) reported that involvement in paid work that was viewed as a positive experience served as a buffer, and Li (2007) reported that these benefits may also extend to volunteer experiences. In fact, she reported that the widowed were more likely to pursue volunteer activities and that these activities helped protect them from depressive symptoms. The more they volunteered, the greater their self-efficacy. Indeed, self-efficacy seems to be important when it comes to coping with bereavement in that self-efficacy in the domains of interpersonal, instrumental, social support, financial, physical health, nutritional, and spiritual health was associated with health-related quality of life, self-esteem, and life satisfaction (Fry, 2001).

Specific to AR, Kricos, Erdman, Bratt, and Williams (2007) have shown that the number and/or type of life events that a person has experienced impacts adherence to hearing aid use, such that nonusers of hearing aids reported more life events that decreased their use of hearing aids than hearing aid users. The events most associated with decreased hearing aid use were nonworking hearing aids, change in job status, death of spouse, and loss of independence. Note, however, that death of a family member other than a spouse, or health issues, either personal or of family members/close friends, did not impact hearing aid use.

Impacts and Recommendations

Spousal bereavement has the potential to negatively impact AR through decreased motivation to participate socially, decreased need to communicate, and feelings of depression. It may be inappropriate or of limited effectiveness to focus on AR immediately after bereavement. The potential impediments to successful AR following the death of a spouse may highlight the need for counseling and/or support from a bereavement specialist, perhaps prior to, or concurrent with, AR. The audiologist should look for signs of depression and refer to a mental health counselor whenever signs are suspected. On the other hand, many individuals are resilient and it should not be surprising if they actively pursue AR. As reported by Norris and Murrell (1990), some bereaved individuals are more likely to participate in new interests than other groups of older individuals. An assessment of listening needs is therefore recommended. If, however a newly widowed patient is not ready to accept hearing aids, the audiologist should not be discouraged. Such a situation does, however, underscore the need for additional support as the patient enters into AR, through extra follow-up efforts in the form of additional appointments or phone calls. It is further suggested that the patient be strongly encouraged to connect with a local hearing loss support group. In addition to providing hearing-loss related support, it may also help the patient establish new social networks and opportunities. Grief can also impact cognitive function, such as attention and memory (Ward, Mathias, & Hitchings, 2007), thus having informational materials on hand for patients to reread at home is important.

Summary

It is clear from the above review of the literature that there are many factors that should be considered when working with older adults presenting with peripheral and central auditory dysfunction. An overriding consideration is that all rehabilitative tools, whether these are assistive technologies, informational materials, communication strategy advice or training programs, must be accessible, usable and understandable to the older patient. That is, patients should feel that they are able to use the materials, that the clinician is accessible for follow-up questions, and that the rehabilitation they are receiving is tailored directly to their needs. It is well established that better outcomes are achieved in terms of patient compliance (Hamann, Cohen, Leucht, Busch, & Kissling, 2007; Ludman et al., 2003; Schoenthaler, Schwartz, Wood, & Stewart, 2012; Von Korff et al., 2003), and satisfaction (Loh et al., 2007), when the patient and clinician work together to select an intervention, and when the patient believes he or she can be successful with the intervention (Ludwig, Tadayon-Manssuri, Strik, & Moggi, 2012; Somers, Wren, & Shelby, 2012). The suggestions above take these factors into consideration in order to optimize the likelihood of obtaining successful AR outcomes for older individuals.

References

Aber, C. (1992). Spousal death, a threat to women's health: Paid work as a "resistance resource." *Image—The Journal of Nursing Scholarship, 24,* 95–99.

Agnew, J., Dorn, C., & Eden, G. (2004). Effect of intensive training on auditory processing and reading skills. *Brain and Language, 88,* 21–25.

Agrawal, Y., Platz, E., & Niparko, J. (2008). Prevalence of hearing loss and differences by demographic charateristics among U.S. adults. *Archives of Internal Medicine, 168,* 1522–1530.

American Academy of Audiology. (2010). *Diagnosis, treatment and management of children and adults with central auditory processing disorder* [Clinical practice guidelines]. Retrieved from http://www.audiology.org/resources/documentlibrary/Documents/CAPDGuidelines 8-2010.pdf

Anand, J., & Court, I. (1989). Hearing loss leading to impaired ability to communicate in residents of homes of the elderly. *British Medical Journal, 298,* 1429–1430.

ASHA Working Group on Auditory Processing Disorders. (2005). *(Central) auditory processing disorders. American Speech-Language-Hearing Association.* Retrieved from http://www.asha.org/NR/rdonlyres/8404EA5B-8710-4636-B8C4-8A292E0761E0/0/v2TR_CAPD.pdf

Bainbridge, K., Hoffman, H., & Cowie, C. (2008). Diabetes and hearing impairment in the United States: Audiometric evidence from the National Health and Nutrition Examination Survey 1999 to 2004. *Annals of Internal Medicine, 149,* 1–10.

Barnett, S., & Franks, P. (1999). Deafness and mortality: Analysis of linked data from National Health Interview Survey and National Death Index. *Public Health Report, 114,* 330–336.

Baumfield, A., & Dillon, H. (2001). Factors affecting the use and perceived benefit of ITE and BTE hearing aids. *British Journal of Audiology, 35,* 247–258.

Bellis, T. (2006, October 25–29). *Intervention for (C)APD.* Paper presented at the Canadian Academy of Audiology, Calgary, Canada.

Berry, A., Zanto, T., Clapp, W., Hardy, J., Delahunt, P., Mahncke, H., & Gazzaley, A. (2010). The influence of perceptual training on working memory in older adults. *PLoS One, 5,* e11537.

Birkmire-Peters, D., Peters, L., & Whitaker, L. (1999). A usability evaluation for telemedicine medical equipment: A case study. *Telemedicine Journal, 5,* 209–212.

Boi, R., Racca, L., Cavallero, A., Carpaneto, V., Racca, M., Dall Acqua, F., . . . Odetti, P. (2012). Hearing loss and depressive symptoms in elderly patients. *Geriatrics Gerontology International, 12,* 440–445.

Boothroyd, A. (2004). Hearing aid accessories for adults: The remote FM microphone. *Ear and Hearing, 25,* 22–33.

Boothroyd, A. (2008). CasperSent: A program for computer-assisted speech perception testing and training at the sentence level. *Journal of the Academy of Rehabilitative Audiology, 41,* 31–52.

Bowling, A. (2009). Predictors of mortality among a national sample of elderly widowed people: Analysis of 28-year mortality rates. *Age and Ageing, 38,* 527–530.

Brant, L., & Pearson, J. (1994). Modeling the variability in longitudinal patterns of aging. In D. Crews & R. Garruto (Eds.), *Biological anthropology and aging* (pp. 374–393). New York, NY: Oxford.

Brayn, K., Axelrod, L., Maxim, J., Bell, L., & Jordan, L. (2002). Working with older people with communication difficulties: An evaluation of care worker training. *Aging and Mental Health, 6,* 248–254.

Briner, W., & Willott, J. (1989). Ultrastructural features of neurons in the C57BL/6J mouse anteroventral cochlear nucleus: Young mice versus old mice with chronic presbycusis. *Neurobiology of Aging, 10,* 259–303.

Brooks, D., & Hallam, R. (1998). Attitudes to hearing difficulty and hearing aids and the outcome of audiological rehabilitation. *British Journal of Audiology, 32,* 217-226.

Buckner, R. (2004). Memory and executive function in aging and AD: Multiple factors that cause decline and reserve factors that compensate. *Neuron, 44,* 195–208.

Burk, M., & Humes, L. (2008). Effects of long-term training on aided speech-recognition performance in noise in older adults. *Journal of Speech and Hearing Research, 51,* 759–771.

Burk, M., Humes, L., Amos, N., & Strauser, L. (2006). Effect of training on word-recognition performance in noise for young normal-hearing and older hearing-impaired listeners. *Ear and Hearing, 27,* 263–278.

Caffrey, C., Sengupta, M., Park-Lee, E., Moss, A., Rosenoff, E., & Harris-Kojetin, L. (2012). *Residents living in residential care facilities: United States, 2010.* Hyattsville, MD: National Center for Health Statistics.

Canlon, B., Illing, R., & Walton, J. (2010). Cell biology and physiology of the aging central auditory pathway. In S. Gordon-Salant, R. Frisina, A. Popper, & R. Fay (Eds.), *The aging auditory system* (pp. 39-74). New York, NY: Springer.

Capella-McDonnall, M. (2005). The effects of single and dual sensory loss on symptoms of depression in the elderly. *International Journal of Geriatric Psychiatry, 20,* 855–861.

Carmeli, E., Partish, H., & Coleman, R. (2003). The aging hand. *Journals of Gerontology: Medical Sciences, 58A,* 2146–2152.

Carson, A. (2005). "What brings you here today?" The role of self-assessment in help-seeking for age-related hearing loss. *Journal of Aging Studies, 19,* 185–200.

Caspary, D., Milbrandt, J., & Helfert, R. (1995). Central auditory aging: GABA changes in the inferior colliculus. *Experimental Gerontology, 30,* 349–360.

Center for Medicare Education. (2006). http://www.futureofaging.org/PublicationFiles/V1N2.pdf

Centers for Disease Control and Prevention. (2010). Prevalence of doctor-diagnosed arthritis and arthritis-attributable activity limitation—United States, 2007–2009. *Morbidity and Mortality Weekly Report, 59,* 1261–1265.

Chaves, M., Camozzato, A., Eizirik, C., & Kaye, J. (2009). Predictors of normal and successful aging among urban-dwelling elderly Brazilians. *Journal of Gerontology Series B: Psychological Sciences and Social Sciences, 64,* 597–602.

Chisolm, T., & Arnold, M. (2012). Evidence about effectiveness of aural rehabilitation programs for adults. In L. Hickson & L. Wong (Eds.), *Evidence-based practice in audiology: Evaluating interventions for children and adults with hearing impairment.* San Diego, CA: Plural.

Chisolm, T, Noe, C, McArdle, R, & Abrams, H. (2007). Evidence for the use of hearing assistive technology by adults: The role of the FM system. *Trends in Amplification, 11,* 73–89.

Cohen-Mansfield, J., & Taylor, J. (2004a). Hearing aid use in nursing homes. Part 1: Prevalence rates of hearing impairment and hearing aid use. *Journal of the American Directors Association, 5,* 283–288.

Cohen-Mansfield, J., & Taylor, J. (2004b). Hearing aid use in nursing homes. Part 2: Barriers to effective utilization of hearing aids. *Journal of the American Directors Association, 5,* 289–296.

Convery, E., Keidser, G., Dillon, H., & Hartley, L. (2011). A self-fitting hearing aid: Need and concept. *Trends in Amplification, 15,* 157–166.

Cooper, J., & Gates, G. (1991). Hearing in the elderly: The Framingham cohort 1983–1985. Part II: Prevalence of central auditory processing disorders. *Ear and Hearing, 12,* 304–311.

Cox, R. M., & Alexander, G. C. (1995). The abbreviated profile of hearing aid benefit. *Ear and Hearing, 16,* 176–186.

Cox, R. M., Schwartz, K. S., Noe, C. M., Alexander, G. C. (2011) Preference for one or two hearing aids among adult patients. *Ear and Hearing, 32,* 181–197.

Craik, F. (2000). *Handbook of aging and cognition II.* Mahwah, NJ: Erlbaum.

Crews, J., & Campbell, V. (2004). Vision impairment and hearing loss among community-dwelling older Americans: Implications for health and functioning. *American Journal of Public Health, 94,* 823–829.

Cruickshanks, K., Klein, R., Klein, B., Wiley, T., Nondahl, D., & Tweed, T. (1998). Cigarette smoking and hearing loss: The epidemiology of hearing loss study. *Journal of the American Medical Association, 279,* 1715–1719.

d'Epinay, C., Cavalli, S., & Guillet, L. (2009-2010). Bereavement in very old age: Impact on health and relationships of the loss of a spouse, a child, or a close friend. *Omega (Wesort), 60,* 301–325.

Desai, M., Pratt, L., Lentzner, H., & Robinson, K. (2001). *Trends in vision and hearing among older Americans.* Centers for Disease Control and Prevention. National Center for Health Statistics.

Dillon, H., James, A., & Ginis, J. (1997). The Client Oriented Scale of Improvement (COSI) and its relationship to several other measures of benefit and satisfaction provided by hearing aids. *Journal of the American Academy of Audiology, 8,* 27–43.

Ding, D., Allman, B. L., & Salvi, R. (2012). Review: Ototoxic characteristics of platinum antitumor drugs. *Anatomical Record (Hoboken), 295,* 1851–1867.

Dröes, R., van der Roest, H., van Mierlo, L., & Meiland, F. (2011). Memory problems in dementia: Adaptation and coping strategies and psychosocial treatments. *Expert Reviews Neurotherapy, 11,* 1769–1781.

Ebert, D. A., & Heckerling, P. (1995). Communication with deaf patients: Knowledge, beliefs, and practices of physicians. *Journal of the American Medical Association, 273,* 227–229.

Echt, K. (2002). Designing web-based health information for older adults: Visual considerations and design directives. In R. Morrell (Ed.), *Older adults, health information, and the World Wide Web* (pp. 61–87). Mahwah, NJ: Erlbaum.

Echt, K., Smith, S., Backscheider Burridge, A., & Spiro, A. I. (2010). Longitudinal changes in hearing sensitivity among men: The Veterans Affairs Normative Aging Study. *Journal of the Acoustical Society of America, 128,* 1992–2002.

Edwards, J., Delahunt, P., & Mahncke, H. (2009). Cognitive speed of processing training delays driving cessation. *Journal of Gerontology Series A: Biological Sciences and Medical Sciences, 34,* 1262–1267.

Edwards, J., Myers, C., Ross, L., Roenker, D., Cissell, G., McLaughlin, A., & Ball, K. K. (2009). The longitudinal impact of cognitive speed of processing training on driving mobility. *Gerontologist, 49,* 485–494.

Elwert, F., & Christakis, N. (2008). The effect of widowhood on mortality by the causes of death of both spouses. *American Journal of Public Health, 98,* 2092–2098.

Erber, N. (2003). Use of hearing aids by older people: Influence of non-auditory factors (vision, manual dexterity). *International Journal of Audiology, 42*(Suppl. 2), S21–S25.

Erdman, S., & Demorest, M. (1998). Adjustment to hearing impairment II: Audiologic and demographic correlates. *Journal of Speech, Language, and Hearing Research, 41,* 123–136.

Evans, P., & Halliwell, B. (1999). Free radicals and hearing. Cause, consequence, and criteria. *Annals of the New York Academy of Sciences, 884,* 19–40.

Fabry, D. (1996). *Remote hearing aid fitting applications.* Paper presented at the 8th Annual Mayo Clinic Audiology Videoconference, Mayo Center, Rochester, MN.

Feeney, M., & Sanford, C. (2004). Age effects in the human middle ear: Wideband acoustical measures. *Journal of the Acoustical Society of America, 116,* 3546–3558.

Fischel-Ghodsian, N. (2003). Mitochondrial deafness. *Ear and Hearing, 24,* 303–313.

Fry, P. (2001). Predictors of health-related quality of life perspectives, self-esteem, and life satisfactions of older adults following spousal loss: An 18-month follow-up study of widows and widowers. *Gerontologist, 41,* 787–798.

Fuente, A., & McPherson, B. (2006). Organic solvents and hearing loss: The challenge for audiology. *International Journal of Audiology, 45,* 367–381.

Garahan, M., Waller, J., Houghton, M., Tisdale, W., & Runge, C. (1992). Hearing loss prevalence and management in nursing home residents. *Journal of the American Geriatrics Society, 40,* 130–134.

Garfein, A., & Herzog, A. (1995). Robust aging among the young-old, old-old, and oldest-old. *Journal of Gerontology: Psychological Sciences, 50,* S77–S87.

Garstecki, D., & Erler, S. (1996). Older adult performance on the communication profile for the hearing impaired. *Journal of Speech and Hearing Research, 39,* 28–42.

Gatehouse, S. (1999). Glasgow Hearing Aid Benefit Profile: Derivation and validation of a client-centered outcome measure for hearing-aid services. *Journal of the American Academy of Audiology, 10,* 80–103.

Gates, G., Anderson, M., McCurry, S., Feeney, P., & Larson, E. (2011). Central auditory dysfunction as a harbinger of Alzheimer dementia. *Archives of Otolaryngology-Head and Neck Surgery, 137,* 390-395.

Gates, G., Beiser, A., Rees, T., D'Agostino, R., & Wolf, P. (2002). Central auditory dysfunction may precede the onset of clinical dementia in people with probable Alzheimer's disease. *Journal of the American Geriatric Society, 50,* 482–488.

Gates, G., Cobb, J., D'Agostino, R., & Wolf, P. (1993). The relation of hearing in the elderly to the presence of cardiovascular disease and cardiovascular risk factors. *Archives of Otolaryngology-Head and Neck Surgery, 119,* 156–161.

Gates, G., Couropmitree, N., & Myers, R. (1999). Genetic associations in age-related hearing thresholds. *Archives of Otolaryngology-Head and Neck Surgery, 125,* 654–659.

Gates, G., Gibbons, L., McCurry, S., Crane, P., Feeney, M., & Larson, E. (2010). Executive dysfunction and presbycusis in older persons with and without memory loss and dementia. *Cognitive and Behavioral Neurology, 23,* 218–223.

Gates , G., Schmid, P., Kujawa, S., Nam, B., & D'Agostino, R. (2000). Longitudinal threshold changes in older men with audiometric notches. *Hearing Research, 141,* 220–228.

Gleich, O. (1994). The distribution of N-acetyl-galactosamine in the cochlear nucleus of the gerbil revealed by lectin binding with soybean agglutinin. *Hearing Research, 78,* 49–57.

Glorig, A., & Davis, H. (1961). Age, noise, and hearing loss. *Annals of Otology, Rhinology, and Laryngology, 70,* 556–571.

Golding, M., Carter, N., Mitchell, P., & Hood, L. (2004). Prevalence of central auditory processing (CAP) abnormality in an older Australian population: The Blue Mountains Hearing Study. *Journal of the American Academy of Audiology, 15,* 633–642.

Gordon-Salant, S., & Fitzgibbons, P. (2001). Source of age-related recognition difficulty for time-compressed speech. *Journal of Speech, Language, and Hearing Research, 44,* 709–719.

Gordon-Salant, S., Lantz, J., & Fitzgibbons, P. (1994). Age effects on measures of hearing disability. *Ear and Hearing, 15,* 262–265.

Gough, K., & McKim, H. (1986, November). Staff observations help assess residents' hearing handicap. *Dimensions,* 42–44.

Grady, C., & Craik, F. (2000). Changes in memory processing with age. *Current Opinion in Neurobiology, 10,* 224–231.

Gregoire, J., & Van der Linden, M. (1997). Effects of age on forward and backward digit spans. *Aging Neurophyschology and Cognition, 4,* 140–149.

Guimaraes, P., Frisina, S., Mapes, F., Tadros, S., Frisina, D., & Frisina, R. (2006). Progestin negatively affects hearing in aged women. *Proceedings of the National Academy of Sciences, 103,* 246–249.

Hamann, J., Cohen, R., Leucht, S., Busch, R., & Kissling, W. (2007). Shared decision making and long-term outcome in schizophrenia treatment. *Journal of Clinical Psychiatry, 68,* 992–997.

Hart, C., Hole, D., Lawlor, D., Smith, G., & Lever, T. (2007). Effect of conjugal bereavement on mortality of the bereaved spouse in participants of the Renfrew/Paisley

Study. *Journal of Epidemiology and Community Health, 61*, 455–460.

Haug, H., & Eggers, R. (1991). Morphometry of the human cortex cerebri and corpus striatum during aging. *Neurobiology of Aging, 12*, 336–338.

Head, D., Buckner, R., Shimony, J., Williams, L., Akbudak, E., Conturo, T., . . . Snyder, A. Z. (2004). Differential vulnerability of anterior white matter in nondemented aging with minimal acceleration in dementia of the Alzheimer type: Evidence from diffusion tensor imaging. *Cerebral Cortex, 14*, 410–423.

Hedden, T., & Gabrieli, J. (2005). Healthy and pathological processes in adult development: New evidence from neuroimaging of the aging brain. *Current Opinions in Neurology, 18*, 740–747.

Hederstierna, C., Hultcrantz, M., Collins, A., & Rosenhall, U. (2007). Prevalence of hearing loss, audiometric configuration and relation to hormone replacement therapy. *Acta Oto-Laryngologica, 127*, 149–155.

Heinrich, A., & Schneider, B. (2011). The effect of presentation level on memory performance. *Ear and Hearing, 32*, 524–532.

Helzner, E., Cauley, J., Pratt, S., Wisniewski, S., Zmuda, J., Talbott, E., . . . Newman, A. B. (2005). Race and sex differences in age-related hearing loss: The Health, Aging and Body Composition Study. *Journal of the American Geriatric Society, 53*, 2119–2127.

Hetu, R., Jones, L., & Getty, L. (1993). The impact of acquired hearing impairment on intimate relationships: Implications for rehabilitation. *Audiology, 32*, 363–381.

Hudakova, A., & Hornakova, A. (2011). Mobility and quality of life in elderly and geriatric patients. *International Journal of Nursing and Midwifery, 3*, 81–85.

Humes, L., Burk, M., Strauser, L., & Kinney, D. (2009). Development and efficacy of a frequent-word auditory training protocol for older adults with impaired hearing. *Ear and Hearing, 30*, 613–627.

Humes, L., Dubno, J., Gordon-Salant, S., Lister, J., Cacace, A., Cruickshanks, K., . . .

Wingfield, A. (2012). Central presbycusis: A review and evaluation of the evidence. *Journal of the American Academy of Audiology, 23*, 635–666.

Humes, L., Wilson, D., & Humes, A. (2003). Examination of differences between successful and unsuccessful elderly hearing aid candidates matched for age, hearing loss and gender. *International Journal of Audiology, 42*, 432–441.

Iontov, A., & Shefer, V. (1984). The morphological basis of age-induced memory changes. *Neuroscience and Behavioral Physiology, 14*, 349–353.

Jacobs, P., Silaski, G., Wilmington, D., Gordon, S., Helt, W., McMillan, G., . . . Dille, M. (2012). Development and evaluation of a portable audiometer for high-frequency screening of hearing loss from ototoxicity in homes/clinics. *IEEE Transactions on Biomedical Engineering, 59*, 3097–3103.

Jacobson, M., Kim, S., & Romney, J. (2003). Contralateral suppression of distortion-product otoacoustic emissions declines with age: A comparison of findings in CBA mice with human listeners. *Laryngoscope, 113*, 1707–1713.

Jagger, C., & Sutton, C. (1991). Death after marital bereavement—is the risk in increased? *Statistics in Medicine, 10*, 395–404.

Jee, J., Wang, J., Rose, K., Lindley, R., Landau, P., & Mitchell, P. (2005). Vision and hearing impairment in age care clients. *Ophthalmic Epidemiology, 12*, 199–205.

Jerger, J. (1972). Audiological findings in aging. *Advances in Otorhinolaryngology, 20*, 115–124.

Jerger, J. (2011). Predicting binaural interference. *Journal of the American Academy of Audiology, 22*, 128.

Jerger, J., Chmiel, R., Florin, E., Pirozzolo, F., & Wilson, N. (1996). Comparison of conventional amplification and an assistive listening device in elderly persons. *Ear and Hearing, 17*, 490–504.

Jerger J., Jerger S., Oliver T., & Pirozzolo F. (1989) Speech understanding in the elderly. *Ear and Hearing 10*, 79–89.

Jerger, J., Silman, S., Lew, H, & Chmiel, R. (1993). Case studies in binaural interference: Converging evidence from behavioral and electrophysiologic measures. *Journal of the American Academy of Audiology, 4,* 122–131.

Jerram, J., & Purdy, S. (2001). Technology, expectations, and adjustment to hearing loss: Predictors of hearing aid outcome. *Journal of the American Academy of Audiology, 12,* 64–79.

Johnson, C., Danhauer, J., & Krishnamurti, S. (2000). A holistic approach model for matching high-tech hearing aid features to elderly patients. *American Journal of Audiology, 9,* 112–123.

Jonsson, R., & Rosenhall, U. (1998). Hearing in advanced age. A study of presbycusis in 85-, 88- and 90-year old people. *Audiology, 37,* 207–218.

Karlsson, K., Harris, J., & Svartengren, M. (1997). Description and primary results from an audiometric study of male twins. *Ear and Hearing, 18,* 114–120.

Kato, J., Hickson, L., & Worrall, L. (1996). Communication difficulties in nursing home residents: How can staff help? *Journal of Gerontological Nursing, 22,* 26–31.

Keithley, E., & Feldman, M. (1979). Spiral ganglion cell counts in an age-graded series of rat cochleas. *Journal of Comparative Neurology, 188,* 429–442.

Keller, B., Morton, J., Thomas, V., & Potter, J. (1999). The effect of visual and hearing impairments on functional status. *Journal of the American Geriatric Society, 47,* 1319–1325.

Kirikae, I., Sato, T., & Shitara, T. (1964). Study of hearing in advanced age. *Laryngoscope, 74,* 205–221.

Kirsch, I., Jungeblat, A., Jenkins, L., & Kolstad, A. (1993). *Adult Literacy in America*: National Center for Education Statistics, U.S. Department of Education.

Kitchel, E. (2006). *Reading, typography and low vision.* Retrieved from http://www.cehd.umn.edu/NCEO/Presentations/presentations.htm

Kochkin, S. (2007). MarkeTrak VII: Obstacles to adult non-user adoption of hearing aids. *Hearing Journal, 60,* 24–50.

Kochkin, S. (2009). MarkeTrak VIII: 25 Year Trends in the Hearing Health Market. *Hearing Review, 16,* 12–31.

Kochkin, S., & Rogin, C. (2000). Quantifying the obvious: The impact of hearing instruments on the quality of life. *Hearing Review, 7,* 6–34.

Kraus, N., McGee, T., Carrell, T., King, C., Tremblay, K., & Nicol, T. (1995). Central auditory system plasticity associated with speech discrimination training. *Journal of Cognitive Neuroscience, 7,* 25–32.

Kricos, P. (2007). Hearing assistive technology considerations for older individuals with dual sensory loss. *Trends in Amplification, 11,* 273–280.

Kricos, P., Erdman, S., Bratt, G., & Williams, D. (2007). Pyschosocial correlates of hearing aid adjustment. *Journal of the American Academy of Audiology, 18,* 304–322.

Krumm, M., Hogarth, B., & Martin, L. (2001, April). *Providing audiology services through a telemedicine medium.* Paper presented at the annual convention of the American Academy of Audiology, San Diego, CA.

Kujawa, S.G., & Liberman, M. C. (2009). Adding insult to injury: Cochlear nerve degeneration after "temporary" noise-induced hearing loss, *Journal of Neuroscience, 229,* 14077–14085.

Kumar, M., Hickey, S., & Shaw, S. (2000). Manual dexterity and successful hearing aid use. *Journal of Laryngology and Otology, 114,* 593–597.

Lähteenmäki, M., & Kaikkonen, A. (2004, September 7th). *Designing for aged people communication needs.* Paper presented at the HCI and the Older Population, Leeds, UK. Retrieved from http://www.dcs.gla.ac.uk/utopia/workshop/lahteenmaki.pdf

Lee, F., Matthews, L., Dubno, J., & Mills, J. (2005). Longitudinal study of pure-tone thresholds in older persons. *Ear and Hearing, 26,* 1–11.

LePrell, C., Yamashita, D., Minami, S., Yamasoba, T., & Miller, J. (2007). Mechanisms of noise-induced hearing loss indicate multiple methods of prevention. *Hearing Research, 226*, 22–43.

Lewis, M., Crandell, C., Valente, M., & Enrietto, J. (2004). Hearing aid accessories for adults: The remote FM microphone. *Journal of the American Academy of Audiology, 15*, 426–439.

Li , C., Wu, W., Jin, H., Zhang, X., Xue, H., He, Y., . . . Zhang, M. (2006). Successful aging in Shanghai, China: Definition, distribution and related factors. *International Psychogeriatrics, 18*, 551–563.

Li, Y. (2007). Recovering from spousal bereavement in later life: Does volunteer participation play a role? *Journal of Gerontology Series B: Psychological Sciences and Social Sciences, 62*, S257–S266.

Lin, F., Ferrucci, L., Metter, E., An, Y., Zonderman, A., & Resnick, S. (2011). Hearing loss and cognition in the Baltimore Longitudinal Study of Aging. *Neuropsychology, 25*, 763–770.

Lin, F., Metter, E., O'Brien, R., Resnick, S., Zonderman, A., & Ferrucci, L. (2011). Hearing loss and incident dementia. *Archives of Neurology, 68*, 214–220.

Ling, L., Hughes, L., & Caspary, D. (2005). Age-related loss of the GABA synthetic enzyme glutamic acid decarboxylase in rate primary auditory cortex. *Neuroscience, 132*, 1103–1113.

Loh, A., Simon, D., Wills, C., Kriston, L., Niebling, W., & Harter, M. (2007). The effects of a shared decision-making intervention in primary care of depression: A cluster-randomized controlled trial. *Patient Education and Counseling, 67*, 324–332.

Ludman, E., Katon, W., Bush, T., Rutter, C., Lin, E., Simon, G., . . . Walker, E. (2003). Behavioural factors associated with symptom outcomes in a primary care-based depression prevention intervention trial. *Psycholoical Medicine, 33*, 1061–1070.

Ludwig, F., Tadayon-Manssuri, E., Strik, W., & Moggi, F. (2012). Self-efficacy as a predictor of outcome after residential treatment programs for alcohol dependence: Simply ask the patient one question! *Alcoholism, Clinical and Experimental Research*. Epub ahead of print. doi:10.1111/acer.12007

Lupsakko, T., Mantyjarvi, M., Kautiainen, H., & Sulkava, R. (2002). Combined hearing and visual impairment and depression in a population aged 75 and older. *International Journal of Geriatric Psychiatry, 17*, 808–813.

Lutman, M., Brown, E., & Coles, R. (1987). Self-reported disability and handicap in the population in relation to pure-tone threshold, age, sex and type of hearing loss. *British Journal of Audiology, 21*, 45–58.

Mahncke, H., Connor, B., Appelman, J., Ahsanuddin, O., Hardy, J., Wood, R., . . . Merzenich, M. (2006). Memory enhancement in healthy older adults using a brain plasticity-based training program: A randomized, controlled study. *Proceedings of the National Academy of Sciences, 103*, 12523–12528.

Mahoney, D. (1992). Hearing loss among nursing home residents. Perceptions and realities. *Clinical Nursing Research, 1*, 317–332.

Maurer, J., & Schow, R. (1995). Audiologic rehabilitation for elderly adults. In R. Schow & M. Nerbonne (Eds.), *Introduction to Audiologic Rehabilitation* (pp. 413–454). Boston, MA: Allyn & Bacon.

McCoy, S., Tun, P., Cox, L., Colangelo, M., Stewart, R., & Wingfield, A. (2005). Hearing loss and perceptual effort: Downstream effects on older adults' memory for speech. *Quarterly Journal of Experimental Psychology. A: Human Experimental Psychology, 58*, 22–33.

Meister, H., Lausberg, I., Kiessling, J., von Wedel, H., & Walger, M. (2002). Identifying the needs of elderly, hearing-impaired persons: The importance and utility if hearing aid attributes. *European Archives of Otorhinolaryngology, 259*, 531–534.

Menec, V. (2003). The relation between everyday activities and successful aging:

A 6-year longitudinal study. *Journal of Gerontology: Social Sciences, 58,* S74–S82.

Merluzzi, F., & Hinchcliffe, R. (1973). Threshold of subjective auditory handicap. *Audiology, 12,* 65–69.

Merzenich, M., Jenkins, W., Johnston, P., Schreiner, C., Miller, S., & Tallal, P. (1996). Temporal processing deficits of language-learning impaired children ameliorated by training. *Science, 271,* 77–81.

Michael, R., & Bron, A. (2011). The ageing lens and cataract: A model of normal and pathological ageing. *Philosophical Transactions of the Royal Society of London, Series B, Biological Sciences, 366,* 1278–1292.

Miller, J., Watson, C., Kewley-Port, D., Sillings, R., Mills, W., & Burleson, D. (2007). SPATS: Speech Perception Assessment and Training System. *Journal of the Acoustical Society of America, 122,* 3063.

Murrell, S., Himmelfarb, S., & Phifer, J. (1988). Effects of bereavement/loss and pre-event status on subsequent physical health in older adults. *International Journal of Aging and Human Development, 27,* 89–107.

Musiek, F. E., Baran, J. A., & Shinn, J., & Jones, R. (2011). *Disorders of the auditory system.* San Diego, CA: Plural Publishing.

National Institute on Deafness and Other Communication Disorders. (2010). *Quick statistics.* Retrieved from http://www.nidcd.nih.gov/health/statistics/Pages/quick.aspx

Nemes, J. (2010). Tele-audiology, a once-futuristic concept, Is growing into a worldwide reality. *Hearing Journal, 63,* 19–20, 22–24.

Newson, R., Beolen, P., Hek, K., Hofman, A., & Tiemeir, H. (2011). The prevalence and characteristics of complicated grief in older adults. *Journal of Affective Disorders, 132,* 231–238.

Nihtilä, E., & Martikainen, P. (2008). Institutionalization of older adults after the death of a spouse. *American Journal of Public Health, 98,* 1228–1234.

Niu, X., Trifunovic, A., Larsson, N., & Canlon, B. (2007). Somatic mtDNA mutations cause progressive hearing loss in the mouse. *Experimental Cell Research, 313,* 3924–3934.

Nomura, K., Nakao, M., & Morimoto, T. (2005). Effect of smoking on hearing loss: Quality assessment and meta-analysis. *Preventive Medicine, 40,* 138–144.

Nondahl , D., Tweed, T,, Cruickshanks, K., Wiley, T., & Dalton, D. (2012). Aging and the 4-kHz air-bone gap. *Journal of Speech Language and Hearing Research, 55,* 1128–1134.

Norris, F., & Murrell, S. (1990). Social support, life events, and stress as modifiers of adjustment to bereavement by older adults. *Psychology and Aging, 5,* 429–436.

Ott, C., Lueger, R., Kelber, S., & Prigerson, H. (2007). Spousal bereavement in older adults: Common, resilient and chronic grief with defining characteristics. *Journal of Mental and Nervous Diseases, 195,* 332–341.

Oxley, J., & Whelan, M. (2008). It cannot be all about safety: The benefits of prolonged mobility. *Traffic Injury Prevention, 9,* 367–378.

Pacala, F., & Yueh, B. (2012). Hearing deficits in the older patient: "I didn't notice anything." *Journal of the American Medical Association, 307,* 1185–1194.

Palmer, C., Adams, S., Bourgeois, M., Durrant, J., & Rossi, M. (1999). Reduction in caregiver-identified problem behaviors in patients with Alzheimer disease post-hearing-aid fitting. *Journal of Speech, Language, and Hearing Research, 42,* 312–328.

Palomar, G., Abdulghani, M., Bodet, A., Andreu, M., & Palomar, A. (2001). Drug-induced ototxicity: Current status. *Acta Oto-Laryngologica, 121,* 569–572.

Parving, A., & Philip, B. (1991). Use and benefit in the tenth decade-and beyond. *Audiology, 30,* 61–69.

Pearson, J., Morrell, C., Gordon-Salant, S., Brant, L., Metter, E., Klein, L., & Fozard, J. L. (1995). Gender differences in a longitudinal study of age-associated hearing loss. *Journal of the Acoustical Society of America, 97,* 1196–1205.

Peel, N. (2011). Epidemiology of falls in older age. *Canadian Journal of Aging*, 1–13. Epub ahead of print.

Plies, J., & Lethbridge-Cejku, M. (2007). *Summary health statistics for US adults: National Health Interview Survey, 2006. Vital Health Stat 10(235), National Center for Health Statistics.* Washington, DC: U.S. Government Printing Office.

Plomp, R., & Mimpen, A. (1979). Speech-reception threshold for sentences as a function of age and noise level. *Journal of the Acoustical Society of America, 66,* 1333–1342.

Pouyatos, B., & Fechter, L. D. (2007). Industrial chemicals and solvents affecting the auditory system. In K. C. M. Campbell (Ed.), *Pharmacology and ototoxicity for audiologists* (pp. 197–210). Clifton Park, NY: Thomson Delmar Learning.

Preusser, D., Williams, A., Ferguson, S., Ulmer, R., & Weinstein, H. (1998). Fatal crash risk for older drivers at intersections. *Accident Analysis and Prevention, 30,* 151–159.

Proud, E., & Morris, M. (2010). Skilled hand dexterity in Parkinson's disease: Effects of adding a concurrent task. *Archives of Physical Medicine and Rehabilitation, 91,* 794–799.

Pujol, R., & Puel, J. (1999). Excitotoxicity, synaptic repair, and functional recovery in the mammalian cochlea: A review of recent findings. *Annals of the New York Academy of Sciences, 884,* 249–254.

Ramachandran, V. (2005). Plasticity and functional recovery in neurology. *Clinical Medicine, 5,* 368–373.

Rantakokko, M., Mänty, M., & Rantanen, T. (2012). Mobility decline in old age. *Exercise and Sport Sciences review.* Epub ahead of print.

Rantanen, T., Guralnik, J., & Ferrucci, L. (2001). Coimpairments as predictors of severe walking disability in older women. *Journal of the American Geriatric Society, 49,* 21–27.

Reuter-Lorenz, P. (2002). New visions of the aging mind and brain. *Trends in Cognitive Sciences, 6,* 394–400.

Reuter-Lorenz, P., Jonides, J., Smith, E., Hartley, A., Miller, A., Marchuetz, C., & Koeppe, R. A. (2000). Age differences in the frontal lateralization of verbal and spatial working memory revealed by PET. *Journal of Cognitive Neuroscience, 12,* 174–187.

Reuter-Lorenz, P., & Lustig, C. (2005). Brain aging: Reorganizing discoveries about the aging mind. *Current Opinion in Neurobiology, 15,* 245–251.

Rosenhall, U., & Sundh, V. (2006). Age-related hearing loss and blood pressure. *Noise and Health, 8*(31), 88–94.

Rubin, G., West, S., Munoz, B., Bandeen-Roche, K., Zeger, S., Schein, O., . . . the SEE Project Team (1997). A comprehensive assessment of visual impairment in a population of older Americans. The SEE Study. Salisbury Eye Evaluation Project. *Investigative Ophthalmology and Visual Science, 38,* 557–568.

Rutter, M., Tizard, J., & Whitmore, K. (1970). *Education, health and behaviour.* London, UK: Longmans.

Rybak, LP (2005). Neurochemistry of the peripheral and central auditory system after ototoxic drug exposure: Implications for tinnitus. *International Tinnitus Journal. 11,* 23–30.

Salthouse, T. (2010). *Major issues in cognitive aging.* New York, NY: Oxford University Press.

Salthouse, T. (2011). Neuroanatomical substrates of age-related cognitive decline. *Psychological Bulletin, 13,* 753–784.

Saunders, G., Cienkowski, K., Forsline, A., & Fausti, S. (2005). Normative data for the Attitudes towards Loss of Hearing Questionnaire. *Journal of the American Academy of Audiology, 16,* 637–652.

Saunders, G., & Forsline, A. (2012). Hearing aid counseling: Comparison of single-session informational counseling with single-session performance-perceptual counseling. *International Journal of Audiology, 51,* 754–764.

Saunders, G., Forsline, A., & Fausti, S. (2004). The Performance-Perceptual Test (PPT) and its relationship to unaided reported handicap. *Ear and Hearing, 25,* 117–126.

Saunders, G., McArdle, R., Chisolm, T., Smith, S., & Wilson, R. (2011, May 23–25). *Auditory training and hearing aid outcome.* Paper presented at the 6th International Adult Aural Rehabilitation Conference, St. Pete Beach, FL.

Schneider, J., Gopinath, B., Karpa, M., McMahon, C., Rochtchina, E., Leeder, S., & Mitchell, P. (2010). Hearing loss impacts on the use of community and informal supports. *Age and Ageing, 39,* 458–464.

Schneider, J., Gopinath, B., McMahon, C., Leeder, S., Mitchell, P., & Wang, J. (2011). Dual sensory impairment in older age. *Journal of Aging and Health, 23,* 1309–1324.

Schneider, J., Gopinath, B., McMahon, C., Teber, E., Leeder, S., Wang, J., & Mitchell, P. (2012). Prevalence and 5-year incidence of dual sensory impairment in an older Australian population. *Annals of Epidemiology, 22,* 295–301.

Schoenthaler, A., Schwartz, B., Wood, C., & Stewart, W. (2012). Patient and physician factors associated with adherence to diabetes medications. *Diabetes Education, 38,* 397–408.

Schow, R. (1982). Success of hearing aid fitting in nursing homes. *Ear and Hearing, 3,* 173–177.

Schulte, B., Gratton, M., & Smythe, N. (1996). *Morphometric analysis of spiral ganglion neurons in young and old gerbils raised in quiet.* Paper presented at the 19th Annual Midwinter Research meeting of the Association for Research in Otolaryngology, St. Petersburg, FL.

Schulz, R., & Beach, S. (1999). Caregiving as a risk factor for mortality: The caregiver health effects study. *Journal of the American Medical Association, 282,* 2215–2219.

Shah, R., Maitra, K., Barnes, L., James, B., Leurgans, S., & Bennett, D. (2012). Relation of driving status to incident life space constriction in community-dwelling older persons: A prospective cohort study. *Journal of Gerontology Series A: Biological Sciences and medical sciences, 67,* 984–989.

Shinn-Cunningham, B., & Best, V. (2008). Selective attention in normal and impaired hearing. *Trends in Amplification, 12,* 283–299.

Shirinian, M., & Arnst, D. (1982) Patterns in the performance-intensity functions for phonetically balanced word lists and synthetic sentences in aged listeners. *Archives of Otolaryngology, 108,* 15–20.

Singh, G., Pichora-Fuller, MK., Hayes, D., von Schroeder, HP., & Carahan, H. (2012). The aging hand and the ergonomics of hearing aid controls. *Ear and Hearing.* Epub ahead of print.

Smith, J. (2012). Toward a better understanding of loneliness in community-dwelling older adults. *Journal of Psychology, 146,* 293–311.

Smith, S., Kricos, P., & Holmes, A. (2001). Vision loss and counseling strategies for the elderly. *Hearing Review, 8,* 42–46, 56.

Smits, C., Kapteyn, T., & Houtgast, T. (2004). Development and validation of an automatic speech-in-noise screening test by telephone. *International Journal of Audiology, 43,* 15–28.

Somers, T., Wren, A., & Shelby, R. (2012). The context of pain in arthritis: Self-efficacy for managing pain and other symptoms. *Current Pain and Headache Reports.* Epub ahead of print.

Stach, B. A., Loiselle, L. H., & Jerger, J. F. (1991). Special hearing aid considerations in elderly patients with auditory processing disorders. *Ear and Hearing, 12*(Suppl. 6), 131S–138S.

Stach, B., Spretnjak, M., & Jerger, J. (1990). The presence of central presbycusis in a clinical population. *Journal of the American Academy of Audiology, 1,* 109–115

Stecker, G., Bowman, G., Yund, E., Herron, T., Roup, C., & Woods, D. (2006). Perceptual training improves syllable identification in new and experienced hearing aid users. *Journal of Rehabilitation Research and Development, 43,* 513–518.

Stephens, S., & Meredith, R. (1990). Physical handling of hearing aids by the elderly.

Acta Otolaryngololgy Supplement, 476, 281–285.

Sullivan, R. (1997). Video otoscopy in audiologic practice. *Journal of the American Academy of Audiology, 8,* 447–467.

Suryadevara, A., Schulte, B., Schmiedt, R., & Slepecky, N. (2001). Auditory nerve gibers in young and aged gerbils: Morphometric correlations with endocochlear potential. *Hearing Research, 161,* 45–53.

Swanepoel, D., Eikelboom, R., Ferrari, D., & Rumkumar, V. (2012, March 28–31). *Tele-Audiology--Bringing Hearing Health to the people (Part 1).* Paper presented at the AudiologyNow! 2012 Conference, Boston, MA.

Sweetow, R., & Palmer, C. (2005). Efficacy of individual auditory training in adults: A systematic review of the evidence. *Journal of the American Academy of Audiology, 16,* 494–504.

Sweetow, R., & Sabes, J. (2006). The need for and development of an adaptive listening and communication enhancement (LACE) program. *Journal of the American Academy of Audiology, 17,* 538–558.

Tarnowski, B., Schmiedt, R., Hellstrom, L., Lee, F., & Adams, J. (1991). Age-related changes in cochleas of Mongolian gerbils. *Hearing Research, 54,* 123–134.

Tárraga, L., Boada, M., Modinos, G., Espinosa, A., Diego, S., Morera, A., . . . Becker, J. T. (2006). A randomised pilot study to assess the efficacy of an interactive, multimedia tool of cognitive stimulation in Alzheimer's disease. *Journal of Neurology, Neurosurgery & Psychiatry, 77,* 1116–1121.

Terry, R., & Katzman, R. (2001). Life span and synapses: Will there be a primary senile dementia? *Neurobiology of Aging, 22,* 347–348.

Thomas, P. (2011). Gender, social engagement, and limitations in late life. *Social Science and Medicine, 73,* 1428–1435.

Thoren, E., Oberg, M., Wanstrom, G., Anderson, G., & Lunner, T. (2012, August 8–12). *Professional online rehabilitation of adult hearing aid users, a randomized controlled trial.* Paper presented at the International Hearing Aid Conference, Lake Tahoe, CA.

Tolson, D., Swan, I., & Knussen, C. (2002). Hearing disability: A source of distress for older people and carers. *British Journal of Nursing, 11,* 1021–1025.

Tomita, M., Mann, W., & Welch, T. (2001). Use of assistive devices to address hearing impairment by older persons with disabilities. *International Journal of Rehabilitation, 24,* 279–290.

Torre, P., Cruickshanks, K., Klein, B., Klein, R., & Nondahl, D. (2005). The association between cardiovascular disease and cochlear function in older adults. *Journal of Speech, Language and Hearing Research, 48,* 473–481.

Tremblay, K, & Kraus, N. (2002). Auditory training induces asymmetrical changes in cortical neural activity. *Journal of Speech, Language, and Hearing Research, 45,* 564–572.

Tremblay, K, Kraus, N, McGee, T, Ponton, C, & Otis, B. (2001). Central auditory plasticity: Changes in the N1-P2 complex after speech-sound training. *Ear and Hearing, 22,* 79–90.

Uchida, Y., Nakashima, T., Ando, F., Nino, N., & Shimokata, H. (2003). Prevalence of self-perceived auditory problems and their relation to audiometric thresholds in a middle-aged to elderly population. *Acta Otolaryngololgy, 123,* 618–626.

Uhlmann, R., Larson, E., Rees, T., Koepsell, T., & Duckert, L. (1989). Relationship of hearing impairment to dementia and cognitive dysfunction in older adults. *Journal of the American Medical Association, 261,* 1916–1919.

Upfold, L., May, A., & Battaglia, J. (1991). Hearing aid manipulation skills in an elderly population: A comparison of ITE, BTE and ITC aids. *British Journal of Audiology, 24,* 101–108.

U.S. Census Bureau. (2008). *U.S. population projections.* Retrieved from http://www.census.gov/population/www/projections/files/nation/summary/np2008-t2.xls

van den Berg, G., Lindenboom, M., & Portrait, F. (2011). Conjugal bereavement effects on health and mortality at advanced ages. *Journal of Health Economics, 30,* 774–794.

Vaughan, D. (1977). Age-related deterioration of pyramidal cell basal dendrites in rat auditory cortex. *Journal of Comparative Neurology, 171,* 501–515.

Vaughan, D., & Vincent, J. (1979). Ultrastructure of neurons in the auditory cortex of ageing rats: A morphometric study. *Journal of Neurocytology, 8,* 215–228.

Volkow, N., Wang, G., Fowler, J., Logan, J., Gatley, S., MacGregor, R., . . . Wolf, A. P. (1996). Measuring age-related changes in dopamine D2 receptors with 11C-raclopride and 18F-N-methylspiroperidol. *Psychiatry Research, 67,* 11–16.

Von Korff, M., Katon, W., Rutter, C., Ludman, E., Simon, G., Lin, E., & Bush, T. (2003). Effect on disability outcomes of a depression relapse prevention program. *Psychsomatic Medicine, 65,* 938–943.

Walden, B., Busacco, D., & Montgomery, A. (1993). Benefit from visual cues in auditory-visual speech recognition by middle-aged and elderly persons. *Journal of Speech and Hearing Research, 36,* 431–436.

Walden, B., Grant, K., & Cord, M. (2001). Effects of amplification and speechreading on consonant recognition by persons with impaired hearing. *Ear and Hearing, 22,* 333–347.

Walton, J., Frisina, R., & O'Neill, W. (1998). Age-related alteration in processing of temporal sound features in the auditory midbrain of the CBA mouse. *Journal of Neuroscience, 18,* 2764–2776.

Wang, H., Turner, J., Ling, L., Parrish, J., Hughes, L., & Caspary, D. (2009). Age-related changes in glycine recptor subunit composition and binding in dorsal cochlear nucleus. *Neuroscience, 160,* 227–239.

Ward, L., Mathias, J., & Hitchings, S. (2007). Relationships between bereavement and cognitive functioning in older adults. *Gerontology, 53,* 362–372.

Watson, G., & Echt, K. (2010). Aging and vision loss. In A. Corn & A. Koenig (Eds.), *Foundations of Low Vision: Clinical and Functional Perspectives* (pp. 871–916). New York, NY: AFB Press.

Willott, J., Milbrandt, J., Bross, L., & Caspary, D. (1997). Glycine immunoreactivity and receptor binding in the cochlear nucleus of C57BL/6J and CBA/CaJ mice: Effects of cochlear impairment and aging. *Journal of Comparative Neurology, 385,* 405–414.

Wilson, C., & Stephens, D. (2002). Reasons for referral and attitudes toward hearing aids: Do they affect outcome? *Clinical Otolaryngology, 28,* 81–84.

Wilson, R., Noe, C., Cruickshanks, K., Wiley, T., & Nondahl, D. (2010). Prevalence and degree of hearing loss among males in Beaver Dam cohort: Comparison of veterans and nonveterans. *Journal of Rehabilitation Research & Development, 47,* 505–520.

Wingfield, A., McCoy, S., Peelle, J., Tun, A., & Cox, L. (2006). Effects of adult aging and hearing loss on comprehension of rapid speech varying in syntactic complexity. *Journal of the American Academy of Audiology, 17,* 487–497.

Wingfield, A., Panizzon, M., Grant, M., Toomey, R., Kremen, W., Franz, C., . . . Lyons, M. (2007). A twin-study of genetic contributions to hearing acuity in late middle age. *Journals of Gerontology Series A: Biological Sciences and Medical Sciences, 62,* 1294–1299.

Wolinsky, F., Mahncke, H., Vander Weg, M., Martin, R., Unverzagt, F., Ball, K., . . . Tennstedt, S. L. (2010). Speed of processing training protects self-rated health in older adults: Enduring effects observed in the multi-site ACTIVE randomized controlled trial. *International Psychogeriatrics, 22,* 470–478.

Working Group on Speech Understanding and Aging. (1988). Speech understanding and aging. *Journal of the Acoustical Society of America, 83,* 859–894.

Wright, K., Smifiklas-Wright, H., Blood, I., & Wright, C. (1997). Dietitians can and should communicate with older adults with hearing and vision impairments and communication disorders. *Journal of the American Dietetic Association, 97,* 172–174.

Wright Willis, A., Evanoff, B., Lian, M., Criswell, S., & Racette, B. (2010). Geographic and ethnic variation in Parkinson disease: A population-based study of U.S. Medicare beneficiaries. *Neuroepidemiology, 34,* 143–151.

Wu, Y., & Bentler, R. (2012). Do older adults have social lifestyles that place fewer demands on hearing. *Journal of the American Academy of Audiology, 23,* 697–711. doi: 610.3766/jaaa.3723.3769.3764.

Yamasoba, T., Someya, S., Yamada, C., Weindruch, R., Prolla, T., & Tanokura, M. (2007). Role of mitochondrial dysfunction and mitochondrial DNA mutations in age-related hearing loss. *Hearing Research, 226,* 185–193.

Yee, W., Cameron, P., & Bailey, M. (2006). Road traffic injuries in the elderly. *Emergency Medicine Journal, 23,* 42–46.

Zafar, H. (1994). *Implications of frequency selectivity and temporal resolution for amplification in the elderly.* (Unpublished doctoral dissertation). Wichita State University, Wichita, KS.

Zanto, T., Toy, B., & Gazzaley, A. (2010). Delays in neural processing during working memory encoding in normal aging. *Neuropsychologia, 48,* 13–25.

Zelinski, E., Spina, L., Yaffe, K., Ruff, R., Kennison, R., Mahncke, H., & Smith, G. E. (2011). Improvement in memory with plasticity-based adaptive cognitive training: Results of the 3-month follow-up. *Journal of the American Geriatric Society, 59,* 258–265.

SECTION 3

Multidisciplinary Perspectives on Assessment and Intervention Across the Spectrum of Related Disorders

CHAPTER 16

ASSESSMENT OF INDIVIDUALS SUSPECTED OR DIAGNOSED WITH CENTRAL AUDITORY PROCESSING DISORDER

A Medical Perspective

DORIS-EVA BAMIOU and VIVIAN ILIADOU

Introduction

The number of scientific papers on central auditory processing has grown exponentially in the last few decades, mirroring the increasing public interest and ongoing vigorous debate about what constitutes central auditory processing disorder (CAPD) as well as a rising clinical demand for diagnosis and management of CAPD (Bellis, Chermak, Weihing, & Musiek, 2013; Dillon & Cameron 2013; Jerger & Martin, 2013; Moore, Rosen, Bamiou, Campbell, & Sirimanna, 2013). There are several consensus statements from professional organizations worldwide (AAA, 2010; ASHA, 2005; BSA, 2011; Nickisch et al., 2007; Nickisch & Schönweiler, 2011) but there is no broad consensus and CAPD was only recently a recognized disorder in a formal diagnostic classification manual such as the ICD-10 (H93.25 Central Auditory Processing Disorder http://www.icd10data.com/ICD10CM/Codes/H60-H95/H90-H94/H93-).

Is a Medical Professional Required for the Assessment of These Patients?

The majority of the consensus statements (AAA, 2010; ASHA, 2005; BSA 2011; Nickisch et al., 2007) emphasize the need for a multidisciplinary assessment and management of individuals with CAPD. The inclusion of a medical professional on the team is also deemed necessary, for several reasons. In some cases across the age span CAPD will arise due to active brain pathology, and occasionally the listening difficulties may be the presenting, or even sole, symptoms for which the patient sought attention (Bamiou et al., 2007, see also case of music patient in Figure 16–1 and case of pediatric brain pathology in Figure 16–2; and Gold Rojiani & Murtaugh, 1997). These cases will require further medical investigations and treatment.

In the pediatric and young adult population, CAPD may overlap with other developmental disorders in a substantial proportion of cases (e.g., Loo, Bamiou, & Rosen, 2012), thus diagnosis and formulation of appropriate intervention will require a good understanding of developmental pediatrics and liaison with other professionals. Other pediatric cases will have ongoing, but intermittent, *glue ear* and CAPD confirmed in

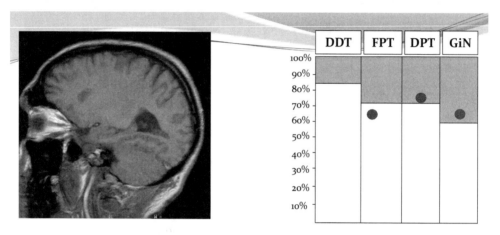

Brain MRI shows a right temporoparietal lesion: This includes the Heschl's gyrus & planum temporale

Right ear tested only: Patient had a congenital left mild to moderate SNHL

Additional non standardized tests conducted:
Consonance/dissonance judgment was abnormal. AEPs to complex sounds: MMN to timbre change with constant pitch was absent (abnormal compared with normal controls The patient could not clap in rhythm to music and could not recognize the emotional content of music.

Figure 16–1. The music patient (Bamiou, unpublished). This 52-year-old male TV/theatre director reported with a minor episode of (resolved) left lower limb weakness. The patient continued playing football after this resolved. His presenting complaints were difficulties with prosody and music perception. He reported that music sounds "out of tune," he cannot judge timbre or pitch, that he is unable to imagine music, or sing in tune. He has had problems judging prosody in his actors and the hearing handicap was perceived by the patient as severe. Neurological examination and cognitive assessment were normal. The patient was sent for central auditory processing tests and brain imaging (MRI). DDT = Dichotic Digits Test; FPT = Frequency Pattern Test; DPT = Duration Pattern Test; GiN = Gaps-In-Noise Test; SNHL = sensorineural hearing loss; AEPs = auditory evoked potentials; MMN = mismatch negativity; MRI = Magnetic resonance imaging.

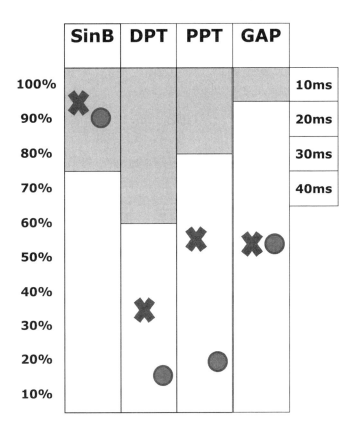

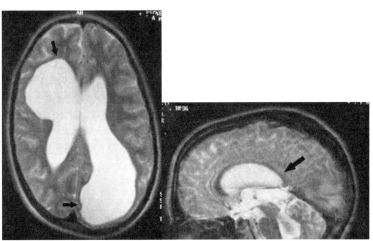

Figure 16–2. Brain pathology in a preterm child (Iliadou et al., 2008). This is the auditory processing evaluation of a 13-year-old girl, preterm at birth with language difficulties, learning difficulties at school and additional listening problems. In terms of identified structural brain pathology on brain MRI, the observed auditory deficits would be compatible with a pressure effect of the large porenchephalic cysts at a brainstem or higher level for the GAP detection test and with the thinning of the corpus callosum for the pattern tests (DPT = Duration Pattern Test; PPT = Pitch (Frequency) Pattern Test; GAP = Gaps-In-Noise Test; SinB = Speech-in-babble; MRI = Magnetic resonance imaging; X = left ear; O = right ear).

the *glue ear-free* intervals or later in life (see also Figure 16–3). These cases will also require monitoring and medical or surgical intervention.

Finally, there are several clinical scenarios that require a careful differential diagnosis. For example, are the child's educational difficulties due to CAPD, or to the presence of undiagnosed and untreated migraine? Is the patient's psychiatric presentation potentially causal (e.g., schizophrenia), or are the psychological/psychiatric difficulties a potential result (Johnston, John, & Kreisman, 2009) or simply concurrent (Davids et al., 2011) with the CAPD, and would treatment affect the clinical presentation

and test results? Is CAPD an early sign of Alzheimer's disease (Gates, Anderson, McCurry, Feeney, & Larson, 2011; Gates, Beiser, Rees, D'Agostino, & Wolf, 2002; Gates et al., 2008) or the result of coexisting cognitive decline (Humes et al., 2012) in an elderly individual?

General Diagnostic Considerations

CAPD may be conceived theoretically as a "mental" disorder defined by the DSM-5 (http://www.dsm5.org/Pages/Default.aspx) as "a clinically significant distur-

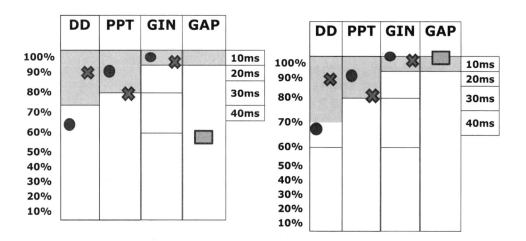

Figure 16–3. Otitis media with effusion case (Iliadou, unpublished). This figure is showing auditory processing evaluation of an 8-year-old boy who had learning difficulties with normal intelligence and history of otitis media with effusion. Following surgery with grommet insertion dichotic digits test results for the right ear are not within normal limits, while still revealing a great difference with the normal dichotic digits results of the left ear. All other auditory processing tests administered were back to normal showing the influence of recurrent episodes of otitis media with effusion left untreated or managed at a later stage in childhood. (DD = Dichotic Digits; PPT = Pitch (Frequency) Pattern Test; GIN = Gaps-In-Noise Test; GAP = Random Gap Detection Test; SNR = signal-to-noise ratio; X = left ear; O = right ear; [] = binaural).

bance in an individual's cognition, emotion regulation, or behavior that reflects a dysfunction in the psychological, biological, or developmental processes underlying mental functioning" and is "usually associated with significant distress in social, occupational, or other important activities" (p. 20). However, the criteria to include such a presentation in the DSM (i.e., assessment to treatment linkages, more than two independent studies demonstrating that this diagnostic category is separate and distinct from other diagnoses, specified diagnostic criteria with more than two empirical studies by independent groups demonstrating a kappa coefficients ≥.70) have not been met in their entirety. CAPD is thus a separate diagnostic entity in ICD-10 with the code H93.25 under the general category disorders of the ear, whereas in the DSM-5 the closest description of CAPD is the subcategory of speech sound disorder (formerly phonological disorder). Diagnostic criteria are not provided in either classification manual, and vary widely, with a recent study identifying at least nine different sets of criteria with a diagnostic rate ranging from 7.3% to 96% (Wilson & Arnott, 2012). There is, however, a clinical need for diagnosis, in order to facilitate communication among professionals, and to guide evidence-based use of existing resources for remediation. The ICD-10 (p. 6) states that "clinicians should record as many diagnoses as necessary to cover the clinical picture" and that "when recording more than one, it is usually best to give one precedence over the others." This will be the *main diagnosis* and it is usually "the disorder that gave rise to the consultation." (p. 6) Thus the first, and fundamental, diagnostic consideration, which is by no means a straightforward one, is to decide and subsequently to be explicit about,

the operational definition and diagnostic criteria adopted for CAPD. Clinicians need to be aware of the several different approaches available to assess this presentation (Jerger, 2009) that may lead to different labels for the same presentation (Dawes & Bishop, 2009) and mindful of the tendency for what James Jerger very aptly terms in his lectures "to the hammer everything looks like a nail."

The second diagnostic consideration involves the selection of auditory processing tests for diagnosis. Exhaustive testing is time consuming and impractical in a clinical setting, whereas the probability of finding chance abnormalities in normal patients rises in proportion to the number of tests employed (Ingraham & Aiken, 1996). The choice of tests should be guided by the clinical history (Griffiths, Bamiou, & Warren, 2010), as symptoms will help formulate a hypothesis about the affected domains that need to be tested. This may be more feasible in neurological patients with discrete brain lesions that lead to specific deficits, such as a pitch disorder, than in the non-neurological pediatric or adult population, for which the body of evidence to facilitate such an approach is not yet available. A hierarchical approach has also been proposed (Dillon, Cameron, Glyde, Wilson, & Tomlin, 2012) that focuses on identification of clinically significant speech in noise difficulties, with a subsequent *master battery* testing identifying areas that require further detailed testing. Identification of risk factors from the history may also help in the choice of tests. For example, masking level difference, which is usually a *low-yield* test, in that it does not identify CAPD in many patients diagnosed by other central auditory tests, possibly because they do not have dysfunction in the lower brainstem (Loo et al., 2012), may be chosen if there is history of glue ear, as this affects MLD (Hall, Grose, Dev, Drake, & Pillsbury, 1998). Other tests sensitive to brainstem pathology may need to be included in the presence of some neurometabolic diseases such as Gaucher's type III (Bamiou, Musiek, & Luxon, 2001). Temporal processing and dichotic listening tests are required for the assessment of presumed central presbycusis, as these domains are reportedly affected in the elderly (Bellis & Wilber, 2001; Gordon-Salant & Fitzgibbons, 1999). Finally, population considerations may also inform test choice, in view of specific deficits known to affect these populations and/or restrictions imposed on testing by the different characteristics and aptitudes of such populations. For example children with language impairments and multilingual individuals will require predominantly nonspeech testing, as speech based testing may reflect language rather than auditory processing competencies (Loo et al., 2012), while patients with dementia will require testing with minimal cognitive load (Goll et al., 2010). A "cookie cutter" diagnostic approach with preset test batteries does not best serve the patient's interests, while a "mix and match" approach, drawing on the available scientific body of evidence and depending on the patient reported symptoms, as well as overall individual's characteristics is called for.

The third diagnostic consideration is whether to base the diagnosis on carefully ascertained and quantified reported symptoms, test deficits, or a combination of both. There are but a few systematic studies describing and quantifying CAPD related symptoms. And while some authors report different weightings of symptoms in CAPD versus other clinical populations (Ferguson, Hall, Riley, & Moore, 2011; Iliadou & Bamiou, 2012)

versus others who have not found such differences (Dawes et al., 2009), it would appear that capd related difficulties are *not* specific for CAPD (AAA, 2010). A diagnosis of CAPD solely based on symptoms or solely based on test results will inevitably lack credibility and provide no framework for intervention. The patient reported symptoms help identify areas of need as well as audiological domains that require testing; the test deficits help define the site of lesion, and also guide the intervention (Griffiths et al., 2010). For example, an auditory neuropathy-related perceptual disorder has a different prognosis and management to that of CAPD, whereas "focal" type test deficits should lead to further neuroradiological investigation. Identification of speech in noise test deficits, which are not necessarily present in all affected individuals with CAPD, will justify the need for a personal FM system in the classroom, while other types of deficit will necessitate targeted training, although admittedly the evidence basis for such training is still only accumulating. See Chapter 3.

The fourth diagnostic consideration involves the need for additional assessments. In general, language (including phonological) and cognitive (including attention and memory) domains need to be assessed, while a potential psychological/psychiatric component should not be overlooked. In the absence of specific guidelines, such assessments may need to be driven by identification of clinical need. Instruments such as the Children's Communication Checklist–2 (CCC-2) (Bishop, 2003) and ADHD questionnaires (e.g., Conners, 1996), as well as screening instruments for anxiety and depression can help identify those in need for further assessment. Additional medical investigations may include imaging, EEG studies, or other laboratory investigations, depending on the clinical presentation (Gold et al., 1997).

Finally, once all this information has been obtained, the process is one of clinical decision making: The clinician will need to think about "outliers" in performance (e.g., a borderline normal test result on a test that should correlate with the patient' reported symptoms in a patient who gives high scores on other tests of auditory processing), factors that may have influenced the clinical presentation (for example limited motivation, short attention span, anxiety, fatigue), but also be aware that potentially the test wise "snapshot" obtained from the patient on a single clinical visit may not be the most representative: factors such as motivation must be considered.

The Diagnostic Process

The diagnostic process includes history taking followed by medical examination, test and laboratory assessment, and other information gathering, formulation of the diagnosis, and communication to the patient.

History: Symptoms and Their Time of Onset

It is useful to first establish what are the parents' main concerns regarding their child. These may not necessarily affect the final diagnosis in that, for example, the presence of parental concerns has low diagnostic sensitivity and specificity for the final diagnosis of sensorineural hearing loss (Hammond, Gold, Wigg, &

Volkmer, 1997) and may be disproportionate to central auditory processing test performance (Dawes & Bishop, 2010). However, establishing concerns may help the clinician understand the parental perspective in order to best engage them when planning and implementing intervention.

In terms of CAPD related symptoms, there are several questionnaire studies in different populations (e.g., Bamiou et al., 2012; Iliadou & Bamiou, 2012; Meister, Von Wedel, & Walger, 2004; Neijenhuis, Stollman, Snik, & Van Den Broek, 2001; Smoski, Brunt, & Tannahill, 1992; Spyridakou, Luxon, & Bamiou, 2012), as well as consensus statements listing the main symptoms of CAPD. The main areas that need to be covered include perception of speech (under different demand situations), music (including pitch difficulties) and environmental sounds; the ability to localize sound; loudness discomfort and perception; as well as the presence of tinnitus and musical hallucinations. Questions that pertain to the patient's memory for speech/song/melody and selective, sustained and divided attention in the auditory domain versus the visual domain are particularly relevant, especially in view of overlap between CAPD with ADHD (Riccio, Hynd, Cohen, Hall, & Molt, 1994). Questionnaires can help both record and quantify these symptoms; however, areas of specific difficulty need to be examined in further detail. It is useful to establish the responder's point of reference for normal (e.g., older siblings of the child, or previous to current experience of the adult) and also to ask for specific examples that illustrate the perceived difficulty within specified contexts. Broader questions about language aptitude and overall communication, including pragmatics, are useful and can also be obtained with a formal questionnaire such as the CCC-2, which may enhance the diagnostic approach (Bishop & McDonald, 2009).

The time course needs to be established: did symptoms have an abrupt onset (e.g., after a cerebrovascular incident or stroke), a more insidious progressive course (indicating e.g., gradual brain degeneration) or have these symptoms been present since early childhood (indicating a *developmental* type CAPD). In addition, was the time of referral due to increased severity of the symptoms, or for example, to increased academic and/or professional demands prompting the individual or their family to seek help? The history should also establish developmental milestones (and listening behaviors of the child in different ages), educational/ occupational history, difficulties experienced in the educational/ professional environment and their context (e.g., how many children there are in the classroom and is it a noisy environment, is the office designed as an open space and what are the noise levels), as well as the support available to the patient. Psychological and psychosocial aspects should also be explored, for differential diagnostic purposes, but also because there is some evidence that the CAPD population has increased difficulties in this domain (Kreisman, John, Kreisman, Hall, & Crandell, 2012) and, such aspects may improve after successful intervention for CAPD (Johnston, John, Kreisman, Hall, & Crandell, 2009). History should also establish the patient's and parent's perception of the affected individual's strengths as well as weaknesses. The next step is to ascertain the presence of additional symptoms and information that will help identify risk factors for this clinical presentation.

CAPD Related Risk Factors: Obtaining a Family History and Medical History

The importance of medical, as well as family history cannot be overemphasized: CAPD may be attributed to a developmental type presentation, but may also be the presenting, or sole, clinical manifestation of potentially life threatening neurological disease. The clinician will need to establish whether any neurological type symptoms have been present since early life (e.g., in the child with neonatal brain hypoxia and cerebral palsy) or more recently (e.g. in the patient with stroke, or the child with a brain tumor). A review of the literature on risk factors for CAPD is provided in the following paragraphs.

A number of different approaches considering etiological classification of CAPD have been proposed over the years. Bamiou et al. (2001) proposed grouping causal factors of CAPD in three main categories: neurological conditions, delayed maturation of the central auditory pathway, and developmental abnormalities. The position statement of the British Society of Audiology (2011) proposed the following three main categories: developmental (including cases that present in childhood with normal audiometry and no other known risk factor), acquired (due to a post-natal event such as neurological trauma or infection), and secondary (in the presence or as a consequence of peripheral hearing impairment). Another classification, by Chermak and Musiek (2011), proposed three different types of CAPD: as a result of frank neurological lesions, neuromaturational lag, and neuroanatomical abnormalities (emphasizing the neurobiological origin of the disorder). The *Guidelines for the Diagnosis, Treatment and Management of Children and Adults with Central Auditory Processing Disorder* by the American Academy of Audiology (AAA, 2010) states that CAPD may be "the result of a number of different etiologies that involve deficits in the function of the central auditory nervous system" (p. 3), emphasize the strong link between "well-defined lesions of the CANS and deficits on behavioral and electrophysiologic central auditory measures" (p. 5), and recognizes "that while there is considerable overlap and possible imprecise use of terms like: cortical deafness, word deafness, auditory agnosia and central deafness; central deafness may define the more fundamental disorder" (p. 5). Finally, Griffiths (2002) included "positive disorders of auditory processing" such as tinnitus and musical hallucinations, in his classification. For the purposes of this chapter, causes of CAPD will be discussed under 6 separate categories, those of developmental disorders, deprivation and plasticity, neurological pathologies, neuropsychiatric disorders, and dementia and central presbycusis.

of CAPD with these disorders or the existence of more global issues manifesting in these disorders that include auditory processing deficits (Moore et al., 2012). There is a tendency to consider auditory sensory processing as mostly bottom-up with a top-down element attributed to cognition. However, evidence exists that this mechanistic view does not account for the dynamic and multilevel interaction of sensory processing and cognition (e.g., Skoe & Kraus, 2010). Cognition may be defined as processing of information entering the brain from the outside world through sensory portals (Cromwell & Panksepp, 2011) and, as a result, processing deficits can impact on information integration from different sensory channels, learning, and attention, and may manifest as communication disorders and/or academic difficulties (Iliadou, 2011). The purpose of testing for CAPD in this pediatric population is to design targeted intervention, and yet as mentioned by Veuillet, Bouilhol, and Thai-Van (2011), " Too rarely to this day, health professionals faced with children with learning difficulties ask whether an APD is present" (p. 236).

Developmental Disorders

Disordered auditory processing may coexist with several developmental disorders, such as autism spectrum disorders (O'Connor, 2012), dyslexia, specific language impairment, learning disabilities (Iliadou, Bamiou, Kaprinis, Kandylis, & Kaprinis, 2009), and attention deficit and/or hyperactivity disorder (ADHD) (Riccio et al., 1994). Several arguments have been postulated as to the causality

Autism Spectrum Disorder

Autism spectrum disorder (ASD) is characterized by impairments in social interactions, communication deficits, and repetitive stereotyped patterns of behavior. Frequently reported sensory symptoms, particularly prevalent in the auditory domain, are not included in the diagnostic criteria (DSM-5). Alcantara, Cope, Cope, and Weisblatt (2012) reported that in a recent analysis of Autism Diagnostic Interview Revised (ADI-R, a structured interview used for diagnosing autism, planning treatment, and distinguishing autism from other developmental disorders [Lord, Rutter, & Couteur, 1994]), 96.8% of children presented with negative auditory reactions to background signals and/or noise hypersensitivity. Individuals with ASD frequently report difficulties perceiving speech in background noise. Individuals with ASD (Alcantara, Weisblatt, Moore, & Bolton, 2004) have similar speech reception thresholds (SRT) as controls in unmodulated background noise, but higher SRTs (by 2–4 dB) in modulated noise. This increment of the SRT is high enough to impact on everyday life communication and academic learning, as well as to interfere with the development of phonological categories in children with an immature central auditory system and/or neurodevelopmental disorders (Talcott et al., 2002). A delay in the development of auditory temporal-envelope processing has also been associated with ASD (Alcantara et al., 2012), and may persist into adulthood, with speech in noise perceptual deficits requiring targeted intervention strategies. The presence of speech in noise perceptual deficits in individuals diagnosed with developmental dyslexia, as well as specific language impairment, indicates that this deficit is not a distinctive feature of the ASD sensory phenotype, but rather a common feature with other developmental disorders. However, in ASD the speech in noise deficit is observed only in the modulated background noise, whereas in developmental dyslexia and specific language impairment it is observed in both modulated and unmodulated background noise (Ziegler, Pech-Georgel, George, & Lorenzi, 2009, 2011). Children with ASD and specifically Asperger's syndrome are less efficient at extracting cues for temporal modulation and this is consistent with abnormalities in processing at the level of the inferior colliculi nuclei of the auditory brainstem and/or increased levels of internal neural noise(Alcantara et al., 2012). It is not yet known if this is the result of abnormal corticofugal modulation of peripheral auditory processing centers or deficiencies in local processes of neural adaptation during critical development periods that lead to changes in subcortical structures, coding, and processing in the ascending auditory pathways.

Developmental Dyslexia

The presence of central auditory processing deficits in the dyslexic population is well established. Researchers have reported deficits in one or more central auditory processing tests in dyslexic subjects (Sharma et al., 2006), or in some cases in subgroups of children with dyslexia (Dawes et al., 2009; Iliadou et al., 2009; Sharma, Purdy, & Kelly, 2009; Veuillet et al., 2011). Deficits across a wide range of auditory processes have been found: gap detection, frequency and amplitude modulation, temporal order and repetition tasks, backward masking and categorical perception of phonemes and nonspeech analogues. A reduction or absence of activity in the left hemisphere temporoparietal cortex is reported in children and adults with dyslexia of different cultural and linguistic backgrounds (Iliadou & Kaprinis, 2003). Neural processing of rapid auditory stimuli is disrupted in dyslexia as shown by event-related potential and magnetoencephalography (MEG) studies. During phonological processing, dyslexics show activity in posterior language brain areas, while during rapid auditory processing they fail to show activity in left prefrontal brain areas. This atypical processing in frontal and posterior networks suggests that dyslexia may be a disconnection syndrome, and implies white matter disruptions in the brain (Boscariol et al., 2009, 2010, 2011; Galaburda, 1985; Temple, 2002). Disorganization of the white matter in dyslexia was shown with diffusion tensor imaging (DTI), showing correlation between reading ability and the degree to which the left hemisphere language *areas* were disorganized (Klingberg et al., 2000). The proportion of dyslexic individuals that present with CAPD is in the range of 40% to 50%. Until the causality debate is resolved, appropriate testing and subsequent management of dyslexic children should be provided, especially since the coexistence with CAPD is so often encountered.

Specific Language Impairment

Specific language impairment (SLI) is characterized by the failure to develop normal language skills in the absence of neurological impairment, hearing deficit, or abnormal intelligence (Choudhury, Leppanen, Leevers, & Benasich, 2007); however, it is debatable whether subtle neurological deficits are ruled out for all diagnosed cases, and while hearing impairment refers to a permanent hearing loss, it does not take into account past episodes of otitis media with effusion (Cordewener, Bosman, & Verhoeven, 2012). Mismatch negativity studies have shown reduction in both linguistic and nonlinguistic perceptual discrimination abilities in children with SLI at a preconscious level, indicating that there is a relationship between SLI children's nonspeech processing difficulties and phonological deficits (Davids et al., 2011; Kleindeinst & Musiek, 2011).

Deprivation and Plasticity

The term "plasticity" (etymology Greek, *plassein*, to mold, the quality of being plastic or formative, Mosby's Medical Dictionary, 8th edition, 2009 Elsevier) refers to the potential of the central auditory system to adapt to changes in environmental auditory stimuli such that representation of the perceived information is more accurate. Both sensorineural and conductive hearing loss may thus lead to changes in the central auditory nervous system (Takesian, Kotak, & Sanes, 2012; Whitton & Polley, 2011), with the relationship between the time of onset and duration of peripheral hearing loss to the stage of language development being potentially critical for the appearance of CAPD.

From a clinical point of view, a history of recurrent otitis media with effusion —OME—is frequently found in children being evaluated for and diagnosed with CAPD. The presence of long-term conductive hearing loss may lead to anatomical and neurophysiological changes of the CANS: For example, unilateral conductive hearing loss leads to changes of the relative size of neuron dendrites in the medial superior olive (MSO), compromising binaural hearing as a result (Moore, Hartley, & Hogan, 2003; Sanes & Woolley, 2011). Degraded signals due to OME during critical periods of brain development may have adverse effects on the formation of neural circuits that persist long after the middle ear pathology has resolved (Whitton & Polley, 2011). A slow recovery of binaural function has been reported in children with OME following restoration of normal hearing thresholds (Hall, Grose, Dev, & Ghiassi, 1998).Perception of speech in noise may be less accurate in children with past history of otitis media with effusion (Hall et al., 1998). Communication and learning difficulties in children may be influenced by the central auditory processing deficits induced by OME (Golz et al., 2006).

Changes in the CANS may also be the result of sensorineural hearing loss across all age groups. The lifelong regulation of synapse strength permits neural circuits' adaptation to an ever changing environment. Both excitatory and inhibitory connections play a role in this regulation. A decline in the inhibitory synapses may be encountered during development (Kandler, Clause, & Noh, 2009), as well as during aging (Caspary, Ling, Turner, & Hughes, 2008). Chronic deprivation elicits unique effects at inhibitory synapses in the auditory cortex. Inhibitory interneurons, even though outnumbered by the excitatory ones, are associated with the sharpening of the receptive fields as a result of being activated, whereas broadening of the receptive field occurs when they are inactivated. Even a moderate hearing loss leads to a pervasive failure of inhibitory synapses in the auditory cortex to properly mature. This may compromise temporal rates and stimulus selectivity. Developmental hearing loss, while originating in the auditory periphery, causes a pervasive CNS impairment involving synapses and membrane properties. These central changes may explain (at least partly) why children with even a transient hearing loss can suffer long-term behavioral deficits, and why aging may interfere with speech comprehension even in the presence of relatively normal thresholds. An interesting point is that central processing improvement is correlated with stronger GABAergic transmission (Edden, Muthukumaraswamy, Freeman, & Singh, 2009; Gleich et al., 2003; Leventhal et al., 2003). Central effects of conductive hearing loss include: smaller nuclei in the cochlear nucleus and medial nucleus of the trapezoid body together with a decrease in spontaneous activity recorded at the round window, and a reduction in neuronal 2-deoxyglucose uptake (Harrison & Negandhi, 2012).

The case of an 8-year-old boy referred for CAPD evaluation due to academic difficulties is presented in Figure 16–3. He had a fluctuating conductive hearing loss as a result of otitis media with effusion. CAPD assessment before and following surgery (adenoidectomy and grommets insertion) is presented showing an immediate postsurgery temporal processing improvement and a sustained dichotic digits deficit affecting the right ear perception.

Neurological Pathology

Prematurity and Low Birth Weight

Preterm infants may be at high risk for CAPD. A case of a premature child with large porencephalic cysts and thinning of the corpus callosum who was diagnosed with CAPD on the basis of deficits in both the frequency and the duration pattern sequence tests, as well as in the random gap detection (GAP) test is shown in Figure 16–2. The observed auditory processing deficits were compatible with: (1) a pressure effect, starting at the brainstem level due to the presence of porencephalic cysts (explaining the resulting performance on the GAP test) and (2) with the thinning of the corpus callosum influencing the pattern test results as interhemispheric transfer of information is required. The case highlights the fact that preterm children with learning difficulties may suffer from a CAPD in the presence of structural abnormalities that are due to birth and neonatal complications. The corpus callosum is extremely vulnerable to ischemia and hemorrhage occurring in preterm births; it can also be influenced by its position adjacent to the periventricular area, a common site of hemorrhage in infancy. Thinning of the corpus callosum is correlated with a reduced ability to perform timbre and bilateral field comparison tasks (Santhouse et al., 2002), reduced performance on verbal fluency tests (Nosarti et al., 2004), increased laterality index (i.e., right minus left ear performace) in dichotic speech tests (reviewed in Bamiou et al., 2007) and low performance in frequency and duration pattern sequence tests (Iliadou et al., 2008).

Lyme Disease

Lyme disease, an inflammatory disease caused by the bacterium *Borrelia burgdorferi*, has been linked with central auditory processing deficits in both adults and children (Bamiou et al., 2001). Central auditory processing deficits are present within months after manifestation of Lyme disease in children and within months to years in adults. Children present with difficulties in repeating sequences of numbers, in identifying similar pairs of sequential rhythmic beats or in following auditory commands with multiple steps. Adults have gradual, sustained improvement in symptoms, and test results following treatment with 2- or 4-week courses of intravenous ceftriaxone.

Infectious Causes

There is some inconclusive evidence that central auditory processing deficits may be present after bacterial meningitis, and in some cases with normal hearing sensitivity (Bamiou et al., 2001). Central deafness has been associated with herpes simplex encephalitis (Bamiou et al., 2001).

Closed Head Trauma

Bergemalm and Lyxell (2005) administered cognitive tests (of short-term working memory, information processing speed, phonological processing and inference making) and central auditory tests (auditory brainstem evoked responses and speech-based central auditory processing tests) to patients admitted to a Swedish hospital due to closed head injury of sufficient severity to cause closed skull-fracture and/or brain contusion. They reported that 58% (11/19) had CAPD. Penn, Wtermeyer, and Schie (2009) reported that auditory (language) processing, including auditory memory, discrimination, analysis and synthesis, were affected in 72% (72/100) of children who had sustained traumatic brain injury. Bergemalm et al. (2009) reported deficits of sound movement direction in the majority of adults with closed head injury. The site of lesion can vary considerably, including brainstem (Bergelmalm & Lyxell 2005) or atrophy of the posterior corpus callosum resulting in auditory interhemispheric disconnection (Benavidez et al., 1999). Poor correspondence in some cases between test deficits with the structural pathology identified by imaging findings can be due to possible axonal degeneration and plastic changes (Bergemalm et al., 2009).

CANS Tumors

Central auditory processing deficits may also arise due to brain tumors, and in the presence of severe neurological symptomatology, CAPD may be overlooked (Bamiou et al., 2001).

Stroke

Stroke is the most common neurological disorder, and may cause physical as well as cognitive impairment. Stroke may result in disordered auditory processing, that is not reflected or accounted for by audiometric thresholds (e.g., Bamiou et al., 2006, 2012). The clinical presentation will depend on the site and extent of the lesion. This specific population highlights the need for detailed audiological testing of the patient. The test results, in combination with the patient report, might help substantiate a diagnosis of amusia (for example), but with environmental sound recognition intact, or an apperceptive (due to disrupted sensory processing) versus associative (due to loss of meaning) sound agnosia (Griffiths et al., 2010). Following a left-hemisphere stroke, the patient's sound discrimination, especially from the right ear, is impaired for up to 10 days and may resolve 3 to 6 months poststroke, with an ensuing improvement in speech recognition. Over the same time period the amplitude of MMN, elicited by vowel

and duration changes in speech sounds, which is initially diminished, gradually increases over a period of months (Ilvonen et al., 2004). A voxel based high-resolution magnetic resonance imaging study of 210 stroke patients found that structural integrity of a posterior region of the superior temporal gyrus and sulcus predicted both auditory short-term memory capacity and speech comprehension (Leff et al., 2009). In this population, functional deficits will need to be assessed and quantified in order to implement appropriate remediation. A questionnaire study of patients with unilateral cerebrovascular lesions of telencephalic auditory structures found that 49% of these patients reported auditory perceptual problems, with sound localization or in situations with simultaneous speakers (Blaettner, Scherg, & von Cramon, 1989). We found severe functional limitation (z score >3) in sound recognition and localization difficulties reported by nine out of 21 cases with stroke of the CANS, with moderate to strong corrrelation with some of the central auditory processing test results, but not with thresholds (Bamiou et al., 2012). Figure 16–1 illustrates the case of a patient who sought medical attention after stroke because of central auditory processing difficulties. In childhood stroke is rare; however, the auditory deficit may appear dramatic, with no behavioral response to sound (Bamiou et al., 2001; Setzen et al.,1999), despite the presence of normal otoacoustic emissions and ABR (for example in Moyamoya disease).

Demyelinating Disorder

Multiple sclerosis is a well-documented CAPD risk factor, with deficits on ABR and binaural hearing tests (e.g., Levine et al., 1993). In other cases such as the rarer x-linked adrenoleukodystrophy, listening difficulties attributed to central auditory processing deficits may be the presenting symptom in childhood and may still be the only severe symptoms in adult life (Bamiou et al., 2004).

Epilepsy

Central auditory processing deficits in children with Rolandic epilepsy have been documented by means of neurophysiology (Liasis, Bamiou, Boyd, & Towell, 2006), suggesting a disruption within the perisylvian region, and possibly underpinning the observed language impairments (Smith et al., 2012). Patients with temporal lobe epilepsy may have speech recognition impairments in the presence of normal hearing sensitivity, while high incidence of deficits in frequency and duration detection has been reported independent of lesion laterality (Han et al., 2011). MRI documented hippocampal sclerosis in this group of patients correlated with poorer frequency test scores, leading Smith et al. (2012) to suggest that hippocampal sclerosis reflects functional impairment in temporal processing. Another study similarly reported binaural temporal resolution deficits, for which attention appeared to play a minimal if any role, in patients who had mesial temporal lobe sclerosis associated with complex partial seizures (Aravindkumar et al., 2012). The presence of CAPD in patients with temporal lobe epilepsy may be associated with risk factors such as long duration of the epilepsy and presence of hippocampal sclerosis or mesial temporal lobe sclerosis that emphasizes the need for routine central auditory processing testing of this population. Conversely, finding central auditory processing test deficits in such patients should raise suspicion of hippocampal or mesial temporal lobe sclerosis.

Landau-Kleffner Syndrome

Landau-Kleffner syndrome (is a rare neurological disorder characterized by aphasia and an abnormal electroencephalogram (Chermak & Musiek, 2011). Children presenting this syndrome usually develop typically until 3 to 7 years, at which time they present aphasia either gradually or suddenly. Symptoms include loss of language skills and auditory comprehension, and auditory agnosia. Even though there are no clinical seizures in the initial stages, EEG reveals paroxysmal spike-and-wave discharges, unilaterally or bilaterally occurring over the temporal regions. A unilateral dichotic listening deficit contralateral to the site of lesion in the temporal cortex is present in most cases. Case 4 (Figure 16–4) illustrates such an example.

Neuropsychiatric Disorders

In all major neuropsychiatric disorders, cognitive decline exists in the form of a temporofrontal functional deficiency expressed as deficient auditory discrimination and orientation. This dysfunction can be detected by the mismatch negativity (MMN), and its magnetoencephalographic equivalent (supratemporal MMN component) manifests a more widespread brain disorder involving a deficient N-methyl-D-aspartate receptor function, which is shared by these disorders and accounts for most of the cognitive decline (Naatanen, 2011).

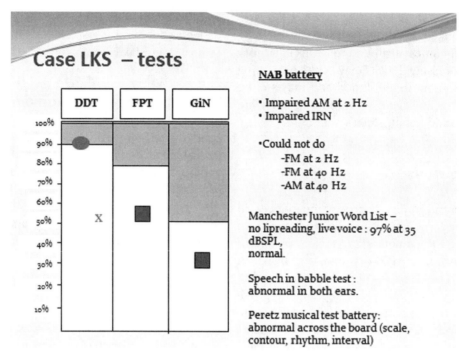

Figure 16–4. The teenager with Landau Kleffner. This 16-year-old right-handed girl reported an episode of meningitis age 15 months with subsequent loss of vocalizing but normal hearing. She had her first word at age 4 to 5 years after intensive speech language input. She started having seizures during the first few years of her life and electroencephalography at age 5 showed epileptiform activity over both hemispheres but dominant on the right and a formal diagnosis of Laudau-Kleffner syndrome (LKS) at age 6 years was made. When seen at age 16 years she still had occasional fits, triggered by stress. Her verbal IQ was significantly lower than her nonverbal IQ She reported very impaired hearing of speech in background noise, very poor recognition of environmental sounds and of music. Pure-tone audiogram, transient otoacoustic emissions, ABR, tympanograms, and acoustic reflexes were bilaterally normal. On environmental sound recognition (on a BBC CD): she missed 4 out of 12 environmental sounds. She had deficits on the Peretz musical test battery as well as on clinical auditory processing tests. (DDT = Dichotic Digits Test; FPT = Frequency Pattern Test; GiN = Gaps-In-Noise Test; NAB = Newcastle Auditory Battery; AM = amplitude modulation; FM = frequency modulation; IRN = iterated rippled noise; X = left ear; O = right ear; [] = binaural).

Schizophrenia

There is evidence of a reduced gray matter volume in the left planum temporale and Heschl's gyrus in schizophrenic patients (Hirayasu et al., 2000) leading to a disappearance of the normally left favoring asymmetry of the temporal lobes or even to the reversal of this asymmetry (Shenton, Dickey, Frumin, & McCarley, 2001). This abnormal brain morphology has been documented even in first episode psychosis, thus excluding the possibility that medication or illness duration may have resulted in these abnormalities.

Central auditory processing deficits have been documented in a large number of studies during the last decade showing deficits for both complex speech stimuli and in basic tone discrimination abilities (Cromwell, Mears, Wan, & Boutros, 2008; Elvevag, McCormack, Brown, Vousden, & Goldberg, 2004; Iliadou et al., 2013; Li, Chen, Yang, Chen, & Tsay, 2002; Ngan et al., 2003; Oades et al., 2006). These abnormal findings cannot easily be attributed to impaired attention, motivation, or cooperation (Rabinowicz, Silipo, Goldman, & Javitt, 2000). Many studies have focused on a particular component of central auditory processing; however, there is one study (McKay, Headlam, & Copolov, 2000) that implemented a clinical diagnostic battery approach to test for CAPD. This study found dysfunction of the right hemisphere and/or dysfunction of the corpus callosum. A more recent study by Turetsky, Bilker, Siegel, Kohler, and Gur (2009) suggested the presence of two discrete neurobiological substrates in schizophrenia, one the early sensory processing deficit and the second a cognitive processing deficit.

Schizophrenia may also be associated with a fundamental deficit in the temporal coordination of information processing in the brain (Tononi & Edelman, 2000) as shown by significantly greater timing variability under both millisecond and several-second timing conditions relative to controls (Carroll, O'Donnell, Shekhar, & Hetrick, 2009). Central auditory processing deficits in first episode psychosis and schizophrenia may result in communication deficits. The MMN, which is generated by a temporofrontal network involved in auditory preperceptual change detection has been examined in schizophrenia, revealing dampening of the frontal involuntary attention-switching component/function (Baldeweg, Klugman, Gruzelier, & Hirsch, 2002) that is correlated with the negative symptoms, such as reduced ability to plan activities, lack of emotion, and loss of motivation and interest in everyday activities (Baldeweg, Klugman, Gruzelier, & Hirsch, 2004). This correlation might actually suggest a causal effect, as the aforementioned dampening function may lead to diminished involuntary attention switches to socially relevant auditory cues such as stress, loudness, changes in speaker voice and change from one speaker to another (Naatanen & Kahkonen, 2009).

Bipolar Disease

Structural and functional auditory cortex abnormalities that may relate to patient's cognitive impairments have been reported in biplor disease (Reite Teale, Rojas, Asherin, & Hernandez, 2009), as well as prolonged MMN peak latencies (Takei et al., 2010) for tone duration and frequency change.

Central Presbycusis

The term presbycusis in Greek literary means elderly hearing (presby = elderly, acusis = hearing). Hearing in the elderly is an interaction of age-related changes in peripheral (cochlear and neural) hearing, central auditory processing, and cognitive processing (Pichora-Fuller, 2003; Tobias et al., 1998). There are several theoretical frameworks to explain the interplay of perception, cognition and aging. These include the common cause hypothesis (i.e., declines are due to widespread neural degeneration), the cognitive load on perception hypothesis (i.e., cognitive decline leads to perceptual decline), a deprivation hypothesis (i.e., permanent reduced auditory input leads to reduced cognitive performance) and the information degradation hypothesis (i.e., reduced temporary auditory input leads to cognitive performance decline). These hypotheses are not mutually exclusive, however (Baltes & Lindeberger, 1997).

The term *central presbycusis* refers to age-related central auditory processing dysfunction that is characterized by deficits in temporal processing and speech recognition (Gordon-Salant & Fitzgibbons, 2001) and interhemispheric transfer (Bellis & Wilber, 2001). Listening for speech is more effortful in the elderly, who show reduced activation in auditory cortex, and increased activation in working memory and attention-related cortical areas, with this latter activation positively correlated with behavioral speech in noise performance (Wong et al., 2009). Auditory distractibility may also be increased (Stevens, Hasher, Chiew, & Grady, 2008). Gates et al. (2010) suggested that candidate anatomic area(s) that may be involved in central presbyacusis include those where auditory association pathways and executive function overlap, and recommended that elderly patients with substantial central auditory dysfunction should be referred for neurologic evaluation, as well as neuropsychologic assessment. Working memory and executive function testing should be considered to rule out cognitive decline when testing the elderly for central presbyacusis (Humes et al., 2012).

Dementia

A prospective collaborative study with the Framingham Heart Study revealed the presence of central auditory speech processing deficits as a possible early manifestation of probable Alzheimer's disease (Gates, Beiser, Rees, D'Agostino, & Wolf, 2002). Testing for CAPD in patients with dementia provides evidence of central auditory processing deficits in verbal and nonverbal tests of the CAPD battery. Interpretation of results should be made with caution as cognitive factors may play a greater or lesser role (Iliadou & Kaprinis, 2003). A more recent study (Goll et al., 2010) proposed that core deficits of nonverbal sound processing, which are modality specific (i.e., more pronounced than visual processing deficits) may underpin the primary progressive nonfluent aphasia type of dementia, thus showing a distinct clinical phenotype relative to semantic dementia, in which auditory deficits are more prominent in the perceptive and semantic level. Central auditory processing dysfunction has been documented to a lesser degree in mild cognitive impairment and to a greater degree in Alzheimer's disease using an assessment largely based on dichotic evaluation (Idrizbegovic et al., 2011). Recent research in the areas of dementia and central auditory processing points to the need for implementing central auditory processing evaluation in older adults with hearing complaints (Gates et al., 2008). This assessment should be individualized in order to identify areas of need that will require further input relative to hearing and cognition.

Medical Examination

A thorough case history interview should be followed by examination. This will be guided by the history; however, in general the examination will include otoscopy (e.g., for signs of glue ear or previous surgery), neuro-otological examination of eye movements and cranial nerves, and additional neurological/neurodevelopmental examination.

Audiological Tests

It is beyond the scope of this chapter to discuss central auditory processing tests as part of the diagnostic evaluation. However, it is important to reiterate that baseline tests are needed to assess thresholds, and outer/middle and inner ear/auditory nerve function, followed by specific tests of central auditory processing. Such tests should include both speech and nonspeech stimuli, tap into different auditory processes, and be chosen on the basis of the patient's reported symptoms and other considerations, as discussed in previous paragraphs. See Volume 1 of this Handbook for in depth discussions of behavioral and electrophysiological tests of central auditory processing.

Additional Investigations

The delineation of additional assessments such as speech and language and cognitive evaluations also are beyond the scope of this chapter. (The reader is referred to Chapters 17 and 18.) This section focuses on investigations that can only be requested by a physician. These include neuroimaging, electroencephalography, or other medical (e.g., blood) investigations and will depend on the findings from the history and medical examination.

Structural neuroimaging (i.e., brain MRI) may be indicated in the following.

- In the presence of focal test findings that would be compatible with a discrete brain lesion (see Musiek & Baran, 1999), when the constellation of test findings is indicative of auditory nerve pathology, or in the presence of asymmetric hearing loss.

- In the case of other developmental disorders that can be associated with abnormal brain structure. For example, structural brain anomalies have been found in children with SLI in Broca's area, with a reduction of volume of the left posterior perisylvian region, and with a volume decrement and absence of a left asymmetry of the planum temporale (Bishop, 2000; Gauger, Lombardino, & Leonard, 1997). Ullman and Pierpont (2005) provided evidence for involvement of Broca's area within the frontal cortex, and caudate nucleus involvement within basal ganglia, and proposed that SLI can largely be explained by the abnormal development of brain structures composing a network of interconnecting structures rooted in fronto-basal-ganglia circuits. Dyslexia has been associated with increased white matter gyral abnormalities, possibly due to increased folding of the cortex in dyslexics (Casanova, El-Baz, Giedd, Rumsey, & Switala, 2010).

Patient symptoms and associated features, as well as their time course, will help decide the need for scanning when neurological pathology is suspected. Stroke is associated with a wide range of symptoms and signs that may include facial/limb weakness, dysarthrias, vision loss, headaches, and vertigo, and as illustrated in Figure 16–4 may first present to the audiology clinic. Congenital structural brain disorders associated with central auditory processing deficits also need to be considered at times. These include the syndrome of congenital aniridia due to mutations in the PAX6 gene and the bilateral perisylvian microgyrias. Autosomal dominant aniridia is due to a mutation in the PAX6 gene in 85% of cases, and associated with interhemispheric transfer central auditory processing deficits and listening difficulties, and MRI abnormalities of the corpus callosum /anterior commissure (Bamiou et al., 2004, 2007). Bilateral perisylvian polymicrogyria is a developmental brain malformation that is characterized on MRI by the presence of hypoplastic gyri around the sylvian fissure. Clinical features include pseudobulbar signs such as drooling, poor swallowing, palatal dysfunction, as well as dysarthria, epilepsy, specific language impairment, reading disabilities and central auditory processing deficits (Boscariol et al., 2010). As previously discussed, imaging may identify brain pathology in cases with previous history of prematurity (see Figure 16–2), whereas in cases with epilepsy, hippocampal sclerosis is an MRI finding that correlates with the presence of central auditory processing deficits (Han et al., 2011). Sometimes test findings are consistent with more diffuse pathology (Bamiou et al, 2007; Bamiou et al., 2000; Iliadou et al., 2008). A high clinical index of suspicion thus needs to be maintained.

Clinical Decision Making for Diagnosis

The diagnosis and subsequently the management plan will be formulated by means of an evidence-based practice approach. Such an approach will consider in equal parts the client's characteristics needs and preferences, as well as the best available scientific evidence relevant to the particular client (defined as "research findings derived from the systematic collection of data through observation and experimentation and the formulation of questions and testing of hypotheses," p. 8), and consideration of the resources, environment, and organizational context (Satterfield et al., 2009). The diagnostic process is seldom a straightforward one. Some examples to illustrate frequent diagnostic challenges include:

- The child with autism spectrum disorder (ASD). Audiology practices may not accept such referrals for CAPD assessment, as some of these children may not cooperate with even a minimal set of tests. However, these children may come to the physician's attention, as the family and other involved professionals seek a better understanding of the child's needs. Although it may not be possible to obtain any more information than a report of the child's auditory and other behaviors, it is important to understand the level of parental resolution (i.e., acceptance regarding this diagnosis). Parental emotional resolution correlates with better parenting (i.e., cognitive interaction) that is in turn associated with better long term communication skills of the child (Wachtel & Carter, 2008). Attempts to examine the presence of CAPD needs to be carefully considered: is there evidence and will it help the management plan, or is it sought to reinforce parental denial?
- The learning disabled (LD) child/ adult. Similar considerations apply as for ASD. The individual with LD

who is testable may not always show central auditpry processing deficits (e.g., Iliadou, 2011; Iliadou et al., 2009). In the presence of central auditory processing test deficits, the physician will need to decide if these are on par with the client's developmental (rather than chronological) age, or over and above, indicating the need for appropriate remediation.

- The musically trained patient with acquired CAPD. Musically trained normal subjects are reported to have better central auditory processing skills than the rest of the population (Parbery-Clark, Skoe, & Kraus, 2009); therefore, the physician needs to consider whether within or near normal, but less than excellent central auditory processing test performance constitutes an impairment or not.

- Also posing challenge is the individual with a high IQ, at any age, who reports listening difficulties, but gives excellent test results, with an exception of one or two "borderline" normal findings. The physician will need to decide whether this presentation is due to a false positive or chance effect, or whether the higher cognitive aptitudes led to the observed ceiling results. Careful consideration of what the reported listening difficulties are, if these align with reported test deficits, and whether further testing adapted to assess the patient's symptoms may be useful (e.g., Davis, Martin, Jerger, Greenwald, & Mehta, 2012).

- Testing central auditory processing in a patient with ADHD should be undertaken in that individual's medicated state. The physician, in consultation with other members of the team, need to determine whether auditory deficits are dissociated from visual ones, or if both modalities are involved, are due to a supramodal higher order deficit rather than a CAPD (Nickish & Schönweiler, 2011). See Chapter 20 of Volume 1 of this Handbook for discussion of differential diagnosis of CAPD and ADHD.

The physician will need to decide if the reported symptoms and results of the multidisciplinary evaluations suggest CAPD. The physician will also need to identify the cause of CAPD (if possible) and the need for additional medical treatment (e.g., for Lyme disease, or microvascular ischemia of the brain). Other identified conditions (e.g., depression) must also be addressed. An explanation of the diagnosis, including uncertainties and ambiguities, will need to be provided to the patient and the family, and a multidisciplinary management plan as needed and agreed upon, must be implemented. Evidence-based practice principles, teaming, and review of ongoing scientific developments are key to the success of this collaborative process.

References

AAA (American Academy of Audiology). (2010). *Diagnosis, treatment and management of children and adults with central auditory processing disorder.* Retrieved from http://www.audiology.org/resources/documentlibrary/Documents/CAPD%20Guidelines%208-2010.pdf

Alcántara, J. I., Cope, T. E., Cope, W., & Weisblatt, E. J. (2012). Auditory temporal-envelope processing in high-functioning children with autism spectrum disorder. *Neuropsychologia, 50,* 1235–1251.

Alcántara, J. I., Weisblatt, E. J. L., Moore, B. C. J., & Bolton, P. F. (2004). Speech-in-noise perception in high-functioning individuals with autism or asperger's syndrome. *Journal of Child Psychology and Psychiatry and Allied Disciplines, 45,* 1107–1114.

American Psychiatric Association. (2013). *Diagnostic and statistical manual of mental disorders* (5th ed.). Washington, DC: Author.

Aravindkumar, R., Shivashankar, N., Satishchandra, P., Sinha, S., Saini, J., & Subbakrishna, D. K. (2012). Temporal resolution deficits in patients with refractory complex partial seizures and mesial temporal sclerosis (MTS). *Epilepsy and Behavior, 24,* 126–130.

ASHA (American Speech-Language-Hearing Association). (2005). *Central auditory processing disorders.* Retrieved from http://www.asha.org/members/deskref-journals/deskref/default

Baldeweg, T., Klugman, A., Gruzelier, J. H., & Hirsch, S. R. (2002). Impairment in frontal but not temporal components of mismatch negativity in schizophrenia. *International Journal of Psychophysiology, 43,* 111–122.

Baldeweg T., Klugman A., Gruzelier J., & Hirsch S. (2004). Mismatch negativity potentials and cognitive impairment in schizophrenia. *Schizophrenia Research, 69,* 203–217.

Baltes P. B., & Lindenberger U. (1997). Emergence of a powerful connection between sensory and cognitive function across the adult life span: a new window to the study of cognitive aging? *Psychology and Aging, 12,* 12–21.

Bamiou, D. E., Liasis, A., Boyd, S., Cohen, M., & Raglan, E. (2000). Central auditory processing disorder as the presenting manifestation of subtle brain pathology. *Audiology, 39,* 168–172.

Bamiou, D., Musiek, F. E., & Luxon, L. M. (2001). Aetiology and clinical presentations of auditory processing disorders —a review. *Archives of Disease in Childhood, 85,* 361–365.

Bamiou, D. E., Musiek, F. E., Jones S., Davies, R. A., Rudge, P., Luxon, L. M. (2004). An unusual case of X-linked adrenoleukodystrophy with auditory processing difficulties as the first and sole clinical manifestation. *Journal of the American Academy of Audiology, 15,* 152–160.

Bamiou, D., Musiek, F. E., Stow, I., Stevens, J., Cipolotti, L., Brown, M. M., & Luxon, L. M. (2006). Auditory temporal processing deficits in patients with insular stroke. *Neurology, 67,* 614–619.

Bamiou, D., Werring, D., Cox, K., Stevens, J., Musiek, F. E., Brown, M. M., & Luxon, L. M. (2012). Patient-reported auditory functions after stroke of the central auditory pathway. *Stroke, 43,* 1285–1289.

Bamiou, D. E., Free, S., Sisodiya, S., Musiek, F. E., Chong, W. K., Gadian, D., Williamson, K., . . . Luxon, L. M. (2007). Auditory interhemispheric transfer deficits, hearing difficulties, and brain magnetic resonance imaging abnormalities in children with congenital aniridia due to PAX6 mutations. *Archives of Pediatrics and Adolescent Medicine, 161,* 463–469.

Bamiou, D. E., Sisodiya, S., Musiek, F. E, & Luxon, L. M. (2007). The role of the interhemispheric pathway in hearing. *Brain Research Review, 56,* 170–182.

Baran, J. A., & Musiek, F. E. (1999). Behavioral assessment of the CANS In F. E. Musiek & W. F. Rintelmann (Eds.), *Contemporary perspectives in hearing assessment.* Needham Heights, MA: Allyn & Bacon.

Bellis, T. J., & Wilber, L. A. (2001). Effects of aging and gender on interhemispheric function. *Journal of Speech, Language, and Hearing Research. 44,* 246–263.

Bellis, T. J., Chermak, G. D., Weihing, J., & Musiek, F. E. (2013). Comments on: Moore, D., Rosen, S., Bamiou, D-E., Campbell, N., & Sirimanna, T. (2013). Evolving concepts of developmental auditory processing disorder (APD): A British Society of Audiology APD Special Interest Group "white paper." *International Journal of Audiology, 52,* 3–13.

Benavidez, D. A., Fletcher, J. M., Hannay, H. J., Bland, S. T., Caudle, S. E., Mendelsohn, D. B., . . . Levin, H. S. (1999). Corpus callosum damage and interhemispheric transfer of information following closed head injury in children. *Cortex, 35*, 315–336.

Bergemalm, P., Hennerdal, S., Persson, B., Lyxell, B., & Borg, E. (2009). Perception of the acoustic environment and neuroimaging findings: A report of six cases with a history of closed head injury. *Acta Oto-Laryngologica, 129*, 801–808.

Bergemalm, P., & Lyxell, B. (2005). Appearances are deceptive? Long-term cognitive and central auditory sequelae from closed head injury. *International Journal of Audiol*ogy, *44*, 39–49.

Bishop, D. V. M. (2000). How does the brain learn language? insights from the study of children with and without language impairment. *Developmental Medicine and Child Neurology. 42*, 133–142.

Bishop, D. V. M. (2003). *The Children's Communication Checklist–second edition* (CCC-2). London, UK: Psychological Corporation.

Bishop, D. V., & McDonald, D. (2009). Identifying language impairment in children: Combining language test scores with parental report. *International Journal of Language and Communication Disorders, 44*, 600–615.

Blaettner, U., Scherg, M., & von Cramon, D. (1989). Diagnosis of unilateral telencephalic hearing disorders. Evaluation of a simple psychoacoustic pattern discrimination test. *Brain, 112*, 177–195.

Boscariol, M., Garcia, V. L., Guimarães, 0C. A., Hage, S. R. V., Montenegro, M. A., Cendes, F., & Guerreiro, M. M. (2009). Auditory processing disorders in twins with perisylvian polymicrogyria. *Arquivos De Neuro-Psiquiatria, 67*, 499–501.

Boscariol, M., Garcia, V. L., Guimarães, C. A., Montenegro, M. A., Hage, S. R., Cendes, F., & Guerreiro, M. M. (2010). Auditory processing disorder in perisylvian syndrome. *Brain Development, 32*, 299–304.

Boscariol, M., Guimarães, C. A., de Vasconcellos Hage, S. R., Garcia, V. L., Schmutzler, K. M. R., Cendes, F., & Guerreiro, M. M. (2011). Auditory processing disorder in patients with language-learning impairment and correlation with malformation of cortical development. *Brain and Development, 33*, 824–831.

BSA (British Society of Audiology). (2011). *Auditory processing disorder (APD)*. Position statement. Retrieved from http://www .thebsa.org.uk/images/stories/docs/BSA_ APD_PositionPaper_31March11_FINAL .pdf

Carroll, C. A., O'Donnell, B. F., Shekhar, A., & Hetrick W. P. (2009). Timing dysfunctions in schizophrenia span from millisecond to several-second durations. *Brain Cognition, 70*, 181–190.

Casanova, M. F., El-Baz, A. S, Giedd, J., Rumsey, J. M., & Switala, A. E. (2010). Increased white matter gyral depth in dyslexia: Implications for corticocortical connectivity. *Journal of Autism and Developmental Disorders, 40*, 21–29.

Caspary, D. M., Ling, L., Turner, J. G., & Hughes, L. F. (2008). Inhibitory neurotransmission, plasticity and aging in the mammalian central auditory system. *Journal of Experimental Biology, 211*, 1781–1791.

Chermak, G. D., & Musiek, F. E. (2011). Neurological substrate of central auditory processing deficits in children. *Current Pediatric Reviews, 7*, 241–251.

Choudhury, N., Leppanen, P. H. T., Leevers, H. J., & Benasich, A. A. (2007). Infant information processing and family history of specific language impairment: Converging evidence for RAP deficits from two paradigms. *Developmental Science, 10*, 213–236

Conners, C. K. (1996). *Conners' Rating Scales–revised (CRS-S)*. London, UK: Psychological Assessment Resources.

Cordewener, K. A. H., Bosman, A. M. T., & Verhoeven, L. (2012). Specific language impairment affects the early spelling process cess quantitatively but not qualitatively.

Research in Developmental Disabilities, 33, 1041–1047.

Cromwell, H. C., Mears, R. P., Wan L., & Boutros, N. N. (2008). Sensory gating: A translational effort from basic to clinical science. *Clinical EEG and Neuroscience, 39,* 69–72.

Cromwell, H. C., & Panksepp, J. (2011). Rethinking the cognitive revolution from a neural perspective: How overuse/misuse of the term 'cognition' and the neglect of affective controls in behavioral neuroscience could be delaying progress in understanding the BrainMind. *Neuroscience and Biobehavioral Reviews, 35,* 2026–2035.

Davids, N., Segers, E., van den Brink, D., Mitterer, H., van Balkom, H., Hagoort, P., & Verhoeven, L. (2011). The nature of auditory discrimination problems in children with specific language impairment: An MMN study. *Neuropsychologia,* 49, 19–28.

Davis, T., Martin, J., Jerger, J., Greenwald, R., & Mehta, J. (2012). Auditory-cognitive interactions underlying interaural asymmetry in an adult listener: A case study. *International Journal of Audiology, 51,* 124–134.

Dawes, P., & Bishop, D. (2009). Auditory processing disorder in relation to developmental disorders of language, communication and attention: A review and critique research report. *International Journal of Language and Communication Disorders, 44,* 440–465.

Dawes, P., & Bishop, D. V. (2010) Psychometric profile of children with auditory processing disorder and children with dyslexia. *Archives of Disease in Childhood, 95,* 432–436.

Dawes, P., Sirimanna, T., Burton, M., Vanniasegaram, I., Tweedy, F., & Bishop, D. V. M. (2009). Temporal auditory and visual motion processing of children diagnosed with auditory processing disorder and dyslexia. *Ear and Hearing, 30,* 675–686.

Dillon, H., & Cameron, S. (2013). Comments on: Moore, D., Rosen, S., Bamiou, D-E., Campbell, N., & Sirimanna, T. (2013). Evolving concepts of developmental auditory processing disorder (APD): A British Society of Audiology APD Special Interest Group "white paper." *International Journal of Audiology, 52,* 3–13.

Dillon, H., Cameron, S., Glyde, H., Wilson, W., & Tomlin, D. (2012) An opinion on the assessment of people who may have an auditory processing disorder. *Journal of the American Academy of Audiology, 23,* 97–105.

Edden, R. A. E., Muthukumaraswamy, S. D., Freeman, T. C. A., & Singh, K. D. (2009). Orientation discrimination performance is predicted by GABA concentration and gamma oscillation frequency in human primary visual cortex. *Journal of Neuroscience, 29,* 15721–15726.

Elevåg B., McCormack T., Brown G. D. A., Vousden J. I., & Goldberg T. E. (2004). Identification of tone duration, line length, and letter position: An experimental approach to timing and working memory deficits in schizophrenia. *Journal of Abnormal Psychology, 113,* 509–521.

Ferguson, M. A., Hall, R. L., Riley, A., & Moore, D. R. (2011). Communication, listening, cognitive and speech perception skills in children with auditory processing disorder (APD) or specific language impairment (SLI). *Journal of Speech, Language, and Hearing Research, 54,* 211–227.

Galaburda, A. M., Sherman, G. F., & Rosen, G. D. (1985). Developmental dyslexia: Four consecutive patients with cortical anomalies. *Annals of Neurology, 18,* 222–233.

Gates, G. A., Anderson, M. L., Feeney, M. P., McCurry, S. M., & Larson, E. B. (2008). Central auditory dysfunction in older persons with memory impairment or Alzheimer dementia. *Archives of Otolaryngology: Head and Neck Surgery, 134,* 771–777.

Gates, G. A., Beiser, A., Rees, T. S., D'Agostino, R. B., & Wolf, P. A. (2002) Central auditory dysfunction may precede the onset of clinical dementia in people with probable Alzheimer's disease. *Journal of the American Geriatrics Society, 50,* 482–488.

Gates, G., Anderson, M., McCurry, S., Feeney, P., & Larson, E. (2011). Central auditory dysfunction as a harbinger of Alzheimer dementia. *Archives of Otolaryngology: Head and Neck Surgery, 137*, 390–395.

Gates, G. A., Gibbons, L., McCurry, S., Crane, P., Feeney, M. P., & Larson, E. (2010). Executive dysfunction and presbycusis in older persons with and without dementia. *Cognitive and Behavioral Neurology, 23*, 218–223.

Gauger, L. M., Lombardino, L. J., & Leonard, C. M. (1997). Brain morphology in children with specific language impairment. *Journal of Speech, Language, and Hearing Research, 40*, 1272–1284.

Gleich, O., Hamann, I., Klump, G. M., Kittel, M., & Strutz, J. (2003). Boosting GABA improves impaired auditory temporal resolution in the gerbil. *NeuroReport, 14*, 1877–1880.

Gold, M., Rojiani, A., & Murtaugh, R. (1997). A 66-year-old woman with a rapidly progressing dementia and basal ganglia involvement. *Journal of Neuroimaging, 7*, 171–175.

Goll, J. C., Crutch, S. J., Loo, J. H., Rohrer, J. D., Frost, C., Bamiou, D.E., & Warren, J. D. (2010). Non-verbal sound processing in the primary progressive aphasias. *Brain, 133*, 272–285.

Golz, A., Westerman, S. T., Westerman, L. M., Gilbert, D. A., & Netzer, A. (2006). Does otitis media in early childhood affect reading performance in later school years? *Otolaryngology-Head and Neck Surgery, 134*, 936–939.

Gordon-Salant, S., & Fitzgibbons, P. J. (1999). Profile of auditory temporal processing in older listeners. *Journal of Speech, Language, and Hearing Research, 42*, 300–311.

Gordon-Salant, S., & Fitzgibbons, P. J. (2001). Sources of age-related recognition difficulty for time-compressed speech. *Journal of Speech, Language, and Hearing Research, 44*, 709–719.

Griffiths, T. D. (2002). Central auditory processing disorders. *Current Opinion in Neurology, 15*, 31–33.

Griffiths, T. D., Bamiou, D. E., & Warren, J. D. (2010). Pathology of the central auditory system and its treatment: Neurological aspects and clinical consequences of central lesions. In A. Palmer & A. Rees (Eds.), *OUP handbook of auditory science. The auditory brain* (Vol. 2) Oxford, UK: Oxford University Press.

Hall, J. W, Grose, J. H., Dev, M. B., Drake, A. F., & Pillsbury, H. C. (1998). The effect of otitis media with effusion on complex masking tasks in children. *Archives of Otolaryngology: Head and Neck Surgery, 124*, 892–896.

Hall, J. W. III, Grose, J. H., Dev, M. B., & Ghiassi, S. (1998). The effect of masker interaural time delay on the masking level difference in children with history of normal hearing or history of otitis media with effusion. *Ear and Hearing, 19*, 429–433.

Hammond, P. D., Gold, M. S., Wigg, N. R., & Volkmer, R. E. (1997). Preschool hearing screening: Evaluation of a parental questionnaire *Journal of Paediatrics and Child Health, 33*, 528–530.

Han, M. W., Ahn, J. H., Kang, J. K., Lee, E. M., Lee, J. H., Bae, J. H., & Chung, J. W. (2011). Central auditory processing impairment in patients with temporal lobe epilepsy. *Epilepsy and Behavior, 20*, 370–374.

Harrison, R. V., & Negandhi, J. (2012). Resting neural activity patterns in auditory brainstem and midbrain in conductive hearing loss. *Acta Oto-Laryngologica, 132*, 409–414.

Hirayasu Y., McCarley R. W., Salisbury D. F., Tanaka S., Kwon J. S., Frumin, M., . . . Shenton, M. E. (2000). Planum temporale and Heschl gyrus volume reduction in schizophrenia: A magnetic resonance imaging study of first-episode patients. *Archives of General Psychiatry, 57*, 692–699.

Humes, L. E., Dubno, J. R., Gordon-Salant, S., Lister, J. J., Cacace, A. T., Cruickshanks, K. J., . . . Wingfield, A. (2012). Central presbycusis: A review and evaluation of the evidence. *Journal of the American Academy of Audiology, 23*, 635–666.

ICD-10 (International Classification of Diseases, 10th ed.). *H93.25 Central auditory processing disorder.* Retrieved from http://www.icd10data.com/ICD10CM/Codes/H60-H95/H90-H94/H93-

Idrizbegovic, E., Hederstierna, C., Dahlquist, M., Kämpfe Nordström, C., Jelic, V., & Rosenhall, U. (2011) Central auditory function in early Alzheimer's disease and in mild cognitive impairment. *Age and Ageing, 40,* 249–254.

Iliadou, V. (2011). Auditory processing disorder. *Current Pediatric Reviews, 73,* 212–213.

Iliadou, V., Apalla, K., Kaprinis, S., Nimatoudis, I., Kaprinis, G., & Iacovides, A. (2013). Is central auditory processing disorder present in psychosis? *American Journal of Audiology.* Advance online publication. doi:10.1044/1059-0889(2013/12-0073)

Iliadou, V., & Bamiou, D. E. (2012). Psychometric evaluation of children with auditory processing disorder (APD): Comparison with normal-hearing and clinical non-APD groups. *Journal of Speech, Language, and Hearing Research, 55,* 791–799.

Iliadou, V., Bamiou, D., Kaprinis, S., Kandylis, D., Vlaikidis, N., Apalla, K., . . . St. Kaprinis, G. (2008). Auditory processing disorder and brain pathology in a preterm child with learning disabilities. *Journal of the American Academy of Audioliology, 19,* 557–563.

Iliadou, V., Bamiou, D. E., Kaprinis, S., Kandylis, D., Kaprinis, G. (2009) Auditory processing disorders in children suspected of learning disabilities—a need for screening? *International Journal of Pediatric Otorhinolaryngology, 73,* 1029–1034.

Iliadou, V., & Kaprinis, S. (2003). Clinical psychoacoustic in Alzheimer's disease central auditory processing disorders and speech deterioration. *Annals of General Psychiatry, 2*(1), 12.

Ilvonen, T., Kujala, T., Kozou, H., Kiesiläinen, A., Salonen, O., Alku, P., & Näätänen, R. (2004). The processing of speech and non-speech sounds in aphasic patients as reflected by the mismatch negativity (MMN). *Neuroscience Letters, 366,* 235–240.

Ingraham, J. L., & Aiken, C. B. (1996). An empirical approach to determining criteria for abnormality in test batteries with multiple measures. *Neuropsychology, 10,* 120–124.

Jerger, J. (2009). The concept of APD: A brief history. In A. T. Cacace & D. J. McFarland (Eds.), *Controversies in central auditory processing disorder* (pp. 1–13). San Diego, CA: Plural.

Jerger, J., & Martin, J. (2013). Comments on: Moore, D., Rosen, S., Bamiou, D-E., Campbell, N., & Sirimanna, T. (2013). Evolving concepts of developmental auditory processing disorder (APD): A British Society of Audiology APD Special Interest Group "white paper." *International Journal of Audiology, 52,* 3–13.

Johnston, K. N., John, A. B., Kreisman, N. V., Hall, J. W., & Crandell, C. C. (2009). Multiple benefits of personal FM system use by children with auditory processing disorder (APD). *International Journal of Audiology, 48,* 371–383.

Kandler, K., Clause, A., & Noh, J. (2009). Tonotopic reorganization of developing auditory brainstem circuits. *Nature Neuroscience, 12,* 711–717.

Kleindeinst, L., & Musiek, F. E. (2011). Do frequency discrimination deficits lead to specific language impairments? *Hearing Journal, 64,* 10–11.

Klingberg, T., Hedehus, M., Temple, E., Salz, T., Gabrieli, J. D., Moseley, M. E., & Poldrack, R. A. (2000). Microstructure of temporoparietal white matter as a basis for reading ability: Evidence from diffusion tensor magnetic resonance imaging *Neuron, 25,* 493–500.

Kreisman, N. V., John, A. B., Kreisman, B. M., Hall, J. W., & Crandell, C. C. (2012) Psychosocial status of children with auditory processing disorder. *Journal of the American Academy of Audiology, 3,* 222–233.

Leff, A. P., Schofield, T. M., Crinion, J. T., Seghier, M. L., Grogan, A., Green, D. W., & Price, C. J. (2009). The left superior temporal gyrus is a shared substrate for auditory short-term memory and speech comprehension: Evidence from 210 patients with stroke. *Brain, 132,* 3401–3410.

Leventhal, A. G., Wang, Y., Pu, M., Zhou, Y., & Ma, Y. (2003). GABA and its agonists improved visual cortical function in senescent monkeys. *Science, 300,* 812–815.

Levine, R. A., Gardner, J. C., Stufflebeam, S. M., Fullerton, B. C., Carlisle, E. W., Furst, . . . Kiang, N. Y. (1993). Binaural auditory processing in multiple sclerosis subjects. *Hearing Research, 68,* 59–72.

Li, C. R., Chen, M., Yang, Y., Chen, M., & Tsay, P. (2002). Altered performance of schizophrenia patients in an auditory detection and discrimination task: Exploring the "self-monitoring" model of hallucination. *Schizophrenia Research, 55,* 115–128.

Liasis, A., Bamiou, D. E., Boyd, S., & Towell, A. (2006). Evidence for a neurophysiologic auditory deficit in children with benign epilepsy with centro-temporal spikes. *Journal of Neural Transmission, 113,* 939–949.

Loo, J. H, Bamiou, D. E., & Rosen, S. (2012). The impacts of language background and language-related disorders in auditory processing assessment. *Journal of Speech, Language, and Hearing Research, 56,* 1–12.

Lord, C., Rutter, M., & Couteur, A. L. (1994). Autism diagnostic interview-revised: A revised version of a diagnostic interview for caregivers of individuals with possible pervasive developmental disorders. *Journal of Autism and Developmental Disorders, 24,* 659–685.

McKay, C. M., Headlam, D. M., & Copolov, D. L. (2000). Central auditory processing in patients with auditory hallucinations. *American Journal of Psychiatry, 157,* 759–766.

Meister, H., Von Wedel, H., & Walger, M. (2004). Psychometric evaluation of children with suspected auditory processing disorders (APDs) using a parent-answered survey. *International Journal of Audiology, 43,* 431–437.

Moore, D. R., Hartley, D. E. H., & Hogan, S. C. M. (2003). Effects of otitis media with effusion (OME) on central auditory function. *International Journal of Pediatric Otorhinolaryngology, 67*(Suppl. 1), S63–S67.

Moore, D. R., Rosen, S., Bamiou, D. E., Campbell, N. G., & Sirimanna, T. (2013). Evolving concepts of developmental auditory processing disorder (APD): A British Society of Audiology APD Special Interest Group "white paper." *International Journal of Audiology, 52,* 3–13.

Naatanen, R., & Kahkonen, S. (2009). Central auditory dysfunction in schizophrenia as revealed by the mismatch negativity (MMN) and its magnetic equivalent MMNm: a review. *International Journal of Neuropsychopharmacology, 12,* 125–135.

Näätänen, R., Kujala, T., Kreegipuu, K., Carlson, S., Escera, C., Baldeweg, T., & Ponton, C. (2011). The mismatch negativity: An index of cognitive decline in neuropsychiatric and neurological diseases and in ageing. *Brain, 134,* 3432–3450.

Neijenhuis, K. A. M., Stollman, M. H. P., Snik, A. F. M., & Van Den Broek, P. (2001). Development of a central auditory test battery for adults. *Audiology, 40,* 69–77

Ngan, E. T. C., Vouloumanos, A., Cairo, T. A., Laurens, K. R., Bates A. T., Anderson, C. M., . . . Little, P. F. (2003). Abnormal processing of speech during oddball target detection in schizophrenia. *NeuroImage, 20,* 889–897.

Nickisch, A., Gross, M., Schönweiler, R., Uttenweiler, V., Am Zehnhoff-Dinnesen, A., Berger, R., Radu, H. J., & Ptok, M. (2007). Auditory processing disorders: Consensus statement by the German Society for Phoniatry and Paedaudiology. *HNO, 55,* 61–72.

Nickisch, A., & Schönweiler, R. (2011). Auditory processing disorders—differential diagnosis: Guidelines of the German Society for Phoniatry and Pedaudiology. *HNO, 59,* 380–384.

Nosarti, C., Rushe, T. M., Woodruff, P. W. R., Stewart, A. L., Rifkin, L., & Murray, R. M. (2004). Corpus callosum size and very preterm birth: Relationship to neuropsychological outcome. *Brain, 127,* 2080–2089.

Oades, R. D., Wild-Wall, N., Juran, S. A., Sachsse, J., Oknina, L. B., & Ropcke, B.

J. (2006). Auditory change detection in schizophrenia: Sources of activity, related neuropsychological function and symptoms in patients with a first episode in adolescence, and patients 14 years after an adolescent illness-onset. *BMC Psychiatry, 6.*

O'Connor, K. (2012). Auditory processing in autism spectrum disorder: A review. *Neuroscience and Biobehavioral Reviews, 36,* 836–854.

Parbery-Clark, A., Skoe, E., & Kraus, N. (2009). Musical experience limits the degradative effects of background noise on the neural processing of sound. *Journal of Neuroscience, 29,* 14100–14107.

Penn, C., Wtermeyer J., & Schie, K. (2009). Auditory disorders in a South African paediatric TBI population: Some preliminary data. *International Journal of Audiology, 48,* 135–143.

Pichora-Fuller, M. K. (2003). Cognitive aging and auditory information processing. *International Journal of Audiology, 42*(Suppl. 2), 2S26–2S32.

Rabinowicz, E. F., Silipo, G., Goldman, R., & Javitt, D. C. (2000). Auditory sensory dysfunction in schizophrenia: Imprecision or distractibility? *Archives of General Psychiatry, 57,* 1149–1155.

Reite, M., Teale, P., Rojas, D. C., Asherin, R., & Hernandez, O. (2009). MEG auditory evoked fields suggest altered structural/functional asymmetry in primary but not secondary auditory cortex in bipolar disorder. *Bipolar Disorders, 11,* 371–381.

Riccio, C. A., Hynd, G. W., Cohen, M. J., Hall, J., & Molt, L. (1994). Comorbidity of central auditory processing disorder and attention-deficit hyperactivity disorder. *Journal of the American Academy of Child and Adolesccent Psychiatry, 33,* 849–857.

Roine, R. O., Kaste, M., & Naatanen, R. (2003). Auditory discrimination after left hemisphere stroke: An MMN follow-up study. *Stroke, 34,* 1746–1753.

Sanes, D. H., & Woolley, S. M. N. (2011). A behavioral framework to guide research on central auditory development and plasticity. *Neuron, 72,* 912–929.

Santhouse, A. M., Ffytche, D. H., Howard, R. J., Williams, S. C. R., Stewart, A. L., Rooney, M., . . . Murray, R. M. (2002). The functional significance of perinatal corpus callosum damage: An fMRI study in young adults. *Brain, 125,* 1782–1792.

Satterfield, J. M., Spring, B., Brownson, R. C., Mullen, E. J., Newhouse, R. P., Walker, B. B., & Whitlock, E. P. (2009). Toward a transdisciplinary model of evidence-based practice. *Milbank Quarterly, 87,* 368–390.

Schönweiler, R., Nickisch, A., & Am Zehnhoff-Dinnesen, A. (2012). Auditory processing and perception disorders: Proposed treatment and management: Guidelines of the German Society for Phoniatry and Pedaudiology. *HNO, 60,* 359–368.

Setzen, G., Cacace, A. T., Eames, F., Riback, P., Lava, N., McFarland, D. J., . . . Kerwood, J. A. (1999). Central deafness in a young child with moyamoya disease: Paternal linkage in a caucasian family: Two case reports and a review of the literature. *International Journal of Pediatric Otorhinolaryngology, 48,* 53–76.

Sharma, M., Purdy, S., & Kelly, A. S. (2009). Co-morbidity of auditory processing, language, and reading disorders. *Journal of Speech, Language, and Hearing Research, 52,* 706–722.

Sharma, A., Purdy, S. C., Newall, P., Wheldall, K., Beaman, R., & Dillon, H. (2006). Electrophysiological and behavioral evidence of auditory processing deficits in children with reading disorder. *Clinical Neurophysiology, 17,* 1130–1144.

Shenton, M. E., Dickey, C. C., Frumin, M., & McCarley, R. W. (2001). A review of MRI findings in schizophrenia. *Schizophrenia Research, 49,* 1–52.

Silman, S., Silverman, C. A., & Emmer, M. B. (2000). Central auditory processing disorders and reduced motivation: three case studies. *Journal of the American Academy of Audiology, 11,* 57–63

Skoe, E., & Kraus, N. (2010). Hearing it again and again: on-line subcortical plasticity in humans. *PLoS One, 5,* e13645.

Smith, A. B., Kavros, P. M., Clarke, T., Dorta, N. J., Tremont, G., & Pal, D. K. (2012). A neurocognitive endophenotype associated with rolandic epilepsy. *Epilepsia, 53,* 705–711

Smoski, W. J., Brunt, M. A., & Tannahill, J. C. (1992). Listening characteristics of children with central auditory processing disorders. *Language, Speech, and Hearing Services in Schools, 23,* 145–152.

Spyridakou, C., Luxon, L. M., & Bamiou, D. E. (2012). Patient-reported speech in noise difficulties and hyperacusis symptoms and correlation with test results. *Laryngoscope, 122,* 1609–1614.

Stevens, W. D., Hasher, L., Chiew, K. S., & Grady, C. L. (2008) A neural mechanism underlying memory failure in older adults. *Journal of Neuroscience, 28,* 12820–12824.

Takei, Y., Kumano, S., Maki, Y., Hattori, S., Kawakubo, Y., Kasai, K., . . . Mikuni, M. (2010). Preattentive dysfunction in bipolar disorder: a MEG study using mismatch negativity. *Progress in Neuropsychopharmacology and Biological Psychiatry, 34,* 903–912.

Takesian, A. E., Kotak, V. C., & Sanes, D. H. (2012). Age-dependent effect of hearing loss on cortical inhibitory synapse function. *Journal of Neurophysiology, 107,* 937–947.

Talcott, J. B., Witton, C., Hebb, G. S., Stoodley, C. J., Westwood, E. A., France, S. J., . . . Stein, J. F. (2002). On the relationship between dynamic visual and auditory processing and literacy skills; results from a large primary-school study. *Dyslexia, 8,* 204–225.

Temple, E. (2002). Brain mechanisms in normal and dyslexic readers. *Current Opinion in Neurobiology, 12*(2), 178–183.

Tobias, J. V., Bilger, R. C., Brody, H., Gates, G. A., Haskell, G., Howard, D., . . . Pickett, J. A. (1988). Speech understanding and aging. *Journal of the Acoustical Society of America, 83,* 859–895.

Tononi, G., & Edelman, G. M. (2000). Schizophrenia and the mechanisms of conscious integration. *Brain Research Reviews, 31,* 391–400.

Turetsky, B. I., Bilker, W. B., Siegel, S. J., Kohler, C. G. & Gur, R. E. (2009). Profile of auditory information-processing deficits in schizophrenia. *Psychiatry Research, 165,* 27–37.

Ullman, M. T., & Pierpont, E. I. (2005). Specific language impairment is not specific to language: The procedural deficit hypothesis. *Cortex. 41,* 399–433.

Veuillet, E., Bouilhol, C., & Thai-Van, H. (2011). Co-morbidity of APD and reading disabilities. *Current Pediatric Reviews, 7,* 227–240.

Wachtel, K., & Carter, A. S. (2008). Reaction to diagnosis and parenting styles among mothers of young children with ASDs. *Autism, 12,* 575–594.

Whitton, J. P., & Polley, D. B. (2011). Evaluating the perceptual and pathophysiological consequences of auditory deprivation in early postnatal life: A comparison of basic and clinical studies. *Journal of the Association for Research in Otolaryngology, 12,* 535–546.

Wilson, W. J., & Arnott, W. (2012). Using different criteria to diagnose CAPD: How big a difference does it make? *Journal of Speech, Language, and Hearing Research, 56,* 63–70.

Wong, P. C., Jin, J. X., Gunasekera, G. M., Abel, R., Lee, E. R., & Dhar, S. (2009). Aging and cortical mechanisms of speech perception in noise. *Neuropsychologia. 47,* 693–703.

Ziegler, J. C., Pech-Georgel, C., George, F., & Lorenzi, C. (2009). Speech-perception-in-noise deficits in dyslexia. *Developmental Science, 12,* 732–745.

Ziegler, J. C., Pech-Georgel, C., George, F., & Lorenzi, C. (2011). Noise on, voicing off: Speech perception deficits in children with specific language impairment. *Journal of Experimental Child Psychology, 110,* 362–372.

CHAPTER 17

COGNITIVE-COMMUNICATIVE AND LANGUAGE FACTORS ASSOCIATED WITH CENTRAL AUDITORY PROCESSING DISORDER

A Speech-Language Pathology Perspective on Assessment and Intervention

DONNA GEFFNER and DEBORAH ROSS-SWAIN

Introduction

Central auditory processing involves many processes that are mediated at different levels of the CANS. Individuals may present with some of the behaviors attributed to central auditory processing disorder (CAPD), which may also include behaviors that overlap with it, specifically those that are associated with other cognitive, linguistic or behavioral disorders (AAA, 2010). Presenting with some of these behaviors would not necessarily indicate that the individual has a CAPD, since many of these symptoms can be attributed to other conditions or disorders, or may coexist with CAPD. CAPD can affect listening, communication, social skills, and academic performance. Given the extensive neurological systems involved in processing information that produce complex behaviors, it is understandable that there would be comorbidity across disorders. It then behooves the audiologist and speech-language pathologist to closely examine the various disorders that can co-occur or be influenced by CAPD and to understand the linkages between brain organization and its dysfunction that result in auditory deficits (AAA, 2010). See Chapter 1 for discussion of comorbidity and brain organization.

There is general consensus among professionals that CAPD can occur with other comorbid conditions that can mirror CAPD. Such *look-alike* disorders include attention deficit/hyperactivity disorder (ADHD), learning disabilities (LD), reading disorders, speech and language disorders, and hearing loss (Emanual, Ficca, & Korzak, 2011). Some children with auditory neuropathy (AN), in particular, tend to demonstrate similar characteristics to those seen in CAPD, thus confounding the process of a differential diagnosis (Rance, 2013). Furthermore, any definitive diagnosis requires a team of experts who, at times, "see different parts of the elephants" (Richard, 2012). Had there been a national consensus defining CAPD, and a respective diagnostic protocol in delineating such, the task would be easier. However, establishing consensus is not an easy task and thus arriving at a given protocol is not always possible, given the myriad of symptoms and overlapping behaviors. It is often these co-occurring conditions that merit the referral of the child for CAPD testing. Clinically, most cases of CAPD will be associated with abnormalities of language, literacy, attention or social skills behaviors. If we conclude that CAPD occurs only in a pure form, then there would not be the other comorbidities to confound it. The fact remains that comorbidity does exist. However, this understanding does not preclude the need to know the primary cause of the child's problem. Is the disorder of CAPD a secondary consequence of ADHD or LD that leads to the other comorbid deficits? Or do these disorders arise from CAPD? In the case of ADHD where the child is unable to focus, he or she will not be able to attend to auditory stimuli, thus leading to poor performance on measures of auditory processing. Likewise, if the problem is CAPD, then the child's ability to pay attention to auditory information wanes when it is too difficult for him or her to process it. Similarly, if a child is experiencing a language impairment and poor auditory/sound discrimination, is the poor auditory discrimination a cause or a consequence of the language

impairment? Careful and thorough multidisciplinary assessment should help to establish causality and should lead to resolution of these questions.

Jerger and Musiek (2000) noted that CAPD may coexist with other disorders, but they do not suggest that the association is necessarily one of simple causation. They indicated that CAPD should be seen as a "discrete entity apart from other childhood problems (Jerger & Musiek, 2002, p. 19). The American Speech-Language Hearing Association (ASHA) Task Force (2005a) stated that CAPD is a deficit in the neural processing of auditory stimuli that may coexist with, but is not the result of, dysfunction in the other modalities (ASHA, p. 3). However, Katz et al. (2002) disagreed, suggesting that CAPD may cause speech and language impairment, dyslexia and ADHD. Cacace and McFarland (2005) argued that associating language and learning problems with deficits in auditory processing cannot be determined because almost all of the research employed acoustic stimuli and not language stimuli. Given the fact that CAPD and LD are both complex and heterogeneous, a simple correspondence between deficits in fundamental auditory processes and language, learning and related sequelae may be nearly impossible to demonstrate (ASHA, 2005a, pp. 3–4). Furthermore, in basic cognitive neuroscience, it is generally understood that there are few entirely compartmentalized areas in the brain that are responsible for a single sensory modality (ASHA, 2005a, p. 3). Other researchers have linked auditory processing with weaknesses in phonological processing—namely, temporal processing or the perception of rapid changes in acoustic information (Tallal & Piercy, 1973), although a functional relationship has yet to be established between auditory perceptual deficits and phonological processing deficits (Troia, 2003). Troia (2003) indicated that the differences between the two are part of a broader pansensory disorder and advocates for "a better grasp of nature of temporal processing and its relationship with cognitive and linguistic skills required for literacy achievement" (p. 32).

According to the British Society of Audiology (BSA, 2005), CAPD is a disorder affecting auditory processing that may co-occur with other cognitive and perceptual impairments. The BSA noted that the same child may be diagnosed with specific language impairment (SLI) by a speech-language pathologist, or diagnosed with CAPD, if tested by an audiologist. Therefore, a child might receive two different diagnoses rather than a diagnosis of one overarching disorder with co-occurring deficits.

According to the ASHA Task Force (2005a), children of school age with CAPD can have difficulties with learning, speech, and language, which include written language, reading and spelling, as well as deficits in social skills and related functions. Furthermore, the impact of the auditory deficit may be different across individuals due to a number of factors, some of which are pansensory, including neuromaturation, presence of a brain injury or neurological disorder, or specific dysfunction of the central nervous system (CNS). Social and environmental factors may play a role as well. Given the variety of factors involved and the pansensory nature of many of these factors (i.e., attention, memory, and language), as well as the multisensory, neural interfacing and integrated processing of sensory data and other information, it is often difficult to establish a direct relationship or a predictive occurrence between CAPD

and other coexisting disorders (ASHA, 2005a). Given the complexity of CAPD, its manifestation across individuals, and the complexity of learning and reading disorders, the nature of the relationship among deficits of central auditory processes and language, learning and related disorders can be difficult to establish. It is important, therefore, to undertake comprehensive assessment to determine the presence of other disorders in an individual diagnosed with CAPD and the impact of such co-occurring disorders for intervention planning and implementation. In particular, it is essential to determine the speech-language-cognitive-communicative behaviors in children and adults with CAPD using appropriate assessment instruments.

The authors of this chapter bring a unique perspective from the point of view of a speech-language pathologist (Deborah Ross-Swain, CCC-SLP) and an audiologist who is also a speech-language pathologist (Donna Geffner, CCC-SP/A). From the combined years of practice, we have observed a common set of language and communicative characteristics that manifest in populations with CAPD. We acknowledge the intricate and interconnected, linguistic and higher cognitive processes involved in processing auditory information. Thus, we also ascribe to the concept that CAPD is not a unimodal function, but rather one that involves several levels of processing within the brain. The framework for processing is so intricate that it involves highly complex synchronization and synthesis of auditory, cognitive and linguistic mechanisms. As Medwesky (2006) noted, spoken language processing involves the concurrent engagement of central auditory processing, cognition, and language mechanisms. This framework leads to a corollary—that trying to crowd too many children with a wide diversity of issues under the same umbrella for some *standard* assessment and treatment can be ineffective. According to Medwetsky (2011), application of any intervention without careful delineation of the sub-populations will result in nonsignificant group effects and thus misrepresent outcomes or benefits of intervention.

In summary, it is known that processing input through the auditory modality engages and is dependent upon other systems within the CNS and includes attention, language, and cognition. There are convergent sensory *tracks*, multisensory neurons and neural interfacing that create the interdependent processing of sensory data (ASHA, 2005a, p. 3). This chapter will describe these systems and their impact and influence on CAPD.

Interaction Among Cognition, Social Skills, and CAPD

Cognition is the general concept of taking in all the modes of knowing, such as perceiving, remembering, imagining, conceiving, judging and reasoning, in the process of knowing (Nicolosi, Harryman, & Kresheck, 2004, p. 74). It involves the ability to understand concepts that include language and the use of language for learning purposes. Utilizing contextual cues and other supports to derive meaning requires an ability to cognitively conceptualize the information, both a *thinking skill* and a measure of intelligence. The individual's mental age and cognitive status (e.g., IQ) can influence that individual's ability to perform complex auditory tasks, making it difficult to

interpret results. In some cases, results may be invalid due to the individual's lack of understanding of the task. In other cases, the cause might be inability to perform the task because of its complexity. Accordingly, it is recommended that a multidisciplinary team partake in the assessment (AAA, 2010). It is recommended that if there is suspected, significant impairment in cognition and that information regarding cognitive/intellectual ability is not available, then a referral to another professional is warranted prior to central auditory testing (AAA, 2010). Given the attention demands needed to complete any behavioral test, as well as some degree of memory and even the minimal language used in central auditory processing evaluations, individuals with reduced cognitive ability may have limited capacity to perform reliably or to their maximum potential on the central auditory test battery, especially if these other deficits are not identified prior to the central auditory evaluation.

Rosen, Cohen, and Vanniasegaram (2010) examined both auditory and cognitive abilities in a group of children *suspected* of having CAPD. They administered a battery of auditory and cognitive tests to 20 children who were reported to have listening problems despite having normal hearing, as well as to a group of 28 matched controls. Of the children suspected of having CAPD, two-thirds showed performance deficits on at least one auditory task. The remaining third, did not display any deficit on any test. All children in the suspected CAPD group performed consistently more poorly on cognitive tasks than the typically developing children; however, no relationship was seen between cognitive test scores and the degree of suspected CAPD. The authors noted that there was no improvement in cognitive scores upon remediation of the auditory skills, which might be expected given the focus of auditory training to improve auditory skills. We would add that it is not clear whether these participants actually presented with CAPD or some other look alike disorder, given their status as *suspected* of CAPD rather than having been diagnosed with CAPD.

In an attempt to investigate the prevalence of cognitive impairment in a population of children suspected of having CAPD, Ferguson, Hall, Riley, and Moore (2011) administered tests of verbal and nonverbal IQ, including digit span to three groups of children: those with the suspected CAPD diagnosis (based on symptoms frequently associated with CAPD as reported by the children's parents), those with an SLI diagnosis, and mainstream school children. Nonsense word repetition, reading sentences and one syllable nonword repetition revealed no significant difference in performance between the children with CAPD and those with SLI. Both of these groups scored consistently lower than the mainstream school children in the areas of cognitive skills, literacy, and language skills. Since the behaviors exhibited by the suspected CAPD and SLI group were so similar, the researchers indicated that the differential diagnosis was based on the children's route of referral rather than on real measurable differences. When Ferguson et al. (2011) compared intelligence, language, literacy, phonology, memory, and speech intelligibility test results with parental reports of listening, behavioral and communication in children suspected of CAPD or SLI, they found that there was no significant difference between the two groups on the majority of measures, further confirming

the researchers' perspective on the co-occurrence of language, communication, and cognitive skill deficits in the CAPD population. Although the authors suggest that CAPD and SLI cannot only co-occur, but that they may be virtually indistinguishable, the current authors must again note the absence of a firm diagnosis in the children purportedly presenting with CAPD: these children were "identified" based on parental reports of basic symptoms typical of CAPD. In this case, it was based on symptoms acceptable in the United Kingdom, which is known to have a wide disparity in approaches to the diagnosis of CAPD. Ferguson et al. (2011) also cited other disorders with overlapping symptoms such as those found in inattentiveness, distractibility, language difficulties, reading difficulties, and autism spectrum disorder (ASD).

The relationship between audition and cognition is not entirely clear. Beck and Clark (2009) noted that the relationship between audition and cognition is interdependent and symbiotic and stated that as cognition declines, audition becomes more important, whereas as audition declines, cognition becomes more important. Clearly, cognitive-communicative and language deficits co-occurring in a child with CAPD can impact that child's social skills. A child's slower processing rate, the need for repetition of simple questions, and trouble following complex directions prevent him or her from keeping up with peers. Even responding to a quip or sarcastic remark may be too difficult a task for such a child. The child may not be able to pick up on nuances, sarcasm, or understand puns. As a result of these difficulties, the child may feel removed from classmates and same-age peers and resort to playing with younger children.

A study of the social well-being of children with CAPD was conducted by Kreisman, John, Kreisman, Hall, and Crandell (2012). They investigated a group of children with CAPD and an age-matched control group of children with no history of hearing problems. Data collected from primary caretakers, and the children themselves, revealed that children in the CAPD group presented more significant emotional problems. Parents of these children reported a higher incidence of psychosocial difficulties than reported by parents of children in the control group. Their findings indicate that children with CAPD experience more emotional and social problems than their typically developing peers.

Communicative Factors

It is generally accepted that an individual child must have adequate receptive and expressive language skills to perform on verbal tests of central auditory processing (AAA, 2010). However, many of the youngsters (and some adults) being tested for CAPD also present with language disorders. It is important to consider the level of language function of the child being tested, since many of the central auditory tests involve verbal directions, use verbal stimuli, and require a verbal response. If verbal central auditory tests are employed, it requires a skilled audiologist to tease out the impact of a language disorder on central auditory test measures. The presence of language and/or communication difficulties should be known to the audiologist prior to assessing the individual's central auditory processing.

Comorbidity of Literacy Issues, Language Disorders, and CAPD

There is a high prevalence of language and reading difficulties (and dyslexia) among children with CAPD (Chermak & Musiek, 1997; Giraud & Ramus, in press; Tallal, 2004). Some researchers have even suggested that auditory processing deficits are pansensory and underlie language and reading difficulties (Stein, 2001). Boscariol, Guimaraes, Hage, Cendes, and Guerrieiro (2010) produced evidence of an anatomical correlate with dyslexia and cortical malformation in the perisylvian polymicrogyria. They concluded that children with developmental dyslexia may present with temporal auditory processing disorders with underlying cortical malformations as a substrate of these disorders. In some other cases, the relationship is not exact but rather reflective of different etiologies of the language impairment and therefore not causally related. Early onset central auditory processing deficits may affect how phonological representations are established, leaving a lasting impairment even when the auditory deficits lessen with age. This is one reason that it has been suggested that electrophysiological measures of central auditory processing, such as those proposed by Kraus and Nicol (2005), are incorporated to help establish the presence of CAPD as early as possible in these populations. The interdependence of language, cognition, and auditory processing and the frequent comorbidity of language impairment, attention and memory deficits, and CAPD, led Chermak et al. (2007) to suggest the use of broadly based interventions including bottom-up and top-down strategies in intervention for CAPD. Many of the latter strategies are reviewed in this chapter.

Some audiologists and reading specialists suggest that the ability to process phonemes and develop phonological awareness skills is an auditory ability. However, language specialists would argue that it is the phonology of language that contributes to the ability to process phonemes and develop phonemic awareness skills. For many, including the authors of this chapter, phonological awareness is considered an auditory skill. In fact, the British Association of Audiology has included phonological awareness in their definition and interpretation of CAPD. Many studies have attempted to find the linkage between audition of phonemes and ultimate reading decoding ability. Investigators have proposed temporal processing as the mediating factor (Debonnis & Moncrieff, 2008). They argue that temporal processing of rapid changes in acoustic information is the underlying impairment of children with weak phonological processing skills and reading deficits.

Phonemic awareness, a major component of phonological awareness, is the ability to isolate and manipulate sounds and is a key factor in learning to read. Sharma et al. (2006) investigated the comorbidity of auditory processing deficits in children with reading disorders, using a battery of behavioral tests along with an electrophysiological measure (the mismatch negativity potential or MMN). They reported a significant co-occurrence, citing a combination of deficits on frequency patterns (Frequency Pattern Test), and absent or small /ga/-evoked MMN. The reading disordered group performed more poorly than con-trols for most tests in the reading and central auditory processing test battery. All children with reading disorders failed at least one behavioral test of auditory processing and that group had significantly smaller /ga/-evoked MMN than the control group. Sharma, Purdy, and Kelly (2009) found that nearly half of the children diagnosed with CAPD had reading and/or language disorders. Because of the significant linkage among the three disorders, the authors stressed the importance of assessing language before making a diagnosis of CAPD. Sharma et al. (2009) concluded that of the children tested, 72% presented with CAPD. More children presented CAPD with a comorbid reading disorder or a language impairment than CAPD, reading disorder or language impairment alone: nearly half of the children (47%) had problems in all three areas and only a small percentage had problems in only one area. Only 4% of the children studied presented CAPD alone. The authors concluded that language impairment and reading disorders commonly co-occur with CAPD. Although attention and memory are linked to the performance on some auditory performance tasks, it only explained a small of amount of the variance found in the auditory scores. In fact, in a few children, attention deficits occurred in the absence of auditory, reading and language deficits, suggesting that at least attention deficits of a certain severity is needed to demonstrate any underlying link between central auditory processing, reading and language impairment. The authors suggested that perhaps the link is perceptual learning as Moore, Amitay, and Hawkey (2003) suggested.

Kleindienst and Musiek (2011) reviewed five studies looking at the relationship of frequency discrimination in children with SLI. These studies (Davids et al. 2010; Hill, Hogben, & Bishop, 2005; Mengler, Hogben, Michie, & Bishop, 2005; McArthur & Bishop, 2004; Nickisch & Massinger, 2009) incorporated behavioral and electrophysiological measures and revealed findings that suggested significant deficits in frequency discrimination in children with SLI. The results of these studies support the hypothesis of a probable auditory component present in youngsters with SLI, with deficits in frequency discrimination as a possible early indicator of a language impairment. Further, mean frequency discrimination thresholds differed in children from that obtained by children with average language development, with differences increasing as the children aged. Davids et al.'s (2010) study demonstrated that children with SLI do not show a MMN to linguistic or nonlinguistic contrasts, further supporting the hypothesis that frequency discrimination difficulties could be related to nonspeech processing problems. Such findings as in these five studies have great potential in the treatment for children with SLI.

Literacy and CAPD

It is well understood that when children struggle to read in the primary grades, they will more likely continue to manifest reading problems as they progress through their school careers (Astrom, Wadsworth, & DeFries, 2007). One of the important findings in the last several years is the relationship between reading skill, phonological awareness (i.e., the understanding of the structure of language and the syllables and phonemes that form words [Catts, 1991]) and early

reading ability. Early phonological awareness of syllable and rhyme emerges as part of natural language acquisition processes (Ziegler & Goswami, 2005). This skill in turn predicts how rapidly children will acquire letter sound units or phonemic awareness as letters are taught (Ziegler & Goswami, 2005). Such ability to acquire this letter knowledge has been found to account for 40% to 60% of the variance in kindergartner's subsequent reading achievement (Scanlon & Vellutino, 1996). In their study of 88 children between the ages of 3 and 6 years old, Corriveau, Goswami, and Thomson (2010) administered a battery of psychometric tests including phonological awareness measures, intelligence, verbal knowledge, receptive language, riddles, and early reading ability to young children. Psychoacoustic tasks including an amplitude rise-time discrimination task, and intensity discrimination, and a sweep frequency discrimination task also were administered. Results from both cross-sectional and longitudinal analysis suggested that early auditory rise time sensitivity in developing phonological awareness also is important in the development of rhyme awareness. Corriveau et al.'s hypothesis that central auditory processing skills, especially those that focus on sensitivity to the speech envelope, are highly correlated with reading precursor skills in children between the ages of 3 and 6 years. Performance on the rise time discrimination task was strongly associated with rhyme awareness and with initial phoneme detection and identification of sound. Sweep frequency discrimination and intensity discrimination correlated with rhyme awareness. The strongest relationships were between both rise time and frequency discrimination and rhyme awareness. They concluded that "[t]hus auditory processing influences reading acquisition through its effects on a children's ability to extract phonological information from the speech stream" (Corriveau et al., 2010, p. 380).

The findings of Corriveau et al. (2010) are similar to other studies that also reported associations between basic central auditory processing abilitiy (e.g., rise time) and other measures of early literacy. For example, Boets, Wouters, Wieringen, De Smedt, and Ghesquire (2008) found that phonological awareness was a unique predictor of reading and spelling abilities. Similarly, Miller and Wagstaff (2011) found no group mean differences on any of the 18 behavioral variables examined between children who received a diagnosis of CAPD from an audiologist and children who received services for language impairments but did not have a CAPD diagnosis. There was no difference on tasks that measured auditory processing, grammar and vocabulary, reading fluency, verbal and nonverbal working memory, motor speech, and attention functions as reported by parents. When laboratory testing was used to establish those children affected or unaffected with SLI and CAPD, the multivariate test produced four group mean differences for the SLI/not SLI comparison and two group mean differences for the CAPD/not CAPD comparison. On average, the children who met the test-based criterion for APD had lower scores on cube design and reading fluency than did children who did not meet the criterion. For children who met the test-based criterion of SLI had poor performance on nonword repetitions, spatial working memory and two auditory processing tests than did children who did not meet the criterion. The performance of children affected with SLI differed significantly from those unaffected with SLI on the four variables used to classify SLI, as well as in nonword repetition, Dichotic Digits Left, the SSW test, and Spatial Working Memory. The authors implied that different sets of variables distinguish the affected and unaffected groups for SLI and CAPD, but such group differences are not straightforward (p. 14). Nevertheless, the behavioral patterns of children with CAPD and SLI were similar. Of the 75% of the sample identified with CAPD, 31% were also affected by SLI, evidence that CAPD is seen in a population of dyslexics and SLI.

As one reviews these studies, it becomes clear that central auditory processing, which may not be a direct predictor of a reading impairment, but it may be an important precursor to decoding and phonological awareness, both early reading skills. Having the ability to predict early precursors of reading ability or those at risk for reading failure also is of value in developing early intervention programs. For example, Thomson, Cheah, and Goswami (2012) found that a six-week intervention program targeted towards improving rise time discrimination led to improved rhyming skills in normal children. Because rhyming skill ability has been demonstrated to predict reading ability (Thomson et al., 2012), it was expected that the group of children who had received the rise time discrimination training also would demonstrate improved reading ability and such training would be more effective at the pre-school level when pre-reading skills are emerging. In their study comparing the efficacy of two auditory processing interventions for developmental dyslexia based on rhythm and phonetic training in a six-week program, Thomson, Leong, and Goswami (2012) found that both rhythmic intervention and phonemic intervention led to significant gains on phonological awareness with medium- to large-effect sizes on literacy outcome measures. Although gains were non-significant when compared to the controls, the data suggest that rhythmic training plays an important role in developing phonological skills critical for literacy acquisition. Further, the authors suggested that combining both prosodic-rhythmic and phonemic cues in auditory training programs may be advantageous for children with developmental dyslexia.

Billiet and Bellis (2011) reported that about 30% of children with language-based learning problems present abnormal brainstem timing and difficulty with linguistic labeling on nonverbal acoustic contours. They compared performance of children with dyslexia with and without abnormal brainstem timing (in response to simple speech stimuli) and a control group of children with no history of learning or related disorders on behavioral tests of central auditory function. They reported that all children with dyslexia with normal brainstem timing met criteria for CAPD diagnosis on the basis of the behavioral tests; however, very few of the children with dyslexia with abnormal brainstem timing met criteria for CAPD diagnosis. They explained that it is possible that the behavioral measures reflected different processes, mechanisms, and regions of the CANS; therefore, some children with dyslexia might exhibit abnormal brainstem transcription of speech stimuli whereas others may exhibit deficits at the cortical level in processes that are not necessarily reliant on precise brainstem timing (e.g., binaural integration, binaural separation, auditory closure, temporal patterning).

They concluded that central auditory assessment is crucial for children with dyslexia, and emphasized the importance of both behavioral and electrophysiological approaches.

Language and CAPD

It is generally understood that children with CAPD present deficits in understanding speech in the presence of background or competing noise, or in otherwise poor acoustic environments (e.g., reverberant). In addition, they present related deficits including, misunderstanding messages; responding inappropriately; needing frequent repetition; having delayed response to others; having difficulty following auditory directions; localizing sounds; exhibiting poor musical ability; and having associated spelling, learning and reading problems (ASHA, 2005a). (See Chapter 4 for discussion of room acoustics.)

Since the early 1970s, considerable evidence has accumulated to suggest a causal link between central auditory processing deficits and SLI (Tallal & Piercy, 1973). Studies investigating neuropathologies in developmental dysphasia identified structural abnormalities of the auditory cortex, suggesting that a central auditory processing deficit may be a crucial component of a language impairment (Tallal, Miller, & Fitch, 1993). Witton's work (2010) supports the accumulating evidence that CAPD is over-represented in populations with dyslexia and SLI. The issue raised is whether the comorbidity is causal or associative. CAPD also is seen in a sample of children diagnosed with non-verbal learning disability (Keller, Tillery, & McFadden, 2006). Sixty-one percent of their population met the diagnostic criteria for CAPD. Dawes, Bishop, Sirimanna, and Damiou (2008) also reported this same trend in their population of children with autism.

Cortical malformations in auditory regions of the brain have been described in children with CAPD and language-learning impairment (Boscariol et al., 2011). Comparing three groups of children (group 1 with language-learning impairment and polymicrogyria; group 2 with language-learning impairment and normal MRIs; and the control group [3] of normal children), Boscariol et al. (2011) reported that Groups 1 and 2 showed abnormalities on central auditory processing tests (i.e., gap detection, dichotic digits), with group 1 demonstrating greater performance deficits than group 2. Thus, cortical malformation in auditory regions of the brain correlates with poor performance on auditory processing tasks and the presence of language-learning impairment.

Receptive and Expressive Language Skills

Certain language-related behaviors seen in children with CAPD (e.g., inability to organize and express one's thoughts, deficits in interpreting and responding to social cues; remembering lengthy directions, getting to the point in conversation, and answering open ended questions) should trigger a language evaluation. Geffner (2007, p. 75) included the inability to infer, interpret and make predictions about language as components of receptive language disorders. Such deficits may lead to metalinguistic difficulties with nonliteral language (e.g., understanding jokes, humor, sarcasm, puns, and nuances of the spoken message), inferential language, ambiguous language, figures of speech, and resultant failure to interpret the implied message correctly. This leaves the impression that the person is *very literal* in his or her thoughts and is unable to *see the forest from the trees*, or unable to *connect the dots*, suggesting an imbalance between understanding abstract versus concrete language, reflective of or mistaken for a nonverbal learning disability (NLD). See discussion of metalinguistics below.

Deficits in spoken language comprehension are caused by a number of factors and are often mistaken for CAPD. Many clinicians assume that if the child cannot follow directions, understand what is being said, frequently asks *what?*, mishears words, or needs directions repeated, then the child has CAPD, when in fact the child may have a receptive language impairment. It can be difficult to determine the relative impact of language limitations versus central auditory processing deficits that contribute to the diagnosis using currently available assessment tools. Sharma et al. (2009) found most children with CAPD showed difficulty following directions, recalling sentences, formulating sentences and forward number repetition (a memory task). In fact, 75% of her population presented a comorbid language impairment with language scores falling below the 10th percentile or standard scores (SS) of 80.

Expressive language problems may include difficulty getting to the point succinctly, accessing readily available vocabulary (word retrieval problems), knowing what to say in social situations, and using vague language. Clinically, it has been observed that children with CAPD are not as facile expressively. It is difficult for these youngsters to explain, give details, extract relevant from irrelevant information, repeat a story in sequential order, and retrieve the words they want to say, often replacing it with "thing," "thingy," or "stuff."

Effective narrative discourse skills have been reported to be an area of weakness in children with deficient expressive language skills. These skills enable a child to verbally describe remote or current events that require organization, sequential order and clarity with regard to vocabulary, semantics and linguistic decisions. A youngster with CAPD and language deficits may talk incessantly without *getting to the point*, partly due to poor organization of thought and his or her difficulty retrieving words. Word retrieval is often reported by parent informants as an area of deficit in children diagnosed with CAPD.

Metalinguistic Skills and CAPD

Metalinguistics refers to the self-awareness of language. Metalingusitic skills develop between the ages of 5 to 10 years. According to Baran (2013), there is not a single metalinguistic skill but rather several skills that collectively form the basis for what is revered to as "language awareness." Metalinguistic skills are cognitive-linguistic processes that enable individuals to use critical thinking skills to analyze language. These cognitive-linguistic processes enable individuals to "not only make judgments about the accuracy of the linguistic code and the appropriate (or inappropriate) use of language both in terms of form and function, but they also provide the listener with the ability to talk about language in meaningful

ways" (Baran, 2013, p. 303). Development and mastery of metalinguistic skills enable an individual to understand and use humor, idioms, multiple word meanings, inferences and figurative language.

Metalinguistic skills are essential in oral communication particularly in a social context. These skills enable a communicator to initiate and maintain a social conversation, such as discussing a television show, movie or video game, where both speakers are engaged with the content of the message as well as the mechanics. Children with CAPD can be at risk for having metalinguistic skill weaknesses that will interfere with speaking, listening and learning. Metalinguistic awareness involves the knowledge and ability to manipulate the structural aspects of language independently from the meaning conveyed by the message itself. It involves the ability to focus on language as an entity, to problem solve, predict outcomes and understand underlying meaning. Children with CAPD typically experience some degree of language impairment that might include metalinguistic skill weaknesses (Wallach, 2008). Children with CAPD often do not understand the nuances that are implied within a spoken message. They may interpret spoken language literally and miss the implied message and even the intent conveyed by the tone of voice of the speaker.

As higher order language skills, metalinguistic skills require the ability to go beyond the typical conventional meaning of language. Figurative language forms (e.g., metaphors, proverbs) appear more frequently in oral and written language, beginning at the time of middle and upper elementary school years. Semantic development further grows in vocabulary size and depth of word knowledge that includes an understanding of double meaning words and literate lexicon. In addition, written language develops as the student becomes a mature reader. With this comes the demand for synthesizing new information for a variety of print materials that require the student to organize, assimilate new information, make inferences for comprehension (predict what's coming next, understand what is not explicitly stated), summarize, and search for information from memory. It is in these areas that youngsters with CAPD may falter (Tazeau & Hamaguchi, 2013; Wallach, 2008). Such challenges appear when the youngster approaches middle school, at the time that such language forms emerge. During adolescence, development continues in conversational maturity, utterance length and comprehension of complex sentences and linguistic cohesion, along with semantic (vocabulary) growth. Included in this developmental process is metacognitive/executive functioning. For some youngsters with CAPD, a language impairment was never identified. However, as they advance in grade level, the greater demands made on their higher order thinking skills require more sophisticated language. Children with CAPD may not be as proficient in these more sophisticated areas of language processing as the typical middle/high school student, although they might not be diagnosed with a language deficit.

Metacognitive Skills and CAPD

Metacognitive abilities involve an awareness of one's own problem-solving abilities and include self-regulation behaviors that are used to guide, monitor and evaluate the outcome of one's behavior (Roth & Worthington, 2011). Such skills involve planning, attending selectively to a situation or event, shifting focus and attention when needed, inhibiting behavioral impulses, setting goals and priorities to effectuate a plan, organizing one's behavior and work output, evaluating one's work and revising or repairing it to meet goals, and using time efficiently in order to meet deadlines and plan of action. Students show improvement in executive function at about the fourth grade at which time they become more strategic learners. Metacognition is an higher order ability in that the *meta* strategies must be involved from the outset of the task and require task analysis and planning (Roth & Worthington, 2011, p. 199). Given the fact that metacognitive tasks are mediated through language and language must be proficient in order to effectuate these strategies, youngsters with comorbid CAPD and language deficits may experience difficulties with metacognitive functions.

Students typically impose *self-talk* strategies throughout their day to reiterate their task assignment, think about the assignment, why they are doing it, how they are doing it, and how they need to make changes in their strategies to meet their goals. It is no wonder that deficits in executive function, as cited in the literature (Chermak, Tucker, & Siekel, 2002) are present in this population. Although not a prominent characteristic of CAPD, but more so if the youngster also has a comorbid ADHD, executive function skills can be deficient in CAPD and require attention and assessment. (See Chapter 10 for discussion of intervention for metalinguistic and metacognitive deficits in individuals with CAPD.)

Working Memory and CAPD

Baddeley and Hitch (1974) introduced the term working memory and described its effects on the processing of information. Working memory is the capacity to hold or store and manipulate units of information in short-term memory. Schwartz (2011) described working memory as "the neural structures and cognitive processes that maintain the accessibility of information for short periods of time in an active conscious state" (p. 59). Working memory enables listeners to process and store auditory information for successful listening, communication and learning. Since working memory supports most, if not all, sensory and linguistic processes, it is important to ascertain the status of working memory in children and adults with CAPD. Not surprisingly, Bamiou et al. (2004) reported working memory deficits in a child with a PAX 6 genetic mutation and CAPD. See Chapter 10 for discussion of the role of working memory in comprehensive intervention for CAPD.

Baddeley (1986) proposed that working memory is composed of three distinct components: the central executive, the phonological loop and the visuospatial sketchpad. Of these three, the component that has been identified as the most important in the many aspects of language processing (e.g., vocabulary acquisition and mastery, speech production and expression, language comprehension) is the phonological loop (Schwartz, 2011). Wentworth (2009) noted that the phonological loop is usually referred to as auditory working memory and that relevant auditory information is held in this auditory store while cognitive and language activities are com-

pleted (e.g., reading comprehension, a sequential math problem, following sequential directions). When information is presented through the auditory modality one must actively rehearse what is heard because the information rapidly decays after one to two seconds (Wentworth, 2009). In order to rehearse, one must then use selective attention to filter irrelevant sounds in order to attend to the significant information at hand (Wentworth, 2009). Wentworth argued that if auditory working memory is weak, then one will experience difficulty listening to and selecting appropriate information. According to Wentworth (2009), the behavioral profile of a child with weak auditory working memory includes inattention, distraction, forgetting what was learned, forgetting instructions, not completing tasks, making careless mistakes and having difficulty in solving problems.

Individuals with CAPD frequently exhibit behaviors that may be related to their underlying perceptual deficits or perhaps to an associated working memory (or language processing) deficit. These behaviors include: (1) the need for information to be repeated or rephrased; (2) difficulty following age-level appropriate instructions; (3) difficulty remembering instructions; (4) difficulty comprehending auditory information; (5) use of "uhs" and "ums" fillers; and (6) difficulty with short-term memory (Geffner & Ross-Swain, 2013)

According to Schwartz (2011), working memory is generally considered to have a limited capacity or number "items" or "units" that can be stored for immediate recall. Miller (1956) argues that the capacity of working memory in humans is seven units of information in adults with varying capacity from person to person. Factors affecting capacity include education, cognitive development, speech-language development and skill mastery, social milieu, and physical status. Weaknesses with working memory capacity can affect successful processing of input for communication and learning. Heinrich and Schneider (2011) found that a high presentation level of distorted words can adversely affect memory, even when intelligibility is controlled, particularly for older listeners.

A number of linguistic variables affect working memory capacity. Pronunciation time refers to the amount of time that is needed to say aloud the items being rehearsed in working memory. The limit on working memory capacity is the number of words that can be said or pronounced, either subvocally or aloud, in approximately 1.5 seconds (Schweickert & Boruff, 1986). Word length effect is another variable affecting working memory capacity. Single syllable words take less time to produce than longer words, thereby placing less demand on working memory. The longer the word(s), the more demand on working memory, contributing to constraints and limitations for remembering input stimuli or information. Vocabulary familiarity is another consideration for chunking skill ability. Less familiar vocabulary will impose further constraints and limitations whereas more familiar words will be easier to chunk and retain. Taken together, these influences suggest several intervention strategies in a comprehensive approach for individuals with CAPD. Vocabulary building to increase the number of familiar words and decrease the number of words less familiar to the listener is one such strategy. See Chapter 10 for discussion of this strategy.

Auditory working memory capacity is critical for a child's academic success.

Reading, reading comprehension and math skill acquisition and mastery rely on age level appropriate working memory skills. Schwartz (2011) noted that working memory enables the reader to hold (in memory) the words and ideas in a sentence so as to understand the information without having to stop and start. Daneman and Carpenter (1980) concluded that the better a child's working memory skills, the better that child's reading accuracy, reading fluency, and understanding.

The effects of working memory capacity on verbal fluency have been investigated. Engle (2002) asserted that individuals with effective working memory capacity demonstrated more fluent verbal skills with fewer "uhs" or "ums." The use of these filler words typically reflects difficulty with access to readily available vocabulary, word finding, or semantic organization. Engle argued that individuals with larger working memory capacities demonstrated expressive communication skills with fewer hesitations and pauses. To test his assertion, Engle and his colleagues investigated two populations of students differing in working memory capacity. The results of the investigation indicated that the group with the higher working memory capacity was able to generate more responses to a category member recall task within a limited time frame than those with lower working memory scores.

The foregoing demonstrates the importance of working memory and its likely role in supporting central auditory processing. Since individuals with CAPD demonstrate behaviors that suggest possible working memory deficits, the extent to which working memory affects the processing of auditory input must be carefully evaluated and interpreted in order to best plan and implement comprehensive intervention. Moreover, even when a child with CAPD's working memory capacity is not below age-appropriate levels, it may be useful to attempt to strengthen working memory to buttress auditory processes, as argued by Chermak in Chapter 10.

Many contemporary standardized assessment batteries enable clinicians and educators to determine working memory capacity or skills. The primary method of assessing working memory/immediate memory skills is digit, word, and sentence repetition tasks. These tasks require a person to repeat a set of digits, words, or sentences of increasing length and complexity, forward and backward. The results of these types of tasks can provide information relative to the status of one's working memory capacity and potential effects on learning and communication. (See Chapter 18 for further discussion of working memory and CAPD and ADHD.)

Attention and CAPD

It is known that CAPD negatively impacts speech perception, academic performance and on task behavior, the latter confirming its impact on attention (Crandall & Smaldino, 2000). ADHD is one of the most prevalent chronic health disorders affecting school-age children (Berger, 2011). Evidence supports the high comorbidity of CAPD with ADHD. Riccio, Cohen, Garrison, and Smith (2005) found that children children with CAPD and ADHD are often more distracted in background noise and have poor discrimination in noise (Baquet, Geffner, & Martin, 2012; Geffner, Lucker, & Koch, 1996) and greater sensitivity to noise

(Lucker, Geffner, & Koch, 1996). Effat, Tawfik, Hussein, Azzam, and El Eraky (2011) found that the most affected abilities in people with comorbid CAPD and ADHD are auditory temporal processing, temporal ordering/sequencing, and temporal resolution. DaParma, Geffner, and Martin (2011) reported a high probability of symptoms that mirrored auditory processing deficits in their children with ADHD. Thus, it would be appropriate to utilize a screen of attention in the central auditory processing evaluation. The reader is referred to Chapter 20 in Volume 1 of this Handbook for discussion of differential diagnosis of CAPD and ADHD. Moreover, children with CAPD and those with ADHD present a number of overlapping behavioral characteristics, including poor speech discrimination in noise, and difficulties comprehending spoken language (Baquet, Geffner, & Martin, 2012; Chermak, Tucker, & Seikel, 2002; DaParma, Geffner, & Martin, 2011). Given the overlapping symptomatology (Chermak et al., 2002), it behooves the clinical team to differentially diagnose these conditions and when they are found to present comorbidly, to design appropriate intervention. Intervention for a child with both CAPD and ADHD might involve working on executive function, speech discrimination, comprehension of spoken language, metalinguistics, and working memory. See Chapter 18 for a neuropsychological perspective on assessment of attention.

Assessment of Attention

Assessment of attention typically has involved questionnaires completed by the parent, teacher and often the individual.

One of the more common questionnaires is the Brown ADD Rating Scales (Brown, 2001), which is normed for different age groups, from 3 years through adults, and can be used as a component of a comprehensive assessment, as well as a measure of effectiveness of treatment for ADHD. The rating scales include 40 items that assess five clusters of ADHD-related executive function impairments, such as: organizing, prioritizing and activating to work; focusing, sustaining, and shifting attention to tasks; regulating alertness, sustaining effort and processing speed; managing frustration and modulating emotions; and utilizing working memory and accessing recall. Versions for the younger population of children ages 2 to 12 include a sixth cluster to assess problems in monitoring and self-regulation.

Other instruments to measure attention include the *Test of Everyday Attention for Children*, (*TEA-Ch*; Manly, Robertson, Anderson, & Nimmo-Smith, 1998), which assesses the capacities of children in the following areas: selectively attend, sustain attention, divide attention, switch attention from one task to another, and withhold verbal and motor responses. The *ADHD Rating Scale* from The Foundation for Medical Practice Education (http://www.fmpe.org), which uses as its source the APA DSM-IV-TR edition guidelines (February, 2008), is based on a Likert scale of behaviors that occur always, often, somewhat, rarely or never, designed for the school and for the home. The *ADDES Scale–Third Edition* (McCarney & Arthaud, 2004), is a questionnaire with subscales for inattentive and hyperactive-impulsive behaviors with two versions: for the school, and home to be used by educators, school and private psychologists, pediatricians and other medical personnel. The ADDES

Scale, compared to the Conners' Rating Scale, indicated concurrent validity. The companion *Attention Deficit Disorders Intervention Manual–Second Edition (ADDIM)* includes goals, objectives, and intervention strategies for all behaviors measured by the scale. *Conners' AD/HD Rating Scales–Revised* (Conners, 2012) continues to be a widely used questionnaire, citing behaviors consistent with the DSM-IV-TR characteristics. It has two forms for teacher and parent to complete.

Other questionnaires for children include the *ADD-H Comprehensive Teacher's Rating Scale* and *Parent Form: ACTeRS* (Ullman, Sleator, & Sprague, 1988), which contains both versions to assess attention, hyperactivity, social skills and oppositional behavior in children and adolescents ages 6 to 14. Each form contains 24 items and takes 5 to 10 minutes to complete. It can be used for screening or to measure response to treatments. The *Swanson Nolan and Pelam Rating Scale–4th Edition–Revised* (*SNAP-IV-R*), useful with children and adolescents ages 6 to 18, contains 90 items and takes 10 minutes to complete (Swanson, Nolan, & Pelam, 1992). It includes symptoms of AD/HD along with Oppositional Defiant Disorders and Aggression. It is Free online at http://www.adhd.net/. The *Parent and Teacher Form of the Vanderbilt ADHD Diagnostic Parent Rating Scale* is also free and available online in PDF format containing 55 items for parents and 43 items for teachers, designed for children ages 6 to 12. Rating scales are listed for symptoms and impairment in academic and behavioral performance in the home, school and social settings. Continuous Performance Tests like the *Conners' Continuous Performance Test-II*, and *Test of Variables of Attention* (*TOVA*; Greenberg, 2011) are becoming more popular as they provide more direct measures of attention and impulsivity. The *Integrated Visual and Auditory Continuous Performance Test* (*IVA CPT*; Tinius, 2003) is another direct test of attention, which gives a measure of both auditory and visual attention which is helpful in differentiating CAPD from a pansensory ADHD.

Assessment of Cognition and Language in Individuals With CAPD

It requires skilled clinicians working as a multidisciplinary team to evaluate the potential of comorbid and co-occurring disorders of language, literacy, memory, attention in the child with CAPD. The team assesses the impact of each on the child's auditory processing skills and to sort out what is truly a CAPD as opposed to another look-alike condition, or perhaps, simply a combination of several conditions. Given the comorbidity discussed above and the bidirectional relationships among CAPD and listening, language, memory, and attention, a multidisciplinary test battery administered by a multidisciplinary team is necessary to completely assess and describe an individual's functional deficits in a variety of settings, including the classroom, and identify multidisciplinary intervention strategies. The SLP is uniquely qualified to delineate the cognitive/communicative and speech-language factors that may be associated with CAPD (ASHA, 2005c) and is a pivotal member of the team. Functional abilities related to auditory skills such as those seen in language processing, phonological awareness, and academic skills should be considered.

Brain imaging tools have been widely used to study cognition, language, and auditory processing in a number of different populations (Friederici, 2009; Minagawa-Kawai et al., 2011; Yeatman, Ben-Schacher, Glover, & Feldman, 2010). Moncrieff, McColl, and Black (2008) linked differences in the functional magnetic resonance imaging (fMRI) hemodynamic response recorded from reading disabled children with a unilateral dichotic listening deficit when the children were told to listen with their right ear. Such studies could provide standards for brain activation patterns during various auditory processing tasks. Hornickel and Kraus (2012) reported that speech-evoked ABR (cABR) is a reliable procedure for research and clinical assessment of auditory functions, particularly for auditory-based communication skills (p. 28). This objective measure allows for reliable test/retest data and seems to predict speech-in-noise perception and reading abilities (Kraus & Hornickel, 2013). It can also be used to demonstrate changes in sensory function and consequences of training (Kraus & Hornickel, 2013). See Chapters 3, 7, and 17 in Volume 1 of this Handbook for discussion of the use of these procedures in research and clinical diagnosis.

The SLP's assessment does not result in a diagnosis of CAPD, but a means of providing information on specific skills that may include auditory association/receptive vocabulary, word discrimination, auditory memory, phonemic awareness/phonological processing, auditory closure, auditory cohesion, and auditory/language comprehension (California Speech-Language and Hearing Association-CSHA Task Force document, 2004; Ross-Swain, 2013). The testing provides information on such skills as expressive vocabulary, word retrieval, syntax, grammar, metalinguistic skills, and nonliteral and narrative language skills.

In a perfect situation, the audiologist and SLP work collaboratively to assess each child referred for testing, interpret findings and make recommendations for intervention. However, accessibility and resources can preclude collaborative or multidisciplinary assessment. It is not uncommon for school districts to have limited or no access to audiologists who can administer comprehensive central auditory processing testing. However, most all school districts do have SLPs who can administer appropriate testing that can provide the necessary information relative to cognitive-communication and language factors that are commonly associated with CAPD. The reader is referred to Chapter 5 for a discussion of school policies, process, and services for children with CAPD.

In order to select appropriate assessment batteries the SLP should consider the specific areas of assessment. Richard (2012) and Medwetsky (2011) referred to processing as a continuum or an integration of skills. These skills would include auditory processing; spoken language processing, to include phonemic and language processing; and information processing and executive functioning. With this model in mind, the SLP would select an assessment battery that would provide a multidisciplinary team with information relative to cognitive-communication and language skills affecting a child's ability to communicate, learn and socialize, relative to age-level norms and expectations. Such testing to differentiate central auditory processing deficits from spoken language processing deficits would include language measures such as: receptive vocabulary, word discrimination, auditory

memory, phonemic awareness/phonological processing, auditory closure, auditory cohesion, and auditory/language comprehension, expressive vocabulary, word retrieval, syntax, grammar, metalinguistic skills, and nonliteral and narrative language skills (California Speech Language and Hearing Association [CSHA] Task Force, 2004).

Red flags to alert the SLP clinician to refer a child for central auditory testing might be suggested by poor auditory comprehension, discrepancies between receptive and expressive language, and delayed processing speed (i.e., the child needs more time ("wait time") to respond). The SLP may begin with cognitive-communicative assessment with language screening tools to guide the assessment process, as described below.

Screening Instruments

Screening instruments have been developed to assist audiologists, SLPs and educators in decision making relative to comprehensive testing. These screening instruments will assist in not only determining if comprehensive testing is necessary, but also which specific standardized batteries should be included in the assessment. Since the impetus for testing is suspected CAPD, the following screening tools are useful in assisting and obtaining initial information related to auditory-language processing:

1. *The Listening Inventory (TLI)* (Geffner & Ross-Swain, 2006): *TLI* is a validated criterion-referenced instrument designed for use by SLPs, audiologists, teachers, and special educators to identify at-risk children between the ages of 4 years

through 17 years. *TLI* provides a rating scale for rating 110 behaviors in six categories that are often associated with auditory processing skill weaknesses. The categories include: Linguistic Organization (LO), Decoding and Language Mechanics (DL), Attention and Organization (AO), Sensory-Motor (SM), Social and Behavioral (SB), and Auditory Processes (AP).

2. *The Auditory Skills Assessment (ASA)* (Geffner & Goldman, 2010) is a screening instrument normed on children aged 3 to 6 through 6 to 11 years who are deemed to be at-risk for a CAPD. Subtests include: Speech Discrimination Domain, Phonological Awareness Domain, and Nonspeech Processing Domain. The ASA is an efficient and reliable indicator of a child's auditory skills that can be used for early identification and intervention for this population of children. The six sections of the ASA provide data on speech discrimination, phonological awareness, and nonspeech processing.

3. *The SCAN-3:C* (Keith, 2009) was developed for use by SLPs, audiologists, neuropsychologists, and educational diagnosticians. The SCAN-3:C offers three screening subtests, four diagnostic subtests, and three supplementary subtests and is intended for use with children 5 through 12 years of age. The *SCAN-3:A* is standardized on ages 13 through adults, age 55, and also has screening tests. See Chapter 10 of Volume 1 of the Handbook for audiological screening for CAPD.

Assuming that the results of the screening indicate further testing is appropriate, the SLP faces the daunting task of determining that standardized instruments would provide the multidisciplinary team with the most comprehensive information. There are literally hundreds of standardized measures that are available to SLPs to assess cognitive-communicative and language skills associated with CAPD. The SLP is encouraged to consider the specific skill categories warranting more comprehensive testing before selecting a battery of instruments to administer. According to the California Speech-Language and Hearing Association Task Force on Guidelines for Auditory Processing Disorder (2004) the following skills categories should be considered: receptive and expressive vocabulary skills, auditory perception and discrimination, auditory memory, phonemic awareness, auditory closure, auditory comprehension, and cohesion and word retrieval.

The following section provides a partial list of commercial standardized batteries that are available to be used to assess the aforementioned skill areas. The reader is cautioned that a clinician should evaluate the extent to which a particular cutoff score is effective for distinguishing normal from impaired language in a specific test that has been selected for use. Applying arbitrary low cutoff scores for diagnosing the presence or absence of a language impairment may not be the only method to use when identifying children. Although applying low cut off scores is common in clinical practice and research, we do not know whether such a cut off provides accurate evidence for such a disorder (Spaulding, Plante, & Farinella, 2006). Interestingly, only a few tests studied by these researchers contain primary evidence to support test sensitivity and specificity for diagnostic use.

Receptive and Expressive Language

1. The Clinical Evaluation of Language Function–Fourth Edition (CELF-4; Semel, Wiig, & Secord, 2003): The CELF-4 determines language strengths and weaknesses. It provides Receptive Language and Expressive Language scores, and additional composite scores: Language Structure, Language Content, Language Content and Memory, and Working Memory.
2. The Test of Language Development–4th Edition (TOLD-P:4; Hammill & Newcomer, 2008) (Subtest 1): The TOLD-P:4 assesses spoken language in young children. Professionals can use the TOLD-P:4 to: (1) identify children who are significantly below their peers in oral language proficiency, (2) determine their specific strengths and weaknesses in oral language skills, (3) document their progress in remedial programs, and (4) measure oral language in research studies.

Receptive and Expressive Vocabulary

1. The Peabody Picture Vocabulary Test™–4th Edition (PPVT™-4; Dunn & Dunn, 2007): The PPVT-4 measures receptive single-word vocabulary.
2. The Receptive One Word Picture Vocabulary Test-4 (ROWPVT-4; Martin & Brownell, 2010): The ROWPVT-4 tests an individual's ability to match a spoken word with an image of an object, action, or concept. The tests target the ability to understand the meaning of words spoken and name what is depicted on a test plate without context.

3. The Expressive One Word Picture Vocabulary Test–4th Edition (EOWPVT-4) (Martin & Brownell, 2010): The EOWPVT-4 tests an individual's ability to name, with one word, objects, actions, and concepts when presented with color illustrations. The tests target the ability to understand the meaning of words spoken and name what is depicted on a test plate without context.
4. The Comprehensive Receptive and Expressive Vocabulary Test–Revised (CREVT-2; Wallace & Hammill, 2002): The CREVT-2 identifies students who are significantly below their peers in oral vocabulary proficiency. It measures discrepancies between receptive and expressive vocabulary and documents progress in oral vocabulary development resulting from intervention. It measures oral vocabulary for research studies.

Auditory-Language Perception and Discrimination

1. The Lindamood Auditory Conceptualization Test–Third Edition (LAC-3; Lindamood & Lindamood, 2004): The LAC-3 is an individually administered, norm-referenced assessment that measures an individual's ability to perceive and conceptualize speech sounds using a visual medium.
2. The Test of Auditory Processing Skills–Third Edition (TAPS-3; Martin & Brownell, 2005): The TAPS-3 battery can assist in diagnosing auditory-language processing difficulties, imperceptions of auditory modality, language problems, and/or learning disabilities in both children and teens.

3. The Test of Language Development-Fourth Edition (TOLD-P:4; Hammill & Newcomer, 2008): The TOLD-P:4 assesses spoken language in young children. Professionals can use the TOLD-P:4 to (1) identify children who are significantly below their peers in oral language proficiency, (2) determine their specific strengths and weaknesses in oral language skills, (3) document their progress in remedial programs, and (4) measure oral language in research studies.

4. Auditory Skills Assessment (ASA, Geffner & Goldman, 2010): The ASA provides a tool for early identification of young children who might be at risk for auditory skill deficits and/or early literacy skill difficulties.

Auditory Memory

1. The Auditory Processing Abilities Test (APAT; Ross-Swain & Long; 2004) (Subtests 2, 6, and 9): The APAT is used in the identification of children who are at risk for CAPD or who may experience auditory processing skill deficits. The APAT yields scores in the following areas: global auditory processing, auditory discrimination, auditory memory, auditory sequential memory, auditory association, and auditory cohesion.

2. The Comprehensive Test of Phonological Processing (CTOPP; Wagner, Torgesen & Rashotte, 1999) (Subtest III): The CTOPP is used to identify individuals who need help in developing phonological skills. The three subtests include: Phonological Awareness Quotient (PAQ), which measures an individual's awareness and access to the phonological structure of oral language; Phonological Memory Quotient (PMQ), which measures an individual's ability to code information phonologically for temporary storage in working or short-term memory; and Rapid Naming Quotient (RNQ), which measures the individual's efficient retrieval of phonological information from long-term or permanent memory, as well as the ability to execute a sequence of operations quickly and repeatedly.

3. The Test of Language Development-Primary–Fourth Edition (TOLD-P:4) (Subtest V).The TOLD-P-4 assesses spoken language in young children. It is well constructed, reliable, practical, research-based, and theoretically sound. Professionals can use the TOLD-P:4 to: (1) identify children who are significantly below their peers in oral language proficiency, (2) determine their specific strengths and weaknesses in oral language skills, (3) document their progress in remedial programs, and (4) measure oral language in research studies.

4. The Token Test for Children–Second Edition (TTFC-2; McGhee, Ehrer, & DiSimoni, 2007): The Token Test for Children–Second Edition (TTFC-2) is a reliable and effective screening measure for assessing receptive language in children ages 3 years 0 months to 12 years 11 months.

5. The Test of Auditory Processing Skills–Third Edition (TAPS-3;) (Subtests of Number Memory Forward; Number Memory Reversed; Word Memory and Sentence Memory)

Phonemic Awareness

1. The Auditory Processing Abilities Test (APAT) Subtest 1: The APAT is a nationally standardized, norm-refer-

enced auditory processing battery. It may be used in the identification of children who are at risk for or who may have central auditory processing deficits. The APAT was developed using a model based on a heirarchy of auditory processing skills that are basic to listening and processing spoken language. These skills range from sensation to memory to cohesion. The APAT is comprised of 10 subtests that quantify a child's performance in various areas of auditory processing. The APAT provides composite index scores as well as individual subtest scores: Global Index reflecting overall auditory processing efficiency, Linguistic Processing Index, and Auditory Memory Index. Optional analyses allow further examination of Linguistic Processing tasks (yielding indices for discrimination, sequencing, and cohesion) and Memory tasks (yielding indices for immediate recall, delayed recall, sequential recall, and cued recall). The battery is designed primarily to be used by speech-language pathologists but may also be used by other professionals such as learning disabilities specialists, psychologists, and resource specialists. The APAT is individually administered and can be completed and scored in less than 45 minutes. It yields scaled scores and percentile ranks for subtests and standard scores and percentile ranks for the composites. Age equivalents are also available for all areas assessed.

2. The Comprehensive Test of Phonological Processing (CTOPP) Subtests 1, 2, 8, 10, 1, and 12: The CTOPP is a comprehensive instrument designed to assess phonological awareness, phonological memory, and rapid naming. People with deficits in one or more these areas may have more difficulty reading than those who do not. The CTOPP was developed to aid in the identification of who may benefit from kindergarten all the way through to college who may benefit from instructional activities to enhance their phonological skills.

3. The Lindamood Auditory Conceptualization Test-Third Edition (LAC-3): The LAC-3 is an individually administered, norm-referenced assessment that measures an individual's ability to perceive and conceptualize speech sounds using a visual medium. Because of the importance of these auditory skills to reading, the results are helpful for speech-language pathologists, special educators, and reading specialists. The LAC-3 also measures the cognitive ability to distinguish and manipulate sounds, which success in reading and spelling requires. This third edition of the LAC has been improved considerably. Three new categories of items that relate to multisyllabic processing have been added. The availability of standard scores for the LAC-3 total score is a desirable new feature.

4. The Phonological Awareness Test (PAT-2; Robertson, 2007): This test assesses all the pre-reading skills that are early indicators of reading success. Use it to identify children who lack explicit phonological knowledge and have difficulty acquiring sound/symbol correspondences in words.

5. The Test of Auditory Processing Skills–Third Edition (TAPS-3) Subtests of Phonological Segmentation and Phonological Blending: The TAPS-3 battery can assist in diagnosing auditory-language processing

difficulties, imperceptions of auditory modality, language problems, and/or learning disabilities in both children and teens. Subtests 2 and 3 assess phonological processing/phonemic awareness skills.

Auditory Closure

1. The Comprehensive Assessment of Spoken Language (CASL) (Carrow-Woolfolk, E., 1999). Subtest of Meaning from Context: The CASL assessment provides a measure of delayed language, spoken language disorders, dyslexia, and aphasia. The CASL provides a precise picture of language processing skills and structural knowledge, allowing you to document development from pre-school through the post secondary years. This test battery consists of 15 tests that measure language processing skills—comprehension, expression, and retrieval—in four language structure categories: Lexical/Semantic, Syntactic, Supralinguistic, and Pragmatic.
2. Test of Language Competence (TLC) (Wiig & Secord, 1989) Subtest 3: The TLC measures metalinguistic higher level language functions. Subtests include Ambiguous Sentences, Listening Comprehension: Making Inferences, Oral Expression: Recreating Speech Acts, Figurative Language, and a supplemental memory subtest.
3. SCAN-3 for Children (SCAN-3) (Keith, 2009) Subtest 1: The SCAN-3 is used to assess a auditory processing deficits in children 5 to 12 years old. The SCAN-3's subtest "Filtered Speech" is a measure of auditory closure, as

the subject has to fill in the gaps for the extracted frequencies to render the word intelligible.

Auditory Cohesion and Comprehension

1. The Auditory Processing Abilities Test (APAT) Subtests 7, 8, and 10 (See above.)
2. The Clinical Evaluation of Language Fundamentals–Fourth Edition (CELF-4) Subtests of Linguistic Concepts, Sentence Structure, Understanding Concepts and Following Directions and Understanding Spoken Paragraphs
3. The Comprehensive Assessment of Spoken Language (CASL) Subtests of Sentence Comprehension, Paragraph Comprehension, Nonliteral Language, Ambiguous Sentences and Inference
4. The Listening Test (Barrett, Huisingh, Bowers, Logiudice, & Orman, 1992): The Listening Test assesses listening behaviors that reflect classroom listening situations. Subtests include Main Idea, Details, Concepts, Reasoning, and Story Comprehension. Includes a Classroom Listening Scale for the classroom teacher to rate the student's listening performance in the classroom in comparison to classmates.
5. The Test of Auditory Processing Skills–Third Edition (TAPS-3) Subtests of Auditory Comprehension and Auditory Reasoning
6. The Test of Language Competence (TLC) Subtests 1 and 4 (See above for test description.)
7. The Token Test for Children–2nd Edition (TTFC-2) (See above for test description.)

Word Retrieval

1. The Clinical Evaluation of Language Fundamentals–Fourth Edition (CELF-4) Subtests such as Word Associations and Rapid Automatic Naming are two supplemental tests that are criterion referenced based on the timing and error score of a subject naming colors and shapes in rows on a page.
2. The Comprehensive Assessment of Spoken Language (CASL) Subtests of Antonyms, Synonyms, and Sentence Completion
3. The Comprehensive Test of Phonological Processing (CTOPP) Subtests IV, VI, VII, and IX
4. The Test of Word Finding-Second Edition (TOWF-2) (German, 1999): TWF-2 is a nationally standardized, individually administered diagnostic tool for the assessment of children's word finding skills.

Metalinguistics

The following are suggested standardized batteries that can be used to obtain clinically and functionally useful information relative to a child's metalinguistic skills and the potential effects on listening, communicating and learning.

1. The Comprehensive Assessment of Spoken Language (CASL; Carrow-Woolfolk, 1999): Designed to measure the processes of comprehension, expression, and retrieval in four language categories: Lexical/Semantic, Syntactic, Supralinguistic, and Pragmatic. Specific subtests include: Test of Inference, Test of Nonliteral Language, Meaning from Context, and Ambiguous Language.
2. Test of Language Competence (TLC) (Wiig & Secord, 1989): Designed to assess and measure metalinguistic competence in semantics, syntax, and pragmatics and assess emerging metalinguistic abilities and linguistic strategy acquisition.

Summary

Although the diagnosis of CAPD is the responsibility of the audiologist, the SLP plays an integral role in assessing skills in the spoken language and information processing domains. The results of a comprehensive assessment can enable the SLP to identify specific skill weaknesses in each of these areas and assist the multidisciplinary team in determining how these weaknesses may be affecting a child's success in the classroom. Bellis (2003) asserted that the results of all testing should be related to the communicative, behavioral and academic performance of the child so that a multidisciplinary intervention and management program can be developed and implemented that will target functional outcomes. The input from all team members can assist in developing a plan for a child's social and academic success.

Treatment/Intervention

Given the multitude of functions potentially affected by CAPD and the complexity of the neurophysiologic substrates that are involved in processing, as well as the frequently observed comorbidities and co-occurring behaviors seen in CAPD, a comprehensive, multidisciplinary approach must be taken to intervention.

Such an approach has typically been segmented into *top-down* or *bottom-up* treatment protocols. Given the potential impact of CAPD on listening, communication and academic performance, and given the comorbidity with language, learning and reading disorders, intervention should include a broad spectrum of activities to address the child's areas of weaknesses. Such intervention should be considered early (especially if the child is at risk) to take advantage of brain neuroplasticity in order to reduce the functional deficits that can accompany CAPD and its impact on language and learning. Such intervention should also be considered for the classroom and home environment to ensure generalization of skills.

According to ASHA (2005a), the two approaches: bottom-up and top-down address auditory training, environmental manipulation, and compensatory approaches.

A bottom-up approach would be stimulus driven, to include auditory training and direct skills remediation to reorganize the CANS. Environmental modifications to improve the listening environment, such as use of an FM system, also is a bottom-up approach. The use of an FM system, either for classroom (sound field) enhancement or as a personal unit, has evidence-based data to support its usefulness and effectiveness (see Chapter 12). A top-down approach utilizes *central resources* such has language strategies, and metacognitive and cognitive strategies, along with educational interventions and accommodations. (See Chapters 1, and 7–14.)

Compensatory Strategies

The SLP is instrumental to top-down therapies. Compensatory strategies involve teaching the individual to self-advocate, ask for clarification, remove oneself from a noxious environment whereby it is too noisy to communicate or hear, and ask the speaker to slow down or repeat what was said. All this can be accomplished in training, but the client should be encouraged to develop advocacy skills. Many children fail to ask for help and simply let the message go by. It is said in a Chinese proverb, "Once the word leaves the mouth the fastest horse can't catch it." We must instruct the youngster, that they need to run after it-by using compensatory strategies.

Direct Treatment

Direct treatment complements environmental alteration and compensatory strategy instruction. We must use evidence-based protocols to address specific deficiencies (e.g., auditory figure-ground listening, phonological awareness, temporal processing, auditory discrimination, auditory integration) and the various auditory-linguistic deficits associated with the disorder. Such auditory-linguistic areas may include and/or be influenced by: vocabulary, language formulation, narrative discourse, metalinguistics, comprehension of spoken and written language, auditory working memory, following directions, syntactical formulation, understanding the relevant from the irrelevant, getting to the point, organizing one's thoughts, and retrieving words for fluency. Reading is another area that should be addressed by reading specialists and SLPs, particularly when concentrating on phonological awareness skills. Other concomitant problems should involve a team of clinicians to address social language issues (pragmatics), behaviors, learning and memory, executive function and organization. See Chapter 2 for discussion of evidence-based practice and treatment efficacy.

Activities or games may be played to stimulate vocabulary growth, including word association, synonyms, category names and semantic cues to generate retrieval. Narrative discourse can be encouraged by instructing the student to use cuing questions to construct stories and use graphic organizers (i.e., Write out Loud, Draft Builder, such as those found in Kidspiration, Inspiration and Solo 6 (http://www.donjohnston.com). Use of technology to help develop language structures can be effective and motivating. The preceding suggestions apply to written discourse as well. Expository writing can be improved by teaching the youngster to organize his thoughts and sequence them in a logical manner using the concepts of setting, problem, action, or beginning middle and end, or who, what, where, when, and why. Punctuation, spelling and syntax needs tending to, which can be accomplished by spelling improvement programs (SPELL-2; Masterson, Apel, & Wasowicz, 2006) and use of the computer's spell and grammar check. In training, the youngster with CAPD needs to develop skills of observing, describing, hypothesizing, generalizing, predicting outcomes explaining events in a cohesive organized manner, preparing for alternative choices, inferring, and using language appropriately. Executive functions of organization, time management and attention should be considered as well.

Regardless of one's role in the screening, evaluation, or intervention processes, it is crucial that all work in a team effort so that all the concomitant aspects of CAPD are addressed and managed appropriately in the home, school, and community setting. For additional discussion of treatment approaches and specific protocols, the reader is referred to other texts (i.e., Masters, Stecker & Katz, *Central Auditory Processing Disorders Mostly Management*, 1998; Geffner and Swain, *Auditory Processing Disorders: Assessment, Management and Treatment, 2nd Edition*, 2012), as well as the other chapters in this Handbook.

References

Aithal, V., Yonovitz, A., & Aithal, S. (2006). Tonal masking level differences in Aboriginal children: Implications for binaural interaction, auditory processing disorders and education. *Australian and New Zealand Journal of Audiology, 28*, 31–40.

American Academy of Audiology (AAA). (2011). *Guidelines for the diagnosis, treatment and management of children and adults with central auditory processing disorder.* Retrieved from http://www.audiology.org/resources/documentlibrary/documents/capd%20guidelines%208-2010.pdf

American Psychiatric Association. (1987). *Diagnostic and statistical manual of mental disorders* (3rd ed.). Washington, DC: Author.

American Psychiatric Association. (2000). *Diagnostic and statistical manual of mental disorders* (4th ed., Text rev.). Washington, DC: American Psychiatric Association.

American Speech-Language Hearing Association. (2005a). *(Central) auditory processing disorders* [Task Force Technical Report]. Retrieved from http://www.asha.org/policy/TR2005-00043.htm

American Speech-Language Hearing Association. (2005b). *(Central) auditory processing disorders—the role of the audiologist* [Position Statement]. Retrieved from http://www.asha.org/docs/html/PS2005-00114.html

American Speech-Language-Hearing Association. (2005c). *SLP preferred practice patterns.* Retrieved from http:/www.asha .org/members/deskref-journals/deskref/ default

American Speech-Language Hearing Association Working Group on Classroom Acoustics. (2005). *Guidelines for addressing acoustics in educational setting.* Retrieved from www.asha.org/docs/html/gl2005-0023.html#sec1.1

Astrom, R., Wadsworth, S. J., & DeFries, J. (2007). Etiology of the stability of reading difficulties: The longitudinal twin study of reading disabilities. *Twin Research and Human Genetics, 10,* 434–439.

Baddeley, A.D. (1986). *Working memory.* London, UK: Oxford University Press.

Baddeley, A. D., & Hitch, G. J. (1974). Working memory. *The psychology of learning and motivation, 8,* 47–89.

Baquet, J., Geffner, D., & Martin, N. (2012). *Prevalence of speech-in-noise deficits in children with AD/HD.* Unpublished manuscript.

Baran, J.A. (2013) Metalinguistic skills, strategies, and approaches. In D. Geffner & D. Ross-Swain (Eds.), *Auditory processing disorders: Assessment, management, and treatment* (pp. 469–495). San Diego, CA: Plural.

Barrett, M., Huisingh, R., Bowers, C., LoGiudice, C., & Orman, J. (1992). *The listening test.* East Moline, IL: LinguiSystems.

Beck, D. L., & Clark, J. L. (2009). Audition matters more as cognition declines: Cognition matters more as audition declines. *Audiology Today, 21,* 48–59.

Bellis, T. J. (2003). Auditory processing disorders: It's not just kids who have them. *Hearing Journal, 56,* 10.

Berger, I. (2011). Using technology in the diagnosis of attention-deficit/hyperactivity disorder. *Journal of Ergonomics, 1,* e102.

Billiet, C. R., & Bellis, T. J. (2011). The relationship between brainstem temporal processing and performance on tests of central auditory function in children with reading disorders. *Journal of Speech, Language, and Hearing Research, 54,* 228–242.

Boets, B., Wouters, J., van Wieringen, A., De Smedt, B., & Ghesquire, P. (2008). Modeling relations between sensory processing, speech perception, orthographic and phonological ability, and literacy achievement. *Brain and Language, 106,* 29–40.

Boscariol, M., Guimaraes, C. A., Hage, S. R., Cendes, F., & Guerreiro, M. M. (2010). Temporal auditory processing: Correlation with developmental dyslexia and cortical malformation. *Pro Fono, 22,* 537–542.

Boscariol, M., Guimaraes, C. A., Hage, S. R., Garcia, V. L., Schmutzler, K. M., Cendes, F., & Guerreiro, M. M. (2011). Auditory processing disorder in patients with language-learning impairment and correlation with malformation of cortical development. *Brain Development, 33,* 824–831.

Boothroyd, A., & Nittrouer, S. (1988). Mathematical treatment of context effects in phoneme and word recognition. *The Journal of the Acoustical Society of America, 84,* 101–114.

British Society of Audiology. (2005). *Working definition of APD.* Retrieved from http:// www.thebsa.org.uk/apd/Home.htm# working%20dcf

Brown, T. E. (2001). *Brown ADD rating scales for children, adolescents, and adults.* San Antonia, TX: PsychCorp.

Cacace, A. T., & MacFarland, D. J. (2005). The importance of modality specificity in diagnosing central auditory processing disorder. *American Journal of Audiology, 14,* 112–123.

California Speech-Language and Hearing Association. (2004). *Guidelines for the diagnosis and treatment for auditory processing disorders.* Position paper.

Carrow-Woolfolk, E. (1999). *Comprehensive assessment of spoken language.* Circle Pines, MN: American Guidance Service.

Catts, H. (1991). Facilitating phonological awareness: Role of speech-language pathologists. *Language, Speech, and Hearing Services in Schools, 22,* 196–203.

Chermak, G. D., & Musiek, F. (1997). *Central auditory processing disorders (New perspectives).* (p. 374). San Diego, CA: Singular.

Chermak, G. D., & Musiek, F. E. (Eds.). (2007). *Handbook of (central) auditory processing disorder: Comprehensive intervention* (Vol. 2). San Diego, CA: Plural.

Chermak, G. D., Tucker, E., & Seikel, J. A. (2002). Behavioral characteristics of auditory processing disorder and attention-deficit hyperactivity disorder: Predominantly inattentive type. *Journal of the American Academy of Audiology, 13,* 332–338.

Conners, K. (2012). *Conners' AD/HD Rating Scales–Revised (CRS-R).* San Antonio, TX: Pearson Assessments.

Corriveau, K. H., Goswami, U., & Thomson, J. M. (2010). Auditory processing and early literacy skills in a preschool and kindergarten population. *Journal of Learning Disabilities, 43,* 369–382.

Cowan, N. (2001). The magical number 4 in short-term memory: A reconsideration of mental storage capacity. *Behavioral and Brain Sciences, 24,* 87–185.

Crandall, C. C., & Smaldino, J. J. (2000). Classroom acoustics for children with normal hearing and with hearing impairment. *Language, Speech, and Hearing Services in Schools, 31,* 362–370.

Daneman, M., & Carpenter, P.A. (1980). Individual differences in working memory and reading. *Journal of Verbal Learning and Verbal Behavior, 19,* 450–466.

DaParma, A., Geffner, D., & Martin, N. (2011). Prevalence and nature of language impairment in children with attention deficit/hyperactivity disorder. *Contemporary Issues in Communication Science and Disorders, 38,* 119–125.

Davids, N., Segers, E., Van Den Brink, D., Mitterer, H., Van Balkom, H., Hagoor, P., & Verhoeven, L. (2010). The nature of auditory discrimination problems in children with specific language impairments: An MMN Study. *Neuropsychologia, 49,* 19–28.

Dawes, P., Bishop, D.V., Sirimanna, T., & Damiou, D.E. (2008). Profile and etiology of children diagnosed with auditory processing disorder (APD). *International Journal of Pediatric Otorhinolaryngology, 72,* 483–489.

DeBonis, D. A., & Moncrieff, D. (2008). Auditory processing disorders: An update for speech-language pathologists. *American Journal of Speech Language Pathology, 17,* 4–18.

Dunn, L. M., & Dunn, L. M. (2007). *Peabody Picture Vocabulary Test–Fourth Edition.* Circle Pines, MN: American Guidance Service.

Effat, S., Tawfik, S., Hussein, H., Assam, H., & El Eraky, S. (2011). Central auditory processing in attention deficit hyperactivity disorder: An Egyptian study. *Middle East Current Psychiatry, 18,* 245–252.

Emanuel, D. C., Ficca, K. N., & Korczak, P. (2011). Survey of the diagnosis and management of auditory processing disorder. *American Journal of Audiology, 20,* 48–60.

Engle, R. W. (2002). Working memory capacity as executive attention. *Current Directions in Psychological Science, 11,* 19–33.

Ferguson, M. A., Hall, R. L., Riley, A., & Moore, D. R. (2011). Communication, listening, cognitive and speech perception skills in children with auditory processing disorder (APD) or specific language impairment (SLI). *Journal of Speech, Language and Hearing Research, 54,* 211–227.

Friederici, A. D. (2009). Pathways to language: Fiber tracts in the human brain. *Trends in cognitive sciences, 13,* 175–181.

Geffner, D. (2013). *Central auditory processing disorders: definition, description, and behaviors.* In D. Geffner & D. Ross-Swain (Eds.), *Auditory processing disorders: Assessment, management, and treatment* (pp. 59–89). San Diego, CA: Plural.

Geffner, D., & Goldman, R. (2010). *Auditory skills assessment.* Minneapolis, MN: Pearson.

Geffner, D., Lucker, J. R., & Koch, W. (1996). Evaluation of auditory discrimination in children with ADD and without ADD. *Child Psychiatry and Human Development, 26,* 169–180.

Geffner, D., & Ross-Swain, D. (2006). *The Listening Inventory.* Novato, CA: Academic Therapy.

Geffner, D. & Ross-Swain, D. (2013). *Auditory processing disorders: Assessment, management, and treatment* (2nd ed.). San Diego, CA: Plural.

German, D. J. (1999). *Test of word finding* (2nd ed.). Austin, TX: ProEd.

Giraud, A. L., & Ramus, F. (in press). Neurogenetics and auditory processing in developmental dyslexia. *Current Opinion in Neurobiology.*

Greenberg, L. M. (2011). *The Test of Variables of Attention (Version 8.0)* [Computer software]. Los Alamitos: TOVA Company.

Hamaguchi, P. M. (2013). Metacognitive therapy approaches. In D. Geffner & D. Swain (Eds.), *Auditory processing disorders: Assessment, management, and treatment* (pp. 431–446). San Diego, CA: Plural.

Hammill, D. D., & Newcomer, P. L. (2008). *The Test of Language Development–primary fourth edition.* Austin, TX: Pro-Ed.

Heinrich, A., & Schneider, B. A. (2011). The effect of presentation level on memory performance. *Ear and Hearing, 32,* 524–532.

Hill, P. R., Hogben, J. H., & Bishop, D. M. (2005). Auditory frequency discrimination in children with specific language impairments: A longitudinal study. *Journal of Speech, Language, and Hearing Research, 48,* 1136–1146.

Hornickel, J., & Kraus, N. (2012). cABR can predict auditory-based communication skills. *Hearing Journal, 65,* 28–30.

Iliadou, V., & Bamiou, D. E. (2012). Psychometric evaluation of children with auditory processing disorder (APD): Comparison with normal-hearing and clinical non-APD groups. *Journal of Speech, Language, and Hearing Research, 55,* 791–799.

Jerger, J., & Musiek, F. (2000). Report of the consensus conference on the diagnosis of auditory processing disorders in school-aged children. *Journal of the American Academy of Audiology, 11,* 467–474.

Jerger, J., & Musiek, F. (2002). On the diagnosis of auditory processing disorder: A reply to "clinical and research concerns regarding Jerger and Musiek (2000) APD recommendations." *Audiology Today, 14,* 19–21.

Katz, J., Johnson, C., Tillery, K. L., Bradham, T., Brander, S., Delagrange, T., . . . Stecker, N. A. (2002). *Clinical and research concerns—regarding Jerger and Musiek (2000) APD Recommendations.* Retrieved from http://audiologyonline.com/articles/pf_article_detail.asp?article_id=341

Keith, R.W. (2000). *Random Gap Detection Test.* San Antonio, TX: Auditec.

Keith, R. W. (2009). *SCAN-3 for Children: Tests for auditory processing disorders.* San Antonio, TX: Pearson.

Keller, W. D., Tillery, K. L., & McFadden, S. L. (2006). Auditory processing disorder in children diagnosed with nonverbal learning disability. *American Journal of Audiology, 15,* 108.

Kraus, N., & Hornickel, J. (2013). cABR: A biological probe of auditory processing. In D. Geffner & D. Swain (Eds.), *Auditory processing disorder: Assessment, management, and treatment* (pp. 283–299). San Diego, CA: Plural.

Kraus, N., & Nicol, T. (2005) How can the neural encoding and perception of speech be improved? *Plasticity and signal representation in the auditory system* (pp. 259–270). New York, NY: Springer.

Kreisman, N. V., John, A. B., Kreisman, B. M., Hall, J. W., & Crandell, C. C. (2012). Psychosocial status of children with auditory processing disorder. *Journal of the American Academy of Audiology, 23,* 222–233.

Lindamood, P. C., & Lindamood, P. (2004). *Lindamood auditory conceptualization test.* Austin, TX: Pro-Ed.

Lucker, J. R., Geffner, D., & Koch, W. (1996). Perception of loudness in children with ADD and without ADD. *Child Psychiatry and Human Development, 26,* 181–190.

Martin, N., & Brownell, R. (2005). *Test of Auditory Processing Skills* (3rd ed.). Novato, CA: Academic Therapy.

Martin, N., & Brownell, R. (2010). *The Expressive One Word Picture Vocabulary Test* (4th ed.). Novato, CA: Academic Therapy.

Martin, N., & Brownell, R. (2010). *The Receptive One Word Picture Vocabulary Test* (4th ed.). Novato, CA: Academic Therapy.

Masters, M. G., Stecker, N. A., & Katz, J. (1998). *Central auditory processing disorders: Mostly management.* Needham Heights, MA: Allyn & Bacon.

Masterson, J., Apel, K., & Wasowicz, J. (2006). *SPELL: Spelling Performance Evaluation for Language and Literacy* [Computer software]. Evanston, IL: Learning By Design.

McArthur, G. M., & Bishop, D. M. (2004). Frequency discrimination deficits in people with specific language impairments: Reliability, validity, and linguistics correlates. *Journal of Speech, Language, and Hearing Research, 47*, 527–541.

McCarney, S. B., & Arthaud, T. J. (2004). *Attention Deficit Disorders Evaluation Scale–Third Edition (ADDES-3).* Columbia, MO: Hawthorne Educational Services.

McGhee, R. L., Ehrleer, D. J., & DiSimoni, F. (2007). *The Token Test For Children* (2nd ed.). Austin, TX: Pro-Ed.

Medwetsky, L. (2006, June). Spoken language processing: A convergent approach to conceptualizing (central auditory processing). *ASHA Leader.*

Medwetsky, L. (2011). Spoken language processing model: Bridging auditory and language processing to guide assessment and intervention. *Language, Speech, and Hearing Services in Schools, 42*, 286–296.

Mengler, B. D., Hogben, J. H., Michie. P., & Bishop, D. V. (2005). Poor frequency discrimination is related to oral language disorder in children: A psychoacoustic study. *Dyslexia, 11*, 155–173.

Miller, C. A., & Wagstaff, D. A. (2011). Behavioral profiles associated with auditory processing disorder and specific language impairment. *Journal of Communication Disorders, 44*, 745–763.

Miller, G. A. (1956). The magical number seven, plus or minus two: Some limits on our capacity for processing information. *Psychological Review, 63*, 81–97.

Minagawa-Kawai, Y., van der Lely, H., Ramus, F., Sato, Y., Mazuka, R., & Dupoux, E. (2011).

Optical brain imaging reveals general auditory and language-specific processing in early infant development. *Cerebral Cortex, 21*, 254–261.

Moncrieff, D., McColl, R. W., & Black, J. R. (2000). Hemodynamic differences in children with dichotic listening deficits. *Journal of American Academy of Audiology, 19*, 33–45.

Moore, D. R., Amitay, S., & Hawkey, D. J. (2003). Auditory perceptual learning. *Learning and Memory, 10*, 83–85.

Musiek, F. E. (1983). Assessment of central auditory dysfunction: The Dichotic Digits Test revisited. *Ear and Hearing, 4*, 79–83.

Musiek, F. E. (1994). Frequency (pitch) and duration pattern tests. *Journal of the American Academy of Audiology, 5*, 265–268.

Nickisch, A., & Massinger, C. (2009). Auditory processing in children with specific language impairments: Are there deficits in frequency discrimination, temporal auditory processing or general auditory processing? *Folia Phoniatrica et Logopaedica, 61*, 323–328.

Nicolosi, L., Harryman, E., & Kresheck. J. (2004). *Terminology of communication disorders* (5th ed.). Philadelphia, PA: Lippincott Williams & Wilkins.

Pedigo, T., Pedigo, K., & Scott, V. B. (2006). *Pediatric Attention Disorders Diagnostic Screener (PADDS),* Okeechobee, FL: Targeted Testing.

Rance, G. (2013). Auditory processing in individuals with auditory neuropathy spectrum disorder. In D. Geffner & D. Swain (Eds.), *Auditory processing disorder: Assessment, management, and treatment* (pp. 185–210). San Diego, CA: Plural.

Reddy, L. A., Newman, E., Pedigo, T. K., & Scott, V. (2010). Concurrent validity of the pediatric attention disorders diagnostic screener for children with ADHD. *Child Neuropsychology, 16*, 478–493.

Riccio, C. A., Cohen, M. J., Garrison, T., & Smith, B. (2005). Auditory processing measure: Correlation with neuropsychological measures of attention, memory, and behavior. *Child Neuropsychology: A Journal on Normal and Abnormal Development in Childhood and Adolescence, 11*(4), 363–372.

Riccio, C. A., Waldrop, J. J., Reynolds, C. R., & Lowe, P. (2001). Effects of stimulants on the continuous performance test (CPT): Implications for CPT use and interpretation. *Journal of Neuroscience, 13,* 326–335.

Richard, G. J. (2013). Language processing versus auditory processing. In D. Geffner & D. Swain (Eds.), *Auditory processing disorder: Assessment, management, and treatment* (p. 283–299). San Diego, CA: Plural.

Robertson, C. (2007). *Phonological Awareness Test 2.* East Moline, IL: LinguiSystems.

Rosen, S., Cohen, M., & Vanniasegaram, I. (2010). Auditory and cognitive abilities of children suspected of auditory processing disorder (APD). *International Journal of Pediatric Otorhinolaryngology, 74,* 594–600.

Ross-Swain, D. (2013). The speech-language pathologist's role in the assessment of auditory processing skills. In D. Geffner & D. Swain (Eds.), *Auditory processing disorder: Assessment, management, and treatment* (pp. 251–281). San Diego, CA: Plural.

Ross-Swain, D., & Long, N. (2004). *Auditory Processing Abilities Test.* Novato, CA: Academic Therapy.

Roth, F. P., & Worthington, C. K. (2011). *Intervention resource manual for speech-language pathology* (4th ed.). Clifton Park, NY: Thomson Delmar Learning.

Scanlon, D. M., & Vellutino, F. R. (1996). Prerequisite skills, early instruction, and success in first-grade reading: Selected results from a longitudinal study. *Mental Retardation and Developmental Disabilities Research Reviews, 2,* 54–63.

Schwartz, B. L. (2011). *Memory foundations and applications.* Los Angeles, CA: Sage.

Schweickert, R., & Boruff, B. (1986). Short-term memory capacity: Magic number or magic spell? *Journal of Experimental Psychology: Learning, Memory, and Cognition, 12,* 419–425.

Semel, E., Wiig, E. H., & Secord, W. A. (2003). *Clinical Evaluation of Language Fundamentals* (4th ed.). San Antonio, TX: Psychological Corporation.

Sharma, M., Purdy, S. C., & Kelly, A. S. (2009). Comorbidity of auditory processing, language, and reading disorders. *Journal of Speech, Language, and Hearing Research, 52,* 706–722.

Sharma, M., Purdy, S. C., Newall, P., Wheldall, K., Beaman, R., & Dillon, H. (2006). Electrophysiological and behavioral evidence of auditory processing deficits in children with reading disorder. *Clinical Neurophysiology, 117,* 1130–1144.

Spaulding, T. J., Plante, E., & Farinella, K. A. (2006). Eligibility criteria for language impairment: Is the low end of normal always appropriate? *Language, Speech, and Hearing Services in Schools, 37,* 61–72.

Stein, J. F. (2001). The magnocellular theory of development dyslexia. *Dyslexia, 7,* 12–36.

Swanson, J. M., Nolan, W., & Pelam, W. E. (1992). *Swanson Nolan and Pelam Rating Scale Revised (SNAP-IV-R)* (4th ed.). Irvine, CA: Sage.

Tallal, P. (2004). Improving language and literacy is a matter of time. *Nature Reviews Neuroscience, 5,* 721–728.

Tallal, P., Miller, S., & Fitch, R. H. (1993). Neurobiological basis of speech: A case for the preeminence of temporal processing. *Annals of the New York Academy of Sciences, 682,* 27–47.

Tallal, P., & Piercy, M. (1973). Defects of nonverbal auditory perception in children with developmental aphasia. *Nature, 241,* 468–469.

Tazeau, Y. N., & Hamaguchi, P. M. (2013). Disorders and deficits that co-occur or look like APD. In D. Geffner & D. Swain (Eds.), *Auditory processing disorder: Assessment, management, and treatment* (pp. 91–116). San Diego, CA: Plural.

Thomson, J. M., Cheah, V., & Goswami, U. (2012). *Auditory processing intervention for school-age children with developmental dyslexia: A comparison of speech and non-*

speech approaches. Boston, MA: Harvard University.

Thomson, J. M., Leong, V., & Goswami, U. (2012). *Auditory processing intervention and developmental dyslexia: A comparison of phonemic and rhythmic approaches.* Reading and Writing, 1–23. Netherlands: Springer.

Tinius, T. P. (2003). The integrated visual and auditory continuous performance test as a neuropsychological measure. *Archives of Clinical Neuropsychology, 18,* 439–454.

Troia, G. (2003). Auditory perceptual impairments and learning disabilities: Theoretical and empirical considerations. *Learning Disabilities: A Contemporary Journal, 1,* 27–37.

Ullman, R. K., Sleator, E. K., & Sprague, R. L. (1988). *ADD-H Comprehensive Teacher's Rating Scale* and *Parent Form: ACTeRS.* Torrance, CA: Western Psychological Service.

Wagner, R. K., Torgesen, J. K., & Rashotte, C. A. (1999). *Comprehensive Test of Phonological Processing.* Austin, TX: Pro-Ed.

Wallace, G., & Hammill, D. D. (2002). *Comprehensive Receptive and Expressive Vocabulary Test–Second edition.* Austin, TX: Pro-Ed.

Wallach, G. P. (2008). *Language intervention for school-age students: Setting goals for academic success.* St. Louis, MO: Mosby.

Wentworth, C. (2009). Auditory working memory—what is it, and why is it so important? *Ezine Articles.* Retrieved from http://EzineArticles.com/?expert=Carlene _Wentworth

Wiig, E. H., & Secord, W. (1989). *Test of language competence—expanded edition.* San Antonio, TX: Psychological Corporation.

Witton, C. (2010). Childhood auditory processing disorder as a developmental disorder: The case for a multi-professional approach to diagnosis and management. *International Journal of Audiology, 49,* 83–87.

Yeatman, J. D., Ben-Shachar, M., Glover, G. H., & Feldman, H. M. (2010). Individual differences in auditory sentence comprehension in children: An exploratory event-related functional magnetic resonance imaging investigation. *Brain and language, 114,* 72–79.

Ziegler, J., & Goswami, U. (2005). Reading acquisition, developmental dyslexia, and skilled reading across languages: A psycholinguistic grain size theory. *Psychological Bulletin, 131,* 3–29.

CHAPTER 18

CENTRAL AUDITORY PROCESSING DISORDER AND ATTENTION DEFICIT HYPERACTIVITY DISORDER

A Neuropsychological Perspective

ART MAERLENDER AND LINDSAY HEATH

Introduction

Central auditory processing disorder (CAPD) is defined as "a deficit in the perceptual processing of auditory processing in the central nervous system and the neurobiological activity underlying that process" (ASHA, 2005). This disorder is thought to disrupt the continuous auditory processing of acoustic, phonetic and linguistic information; however, little is known about this symptom cluster from a neuropsychological perspective as neuropsychology as a discipline is largely absent from CAPD research (Bailey, 2010). In children, this disruption has been associated with a variety of functional problems, including difficulties with selective attention,

temporal processing problems, auditory memory, and sound blending (Jerger & Musiek, 2000). In addition, the relationship between auditory-sensory deficits and other known clinical and psychiatric disorders is being identified in schizophrenia, (Iliadou & Iakovides, 2003), Alzheimer's disease (Idrizbegovic et al., 2011), and traumatic brain injury (Fausti, Wilmington, Gallun, Myers, & Henry, 2009). (The reader is directed to Chapter 16 in this volume and Chapter 23 of Volume 1 of the Handbook for discussion of central auditory processing deficits in patients with schizophrenia and other psychiatric disorders.) For example, two studies examining the comorbidity of CAPD and attention deficit hyperactivity disorder (ADHD) demonstrated substantial overlap of clinical profiles, but independence of diagnoses (Chermak, 1996; Riccio, Hynd, Cohen, Hall, & Molt, 1994), possibly because the same etiological factors can affect multiple developmental pathways (Bishop, 2006). Little follow-up work has been completed.

Research to bridge the gap between audiology and psychology has been limited, making it difficult for psychologists to incorporate the putative CAPD construct into their own theoretical frameworks. Because there is overlap in symptoms in ADHD and CAPD, this is a point at which clinical audiology and clinical behavioral neurosciences appear to intersect. Thus, ADHD is an appropriate clinical entity to study in regards to relationships between these disciplines and their different ways of understanding. In this chapter we discuss the clinical entity of ADHD from neurological and behavioral perspectives and then report on studies from our clinical neuropsychology laboratory assessing CAPD from a neuropsychological perspective. Specific inquiry into the relationship between CAPD and ADHD is reported. That work has been previously published (Maerlender, Isquith, & Wallis, 2004; Maerlender, 2005). The literature on ADHD is quite extensive. The discussion presented here is an attempt to synthesize some of the important work that has been done in this area, but it is by no means complete.

The Diagnostic Construct of ADHD

ADHD is a well-characterized, and relatively common behavior disorder of development (American Psychiatric Association, 2013). However, controversies about its diagnostic consistency (i.e., purity) remain. The name of the disorder suggests that it is primarily related to attentional functioning. Because of the similarity in symptom presentation between ADHD and traumatic brain injured patients, a relationship with executive functioning (EF) has long been posited (EF representing those behaviors necessary for planning and carrying out complex behaviors; Barkley, 1997). Willcutt et al. (2005) challenged the idea that EF is a core construct of ADHD because of the moderate effect sizes of EF measures in explaining symptoms of ADHD, and in part because of the typical failure to control for covariates such as IQ and reading ability. However, a good deal of literature confirms that a relationship exists (e.g., see Weyandt, 2005). In fact, one study concluded that many children with ADHD are primarily characterized by executive function weaknesses (Lambek et al., 2010).

Over the past two decades there have been many community-based studies offering estimates of prevalence of ADHD ranging from 2% to 17% (Scahill & Schwab-Stone, 2000). The dramatic differences in these estimates are due to the choice of informant, methods of sampling and data collection, and the diagnostic definition. One review of 303 study articles from several countries reported a worldwide pooled ADHD prevalence of 5.29% (Polancyk et al., 2007). Based on review and the 19 studies reviewed by Scahill, the best estimate of prevalence of ADHD is 5% to 10% in school-aged children.

As a diagnostic category, current conceptualization of ADHD (Diagnostic and Statistical Manual of Mental Disorders [DSM-5]) identifies three primary subtypes (American Psychiatric Association, 2013): symptoms of inattentive behaviors (including difficulty sustaining attention in tasks or play activities, and not seeming to listen when spoken to directly);

hyperactive-impulsive behaviors (excessive motor behaviors, fidgeting and difficulty sitting still), and a combined type. A "sluggish-cognitive tempo" type has also been discussed as a specific subtype of the inattentive type (Hartman, Willcutt, Rhee, & Pennington, 2004). This research subtype is thought to include symptoms of daydreaming, a tendency to become confused, a lack of mental alertness, and physical hypoactivity, though it is not currently a clinically valid diagnostic type.

Besides the presence of specific symptom clusters, other qualitative factors must be documented to diagnose ADHD. Some of the symptoms must be present before the age of 12 in a manner that is inconsistent with normal development. There must be clear indication that the symptoms cause functional impairment; the symptoms must cause impairment across settings in order to rule out the effect of specific environments or demands. The symptoms must also not be better explained by other developmental or psychiatric disorders, such as autism, anxiety or a dissociative disorder (American Psychiatric Association, 2013). While specific neuropsychological tests have been shown to differentiate ADHD from normal controls (Hale, Hoeppner, & Fiorello, 2002; Kelly, 2000; Lovejoy et al., 1999), the clinical diagnosis of ADHD does not require such testing. In fact, the current practice parameter for the assessment and treatment of ADHD states that neuropsychological testing is not mandatory in the diagnosis of ADHD, but may be considered if low general intellectual ability or low academic achievement relative to intellectual ability is suspected (AACAP, 2007). The current standard for diagnosis rests on functional behaviors (across settings) and identified history of problems (to establish the developmental nature of the behaviors).

In addition, the subtyping of ADHD is still open to question. In fact, one of the major questions during the revision of the DSM-5 was how to handle the subtyping of ADHD (Nigg, Tannock, & Rohde, 2010). A major question concerned whether the heterogeneity in presentation of ADHD warrants distinct subtypes and whether this distinction is clinically useful. Though there is a great deal of evidence in support of a distinction between an inattentive-disorganized profile and a hyperactive-impulsive profile (Willcutt et al., 2010), findings related to the differentiation between subtypes have been variable. It has also been noted that subtype presentation does not appear to be stable over time as a child with ADHD may appear primarily inattentive at one point in time and primarily hyperactive at another (Todd et al., 2008). The DSM-5 maintained the ADHD subtyping of the earlier DSM-IV (American Psychiatric Association, 2013).

Nigg (2005) asserts that the issue of heterogeneity of presentation has not been adequately studied, and that most of the neuropsychological literature is focused on the combined subtype (ADHD-combined) that includes symptoms of both inattention and hyperactivity-impulsivity. His study in 2002 (Nigg, Blaskey, Huang-Pollack, & Rappley) assessed 46 children aged 7 to 12 with diagnoses of ADHD-C (Combined type), and 18 children with ADHD-I (Inattentive type) and compared them to 41 community control children. Few differences were found between the ADHD-C and ADHD-I groups and the authors concluded that ADHD-I shared neuropsychological deficits with ADHD-C in the domain of output speed, although boys with ADHD-C differed from boys with ADHD-I in motor inhibition (ADHD-

C being more disinhibited). There was no difference between the girls in this study.

The findings of Nigg et al. (2002) were generally consistent with an earlier study by Chhabildas, Pennington, and Willcutt (2001), who also did not find different neuropsychological profiles in a large sample of children with inattentive, hyperactive-impulsive or combined subtypes of ADHD as compared with controls. That study compared the neuropsychological profiles of children without ADHD (n = 82) and children who met symptom criteria for DSM-IV Predominantly Inattentive subtype (ADHD-I; n = 67), Predominantly hyperactive-impulsive subtype (ADHD-HI; n = 14), and combined subtype (ADHD-C; n = 33) in the areas of processing speed, vigilance, and inhibition. Contrary to their prediction, symptoms of inattention best predicted performance on all dependent measures, and children with ADHD-I and ADHD-C had similar impairment profiles. Children with ADHD-HI were not significantly impaired on any of the dependent measures once subclinical symptoms of inattention were controlled.

The difficulty differentiating ADHD-C and ADHD-I was further explored by Lemiere and colleagues in 2010 (Lemiere et al., 2010). That study utilized laboratory measures, including the Test of Everyday Attention for Children (Heaton, 2010) in order to determine whether such measures could differentiate between the two subtypes. Very few differences between subtypes were noted across tasks, particularly when IQ and age were controlled. Therefore, the authors concluded that the distinction between ADHD-C and ADHD-I is of little value in predicting deficits in everyday attention, as reflected in this set of tests.

Despite the questionable validity, diagnostic nomenclature continues to specify these subtypes in clinical practice. Further, both Clarke, Barry, McCarthy, and Selikowitz (2002) and Stewart, Steffler, Lemoine, and Leps (2001) have provided evidence that both ADHD-C and ADHD-I share similar EEG profiles that are indicative of hypoarousal. Thus, while accepted in clinical practice, the diagnostic descriptions of ADHD and the specificity of its subtypes remain a point of some discussion.

The Neurobiology of ADHD

Although the pathophysiology of ADHD is not completely understood, ADHD is thought to be due to dysfunctional catecholamine neurotransmission (especially norepinephrine and dopamine) in several key brain regions. Catecholamines are involved in attention, various aspects of inhibition and response in the motor system, motivated behaviors, reward systems, and spatial working memory functions (Arnsten, Steere, & Hunt, 1996; Calderon-Gonzalez, 1993). The catecholamines norepinephrine and dopamine are involved in attention-deficit disorders (Himelstein, Newcorn, & Halperin, 2000). Both neurotransmitter systems modulate the transfer of information through different regions of the brain, including the thalamus, prefrontal cortex (PFC), and basal ganglia (Russell, 2002).

Converging evidence from studies of the neuropharmacology, genetics, neuropsychology, and neuroimaging of ADHD imply the involvement of frontostriatal circuitry in ADHD (Durston, 2003; Durston et al., 2003; Sowell et al., 2003;

Tannock, 1998). Although a significant amount of progress has been made investigating the neurobiology of this disorder, its precise etiology still remains unclear. However, although it does appear that poor inhibitory control and the deficits in frontostriatal circuitry associated with it are central to the expression of ADHD, there is evidence to suggest that more posterior cerebral areas are also implicated in this disorder (Castellanos et al., 2002). Anatomical studies suggest widespread reductions in volume throughout the cerebrum and cerebellum. Functional imaging studies suggest that affected individuals activate more diffuse areas than controls during the performance of cognitive tasks (Durston et al., 2003) and differences in the activation of the caudate, frontal lobes, and anterior cingulate have been observed in children with ADHD while completing tasks requiring inhibitory control (Bush et al., 2005).

Quantitative electroencephalogram (qEEG) studies have supported much of the imaging research, and have also identified subcortical structures involved in ADHD, including hippocampal involvement and thalamo-cortico circuits (Chabot et al., 1999). The latter circuits are involved with cognitive control, and thus are important in understanding the neurobiology of ADHD (Luu & Tucker, 2003).

Correlating clinical conditions with cognitive deficits of attention has been a long-standing area of difficulty for researchers. Imaging studies of brain anomalies in ADHD have shed considerable light on the biological bases of ADHD. To be sure, functional differences between ADHD groups and control subjects have been demonstrated, both with functional and structural magnetic resonance imaging (MRI). The link between

response inhibition and frontal lobe functioning in children with ADHD has been well documented in many recent studies (for examples, see Casey et al., 1997, Castellanos et al., 2002; Durston et al., 2003; Rubia et al., 2001; Rubia, Smith, Brammer, Toone, & Taylor, 2005; Schulz et al., 2004; Vaidya et al., 1998; Vaidya et al., 2005). For instance, differential activation of regions such as right frontal lobe and caudate nucleus has been documented (Rubia et al., 2001; Vaidya et al., 2005). Rubia combined specific motor timing and inhibition tasks with fMRI, comparing ADHD and psychiatric control children. They noted that "(t)he impairments in hyperactive children were thus specific to the more demanding inhibition tasks requiring inhibition of discrete motor responses and were not due to generalized impairments in the interruption of automatic activities nor motor timing" (p. 141).

Although the bulk of focus in the attention literature has been on the fronto-striatal circuits, other brain structures have been identified as important in the process of attention. Mirsky et al. (1997) identified brainstem regions (i.e., the mesopontine brainstem reticular formation), as well as other subcortical midline brain regions (i.e., midline thalamus, and reticular nuclei of the thalamus) as critical for sustaining attentional focus. Mirsky asserted that "all patients whose symptoms include disturbances in vigilance or sustained attention, no matter what the diagnosis, share some pathological involvement or disturbance in this corticoreticular system. This would include persons with the diagnosis of ADHD" (Mirsky et al., 1999, p. 171). The brainstem region of the locus coeruleus is known to be the origin of seratonergic neurons, which are closely linked to dopaminergic neurons. Arnsten et al. (1996) argued that diminished brainstem norepinepherine activity and release caused a partial denervation of postsynaptic alpha-2 receptors in the PFC, which in turn disrupts the inhibitory control functions of the PFC. This then produces the deficits in behavioral inhibition characteristic of children with ADHD. Thus, neurophysiological mechanisms originating in the brainstem are also important contributors to the attentional process.

There seems to be agreement that ADHD is characterized by slightly smaller brain volume, involving both gray and white matter (about 4% total brain volume reduction) (Durston, 2003). However, regional enlargements have also been identified. Both Swanson and colleagues (2004) and Durston and colleagues (2003) have identified occipital lobe size increases that are in conjunction with reduced frontal lobe sizes. Sowell and colleagues (2003) found decreased frontal and temporal lobe volume in children with ADHD relative to controls.

As noted, the striatum has been implicated in many studies. The striatum is a part of the basal ganglia, which is a group of neurons in the basal forebrain with rich connections to the premotor frontal areas. These neurons are involved with the modulation of movement, including the force of movement (Parent & Hazrati, 1995; Teicher et al., 2000). In addition, there appears to be a 15% decrease in the size of the posterior cerebellum (Castellanos et al., 2002). The cerebellum also is involved in motor movements; specifically, it appears to be involved in the acquisition and maintenance of motor skills. One function of the cerebellum appears to involve a timing mechanism. Another is for making adjustments to keep movements accu-

rate. Error correction and feedback to the cortex are critical. These structural abnormalities in ADHD do not appear to progress with age. Thus, it is not a degenerative disorder, and some level of accommodative abilities can be obtained (Castellanos et al., 2002).

Sowell and colleagues (2003) observed significant differences in brain structure in the bilateral frontal cortexes of brains of children with ADHD relative to normal children, with reduced regional brain size mainly confined to small areas of the dorsal prefrontal cortexes. Reduced brain size in anterior temporal areas, bilaterally, were also noted in the children with ADHD. In addition, substantial increases were noted in the volume of gray matter in large areas of the posterior temporal and inferior parietal cortexes of children with ADHD, compared with children in the control group. The increased presence of gray matter suggests a decrease in white matter, or connective tissue. There was a statistical trend toward total white matter reduction. These more specific findings indicated smaller and hypofunctional lateral prefrontal cortexes in children with ADHD. The Sowell study (2003) found no differences between boys and girls, although other studies have shown such differences. Durston and colleagues found somewhat similar differences when comparing boys with ADHD and their unaffected siblings (2004).

Given the etiological theories suggesting that ADHD involves a deficit in corticostriatal circuits, particularly circuits modulated by dopamine, Teicher and colleagues (2000) devised a series of functional magnetic resonance imaging (fMRI) experiments to test the hypothesis that the activity of the putamen was related to ADHD symptoms. The putamen is rich in dopaminergic neurons. In their functional imaging studies of ADHD and normal boys, there was significant evidence for deficit in boys with ADHD. In addition, the physiological findings were strongly correlated with the child's capacity to sit still and his accuracy in accomplishing a computerized attention task. They concluded that ADHD symptoms may be closely tied to functional abnormalities in the putamen, which is mainly involved in the regulation of motor behavior.

Willis and Weiler (2005) reviewed the literature on electroencephalography (EEG) and MRI findings in children with ADHD. They concluded that collectively, studies support theories implicating frontal-striatal cortical networks. Unfortunately, they note, these physiological procedures have not yet reached a point where diagnostic utility can be provided.

In addition, a genetic component to ADHD has long been noted. Twin and family studies of ADHD have shown substantial genetic heritability with little or no family environmental effect. Linkage and association studies have consistently implicated the dopamine transporter gene (DAT1: Sharp, McQuillan, & McHugh, 2009). Dopamine and serotonin transporters, as well as the D4 and D5 receptors have also been implicated. (Bobb, Castellanos, Addington, & Rapaport, 2005). However, although twin studies have demonstrated that ADHD is a highly heritable condition, molecular genetic studies point to significant complexity in the genetic architecture of ADHD. Genome-wide scans have provided divergent findings. In contrast, many candidate gene studies have implicated several additional genes in the etiology of the disorder. DRD4, DRD5, DAT, DBH, 5-HTT, HTR1B, and SNAP-25 have also been associated with ADHD, with odds ratios ranging from 1.18 to 1.46. These small odds ratios suggest that the genetic vulnerability to ADHD is mediated by several genes of small effect (Farone et al., 2005).

Thus, a genetic predisposition is well-established as one factor in the etiology of ADHD.

In summary, general consensus about the neurobiology of ADHD appears to include the following: (1) specific regions of the brain that are high in dopamine reception density are smaller in ADHD groups than control groups; (2) there appears to be a frontal-posterior dimension of difference, with ADHD groups having smaller frontal lobes and larger posterior structures (i.e., occipital lobes); and (3) areas that are necessary for the coordination and timing of activities from multiple brain regions have smaller subregions in ADHD groups (i.e., the corpus callosum, cerebellum; Swanson et al., 2004). Pacing of electrical activity (especially theta) implicates hippocampal nuclei, whereas generation of alpha activity suggests thalamic nuclei involvement (Luu & Ticker, 2003). Although a genetic link to ADHD has been established (Bobb et al., 2005; Sharp, McQuillan, & MacHugh, 2009), the precise genetic mechanisms have not been worked out; clearly, dopamine receptors appear to play a role.

ADHD, Attention, and Executive Function

Attention

One of the difficulties in discussing ADHD has been the tendency to conflate the clinical manifestations of the

DSM-IV diagnostic category of ADHD with the cognitive concepts of attention (Swanson et al., 2004). It seems logical that ADHD should be about attention. From a cognitive perspective, attention is a complex neurological phenomenon involving multiple coordinated pathways and structures (e.g., Posner & Peterson, 1990; Posner & Rothbart, 1998). Posner described orienting, alerting, focusing and shifting as key components. Posner's studies demonstrated cortical networks that underlie these functions, which include dorsal parietal, subcortical, and frontal networks.

The term executive function (EF) refers to a collection of inter-related functions that are responsible for purposeful activity that is goal-directed and typically involves some level of problem-solving. EF was originally defined by Luria (1973) as those functions that are involved in the planning, regulation, and verification of an action. Stuss and Benson (1986) described EF as a directive, control-type mechanism that included anticipation, goal selection, planning, monitoring and use of feedback. It has also been described as the set of neurocognitive processes that maintain an appropriate problem-solving set in order to successfully attain future goals (Willcutt et al., 2005). Some of the cognitive abilities included in this domain are self-regulation, set maintenance, response organization and cognitive flexibility (Gioia, Isquith, Guy, & Kenworthy, 2001). However, this term is problematic: Pennington and Ozonoff (1966) stated that the term EF is "provisional and under-specified" (p. 55). Results of studies vary as to the specific measures used, and the operationalization of the term (see for example, Fletcher, 1996). Nevertheless, the term EF enjoys widespread clinical use.

One difficulty in describing "attention" from a sensory perspective is the complexity of attentional processing. As described by Posner (Posner & Peterson, 1990; Posner & Rothbart, 1998), attention is a process and not a site-specific activity. The process of attention serves to connect the individual to the immediate world, with obvious survival (and likely evolutionary) value. The process includes some sort of monitoring or scanning of the environment (awareness), focusing on target stimuli, appropriately processing the information provided, disengaging or shifting to other relevant stimuli (but not irrelevant stimuli), all the while maintaining sufficient cortical arousal to process the information (Posner & Peterson, 1990; Posner & Rothbart, 1998). Much of this process has been well identified in the visual domain. It is noteworthy that only 2 of 32 chapters address audition or auditory processes in Posner's textbook, *The Cognitive Neuroscience of Attention* (2004). However, in clinical studies, temporal lobe processing has been implicated in attentional processing and ADHD (Kelly, 2000; Mirsky, Anthony, Duncan, Ahearn, & Kellem, 1991; Mirsky, Pascualvaca, Duncan, & French, 1999; Posner & Peterson, 1990). An encoding function has been included in these models, based on performance on the auditory Digit Span task (Wechsler Intelligence Scale for Children [Wechsler, 1991] and Wechsler Adult Intelligence Scales [Wechsler, 1981]).

Attention also is a complex process. (Posner refers to it as an "organ system" [2004, p. 3]). Constructs such as "selective" attention and "divided" attention have been well described in the experimental literature (see, for example, Corbetta, Miezin, Dobmeyer, Shulman, & Petersen, 1991; Craik, Govoni, Naveh-

Benjamin, & Anderson, 1996; Luck & Ford, 1998).

Tzourio et al. (1997) confirmed the activation of temporal lobes in a series of selective attention experiments using neuroimaging (positron emission tomography [PET]) and event-related potentials (ERPs). Based on subjects listening to various tonal frequencies, they documented activation in Heschl's gyri and planum temporal cortical areas bilaterally when compared to a resting baseline, with a right > left asymmetry noted. When deviations in stimuli were presented, frontal activation was observed. They concluded that two major networks seemed to be involved during selective auditory attention: a local temporal lobe network, and a frontal network that could mediate the temporal cortex modulation by attention.

Näätänen and colleagues presented data to support the theory that there are two types of selective attention processes in audition (for review, see Näätänen & Ahlo, 2004). One aspect is associated with a "course" selection of sounds (e.g., right versus left and no further discrimination) when stimulus rates are high and focused attention is strong; one process is more similar to the processing of unattended sounds that selects sounds at lower stimulus rates. Selected sounds are gradually matched to what is termed the "attentional trace." This trace is actively maintained in cortical representation. Mismatched sounds are rejected, while matched sounds generate enhanced cortical activity. This attentional trace is formed in the auditory cortex and is composed of actively rehearsed sensory-memory representations. Näätänen and Ahlo (2004) argued that a later response identified in the frontal lobes is generated by the active rehearsal of the attentional trace after each occurrence of an attended sound . Thus, the frontal lobes have an active role in maintaining selective auditory attention.

In studies of lesioned patients, Zatorre and Penhume (2001) concluded that contrary to hypotheses derived from animal studies, human auditory spatial processes are dependent primarily on cortical areas within the right superior temporal cortex. Later experiments on normal adults described activation of posterior temporal lobes and inferior parietal lobes in the auditory identification of spatial cues (Zatorre, Bouffard, Ahad, & Belin, 2002). Thus, the temporal lobe network seems critical for various attentional processes in the auditory modality.

The Neuropsychology of ADHD and Executive Functions

The neuropsychological study of ADHD has been based on the neurological findings, and particularly the work of Posner (Posner & Peterson, 1990; Posner & Rothbart, 1998) and Mirsky and colleagues (1991, 1999). Barkley's description of the role of executive functioning as a hallmark of ADHD has further informed neuropsychology and has led to a great deal of research related to the relationship between ADHD and executive functions. A notable meta-analysis that included 83 studies with a combined total of over 6000 participants found that participants with ADHD demonstrated several executive functioning deficits, including impairments in response inhibition, vigilance, working memory, and planning (Willcutt et al., 2005). Neuropsychological test findings support anatomical and behavioral conclusions, for both attentional and EF deficits, although the specification of diverse sensory processes is still quite crude (see Kelly, 2000, and Perugini, Harvey, Lovejoy, Sanstron, & Webb, 2000). Although diagnostic requirements do not include neuropsychological testing, neuropsychological tests have shown considerable sensitivity to attentional and executive functioning processes (Kelly, 2000; Lovejoy et al., 1999; Muir-Broaddus, Rosenstein, Medinaa, & Soderberg, 2002; Perugini, Harvey, Lovejoy Sanstron, & Webb, 2000).

Mirsky's group (1991, 1999) developed a general neuropsychological model for conceptualizing the components of attention. Neuropsychological test scores obtained from two samples, the first consisting of 203 adult neuropsychiatric patients and normal control subjects, and the second, an epidemiologically based sample of 435 elementary school children, were submitted to a principal components analyses. Each sample yielded similar results with a set of independent elements of attention assayed by different tests. Based on their studies, they proposed a taxonomy of attentive functions that included functions labeled focus, execute, sustain and stabilize, shift, and encode. This taxonomy was based, in part, on the results of a factor analysis of their neuropsychological test data. The tests selected were thought to be especially sensitive to the effects of poor attention. Relevant to our discussion below, the Mirsky group found that variability of reaction time (RT) for the auditory continuous performance test (CPT) (assessing the stabilize function) differentiated the ADHD sample from controls, whereas the Digit Span (reflecting the encode function) did not differentiate groups.

Kelly (2000) submitted neuropsychological results to a factor analysis from a series of 100 children diagnosed with ADHD. He obtained very similar results to Mirsky et al. (1991), with the exception of a factor reflecting impulsivity. Kelly labeled his factors information processing, impulsivity, and sustaining and shifting. Information processing reflected a speed of processing factor that used primarily visual tests, all with time elements. Impulsivity reflected errors made on some of the timed tests; sustaining reflected visual vigilance over time, whereas shifting reflected cognitive flexibility.

Nigg, Blaskey, Huang-Pollack, and Rappley (2002) attempted to differentiate children with DSM-IV attention-deficit/hyperactivity disorder combined (ADHD-C) and inattentive (ADHD-I) subtypes. They administered a battery of neuropsychological tests of EF to 64 boys and girls with ADHD compared to 41 community controls. Both subtypes had deficits on output speed, with one motor response inhibition test differentiating ADHD-C boys from ADHD-I boys. In general, the ADHD-C group demonstrated a deficit in planning. Neither ADHD group had a deficit in interference control per se, although they were slower than controls on one speeded task. Nigg et al. (2002) concluded that children with ADHD-I shared neuropsychological deficits with children with ADHD-C in the domain of output speed; however, in most domains the subtypes did not differ.

Weyandt and Willis (1995) were able to classify 77% of a sample of 115 children using a battery of executive and nonexecutive function tests. Children were identified as either ADHD, developmental language disorder, or nondisabled. Children with ADHD demonstrated significant differences in executive functions relative to the normal controls, but nonexecutive tasks did not differentiate these groups. Only two executive tasks were more impaired in the ADHD group: a visual search and impulse control task, and a planning task. No difference between children with ADHD and language disorder were found on these tests. However, the ADHD group performed more poorly on a maze finding test.

Perugini et al. (2000) compared 21 boys with hyperactive-impulsive or combined types of ADHD to 22 normal controls using a battery of neuropsychological tests (many the same as in the Mirsky and Kelly batteries). Only a visual CPT accurately differentiated the two groups, although a visual speeded sequencing test and the Digit Span test were also sensitive to ADHD. Sensitivity of the CPT was moderate (.62) but strongly specific (.91). These outcomes are somewhat different from other studies of CPTs in that sensitivity is usually higher in the other studies.

Sergeant, Guertz, and Oosterlaan (2002) reviewed tests of EF across several psychiatric disorders including ADHD, oppositional defiant disorder, conduct disorder, higher functioning autism and Tourette syndrome. They noted some specificity of tests for ADHD relative to the other disorders, particularly those requiring behavioral inhibition. Another study by Lambek and associates (2011) that compared a clinical sample of children diagnosed with ADHD and a population sample on a battery of eight EF measures found that, as a group, children with ADHD were significantly more impaired on those measures than children without ADHD. Approximately half of the children with ADHD included in the sample had EF deficits at the individual level.

Although most neuropsychological studies of attention/ADHD in research and clinical practice involve visual CPTs, one exception was a study by Benedict et al. (1998). They were able to adapt a CPT for auditory assessment to be obtained concurrent with fMRI imaging. They also acquired positron emission tomography (PET) scans to corroborate activation patterns. Scans were acquired in normal young adults. They demonstrated that simple attention caused a large region of activation involving the anterior cingulate gyrus and the right anterior/mesial frontal lobe. There were few differences between focused and divided attention. The findings were felt to be consistent with activation of an anterior attention network during auditory attention, without involvement of posterior attention structures. Mirsky et al. (1999) also obtained evidence that the variability of response time to an auditory CPT stimulus differentiated ADHD children from controls.

Barkley and others have noted that the cognitive correlates of ADHD are principally accounted for by deficits in EF (Anderson, 2002; see also Barkley, 1997). The anterior regions of the brain are thought to mediate executive functions. Deficits in EF often follow damage to prefrontal regions (e.g., Stuss & Benson, 1986). Imaging studies have supported these expectations, documenting prefrontal activation in this region while individuals perform EF tasks (e.g., Baker et al., 1996; Morris, Ahmed, Syed, & Toone, 1993).

Significant protective and proactive functionality is associated with well-functioning attentional networks. Barkley's (1997) influential summary and theoretical formulation of ADHD described a model that linked inhibition to executive neuropsychological functions. The four functions identified were: (a) working memory, (b) self-regulation of affect-motivation-arousal, (c) internalization of speech, and (d) reconstitution (behavioral analysis and synthesis).

As discussed previously, response inhibition is seen as a functional hallmark of ADHD. From a neuropsychological perspective, significant findings of (response) inhibitory dyscontrol in children with ADHD-C were noted by Gioia using an executive function rating scale (Gioia et al. 2002). Muir-Broaddus et al. (2002) confirmed findings of EF difficulties on a sample of students with ADHD. Tests of attention span, sustained attention, response inhibition, and working memory were low relative to normative standards. These tests implicated fronto-executive functioning, as well as subcortical functioning relative to the free recall of verbal information. In addition, higher levels of inattention or hyperactivity as assessed from parent reports were associated with poorer performance on neuropsychological tests.

As these dominant neuropsychological theories of ADHD have focused on cognitive impairments associated with deficits in executive functions such as inhibitory control (Nigg, 2005) and working memory (Rapport et al., 2008), they are postulated to be grounded in altered fronto-striatal neural circuits modulated by catecholamine-based neurotransmitters (Arnsten, 2009). However, it seems unlikely that such deficits mediate the link between ADHD and its underlying causes (i.e., genes and environments; Nigg et al., 2005) in any straightforward way (Castellanos et al., 2006). For instance, many children with ADHD appear not to have dysfunctional executive processes, whereas many children without ADHD, either with other disorders or with no disorder at all, do (Willcutt et al., 2005). Even where ADHD and executive dysfunction co-present, the pattern is rather fragmented and variable so that pervasive and severe executive deficit appears quite rare (Nigg et al., 2005).

Typically, executive dysfunction in ADHD is characterized as a fixed, core cognitive deficit that is largely context and state independent (Sonuga-Barke, 1994); however, this is probably an inaccurate characterization. Executive functions are themselves dynamic processes and performance on executive tasks will fluctuate from state-to-state and setting-to-setting (Nigg & Casey, 2005). In keeping with this, context has been shown to play an important role in determining the extent to which performance on executive tasks is deficient in ADHD (cf. Shiels et al., 2008; but see also Shanahan et al., 2008). An alternative class of theoretical constructs has also been used to explain neuropsychological impairment in ADHD. These emphasize the dynamic nature of ADHD and cognitive and performance deficits (Castellanos et al., 2006). As noted by Sonuga-Barke et al. (2010), these may be secondary effects of failures of more deep-seated motivational or energetic systems and processes. Two constructs of this type are delay aversion (DAv), which is described as a preference for small-immediate over large-delayed rewards (Sonuga-Barke et al., 1994) and state regulation (SR), which refers to the impact of reward on performance (van der Meere & Sergeant, 1988). Although a complete explication of the theoretical and empirical evidence for these constructs is not possible here, they are important in that they move ADHD from a strict structural deficit model, to a dynamic model in which structural deficits are manifest in variable outcomes, depending on specific state factors. These two constructs may not be separate, and may represent the same processes from different points of view (experimental paradigms). DAv is postulated to be a function of alterations in the dopamine modulated reward circuits of the brain implicating regions such as orbitofrontal cortex and the ventral striatum (Sonuga-Barke, 2003). It is driven by fundamental neuro-biological alterations in the efficiency with which future rewards are signaled by dopamine within brain reward circuits, which leads to an impulsive drive for immediate reinforcement. SR, on the other hand, has a primary focus on the energetic state of the child with ADHD and they have as their primary goal the explanation of state-specific and context dependent aspects of cognitive performance deficits. In a general sense the SR model of ADHD deficits sees these as being due to failures to properly regulate energy state (arousal/activation) when challenged to do so in suboptimal settings or states.

In summary, although there are difficulties in the definition of ADHD and in operationalizing the constructs of attention and executive functions, there is a large body of literature that implicates poor inhibitory control as a hallmark of ADHD. Inhibitory control is one function of the executive system that is necessary for managing attention and sensory input.

The Relationship of ADHD to CAPD: Empirical Findings

The question of CAPD and ADHD comorbidity has received considerable attention (Chermak, Hall, & Musiek, 1999; Chermak, Somers, & Seikel, 1998; Chermak, Tucker, & Seikel, 2002; Keller & Tillery, 2002; Moss & Sheiffele, 1994; Riccio et al., 1994). In these studies, ADHD was associated with more global disruption of sensory information processing, while CAPD was only associated with disruption of auditory information processing. In fact, one recent study demonstrated that auditory tests alone appear sufficient to differentiate CAPD from supramodal disorders such as ADHD (Bellis, Billiet, & Ross, 2011). This study found that although groups of children with CAPD and ADHD each performed poorer on auditory tasks then a group of healthy controls, intratest comparisons differentiated the CAPD group from the ADHD and healthy control groups. That is, children with CAPD demonstrated a significantly greater humming-labeling differential on a frequency patterns task and a greater right ear advantage on the dichotic digits task. The differentiation has also been based on the observation that not all children with ADHD demonstrate auditory difficulties (Chermak et al., 1999). It should also be noted that ADHD subtype does not appear to be a predictor of auditory dysfunction in children with ADHD (Ghanizadeh, 2009). See Chapter 20 in Volume 1 of the Handbook for discussion of the differential diagnosis of CAPD and ADHD.

Riccio, Cohen, Garrison, and Smith (2005) extended Riccio et al.'s earlier work (1994) to identify relationships between audiometric tests and neuropsychological tests and rating scales for attentional processes. Thirty-six children underwent a neuropsychological test battery and then audiometric testing for CAPD. Correlational analysis revealed only one significant correlation: between the right ear score of the Staggered Spondaic Word (SSW) test (Katz & Smith, 2006) and a memory for sentences test (Clinical Evaluation of Language Fundamentals, 3rd edition, Sentence Repetition)

(Semel, Wiig, & Secord, 1995). They concluded that auditory measures tap some element of auditory memory, and that CAPD and ADHD may be overlapping, but independent disorders. In addition, it appears likely that performance on auditory measures of attention may be poor in a child with undiagnosed CAPD as these tasks are dependent on the auditory processing of the stimulus; therefore, a recent review has suggested that neuropsychologists may best serve their patients if a screening for CAPD is employed to rule out this confounding issue (Bailey, 2010).

In an effort to further explore the differentiation of CAPD and ADHD, Tillery, Katz and Keller (2000) attempted to assess the effects of stimulant medication on 32 children diagnosed with both CAPD and ADHD (though it should be noted that the diagnostic practices for each of these disorders were different at that time from current standards). In a double-blind, placebo-controlled study, they found no effects of methylphenidate on audiometric test scores, whereas scores on an auditory CPT did improve. It has been suggested that perhaps an underlying CAPD may explain why some children diagnosed with ADHD fail to respond to stimulant medications (Riccio, 2005).

The following sections describe results from our neuropsychological laboratory. We completed several studies using psychometric tests that are often used in the characterization of ADHD but that show specificity for identification of CAPD.

Auditory Short-Term Memory and Working Memory

Forward span capacity has a long history in psychology as a measure of auditory short-term, or immediate memory. Although there is much evidence demonstrating that forward and backward span performances and operations are correlated (Daneman & Merikle, 1996; Groeger, Field, & Hammond, 1999), the two span tasks are dissociable (Engle, Tuholski, Laughlin, & Conway, 1999). The forward span process is language related (Paulesu, Frith, & Frackoviak, 1993) and has been described as the "phonological loop" or "articulatory loop" (Baddeley, 1992). This loop theoretically maintains information in short-term or immediate memory store. The digits reversed or backward procedure requires additional processing demands to manipulate the information, scaffolding onto the forward process (Torgesen, 1996). Rudel and Denkla (1974) hypothesized that the digits forward procedure makes greater demands on auditory processes than does the reverse procedure. It was postulated that the reverse procedure utilizes other processing, such as visualization of the numbers.

The need to assess span tasks as separate cognitive functions has long been suggested (Kaplan, Fein, Morris, & Delis, 1991; Rudel & Denckla, 1974). Farrand and Jones (1996) experimentally demonstrated the involvement of different processes in forward versus backward digit recall across several modalities, noting that recall for digits in reverse order was significantly worse than in forward order in both spatial and verbal modalities. Groeger et al. (1999) examined processes underlying forward and reverse auditory, visual and motor span tasks. They found that forward and reverse span performances were highly correlated regardless of presentation modality. Although forward span performance was related to reverse span performance, only reverse span performance was strongly related to other factors, such as general intellectual ability and EF. Hale, Hoeppner, and Fiorello (2002) found that reverse digit span was substantially more predictive of attention and EF than forward digit span, and Reynolds (1997) demonstrated that forward and backward digit span tasks load onto separate factors. In addition to psychometrically based support for separating forward from backward span tasks, functional imaging studies have demonstrated different areas of activation for these tasks, with dorsolateral prefrontal activation obtained during backward span tasks but not for forward span tasks, suggesting greater working memory demand in the former (Larrabee & Kane, 1986).

On the surface, there is considerable overlap in functional demand between one of the most robust tests of CAPD (dichotic listening) and digit span tasks. Both are auditory tasks, frequently presenting numbers for stimuli, and relying on verbal confirmation of the stimuli. While there are significant differences in presentation between the two tasks, some element of short-term memory is required for both. However, the dichotic listening task (Dichotic Digits test; Musiek, 1983), often used in audiological evaluation for CAPD, requires a maximum span of four numbers presented within two seconds. Digit span tasks used in psychometric assessment typically increase the span length with each successful trial and typically present digits at a rate of 1 number per second. Thus, while similar, there are significant differences in processing demands between the two. Reverse digit span tasks likely place the greatest demand on function, requiring mental manipulation in working memory along with increasing reliance on span and on

verbal responses. See Chapter 14 of Volume I of the Handbook for discussion of dichotic listening tests.

Initial Findings

In the first series of studies, archival data of children diagnosed with CAPD was analyzed to demonstrate the relationship of Wechsler Intelligence Scale for Children, 3rd edition (WISC-III) Digit Span (Wechsler, 2004) to CAPD ($n = 74$; Maerlender et al, 2004). Mean Digit Span (DS) scores for children diagnosed with CAPD were compared with DS scores for children evaluated, but who did not meet criteria for diagnosis of CAPD. Analysis of variance revealed a significant difference between groups on DS scores, $F(1, 72) = 7.34, p = .008; \eta2 = 0.092$. Children diagnosed with CAPD had lower DS scores ($M = 7.81, SD = 2.86$) than children who did not meet diagnostic criteria ($M = 9.65, SD = 2.67$). Eighty-one percent (81%) of children with Digit Span scores below 7 (<16th percentile) had positive CAPD diagnoses, whereas only 40% of those not identified as CAPD had scaled scores below 7.

It appeared that poor performance on D S was a robust characteristic of children diagnosed with CAPD. Moreover, children with impaired performance on the Dichotic Digits (DD) test had lower scores on DS than children with normal DD performances, and DS scores were significantly worse for children with bilateral DD performance deficits than for those with only unilateral or no deficits.

A second study from that series analyzed DS and DD data from a cohort of children referred for neuropsychological evaluation ($n = 51$). In this study we did not have diagnostic results, so the independent factor was based on performance on the DD test (Pass Both ears, Fail Left ear; Fail Both ears). Z-scores for maximum forward digit span (DSFm) and maximum backward digit span (DSBm) were entered as dependent variables in a MANOVA with DD group as the between subjects factor. The multivariate test was significant, $F(2, 48) = 8.45$, $p = .001$, $\eta^2 = 0.27$. Examination of the univariate results revealed a significant difference between groups on both DSFm, $F(2, 48) = 6.78$, $p = .003$, $\eta^2 = 0.22$, and DSBm, $F(2, 48) = 3.63$, $p = .043$, $\eta^2 = 0.12$. Planned contrasts revealed a different pattern of performance on DSFm and DSBm by DD performance. For DSFm, both the Fail Both and Fail Left groups had significantly lower scores than the Pass Both group ($p < .01$). Although the Fail Both group was somewhat lower than the Fail Left group, the difference was not significant. For DSBm scores, there was no difference between the Fail Left and Pass Both groups; however, the Fail Both group was significantly lower than the Pass Both group ($p = .023$). Thus, individuals with left ear deficits on a dichotic listening task had lower forward span scores than normal controls, but not lower reverse span scores. Groups with bilateral impairments, however, showed deficits on both forward span and reverse span tasks (Maerlender et al, 2004). Thus, left-ear deficits suggested short-term memory impairment, while bilateral deficits appeared to implicate the larger working memory network.

Series 2: Performance on Neuropsychological Tests by Subjects With CAPD

The previous findings led us to study neuropsychological test results in chil-

dren who had recently undergone CAPD testing. In this second series of studies we hoped to determine the diagnostic utility of specific neuropsychological tests. These data are fully described in Maerlender (2005). Although the neuropsychological battery was primarily composed of auditory tests, two tests related specifically to ADHD also were included: One was a visual CPT (see Perugini et al., 2000 for diagnostic efficiency data), and the other was the Behavioral Rating Inventory of Executive Function (BRIEF; Gioia et al., 2001) rating scale, which has also been shown to have sensitivity to ADHD (Gioia, Isquith, Kenworthy, & Barton, 2002).

Thirty-six consecutive referrals for central auditory processing testing were followed with a battery of neuropsychological tests, although our laboratory received diagnostic information after the neuropsychological battery had been completed. Children who had undergone CAPD evaluations and diagnosis by an expert in CAPD were identified and contacted to participate in the neuropsychological test battery (human subjects approval was obtained). The neuropsychological battery included auditory and visual continuous performance tests (CPTs), as well as many tests thought to measure auditory processes (Table 18–1). Diagnosis of CAPD was based on standard clinical practice of two or more tests showing performance greater than 2 standard deviations below normal.

Test scores were grouped by test, and analyses of variance (MANOVAs) were conducted for each test (i.e., Wechsler Intelligence Scale for Children, 4th ed., WISC-IV, Clinical Evaluation of Language Fundamentals, 3rd ed., CELF-III subtests, etc.) by diagnosis (CAPD vs no CAPD). Five variables were significant ($p < .01$): Digit Span Forward (DSF), Letter Span Non-

Table 18–1. Cognitive Tests Administered

Tests/Subtests
WISC-IV Subtests
Arithmetic
Digit Span Forward (DSF)
Digit Span Reverse (DSB)
Coding (CODE)
Letter Span (Rhyming: LSR; Nonrhyming: LSNR)
CELF-III Subtests
Recalling Sentences (CELFRS)
Listening to Paragraphs
Concepts and Directions (CELFCD)
Comprehensive Test of Phonological Processing (CTOPP)
Rapid Naming (Digits: CTOPPRD; Letters CTOPPRL)
Phonological Awareness (Nonword Blending, Nonword Segmenting)
Continuous Performance Test: Visual & Auditory
Lindamood Auditory Conceptualization Test (LAC) (part 1 only)
Woodcock Johnson III Tests of Cognitive Ability
Sound Blending
Auditory Attention
Incomplete Words
Auditory Perception
Behavioral Rating Inventory of Executive Function (BRIEF)

Rhyming (LSNR), Comprehensive test of Phonological Processing Rapid Digit Naming (CTOPPRD), CELF-III Recalling Sentences (CELFRS), CELF-III Concepts and Directions (CELFCD). Of note, none of the visual or auditory CPT measures, nor the BRIEF scales were significantly different between groups. Three of the five variables demonstrating significance related to short-term memory span (DSF, LSNR, and CELFRS). It was less clear why Concepts and Directions and a rapid naming task would differentiate groups.

To better characterize the diagnostic potential of these subtests, the test scores were entered into several logistic regression analyses (by test grouping). Tests that significantly predicted diagnosis of CAPD within each group were then entered together (forward conditional entry) to identify predictors of CAPD. The results found Digit Span Forward (DSF) to be the best predictor of CAPD from the battery of tests, with all other tests dropping out of the regression. For this sample, DSF had a sensitivity = 85.7%, specificity = 71.4%, positive predictive power = 83%, and negative predictive power = 77%.

In support of the earlier study, DSF and D D showed significant relationships, primarily for left-ear scores. To look at the relative contribution of the most sensitive auditory variables relative to the most robust cognitive variable, DSF, D D—left ear, frequency patterns—right ear and low-pass filtered speech—right ear scores from the CAPD battery were entered into a logistic regression to predict diagnosis. A forward conditional entry was chosen to allow the strongest variables to emerge. Only DSF predicted group membership (β = −0.56499, p = .005), indicating that, in this data set, DSF was a better single predictor of diagnostic group membership than the auditory variables.

Series 3: CAPD and ADHD Findings

Although these studies provided strong support for the role of DSF in identification or corroboration of CAPD, it had not been possible to compare specific clinical groups such as ADHD. In an attempt to answer the specific question of relationships between CAPD and ADHD we were able to obtain and analyze data sets for the same span tasks from the CAPD children above (Series 2) and the ADHD cases from the clinical standardization sample from the WISC-IV database. All children were aged 7 to 14. Cases with positive diagnoses for CAPD from the studies in Series 2 (n = 22; 14 males and 8 females) were combined with the ADHD cases (n = 40; 27 males and 13 females; Wechsler et al., 2004). DSF, DSB, LSR and LSNR were analyzed. Means and standard deviations of the variables appear in Table 18–2.

Between-Group Differences

There was no difference between groups on Verbal IQ [$F(1,58)$ = 3.23, p = .077], and there was no difference in the distribution of gender by diagnostic groups (chi square = 0.094, p = .785). Multivariate analysis of variance of the variables of interest by clinical group found significant differences among all of the variables, $F(1,58)$ = 10.362, p = .000. Univariate results demonstrated significant differences for each, with DSF having the largest effect: DSF, $F(1,58)$ = 33.66, p = 0.000, η^2 = 0.37; DSB, $F(1,58)$ = 22.68, p = 0.000, η^2 = 0.28; LSNR, $F(1,58)$ = 10.66, p = .002, η^2 = 0.16; LSR, $F(1,58)$ = 6.41, p = .014, η^2 = 0.10.

To determine which variable was best at predicting diagnostic membership, the four variables were entered into logistic regression with conditional entry. Of the four variables identified, only DSF func-

Table 18–2. Means (SD) for Span Variables by Diagnostic Group

	CAPD	ADHD
DSF	6.10 (1.77)	10.48 (3.12)
DSB	7.65 (2.64)	11.00 (2.53)
LSNR	7.50 (2.19)	9.88 (2.86)
LSR	7.80 (2.67)	9.88 (3.14)

Notes: ADHD = attention deficit/hyperactivity disorder; *CAPD* = central auditory processing disorder; *DSB* = Digit Span Backward; *DSF* = Digit Span Forward; *LSNR* = Letter Span Nonrhyming; *LSR* = Letter Span Rhyming.

tioned as a significant variable for identifying diagnostic groups (β = -0.900, p = .000). Diagnostic efficiency statistics were quite robust: sensitivity = 90%, specificity = 76%; positive predictive power (PPP) = 88% and negative predictive power (NPP) = 80%. Classification rates are presented in Table 18–3.

Would specific scores on these measures help to differentiate between the two groups? In order to determine cut scores for DSF in identification of diagnoses of CAPD and ADHD, a series of receiver operator characteristics (ROC) curves were fitted to the data for both DSF. Inspection of the test results identified optimal cut scores based on specificity and sensitivity. For differentiating CAPD from ADHD, a DSF scaled score of 7 provided a sensitivity of 0.773 and specificity of 0.875; a scaled score of 8 provided sensitivity of 0.864 and specificity of 0.70. (See Chapter 12 of Volume I of the Handbook for discussion of the importance of sensitivity and specificity for screening and diagnosis.)

Within-Group Differences

The strength of DSF in identifying CAPD in this study is consistent with the previous work. However, DSB has also shown some ability to differentiate groups. The relationship between these two variables is of interest. In all previous studies (including the normative studies of the WISC-IV), there is a strong correlation between DSF and DSB. In this clinical standardization sample, the correlation was r = .622 (p = .000). The question arises: is there a systematic difference in the relationship of DSF and DSR between these two clinical groups? To answer this, we computed paired samples t-tests to determine differences between DSF and DSB, as well as between LSNR and LSR for each of the groups. The difference between DSB and DSF was significantly different for the CAPD group (t (21) = 2.61, p = .01), indicating that, on average (mean = 1.45, SD = 2.61), DSF is significantly lower than DSB in the CAPD sample, but not in the ADHD sample. This difference suggests another possible marker for differentiating the groups.

Summary of Empiric Studies

In two previous series of studies, we demonstrated that DSF was a robust marker of CAPD. In a third study reported here, the earlier findings are supported and extended to differentiating CAPD and ADHD. This combined data set provided a unique opportunity to compare specific test results as they pertain to these diagnostic groups. Significant differences between the two groups for three of four auditory span tasks (i.e., DSF, DSB, LSNR) supports the inference that CAPD and ADHD are indeed independent entities. As predicted, DSF was a robust predictor of group membership between the two diagnostic groups. Furthermore, identification of cut-scores should provide some guidance for helping to differentiate these

Table 18–3. Logistic Regression Classification Rates of Diagnostic Group by DSF Score

Observed	Predicted	
	ADHD	**CAPD**
ADHD	35	5
CAPD	4	16

Notes: ADHD = attention deficit/hyperactivity disorder; *CAPD* = central auditory processing disorder.

two groups. There was also evidence that the absolute difference between DSF and DSB is unique to the CAPD group. It appears that children with CAPD demonstrate consistently weak auditory short-term memory span. The difference between short-term and working memory scores indicates that it is the short-term span that is most impaired.

Conclusions: Relevance to Clinical Practice

The identification of short-term memory impairments as a marker for CAPD is important for clinical practice. Because accurate diagnoses of either ADHD or CAPD cannot be made on one test alone, these findings help to generate hypotheses regarding diagnostic possibilities. It must be noted that at a functional level, an individual's short-term span limits their working memory span. Longer forward spans than backward spans are highly unusual (Wechsler et al., 2004). However, scaled scores are age adjusted and do not accurately reflect the maximum span for any one individual. Thus, a forward span scaled score that is lower than a backward span scaled score may also suggest central auditory difficulties.

The data presented here suggest that, for children with suspected CAPD, a Digit Span forward (DSF) scaled-score of less than eight points may corroborate those suspicions. Furthermore, DSF scaled scores that are more than two scaled-score points lower than the Digit Span backward (DSB) scaled score also raises suspicion of CAPD. In practice, it is important to look for other markers of CAPD versus ADHD. A developmental history that is positive for recurrent,

chronic otitis media, high risk neurologic factors such as prematurity, asphyxia, hyperbilirubinemia, cortical lesion, or vascular changes in the brain can be risk factors (Jerger & Musiek, 2000). Specific functional symptoms can include poor attentiveness, particularly in complex listening environments, and/or difficulty discriminating and retaining auditory information. However, it is important to note that depressed DSF or even the DSF < DSB, even though sensitive in these studies, is probably a nonspecific finding. Hence the use of the efficient central auditory test battery remains the most efficient (sensitive/specific) approach to diagnosing CAPD (ASHA, 2005; Jerger & Musiek, 2000).

These data also suggest that CAPD is an independent entity relative to ADHD, supporting the earlier contention of Chermak (1999) that CAPD is likely a more specific disorder than ADHD in that it involves only one or primarily one sensory modality (AAA, 2010; ASHA, 2005). DSF has been linked to hypoperfusion of the auditory cortex. If, as we suspect, good DSF performance requires intact audiological processes from the peripheral ear to the auditory cortex, it seems reasonable to suspect that DSF is in fact a global indicator of impairment somewhere along the aural pathway, if not the cortex itself. ADHD is known to involve higher level processing that implicates frontal lobes. As the "executive," the frontal lobes depend on accurate information from lower structures and processes. Impairments up to and including the auditory cortex would necessarily impinge on frontal functioning. Thus, executive difficulties (including working memory) are likely secondary effects of more basic sensory dysfunctions. The accurate identification of auditory processing difficulty, whether in the context of ADHD or not, leads to more informed remedial strategies.

Absent a complete central auditory evaluation, recommendations for treatment are based only on symptoms and, therefore, are of questionable value and of uncertain potential for effectiveness. As therapeutic strategies are developed and standardized, it will be interesting to see if short-term auditory span lengths can improve, over and above practice effects. Confirmation through neuroimaging also will be helpful for validating short-term memory as a final common pathway of central auditory impairments. (Rehabilitation approaches for individuals diagnosed with CAPD are described in Sections 2 and 3 of this volume.)

Finally, it is important to reiterate that the clinical practice of reporting only Digit Span (total) scores is a problematic practice. Psychologists are well advised to include both forward and backward scores in their reporting, and to be familiar with the possible implications of low scores.

Acknowledgment. Studies described in this chapter were supported by the Hitchcock Foundation.

References

AACAP. (2007). Practice parameter for the assessment and treatment of children and adolescents with attention-deficit/hyperactivity disorder. *Journal of the American Academy of Child and Adolescent Psychiatry*, *46*(7), 894–921.

AAA (American Academy of Audiology). (2010). *Guidelines for the diagnosis, treatment, and management of children and adults with central auditory processing disorder*. Retrieved from http://www.audiology.org/resources/documentlibrary/Documents/CAPD%20Guidelines%208-2010.pdf

American Psychiatric Association. (2013). *Diagnostic and statistical manual of mental disorders* (5th ed.). Washington, DC: Author.

Anderson, P. (2002). Assessment and development of executive function (EF) during childhood. *Child Neuropsychology*, *8*, 71–82.

Arnsten, A. F., Steere, J. C., & Hunt R. D. (1996). The contribution of alpha 2-noradrenergic mechanisms of prefrontal cortical cognitive function: Potential significance for attention-deficit hyperactivity disorder. *Archives of General Psychiatry*, *53*, 448–448, 455.

ASHA (American Speech-Language-Hearing Association). (2005). *(Central) auditory processing disorders*. Retrieved from http://www.asha.org/members/deskref-journals/deskref/default

Baddeley, A. D. (1992). Working memory. *Science*, *255*, 556-559.

Bailey, T. (2010). Auditory pathways and processes: Implications for neuropsychological assessment and diagnosis of children and adolescents. *Child Neuropsychology*, *15*, 521–548.

Baker, S. C., Rogers, R. D., Owen, A. M., Frith, C. D., Dolan, R. J., Frackowiak, R. S. J., & Robbins, T. W. (1996). Neural systems engaged by planning: A PET study of the Tower of London task. *Neuropsychologia*, *34*, 531–526.

Barkley, R. A. (1997). Behavioral inhibition, sustained attention, and executive functions: Constructing a unifying theory of ADHD. *Psychological Bulletin*, *121*(1), 65–94.

Bellis, T. J., Billiet, C., & Ross, J. (2011). The utlity of visual analogs of central auditory tests in the differential diagnosis of (central) auditory processing disorder and attention deficit hyperactivity disorder. *Journal of the American Academy of Audiology*, *22*, 501–514.

Benedict, R. H. B., Lockwood, A. H., Shucard, J., Shucard, D. W., Wack, D., & Murphy, B. W. (1998). Functional neuroimaging of attention in the auditory modality. *Neuro-Report, 5,* 121–126.

Bishop, D. V. M. (2006). Developmental cognitive genetics: How psychology can inform genetics and vice versa. *Quarterly Journal of Experimental Psychology, 59,* 1153–1168.

Bobb, A. J., Castellanos, F. X., Addington, A. M., & Rapoport, J. L. (2005). Molecular genetic studies of ADHD: 1991 to 2004. *American Journal of Medical Genetics: Neuropsychiatic Genetics, 132,* 109–125.

Bush, G., Valera, E. M., & Seidman, L. J. (2005). Functional neuroimaging of attention-deficit/hyperactivity disorder: A review and suggested future directions. *Biological Psychiatry, 57,* 1273–1284.

Calderon-Gonzalez, R. (1993). Attention deficit disorders spectrum. neurological and neuropsychological basis. *International Pediatrics, 8,* 189–189, 198.

Casey, B. J., Castellanos, F. X., Giedd, J. N., Marsh, W. L., Hamburger, S. D., Schubert, A. B., . . . Rapoport, J. L. (1997). Implication of right frontostriatal circuitry in response inhibition and attention-deficit/hyperactivity disorder. *Journal of the American Academy of Child and Adolescent Psychiatry, 363,* 374–383.

Castellanos, F. X., Lee, P. P., Sharp, W., Jeffries, N. O., Greenstein, D. K., Classsen, L. V., . . . Rapoport, J. L. (2002). Developmental trajectories of brain volume abnormalities in children and adolescents with attention deficit/hyperactivity disorder. *Journal of the American Medical Association, 288,* 1740–1748.

Chabot, R. J., Orgill, A. A., Crawford, G., Harris, M. J., & Serfontein, G. (1999). Behavioral and electrophysiological predictors of treatment response to stimulants in children with attention disorders. *Journal of Child Neurology, 14,* 343–351.

Chermak, G. D. (1996). Central auditory testing. In S. E. Gerber (Ed.), *Handbook of pediatric audiology.* Washington, DC: Gallaudet.

Chermak, G. D., Hall, J. W. 3rd, & Musiek, F. E. (1999). Differential diagnosis and management of central auditory processing disorder and attention deficit hyperactivity disorder. *Journal of the American Academy of Audiology, 10,* 289–303.

Chermak, G. D., Somers, E. K., & Seikel, J. A. (1998). Behavioral signs of central auditory processing disorder and attention deficit hyperactivity disorder. *Journal of American Academy of Audiology, 9,* 78–84.

Chermak, G. D., Tucker, E., & Seikel, J. A. (2002). Behavioral characteristics of auditory processing disorder and attention deficit hyperactivity disorder: Predominantly inattentive type. *Journal of the American Academy of Audiology, 13,* 332–338.

Chhabildas, N., Pennington, B., F., & Willcutt, E. (2001). A comparison of the neuropsychological profiles of the DSM-IV subtypes of ADHD. *Journal of Abnormal Child Psychology, 29,* 529–540.

Clarke, A. R., Barry, R. J., McCarthy, R., & Selikowitz, M. (2002). Children with attention-deficit/hyperactivity disorder and comorbid oppositional defiant disorder: An EEG analysis. *Psychiatry Research, 111,* 181–190.

Corbetta, M., Miezin, F., Dobmeyer, S., Shulman, G., & Petersen, S. (1991). Selective and divided attention during visual discriminations of shape, color, and speed: Functional anatomy by positron emission tomography. *Journal of Neuroscience, 11,* 2383–2402.

Craik, F. I. M., Govoni, R., Naveh-Benjamin, M., & Anderson, N. D. (1996). The effects of divided attention on encoding and retrieval processes in human memory. *Journal of Experimental Psychology: General, 125,* 159–180.

Daneman, M., & Merikle, P. M. (1996). Working memory and language comprehension: A meta-analysis. *Psychonomic Bulletin and Review, 3,* 422–433.

Durston, S. (2003). A review of the biological bases of ADHD: What have we learned from imaging studies? *Mental Retardation and Developmental Disabilities Research Review, 9,* 184–195.

Durston, S., Tottenham, N. T. Thomas, K. M., Davidson, M. C., Eigsti, I. M., Yang, Y., . . . Casey, B. J. (2003). Differential patterns of striatal activation in young children with and without ADHD. *Biological Psychiatry, 53,* 871–878.

Engle, R. W., Tuholski, S. W., Laughlin, J. E., & Conway, A. R. A. (1999). Working memory, short-term memory, and general fluid intelligence: A latent variable approach. *Journal of Experimental Psychology: General, 128,* 309–331.

Farone, S. V., Perlis, R. H., Doyle, A. E., Smoller, J. W., Goralnick, J. J., Holmgren, M. A., & Sklar, P. (2005). Molecular genetics of attention deficit/hyperactivity disorder. *Biological Psychiatry, 57,* 11313–1323.

Farrand, P., & Jones, D. (1996). Direction of report in spatial and verbal serial short-term memory. *Quartery Journal of Experimental Psychology, 20,* 80–115.

Fausti, S. A., Wilmington, D. J., Gallun, F. J., Myers, P. J., & Henry, J. A. (2009). Auditory and vestibular dysfunction associated with blast-related traumatic brain injury. *Journal of Rehabilitation Research and Development, 46,* 797–810.

Fletcher, J. M. (1996). Executive functions in children: Introduction to the special series. *Developmental Neuropsychology, 12,* 1–3.

Ghanizadeh, A. (2009). Screening signs of auditory processing problem: Does it distinguish hyperactivity disorder subtypes in a clinical sample of children? *International Journal of Pediatric Otorhinolaryngology, 73,* 81–87.

Gioia, G., Isquith, P., Guy, S., & Kenworthy, L. (2001). *Behavior rating inventory of executive function (BRIEF) manual.* Odessa, FL: Psychological Assessment Resources.

Gioia, G. A., Isquith, P. K., Kenworthy, L., & Barton, R. M. (2002). Profiles of everyday executive function in acquired and developmental disorders. *Child Neuropsychology, 8,* 121–137.

Groeger, J. A., Field, D., & Hammond, S. M. (1999). Measuring memory span. *International Journal of Psychology, 34,* 359–363.

Hale, J. B., Hoeppner, J. B., & Fiorello, C. A. (2002). Analyzing digit span components for assessment of attention processes. *Journal of Psychoeducational Assessment, 20,* 128–143.

Hartman, C. A., Willcutt, E. G., Rhee, S. H., & Pennington, B. F. (2004). The relation between sluggish cognitive tempo and *DSM-IV* ADHD. *Journal of Abnormal Child Psychology, 32*(5), 491–503.

Heaton, S. C., Reader, S. K., Preston, A. S., Fennell, E. B., Puyana, O. E., Gill, N., & Johnson, J. H. (2001). The test of everyday attention for children (TEA-Ch): Patterns of performance in children with ADHD and clinical controls. *Child Neuropsychology, 7,* 251–264

Himelstein, J., Newcorn, J. H., & Halperin, J. M. (2000). The neurobiology of attention-deficit hyperactivity disorder. *Frontiers in Bioscience, 53,* D461-D461-D478.

Idrizbegovic, E., Hederstierna, C., Dahlquist, M., Kämpfe Nordström, C., Jelic, V., & Rosenhall, U. (2011). Central auditory function in early Alzheimer's disease and in mild cognitive impairment. *Age and Ageing, 40,* 49–54.

Iliadou, V., & Iakovides, S. (2003). Contributions of psychoacoustics and neuroaudiology in revealing correlation of mental disorders with central auditory processing disorders. *Annals of General Hospital Psychiatry, 2.*

Jerger, J., & Musiek, F. (2000). Report of the consensus conference on the diagnosis of auditory processing disorders in school-aged children. *Journal of the American Academy of Audiology, 11,* 467–474.

Kaplan, E., Fein, D., Morris, R., & Delis, D. (1991). *WAIS-R as a neuropsychological instrument.* San Antonio, TX: Psychological Corporation.

Katz, J., & Smith, P. S. (1991). The Staggered Spondaic Word Test: A ten-minute look at the central nervous system through the ears. *Annals of the New York Academy of Sciences, 620,* 233–251.

Keller, W. D., & Tillery, K. L. (2002). Reliable differential diagnosis and effective management of auditory processing and attention deficit hyperactivity disorders. *Seminars in Hearing, 23,* 337–348.

Kelly, T. P. (2000). The clinical neuropsychology of attention in school-aged children. *Child Neuropsychology, 6,* 24–36.

Lambeck, R., Tannock, R., Dalsgaard, S., Trillingsgaard, A., Damm, D., & Thomsen, P. H. (2010). Validating neuropsychological subtypes of ADHD: How do children with and with an executive functioning deficit differ? *Journal of Child Psychology and Psychiatry, 51,* 895–904.

Lambeck, R., Tannock, R., Dlasgaard, S., Trillingsgaard, A., Damm, D., & Thomsen, P.H. (2011). Executive dysfunction in school-age children with ADHD. *Journal of Attention Disorders, 15,* 646–655.

Larrabee, G. J., & Kane, R. L. (1986). Reversed digit repetition involves visual and verbal processes. *International Journal of Neuroscience, 30,* 11–15.

Lemiere, J., Wouters, H., Sterken. C., Lagae, L., Sonuga-Barke, E., & Danckaerts, M. (2010). Are children with ADHD predominantly inattentive and combined subtypes different in terms of aspects of everyday attention? *European Child and Adolescent Psychiatry, 19,* 679–685.

Lovejoy, D. W., Ball, J. D., Keats, M., Stutts, M. L., Spain, E. H., Janda, L., & Janusz, J. (1999). Neuropsychological performance of adults with attention deficit hyperactivity disorder (ADHD): Diagnostic classification estimates for measures of frontal lobe/executive functioning. *Journal of the International Neuropsychological Society, 5,* 222–233.

Luck, S. J., & Ford, M. A. (1998). On the role of selective attention in visual perception. *Proceedings of the National Academy of Sciences, 95,* 825–830.

Luria, A. R. (1973). *The working brain: An introduction to neuropsychology.* New York, NY: Basic Books.

Luu, P., & Tucker, D. M. (2003). Self-regulation and the executive functions: Electrophysiological clues. In A. Zani & A. M. Proverbio (Eds.), *The cognitive electrophysiology of mind and brain* (pp. 199–223). San Diego, CA: Academic.

Maerlender, A. (2010). Short-term memory and auditory processing disorders: Concurrent validity and clinical diagnostic markers. *Psychology in the Schools, 47,* 975–984.

Maerlender, A., Isquith, P., & Wallis, D. (2004). Psychometric and behavioral measures of central auditory function: The relationship of dichotic listening and digit span tasks. *Child Neuropsychology, 10,* 318–327.

Mirsky, A. F., Anthony, B. J., Duncan, C. C., Ahearn, M. B., & Kellam, S. G. (1991). Analysis of the elements of attention: A neuropsychological approach. *Neuropsychology Review (Historical Archive), 2,* 109–145.

Mirsky, A. F., Pascualvaca, D. M., Duncan, C. C., & French, L. M. (1999). A model of attention and its relation to ADHD. *Mental Retardation and Developmental Disabilities Reviews, 5,* 169–176.

Morris R. G., Ahmed S., Syed G. M., & Toone B. K. (1993). Neural correlates of planning ability: Frontal lobe activation during the Tower of London test. *Neuropsychologia, 31,* 1367–1378.

Moss, W. L., & Sheiffele, W. A. (1994). Can we differentially diagnose an attention deficit disorder without hyperactivity from a central auditory processing problem? *Child Psychiatry and Human Development, 25,* 85–96.

Muir-Broaddus, J. E., Rosenstein, L. D., Medina, D. E., & Soderberg, C. (2002). Neuropsychological test performance of children with ADHD relative to test norms and parent behavioral ratings. *Archives of Clinical Neuropsychology, 17,* 671–689.

Musiek, F. E. (1983). Assessment of central auditory dysfunction: The Dichotic Digit Test revisited. *Ear and Hearing, 4,* 79–83.

Näätänen, R., & Alho, K. (2004). Mechanisms of attention in audition as revealed by event-related potentials of the brain. In

M. I. Posner (Ed.), *Cognitive neuroscience of attention* (pp. 194–206). New York, NY: Guilford Press.

Nigg, J. T. (2005). Neuropsychological theory and findings in attention deficit hyperactivity disorder: The state of the field and salient challenges for the coming decade. *Biological Psychiatry, 57*, 1425–1435.

Nigg, J. T., Blaskey, L. G., Huang-Pollack, C. L., & Rappley, M. D. (2002). Neuropsychological executive functions and DSM-IV ADHD subtypes. *Journal of the American Academy of Child and Adolescent Psychiatry, 41*, 59–66.

Nigg, J. T., Tannock, R., & Rohde, L. A. (2010). What is to be the fate of ADHD subtypes? An introduction to the special section on research on the ADHD subtypes and implications for the DSM-V. *Journal of Clinical Child and Adolescent Psychology, 39*, 723–725.

Parent, A., & Hazrati, L.-N. (1995). The functional anatomy of the basal ganglia. II. *Brain Research Review, 20*, 128–154.

Paulesu, E., Frith, C. D., & Frackoviak, R. S. J. (1993). The neural correlates of the verbal component of working memory. *Nature, 362*, 342–345.

Pennington, B. F., & Ozonoff, S. (1996). Executive functions and developmental psychopathology. *Journal of Child Psychology and Psychiatry, 37*, 51–87.

Perugini, A. M., Harvey, E. A., Lovejoy, D. W., Sanstron, K., & Webb, A. H. (2000). The predictive power of combined neuropsychological measures of attention Deficit/Hyperactivity disorder in children. *Child Neuropsychology, 6*, 101–114.

Polancyzk, G., Silva de Lima, M., Horts, B. L., Biederman, J., & Rohde, L. A. (2007). The worldwide prevalence of ADHD: A systematic review and metaregression analysis. *American Journal of Psychiatry, 164*, 942–948.

Posner, M. I. (Ed.) (2004), *Cognitive neuroscience of attention*. New York, NY: Guilford.

Posner, M. I., & Petersen, S. E. (1990). The attention system of the human brain. *Annual Review of Neuroscience, 13*, 25–42.

Posner, M. I., & Rothbart, M. K. (1998). Attention, self-regulation and consciousness. *Philosophical Transactions of the Royal Society of London Biological Sciences, 353*(1377), 1915–1927.

Rapport, M., Alderson, R., Kofler, M., Sarver, D., Bolden, J., & Sims, V. (2008). Working memory deficits in boys with attention deficit/hyperactivity disorder (ADHD): The contribution of central executive and subsystem processes. *Journal of Abnormal Child Psychology, 36*, 825–837.

Reynolds, C. R. (1997). Forward and backward memory span should not be combined for clinical analysis. *Archives of Clinical Neuropsychology, 12*, 29–40.

Riccio, C. A., Cohen, M. J., Garrison, T., & Smith, B. (2005). Auditory processing measures: Correlation with neuropsychological measures of attention, memory and behavior. *Child Neuropsychology, 11*, 363–372.

Riccio, C. A., Hynd, G. W., Cohen, M. J., Hall, J., & Molt, L. (1994). Comorbidity of central auditory processing disorder and attention-deficit hyperactivity disorder. *Journal of the American Academy of Child and Adolescent Psychiatry, 33*, 849–857.

Rubia, K., Smith, A. B., Brammer, M. J., Toone, B., & Taylor, E. (2005). Abnormal brain activation during inhibition and error detection in medication-naive adolescents with ADHD. *American Journal of Psychiatry, 162*, 1067–1075.

Rubia, K., Taylor, E., Smith, A.B., Oksannen, H., Overmeyer, S., & Newman, S. (2001). Neuropsychological analyses of impulsiveness in childhood hyperactivity. *British Journal of Psychiatry, 179*, 138–143.

Rudel, R. G., & Denckla, M. B. (1974). Relation of forward and backward digit span repetition to neurological impairment in children with learning disabilities. *Neurolopsychologia, 12*, 109–118.

Russell, V. A. (2002). Hypodopaminergic and hypernoradrenergic activity in prefrontal cortex slices of an animal model for attention-deficit hyperactivity disorder—the spontaneously hypertensive rat. *Behavior and Brain Research, 130*, 191–196.

Scahill, L., & Schwab-Stone, M. (2000). Epidemiology of ADHD in school-aged children. *Child and Adolescent Psychiatric Clinics of North America, 9*, 541–555.

Schulz, K. P., Fan, J., Tang, C. Y., Newcorn, J. H., Buchsbaum, M. S., Cheung, A. M., & Halperin, J. M. (2004). Response inhibition in adolescents diagnosed with attention deficit hyperactivity disorder during childhood: An event-related fMRI study. *American Journal of Psychiatry, 161*, 1650–1657.

Semel, E., Wiig, E., & Secord, W. (1995). *Clinical Evaluation of Language Fundamentals–Third Edition*. San Antonio, TX: Psychological Corporation.

Sergeant, J. A., Guertz, H., & Oosterlaan, J. (2002). How specific is a deficit of executive functioning for attention-deficit/hyperactivity disorder? *Behavioral and Brain Research, 130*, 3-28.

Sharp, S. I., McQuillan, A., & Gurling, H. (2009). Genetics of attention-deficit hyperactivity disorder (ADHD). *Neuropharmacology, 57*, 590–600.

Sonuga-Barke, E. J. (1994). Annotation: On dysfunction and function in psychological theories of childhood disorder. *Journal of Child Psychology and Psychiatry, 35*, 801–815.

Sonuga-Barke, E. J. S. (2003). The dual pathway model of ADHD. An elaboration of neurodevelopmental characteristics. *Neuroscience and Behavioral Reviews, 27*, 593–604.

Sowell, E. R., Thompson, P. M., Welcome, S. E., Henkenius, A. L., Toga, A. W., & Peterson, B. S. (2003). Cortical abnormalities in children and adolescents with attention-deficit hyperactivity disorder. *Lancet, 363*, 1699–1707.

Stewart, G. A., Steffler, D. J., Lemoine, D. E., & Leps, J. D. (2001). Do quantitative EEG measures differentiate hyperactivity in attention-deficit/hyperactivity disorder? *Child Study Journal, 31*, 103–121.

Stuss, D. T., & Benson, D. F. (1986). *The frontal lobes*. New York, NY: Raven Press.

Swanson, J. M., Casey, J. B., Nigg, J., Catellanos, F. X., Volkow, N. D., & Taylor, E.

(2004). Clinical and cognitive definitions of attention deficits in children with attention deficit/hyperactivity disorder. In M. I. Posner (Ed.), *Cognitive neuroscience of attention*. New York, NY: Guilford.

Tannock, R. (1998). Attention deficit hyperactivity disorder: Advances in cognitive, neurobiological and genetic research. *Journal of Child Psychology and Psychiatry, 39*, 65–99.

Teicher, M. H., Anderson, C. M., Polcari, A., Glod, C. A., Maas, L. C., & Renshaw, P. F. (2000). Functional deficits in basal ganglia of children with attention-deficit/hyperactivity disorder shown *Nature Medicine, 6*, 470–473.

Tillery, K. L., Katz, J., & Keller, W. D. (2000). Effects of methylphenidate (Ritalin) on auditory performance in children with attention and auditory processing disorders. *Jourrnal of Speech, Language, and Hearing Research, 43*, 893–901.

Todd, R. D., Huang, H., Todorov, A. A., Neuman, R. J., Reiersen, A. M., Henderson, C. A., & Reich, W. (2008). Predictors of stability of attention-deficit/hyperactivity disorder subtypes from childhood to young adulthood. *Journal of the American Academy of Child and Adolescent Psychiatry, 47*, 76–85.

Torgesen, J. K. (1996). A model of memory from an information processing perspective: The special case of phonological memory. In G. R. Lyon & N. A. Krasnegor (Eds.), *Attention, memory and executive function* (pp. 157–184). Baltimore, MD: Brookes.

Tzourio, N., El Massioui, F., Crivello, F., Joliot, M., Renault, B., & Mazoyer, B. (1997). Functional anatomy of human auditory attention studied with PET. *NeuroImage, 5*, 63–77.

Vaidya, C. J., Austin, G., Kirkorian, G., Ridlehuber, H. W., Desmond, J. E., Glover, G. H., & Gabrieli, J. D. (1998). Selective effects of methylphenidate in attention deficit hyperactivity disorder: A functional magnetic resonance study. *Proceedings of the National Academy of Sciences, 24*, 14494–14499.

Vaidya, C. J., Bunge, S. A., Dudukovic, N. M., Zalecki, C. A., Elliott, G. R., & Gabrieli, J. D. E. (2005). Altered neural substrates of cognitive control in childhood ADHD: Evidence from functional magnetic resonance imaging. *American Journal of Psychiatry, 162*, 1605–1613.

Van der Meere, J. J., & Sergeant, J. (1988). Controlled processing and vigilance in hyperactivity: Time will tell. *Journal of Abnormal Child Psychology, 16*, 641–655.

Wechsler, D. (1981). *Wechsler adult intelligence scale, revised (WAIS-R) manual.* New York, NY: Psychological Corporation.

Wechsler, D. (1991). *Wechsler Intelligence Scale for Children, 3rd edition manual.* San Antonio, TX: Psychological Corporation.

Wechsler, D., Kaplan, E., Fein, D., Kramer, J., Delis, D., Morris, R., & Maerlender, A. (2004). *Manual for the Wechsler Intelligence Scale for Children, 4th edition, Integrated (*WISC-IV). San Antonio, TX: Psychological Corporation.

Weyandt, L. L. (2005). Executive function in children, adolescents, and adults with attention deficit hyperactivity disorder: Introduction to the special issue. *Developmental Neuropsychology, 27*, 1–10.

Willcutt, E. G., Doyle, A. E., Nigg, J. T., Faraone, S. V., & Pennington, B. F. (2005). Validity of the executive function theory of attention-deficit/hyperactivity disorder: A meta-analytic review. *Biological Psychiatry 57*, 1336–1346.

Willcutt, E. G., Nigg, J. T., Pennington, B. F., Solanto, M. V., Rohde, L. A., Tannock, T., . . . Lahey, B. B. (2012). Validity of DSM-IV attention-deficit/hyperactivity disorder symptom dimensions and subtypes. *Journal of Abnormal Psychology, 121*, 991–1010.

Willis, W. G., & Weiler, M. D. (2005). Neural substrates of attention deficit hyperactivity disorder: Electroencephalagraphic and magnetic resonance imaging evidence. *Developmental Neuropsychology, 27*, 135–182.

Zatorre, R. J., Bouffard, M., Ahad, P., & Belin, P. (2002). Where is "where" in human auditory cortex? *Nature Neuroscience, 5*, 905–909.

Zatorre, R. J., & Penhume, V. B. (2001). Spatial localization after excision of human auditory cortex. *Journal of Neuroscience, 21*, 6321–6328.

CHAPTER 19

CENTRAL AUDITORY PROCESSING DISORDER AND ATTENTION DEFICIT HYPERACTIVITY DISORDER

A Psychological Perspective on Intervention

WARREN D. KELLER and KIM L. TILLERY

There has been an additional six years of clinical work and research since the previous chapter we authored on this topic (Keller & Tillery, 2007), with an emphasis on evidence-based practice in intervening for children and adults with central auditory processing disorders (CAPD). However, the most recent Clinical Policy Bulletin issued by Aetna (2012) continues to maintain that Aetna considers any assessment or therapeutic measure for auditory processing disorder (APD) as experimental due to "insufficient scientific evidence to support the validity of any diagnostic tests and the effectiveness of any treatment for APD (p. 1)." Aetna further discusses that medication is one current approach to treatment, despite research that finds medication contraindicated in the treatment of CAPD (Tillery, Katz, & Keller, 2000). Aetna notes that

their policy on APD is "based upon the limited evidence for APD as a distinct pathophysiologic entity, upon a lack of evidence of established criteria and well validated instruments to diagnose APD and reliably distinguish it from other conditions affecting listening and/or spoken language comprehension, and upon the lack of evidence from well-designed clinical studies proving the effectiveness of interventions for treating APD (p. 3)." Aetna considers that since CAPD co-occurs with many other disorders, it is not a distinct disorder (Aetna, 2012). To add to this confusion, there are some Aetna policies that do indeed reimburse for CAPD evaluations. It is quite disappointing that Aetna ignores the many position statements and guidelines (ASHA, 1995, 2005) including the recent American Academy of Audiology

(AAA, 2010) evidence-based guidelines that argue to the contrary and review the research to support the position statements and guidelines.

Clearly, researchers, clinicians, audiologists, speech and language pathologists, as well as psychologists and other clinical professionals intrigued by differences in how individuals process auditory information continue to have much work ahead of them in establishing CAPD as a distinct clinical entity that is responsive to differential treatment. Previously, we have emphasized the importance of establishing evidence-based treatments for CAPD, treatments that have empirical support for their effectiveness (Keller & Tillery, 2002, 2007). We supported the establishment of empirically supported treatments for CAPD much like the empirically supported treatments that have been established for the treatment of ADHD (Pelham, 1999). We recommended that these same rigorous criteria be established for researchers and clinicians investigating treatments for CAPD in order to advance the validity and clinical utility of the construct and firmly establish CAPD as a distinct clinical entity that could not only be accurately diagnosed but also effectively treated. Such possibilities would provide the necessary data to third-party payers as to the validity of the diagnosis and effective treatment.

What Should CAPD Mean to the Psychologist?

In instructing pediatric residents about neuropsychological assessment and treatment, the first author of this paper would often begin the lecture by presenting a computerized tomography (CT) scan of a brain injured adolescent with the referring question being, "Is the patient capable of driving a motor vehicle?" Although a CT scan can certainly document the existence of a brain injury, the *functional behavioral limitations* accompanying the injury remain unknown without further neuropsychological assessment. Similarly, although a greater number of errors on the left competing condition of dichotic tests may document a particular CAPD subtype (Katz, 1992; Katz & Smith, 1991) or CAPD deficit (Bellis, 1999, 2002; Bellis & Ferre, 1999), it tells us little about the *functional behavioral limitations* accompanying the CAPD. Further neuropsychological assessment, behavioral assessment, speech and language assessment, academic assessment, as well as the observations of parents, teachers, and other caregivers are needed in order to determine the extent to which the inability to process an auditory signal to the left ear in a competing condition is actually impairing, limiting and adversely affecting the quality of an individual's life. Although there has been some discussion of the greater need to document the neurophysiological basis for a CAPD it is our position that the *functional behavioral limitations* of CAPD need to be described in order for the concept to have any validity or clinical utility. Consensus statements (AAA, 2010; ASHA, 1995, 2005) often recommend that an emphasis be placed on describing the functional limitations accompanying impairments in auditory processing. These statements encourage audiologists to continue to document the underlying central auditory nervous system (CANS) dysfunction seen in referred clients, while seeking with other team members to fully explore their listening, communication, learning and social issues.

A disorder is not of clinical significance unless it adversely affects the quality of one's life and has pervasive deleterious effects in several areas of life functioning. One cannot argue that an individual who returns home to check to see if he or she actually unplugged the coffee pot has an anxiety disorder, but if anxiety prevents the individual from developing close interpersonal relationships, prevents the person from remaining at work due to panic, leads them to underachievement due to the fear of failure, induces an excessive fear of risks, then clearly the anxiety becomes debilitating and a disorder. The impairments that individuals with attention deficit hyperactivity disorder (ADHD) experience in a school setting and in their psychosocial development, along with the associated features of anxiety, depression, predisposition to substance use disorders, underachievement, and learning difficulties are well documented.

In over 30 years of clinical practice as a neuropsychologist, the first author continues to encounter clinicians, teachers, school personnel, and other professionals who doubt the reality of CAPD. In our judgment, these doubts stem from the need for additional research to document the *associated features and functional behavioral limitations* associated with CAPD. In order to accomplish this, an audiologist should access the expertise and assessment of others in order to fully determine the extent to which, for example, the inability to process an auditory signal to the left ear while receiving a competing signal to the right ear is exerting functional limitations on the quality of one's life. The assessment of CAPD requires a multidisciplinary approach, based upon a synthesis of information from medical, educational, and developmental histories, behavioral and electrophysiological tests, as well as procedures from neuroimaging, speech and language evaluation, and psychological/cognitive evaluation (Bamiou, Musiek, & Luxon, 2001; Katz, 1992). Unfortunately, one of the downsides of multidisciplinary evaluations is that some professionals will interpret evidence from other professionals as indicative of a disorder bearing a label most familiar to the particular professional. For example, if the child does poorly on a central auditory processing evaluation administered by an audiologist, some speech-language pathologists might question that diagnosis and conclude the child presents a language processing problem. Clearly, professionals must be cautious in interpreting evidence obtained from assessments outside their area of expertise. To do otherwise jeopardizes the purpose and benefits of multidisciplinary evaluations.

In order to provide the best treatment and management once a diagnosis is made, we need to determine the functional limitations associated with the disorder. If audiologic research were able to reliably and validly document particular CAPD subtypes, and their associated comorbidities, this would enhance our understanding and improve effective treatment of CAPD (Keller & Tillery, 2002).

The authors have practiced clinically and have been involved in research during the past fifteen years with the goal of better understanding just what CAPD should mean to the psychologist. The inability to efficiently and correctly process auditory information can sometimes have far-reaching effects on an individual's learning, attention, behavior, and ultimately quality of life.

The associated features of CAPD are becoming more clearly understood. Keller, Tillery, and McFadden (2006) have described some of the associated impairments of CAPD in children with a nonverbal learning disorder (NVLD). While there has been speculation that the prevalence of CAPD may be 3% (Chermak & Musiek, 1997) or 20% (J. Katz, personal communication, 1991), we found that the prevalence of CAPD among a population of children with Nonverbal Learning Disabilities (NVLD) was 61%. Ninety-one percent of the children from this sample evidenced a type of CAPD; namely the tolerance-fading memory (TFM) subtype of CAPD. The criterion to diagnose CAPD was based on a 3 standard deviation test performance from norms for one central auditory processing test or two standard deviations from normal on two central auditory processing tests (ASHA, 2005). A TFM diagnosis is noted when the left competing measure of the dichotic test shows significant errors and the presence of several qualifiers (e.g., a high/low error pattern (missing more errors in the first presented stimuli versus the final stimuli) and/or combining the stimuli to form a new word), and exhibiting difficulty on a speech-in-noise test. We need to continue to substantiate the validity of the proposed subtypes of CAPD (ASHA, 2005); however, it is clear that a multidisciplinary approach will help establish distinct and valid subtypes of CAPD (Keller et al., 2006).

Our previous research efforts have documented some of the associated features that a psychologist may find on psychological assessment in children with CAPD (Keller et al., 2006; Keller & Tillery, 2007). Suppressed performance on working memory subtests such as Digit Span, from the Wechsler Scales and overall weaknesses on measured verbal memory abilities are associated with CAPD. It had been speculated that children evidencing TFM profiles on CAPD evaluations might exhibit weaknesses in short-term memory abilities. In our sample of children with NVLD there were two groups found with or without CAPD. We found those children with CAPD exhibited uniform weaknesses on standardized measures of memory functioning and that their ability to improve their memory with repetition was significantly weaker.

To our knowledge, this was the first time memory deficits have been documented to accompany the TFM subtype of CAPD. It is this type of documentation that is necessary in order to establish the *functional behavioral limitations* of children with CAPD. Once again, a multidisciplinary team assists to comprehensively explore and document functional deficits, since different professionals focus on different areas of disability (e.g., the audiologist focuses on auditory processing and listening, the psychologist focuses on cognition and behavior, and the speech-language pathologist focuses on language and communication. Clearly, CAPD can be associated with a larger range of deficits than just the inability to process auditory signals.

ADHD and Evidence-Based Treatment

It has been recognized for decades that behaviors presented by individuals with ADHD and CAPD overlap and that the some individuals present both conditions (Riccio, 2005). Attention deficit disorder is characterized by impulsivity, hyperactivity and inattention, when inappropriate to the child's chronological age, and is one of the most common childhood disorders (Barkley, 1990, 1998). Some of the associated features of ADHD and the necessity for comprehensive assessment of this disorder have been previously outlined (Keller & Tillery, 2007).

Increasingly in psychology and psychiatry there has been an emphasis upon the use of treatment interventions that have empirical support for their effectiveness (Pelham, Wheeler, & Chronis, 1998). There has been some controversy among academic psychologists and clinicians, with the latter group arguing that clinical research cannot always document some of the subtle positive changes that occur as the result of psychotherapy. Increasingly managed care companies and other third party insurance carriers, as well as consumers of mental health care themselves, have demanded that empirical support be provided for the interventions that are used to treat a variety of mental health disorders, including ADHD (Pelham, 1999). This emphasis on evidence-based practice is consistent with the scientist-practitioner model, or Boulder model, that has been at the core of psychological training and practice for more than 50 years emphasizing an intimate relationship between clinical practice and science (Raimy, 1950).

As early as 1995, the American Psychological Association (APA) Task Force on Promotion and Dissemination of Psychological Procedures developed guidelines for empirically supported treatments for psychosocial interventions for childhood mental disorders (Pelham, 1999). These guidelines stipulated that in order to develop criteria for well-established psychosocial interventions it was necessary to have at least two well-conducted group design studies, conducted by different investigators, showing the treatment to be either superior to pill placebo or alternative treatments, or equivalent to an already established treatment. Random assignment to study comparison groups was required. Criteria could also include a large series of single-case design studies that used both good experimental design and compared the intervention with another treatment. Case studies in and of themselves were deemed inadequate to demonstrate treatment efficacy and establish a treatment approach that would meet the criteria for evidence-based practice. Given these guidelines, a level system for determining the evidence to support a treatment approach was developed. These included: (1) not empirically supported, (2) possibly efficacious, (3) probably efficacious, (4) efficacious, and (5) efficacious and specific. In order for a treatment approach to be efficacious and specific it is necessary for the treatment to be more effective than a no treatment or placebo control group, and to be shown as such in two or more independent studies. Efficacious and specific treatment approaches for ADHD include psychosocial treatments and pharmacological interventions. This has been supported both by the Multimodal Treatment Study of ADHD (MTA Study), as well as by the McMaster University Evidence-Based Practice Center Group (1999). The use of medication as well as psychosocial treatments have been demonstrated to be both efficacious and specific and the use of both treatment approaches in combination yields benefits beyond those in either treatment alone (MTA Cooperative Group, 1999). See Chapter 2 for discussion of evidence-based practice and treatment efficacy.

Psychosocial Treatments

Effective, evidence-based psychosocial treatments for children with ADHD typically include three components: (1) parent training, (2) school intervention, and (3) child interventions (Barkley, 2006). The focus of behavioral treatments include teaching parents behavioral interventions and behavioral management strategies to improve compliance with rules and regulations by focusing on the antecedents to behavior, the specific behaviors that are the focus of change, and the consequences to the child's behavior. Behavioral procedures focus on changing the way parents provide commands to their children and modifying the way parents respond to their children's behavior in order to teach the children new ways of behaving. A significant component of parent training is providing parents instruction in terms of the diagnosis of ADHD, the etiology of the disorder, as well as the components of effective treatment and prognosis. Parents learn to praise appropriate behaviors and to ignore mild inappropriate behaviors. They learn effective management strategies such as time out from positive reinforcement. Parents learn to utilize commands instead of asking questions and learn to be specific with respect to their expectations. Parents learn contingency management strategies so that pleasurable activities for a child are contingent upon the completion of less desirable behaviors. The use of daily charts and token systems with rewards and punishments are learned (Williams, Chacko, Fabiano, & Pelham, 2001).

Effective psychosocial treatments also focus on intervening at the school level by teaching teachers effective classroom management approaches, the implementation of novelty and immediate feedback, and the use of behavioral strategies such as the use of a daily report card as a means of improving the behavior of the child with ADHD (Barkley, 1998, 2000). Clear expectations are provided children with classroom rules and expectations posted. Rules and expectations are posted and made measureable and reinforceable. Teachers are taught to provide children more praise than criticism, and commands are made in clear, specific, manageable manner. Children are provided accommodations in their classrooms with preferential seating, the use of immediate and frequent feedback and frequent breaks with the opportunity to engage in increased physical activity during the course of the school day. Contingency management strategies such as providing recess contingent upon the completion of schoolwork are implemented. The use of daily report cards that target individual behaviors and provide measureable goals are established that also permit regular communication between the teacher and parents. The establishment of behavior charts assures that children are aware of targeted behaviors and the behaviors that need to be extinguished and behaviors that need to be reinforced.

Behavioral treatments also emphasize working with the children themselves in terms of systematically teaching them appropriate social skills, decreasing aggression, developing close interpersonal relations, and building self-efficacy. Child interventions focus on improving problem-solving skills, self-control training, decreasing undesirable and antisocial behaviors, and increasing prosocial behaviors (Pelham, Greiner, & Gnagy, 1997).

Pharmacological Treatments

Individualized medication management is well established as evidence-based treatment for individuals with ADHD with considerable research establishing its effectiveness in well-controlled studies that meet the criteria for empirically supported treatments.

Stimulant medications fall into two categories, methylphenidate products (Ritalin, Focalin, Methylin) and amphetamine products (Adderall, Vyvanse) (Tillery, 2012). If an individual does not respond to an amphetamine-based product then an amphetamine-based medication may be tried and vice versa. Previously, stimulant medications required dosing several times a day given their short duration of effectiveness; however, the newer medications—Adderall XR, Concerta, Metadate, Focalin XR, Ritalin LA, and Vyvanse—have a much longer period of therapeutic effect and more typically require just single dosing (*PDR Consumer Guide to Prescription Drugs*, 2011). For some children who seem to metabolize the medication more quickly, there may be some consideration given to a late afternoon dose of the medication to assist them with after school activities or homework.

The stimulant medications vary with respect to the manner in which they are delivered and with respect to their pharmacokinetics. They can come in pill or a capsule form. Many of the more recent longer acting medications such as Adderall, which is in capsule form, may be opened and spread on pudding or yogurt without compromising the delivery of the medication and its effectiveness. Daytrana is a methylphenidate based medication that is delivered trans-dermally that was first released in 2006. Unlike other stimulant medications that are taken orally, Daytrana is applied to the skin, by a patch, with the medication being released gradually throughout the day. Clinically, Daytrana has become a second line medication for the treatment of ADHD when oral dosing is not tolerated well or with children who have difficulty swallowing pills and capsules. Children often develop a rash or sensitivity in the area where the patch is applied so the location of the patch should be changed regularly and heat should be avoided around the patch as this can affect the delivery of the medication.

Strattera, or atomoxetine, was the first nonstimulant medication approved for the treatment of ADHD. Straterra is a selective norepinephrine reuptake inhibitor and is not a methylphenidate or amphetamine product. Unlike the stimulants that have a rapid onset of effect, Straterra may take up to six weeks or more to obtain a therapeutic effect. Since its approval in 2008, Strattera has not established itself as a first line pharmacological treatment for ADHD, largely due to the greater risk of adverse side effects with the medication. While the typical adverse side effects with the stimulant medications include suppressed appetite, headache, irritability, gastrointestinal upset, increases in heart rate and blood pressure, these effects are short lived as the duration of time it takes the medication to clear the body is relatively short. Strattera, on the other hand, is a longer acting medication and the adverse side effect profile tends to be of greater concern. Strattera has been associated with drug induced liver injury, an increase in suicidal ideation in children, abdominal pain, gastrointestinal complaints, vomiting, nausea, erectile dysfunction, decreased libido, and difficulties with the urogenital system, along with other adverse effects. In general, the adverse side effects associated with Strattera tend to be more serious and of greater concern so that Strattera is typically considered if children have not responded well to a variety of stimulant medications.

Intuniv is yet another nonstimulant medication that was initially approved as a monotherapy to treat ADHD and more recently has been approved as an adjunctive therapy that may be combined with other stimulant medications. Intuniv is an extended release form of guanfacine that has long been used in the treatment for especially hyperaroused, very motorically hyperactive children with ADHD or with children experiencing significant sleep disorders associated with the ADHD. Intuniv is an antihypertensive medication that is believed to have a positive effect on mood regulation, attention, and the regulation of behavior through actions on prefrontal cortical neurons. Intuniv can be adminstered alone or in combination with the stimulant medications and since one of the adverse side effects associated with the medication is lethargy, it can be administered near bedtime to help induce sleep in the hyperaroused ADHD child.

Unlike the stimulants which can be discontinued immediately without adverse effect, Intuniv and other antihypertensive medications used for the treatment of ADHD (Tenex, clonidine, guanfacine) must be discontinued slowly. Nonstimulant medications for ADHD may also be considered when tics occur with the stimulant medications that are commonly used in the treatment of ADHD. Provigil, or modafinil, is an agent that is used in the treatment of narcolepsy, an arousal disorder (Physician's Desk Reference, 2012). While Provigil is indicated to improve the wakefulness of individuals experiencing the excessive daytime sleepiness associated with narcolepsy, its value as an efficacious pharmacological treatment for ADHD is being investigated and the medication is already being used clinically despite limited empirical support.

As our knowledge of ADHD grows, it is expected that we will one day be able to gain an even greater understanding of the disorder so that the specific medication prescribed will be able to be tailored to the specific genetic subtype of ADHD that is diagnosed, improving our capability to provide evidence-based treatments. To the best of our knowledge, there are no data that would suggest long-term negative side effects from the stimulant medications used for children with ADHD, and this would not be surprising given their short-acting effects.

A common question is whether these medications affect performance on central auditory tests. A review of literature shows only two studies in this decade that investigated this question. Cavadas, Pereira, and Mattos (2007) studied the effect of medication when comparing the test performance of one dichotic test in medicated and nonmedicated conditions, finding an improved test performance in the medicated condition of participants with ADHD ($N = 29$) ; however, the test sessions were separated by two to nine months. Thus, the maturation variable was not controlled, the participants were diagnosed with only ADHD, and received one dichotic task in a design without a placebo condition. In contrast, Tillery, Katz, and Keller (2000) used a double-blind, placebo-controlled design and found no effect on auditory processing test performance in a population of children diagnosed with both ADHD and CAPD but did reveal a significant medication effect (p = .004) for the auditory continuous performance test measure of attention. (See below under Differential Interventions for ADHD and CAPD.)

CAPD and Evidence-Based Treatment

The functional impairments associated with CAPD, and its adverse impact on academic, socio-emotional, and long-term development are well documented (AAA, 2010; ASHA, 2005; Chermak, 2002; Chermak, Bellis, & Musiek, 2007.) Considerable evidence has accumulated over the last decade supporting the efficacy of auditory training, FM systems, and related interventions for CAPD (AAA, 2010; ASHA, 2005; Chermak, 2002; Chermak, Bellis, Weihing, & Musiek, 2012). Several recommendations for comprehensive intervention programs have been proposed (Bellis, 2003; Ferre, 2007; Chermak & Musiek, 1997; Musiek, Baran, & Shinn, 2004) and a number of commercially available software programs and print workbooks also are available (Friel-Patti, Loeb, & Gillam, 2001). These programs generally focus on three areas: auditory training, signal enhancement, and central resources training (i.e., metacognition, metalanguage, and cognition). Remediation programs that purport to be useful in the treatment and management of CAPD include: Earobics (Cognitive Concepts, 1997, 1998), Fast ForWord Training Program (Scientific Learning Corporation, 1997), Processing Power (Ferre, 1997), Phonemic Synthesis

Training (Katz & Harmon-Fletcher, 1982), Lindamood Phoneme Sequencing Program (LiPS) (Lindamood-Bell Learning Processes, 1998), and dichotic training (Weihing & Musiek, 2007).

A number of interventions for CAPD have been demonstrated to be effective. Most of the efficacy data have been obtained in support of auditory training (Hayes, Warrier, Nicol, Zecker, & Kraus, 2003; Jirsa, 1992; Kraus & Disterhoft, 1982; Kraus, McGee, Carrell, King, Tremblay, & Nicol, 1995; Merzenich, Grajski, Jenkins, Recanzone, & Perterson, 1991; Merzenich et al., 1996; Miller & Knudsen, 2003; Musiek, Baran, & Pinheiro, 1992; Musiek, Baran, & Shinn, 2004; Russo, Nicol, Zecker, Hayes, & Kraus, 2005; Tallal et al., 1996; Tremblay, 2007; Tremblay & Kraus, 2002; Tremblay, Kraus, Carrell, & McGee, 1997; Tremblay, Kraus, & McGee, 1998; Tremblay, Kraus, McGee, Ponton, & Otis, 2001; Warrier, Johnson, Hayes, Nicol, & Kraus, 2004) and signal enhancement strategies (Blake, Field, Foster, Platt, & Wertz, 1991; Boswell, 2006; Lewis, Crandell, Valente, & Horn, 2004; Crandell, 1998; Rosenberg, 2002; Stach, Loiselle, Jerger, Mintz, & Taylor, 1987). Research has also demonstrated the value of preferential seating, visual cues (i.e., auditory-visual summation) and pre-teaching of information for children with CAPD (Crandell & Smaldino, 2001; Massaro, 1987). Additional research regarding the range of CAPD interventions meeting the strict criteria and highest standards for EBP is needed (i.e., well-designed, randomized controlled trials), as acknowledged by professional organizations representing audiology and others (AAA, 2010; ASHA, 1996, 2005; Bellis & Anzalone, 2008; Chermak, 2001; Cox, 2005; Ferre, 2002). See Chapter 3 for a review of the efficacy of auditory training and related approaches and Chapter 11 for a review of computer-assisted auditory training programs.

Differential Interventions for ADHD and CAPD

Interventions designed to treat and manage children and adults with ADHD focus upon the amelioration of symptomatology associated with the disorder, namely improving sustained attention and concentration, reducing noncompliance, improving school performance, and developing improved social skills. Evidence-based treatments have been shown to be effective in improving performance in all these deficit areas (Pelham, 1999; Pelham et al., 1998).

Prior to developing evidence-based treatments for individuals with CAPD it will be important to designate the specific symptomatology associated with CAPD that we are attempting to address. It is reasonable to assume that not all interventions that are employed for individuals with CAPD will be able to effectively address the range of deficits that may be experienced by this very heterogenous group.

Keller and Tillery (2002) speculated on different treatment approaches that may be effective for individuals with comorbid ADHD and CAPD, as well as approaches that might be helpful for individuals with CAPD alone or ADHD alone. It is without debate that medication is an effective treatment for individuals with ADHD and that these same medications do not appear to be effective treatment for those with CAPD (Tillery et al., 2000). There are no other published studies, since this 2000 study, that employed: (1) a double-blind placebo-controlled design, (2) a large sample population of children with both ADHD (previously diagnosed by a psychologist (six months to seven years prior to the study) and demonstrating consistent evidence that the Ritalin medication was effective for their ADHD and CAPD (a total of 66 children with ADHD were referred for central auditory testing resulting in 36 children diagnosed with CAPD, 32 of whom participated in the study), (3) an attention/impulsive measure (Auditory Continuous Performance Test [ACPT]; Keith, 1994), and (4) a counterbalance of the order of administration of the ACPT and three central auditory processing tests within a 52-day period of participating in the two test sessions: medicated and nonmedicated. The participants ($n = 32$) were randomly assigned to two groups. One group ($n = 16$) first received the placebo condition followed by the medication condition, whereas the other group ($n = 16$) first received the medication condition followed by the placebo condition. The Tillery et al. study began to document treatment approaches that meet the stringent standards for evidence-based treatment.

One may interpret these findings as support for the conclusion that ADHD and CAPD are two distinct clinical entities that often occur comorbidly (Bellis et al., 2012; Chermak, Hall, & Musiek, 1999). If an individual exhibits both of these disorders then he or she should receive evidence-based treatments that have been shown to be effective for ADHD in combination with the evidence-based treatments that have been shown to be effective for CAPD (e.g., auditory and metacognitive training, preferential seating, environmental modifications, self-advocacy, pretutoring, medication management, psychosocial treatments, parent education, behavioral interventions). In the absence of additional research and data examining evidence-based treatments for children exhibiting comorbid CAPD and ADHD, the evidence-based treatments that have been shown to be effective for each disorder should be considered when planning intervention for those with comorbid ADHD and CAPD. See Chapter18 in this Volume and Chapter 20 in Volume 1 of the Handbook for additional perspective on differentiating CAPD and ADHD.

Transdisciplinary Perspective

The critical importance of a transdisciplinary perspective to the understanding, diagnosis, and treatment of CAPD has been encouraged (Keller, 1992, 1998; Keller & Tillery, 2002, 2007; Keller et al., 2006; Tillery, 1998). In addition, we have encouraged the discipline to focus on improving the predictive validity and clinical utility of the concept of CAPD by focusing on the identification of the functional behavioral limitations associated with any diagnosis of auditory processing dysfunction (Keller & Tillery, 2007). It is the functional behavioral limitations that must be the focus of intervention and remediation.

The first author initially became interested in the implications of CAPD after reviewing central auditory processing evaluation where a child was diagnosed with a TFM subtype of CAPD with the audiologist recommending that school personnel should focus on intervention strategies that would allow his presumably stronger visual memory skills to assist him in compensating for his cen-

tral auditory processing dysfunction and therefore improve his learning. Had the audiologist had access to the results of a neuropsychological evaluation, it would have been clear that reliance on visual processing to compensate for the central auditory deficits would not be viable. In fact, the subsequent neuropsychological evaluation, determined that the child was exhibiting a NVLD, which is often characterized by significant weaknesses in visual memory skills (Rourke, 1995). His visual memory skills were at the first percentile and would be of little assistance in improving retention of academic skills if visual memory strategies were to have been utilized as had been recommended by the audiologist. We now know that a substantial portion of children diagnosed with NVLD syndrome can be expected to evidence a TFM profile on the CAPD test battery (Keller et al., 2006). Clearly, this case speaks to the need for communication among the professionals providing the multidisciplinary assessments recommended in the opening paragraphs of this chapter.

Summary

ADHD was first described in the medical literature as early as the 1900s, and our knowledge of the disorder has been increasing exponentially since that time. The use of stimulant medications in the treatment of ADHD has occurred at least since 1935 (Barkley, 1998), and since that time we have been able to delineate both pharmacologic and psychosocial evidence-based treatment approaches. The concept of CAPD was given birth by Helmer Myklebust in the 1950s (Myklebust, 1954), when he and the noted Italian physicians (Bocca, Calearo, & Cassinari, 1954) emphasized that higher level auditory processes must be investigated rather than just peripheral hearing function. Not long after, Katz (1962) developed one of the first dichotic tests to assess the integrity of the central auditory system and the field of CAPD blossomed. (See Chapter 6 for a review of the historical foundations and evolution of the field of CAPD.)

We are continuing to better understand the associated features and functional deficits impacting adversely upon individuals with CAPD. We have been studying ADHD for well over one hundred years and are now beginning to describe empirically supported treatments. Certainly in the next several decades, if we model our research efforts on those utilized for the investigation of ADHD, we will continue to develop more empirically supported customized interventions for CAPD.

A disorder is of clinical significance only if it results in an impairment in life functions. The diagnostic criteria for ADHD include "clear evidence of clinically significant impairment in social, academic, or occupational functioning" (APA, 2013). All too often, this major diagnostic criteria is overlooked. Mere inattention on a continuous performance measure, greater motoric activity in a classroom, or deviations from the norm on a standardized behavioral measure are insufficient criteria to describe a child as having a "disorder" that requires intervention, remediation, and treatment, much less pharmacological intervention. The number of children placed on psychostimulant medications without comprehensive diagnosis is unethical. Diagnosis of ADHD and pharmacologic management should only be considered when a child presents there is a significant impairment in social, academic, or occupational functioning.

In order for a child to be diagnosed as having CAPD, dysfunction and/or deficits in the CANS must be established through electrophysiological/brain imaging methods or inferred from behavioral measures of central auditory processing. The associated functional deficits should guide intervention. It would seem reasonable to determine the extent to which a child's auditory processing differences impact adversely upon language skills, social functioning, and academic or occupational functioning before deciding the appropriate interventions. If there is minimal or no impairment in these areas, then interventions may not be required; however, that does not change the fact that CANS involvement has been demonstrated or has been inferred to be highly probable based on the outcomes of a test battery that has been shown to be both sensitive and specific to CANS dysfunction. Similarly, if a child's inattentiveness in the classroom does not impact adversely upon that child's social functioning or academic performance, psychostimulant medication should not be employed as an intervention.

It is only through the information obtained by the professional team that the audiologist is able to determine the extent to which a child's central auditory processing differences might be impacting his or her social, academic, or occupational functioning and which auditory interventions would be most appropriate.

The social impact of describing a child as having a label of a disorder can affect the way the child is regarded and treated by the parent, and certainly can have an effect on relationships within a family. Labels must only be applied when meeting the criteria specified by the professional associations, based on research. Clinicians, including psychologists, audiologists, and speech-language pathologists, need to focus on the identification of the functional behavioral limitations and assessing the degree to which a child's attentional and behavioral control weaknesses and/or central auditory processing deficits are truly impacting adversely upon that child's social, academic, or occupational functioning before we can begin to develop and implement empirically supported, evidence-based treatments. The continued emphasis that we have placed in our research and clinical work in identifying specific subtypes of CAPD and the functional behavioral limitations, if any, associated with subtypes of CAPD would advance that goal of identification of evidence-based treatments.

References

AAA (American Academy of Audiology). (2010). *Diagnosis, treatment, and management of children and adults with central auditory processing disorder.* Clinical Practice Guidelines.

Aetna. (2012). *Clinical policy bulletin: Auditory processing disorder (APD), 668,* 1–9.

American Psychiatric Association. (2013). *Diagnostic and statistical manual of mental disorders* (5th ed.). Washington, DC: Author.

American Psychological Association Task Force on Promotion and Dissemination of Psychological Procedures. (1995). Training in and dissemination of empirically validated treatments. *Clinical Psychologist, 48,* 2–3.

ASHA (American Speech-Language and Hearing Association). (1995). *Central auditory processing current status of research and implications for clinical practice. A report from the Task Force on Central Auditory Processing.* Rockville, MD: Author.

ASHA. (2005). *(Central) auditory processing disorders. A technical report.* Rockville, MD: Author.

Bamiou, D. E., Musiek, F. E., & Luxon, L. M. (2001). Aetiology and clinical presentations of auditory processing disorders: A review. *Archives Disorders of Children, 85,* 361–365.

Barkley, R. A. (1990). *Attention deficit hyperactivity disorder: A handbook for diagnosis and treatment.* New York, NY: Guilford Press.

Barkley, R. A. (1998). *Attention-deficit hyperactivity disorder: A handbook for diagnosis and treatment* (2nd ed.) New York, NY: Guilford Press.

Barkley, R. A. (2000). *Taking charge of ADHD: The complete, authoritative guide for parents.* New York, NY: Guilford.

Barkley, R. A. (2006). *Attention deficit hyperactivity disorder. A handbook for diagnosis and treatment.* New York, NY: Guilford Press.

Bellis, T. J. (1999). Subprofiles of central auditory processing disorders. *Education Audiology Review, 2,* 9–14.

Bellis, T. J. (2002). Developing deficit-specific intervention plans for individuals with auditory processing disorders. *Seminars in Hearing, 23,* 287–295.

Bellis, T. J. (2003). *Assessment and management of central auditory processing disorders in the educational setting: From science to practice* (2nd ed.) Clifton Park, NY: Thomson Learning.

Bellis, T., & Anzalone, A. (2008). Intervention Approaches for individuals with (central) auditory processing disorder. *Contemporary Issues in Communication Science and Disorders, 5,* 143–153.

Bellis, T., Chermak, G. D., Weihing, J., & Musiek, F. (2012). Efficacy of auditory interventions for central auditory processing disorder: A response to Fey et al. (2011). *Language, Speech, and Hearing Services in Schools, 43,* 381–386.

Bellis, T. J., & Ferre, J. M. (1999). Multidimensional approach to the differential diagnosis of central auditory processing disorders in children. *Journal of American Academy of Audiology, 10*, 319–328.

Blake, R., Field, B., Foster, C., Platt, F., & Wertz, P. (1991). Effect of FM auditory trainers on attending behaviors of learning disabled children. *Language, Speech, and Hearing Services in Schools, 22*, 111–114.

Bocca, E., Calearno, C., & Cassinari, V. (1954). A new method for testing hearing in temporal lobe tumor. *Acta Otolaryngologica, 44*, 219–221.

Boswell, S. (2006). Sound field systems on the rise in school: Improved test scores cited as benefit. *ASHA Leader, 11*, 32–33.

Cavadas, M., Pereira, L. D., & Mattos, P. (2007). Effects of methylphenidate in auditory processing evaluation of children and adolescents with attention deficit hyperactivity disorder. *Arquivos de Neuro-Psiquiatria, 65*, 138–143.

Chermak, G. D. (2001). Auditory processing disorder: An overview for the clinician. *Hearing Journal, 54*, 10–25.

Chermak, G. D. (2002). Deciphering auditory processing disorders in children. *Otolaryngology Clinics of North America, 35*, 733–749.

Chermak, G. D., Baran, J., & Musiek, F. E. (2007). Neurobiology, cognitive science, and intervention. In G. Chermak & F. Musiek (Eds.), *Handbook of central auditory processing disorder* (pp. 3–28). San Diego, CA: Plural.

Chermak, G. D., Hall, J. W., & Musiek, F. E. (1999). Differential diagnosis and management of central auditory processing disorder and attention deficit hyperactivity disorder. *Journal of the American Academy of Audiology, 10*, 289–303.

Chermak, G. D., & Musiek, F. E. (1997). *Central auditory processing disorders: New perspectives*. San Diego, CA: Singular.

Cognitive Concepts. (1997). *Earobics—auditory development and phonics program*. Evanston, IL: Author.

Cognitive Concepts. (1998). *Earobics—step two auditory development and phonics program*. Evanston, IL: Author.

Cox, R. (2005). Evidence-based practice in audiology. *Journal of the American Academy of Audiology, 16*, 408–409.

Crandell, C. (1998). Page ten: Utilizing sound field FM amplication in the educational setting. *Hearing Journal, 51*, 10–19.

Crandell, C., & Smaldino, J. (2001). Acoustical modifications for the classroom. In C. Crandell & J. Smaldino (Eds.), Classroom acoustics: Understanding barriers to learning. *Volta Review, 101*, 33–46.

Ferre, J. M. (1997). *Processing power: A guide to CAPD assessment and management*. San Antonio, TX: Communication Skill Builders.

Ferre, J. M. (2002). Behavioral therapeutic approaches for central auditory problems. In J. Katz (Ed.), *Handbook of clinical audiology* (5th ed., pp.525–531). Philadelphia, PA: Lippincott Williams & Wilkins.

Ferre, J. M. (2007). The ABCs of CAP: Practical strategies for enhancing central auditory processing skills. In D. Geffner & D. Swain (Eds.), *Auditory processing disorders* (pp. 187–205). San Diego, CA: Plural.

Friel-Patti, S., Loeb, D., & Gillam, R. (2001). Looking ahead: An introduction to five exploratory studies of Fast ForWord. *American Journal of Speech-Language Pathology, 10*, 195–202.

Hayes, E. A., Warrier, C. M., Nichol, T. G., Zecker, S. G., & Kraus, N. (2003). Neural plasticity following auditory training in children with learning problems. *Clinical Neurophysiology, 114*, 673–684.

Jirsa, R. E. (1992). The clinical utility of the P3 AERP in children with auditory processing disorders. *Journal of Speech and Hearing Research, 35*, 903–912.

Katz, J. (1962). The use of staggered spondaic words for assessing the integrity of the central auditory system. *Journal of Auditory Research, 2*, 327–337.

Katz, J. (1992). Classification of auditory processing disorders. In J. Katz, N. Stecker,

& D. Henderson (Eds.), *Central auditory processing: A transdisciplinary view* (pp. 81–93). St. Louis, MO: Mosby Year Book.

Katz, J., & Harmon-Fletcher, C. (1982). *Phonemic synthesis program training*. Vancouver, WA: Precison Acoustics.

Katz, J., & Smith, P. (1991). The Staggered Spondaic Word Test: A ten-minute look at the central nervous system through the ears. *Annals of the New York Academy of Sciences, 620*, 233–251.

Keith, R. W. (1994). *ACPT: Auditory Continuous Performance Test*. San Antonio, TX: Psychological Corp.

Keller, W. (1992). Auditory processing disorder or attention deficit disorder? In J. Katz, N. Stecker, & D. Henderson (Eds.), *Central auditory processing: A transdisciplinary view* (pp. 107–114). St. Louis, MO: Mosby.

Keller, W. (1998). The relationship between attention deficit hyperactivity disorder, central auditory processing disorders, and specific learning disorders. In In G. Masters, N. Stecker, & J. Katz (Eds.), *Central auditory processing disorders: Mostly management* (pp. 33–48). Boston, MA: Allyn & Bacon.

Keller, W., & Tillery, K. (2002). Reliable differential diagnosis and effective management of auditory processing and attention deficit hyperactivity disorders. *Seminars in Hearing, 23*, 337–348.

Keller, W., & Tillery, K. (2007). Intervention for individuals with (C)APD and ADHD: A psychological perspective. In G. Chermak & F. Musiek (Eds.), *Handbook of (central) auditory processing disorder: Comprehensive intervention* (Vol. II, pp. 309–324). San Diego, CA: Plural.

Keller, W., Tillery, K. L., & McFadden, S. (2006). Auditory processing disorders in children diagnosed with nonverbal learning disability. *American Journal of Audiology, 15*,108–113.

Kraus, N., & Disterhoft, J. F. (1982). Response plasticity of single neurons in rabbit auditory association cortex during tone-signalled learning. *Brain Research, 246*, 205–215.

Krause, N., Mcgee, T., Carrell, T., King, C., Tremblay, K., & Nicol, T. (1995). Central auditory system plasticity associated with speech discrimination training. *Journal of Cognitive Neuroscience, 71*, 25–32.

Lewis, M. S., Crandell, C., Valente, N., & Horn, J. (2004). Speech perception in noise: Directional microphones versus frequency modulation (FM) systems. *Journal of the American Academy of Audiology, 15*, 424–437.

Lindamood-Bell Learning Processes. (1998). LIPS. Lindamood phoneme sequencing program.

Massaro, D. W. (1987). *Speech perception by ear and eye: A paradigm for psychological inquiry*. Hillsdale, NJ: Lawrence Erlbaum.

McMaster University Evidence-Based Practice Center. (1999). *Treatment of attention-deficit hyperactivity disorder* (Evidence Report/Technology Assessment No. 11, AHCPR Publication no. 99-E018). Rockville, MD: Agency for Health Care Policy and Research.

Merzenich, M. M., Grajski, K., Jenkins, W., Recanzone, G., & Perterson, B. (1991). Functional cortical plasticity: Cortical network origins of representations changes. *Cold Spring Harbor Symposium on Quantum Biology, 55*, 873–887.

Merzenich, M. M., Jenkins, W. M. Johnston, P., Schreiner, C., Miller, S. L., & Tallal, P. (1996). Temporal processing deficits of language-learning impaired children ameliorated by training. *Science, 271*, 77–80.

Miller, G. L., & Knudsen, E. I. (2003, February). Adaptive plasticity in the auditory thalamus of juvenile barn owls. *Journal of Neuroscience, 23*, 1059–1065.

MTA Cooperative Group. (1999). A 14-month randomized clinical trial of treatment strategies for attention-deficit/hyperactive disorder. *Archives General Psychiatry, 56*, 1073–1086.

Musiek, F. E., Baran, J. A., & Pinheiro, M. L. (1992). P300 results in patients with lesions of the auditory areas of the cerebrum. *Journal of the American Academy of Audiology, 3,* 5–15.

Musiek, F. E., Baran, J. A., & Shinn, J. (2004). Assessment and remediation of an auditory processing disorder associated with head trauma. *Journal of the American Academy of Audiology, 15,* 117–132.

Myklebust, H. R. (1954). *Auditory processing disorders in children: A manual for differential diagnosis.* New York, NY: Grune and Stratton.

Pelham, W. E. (1999). Evidence based treatments for childhood disorders: Section initiatives. *Clinical Child Psychology Newsletter, 14,* 1–3.

Pellham, W. E., Greiner, A. R., & Gnagy, E. M. (1997). *Children's summer treatment program manual.* Buffalo, NY: Comprehensive Treatment for Attention Deficit Disorders. Retrieved from http://www .summertreatmentprogram.com

Pellham, W. E., Wheeler, T., & Chronis, A. (1998). Empirically supported psychosocial treatments for attention deficit hyperactivity disorder. *Journal of Clinical Child Psychology, 27,* 190–205.

Physican's desk reference (66th ed.). (2012). Montvail, NJ: Medical Economics.

Physician's desk reference guide to prescription drugs. (2011). Montclair, NJ: PDR Network.

Raimy, V. C. (Ed.). (1950). *Training in clinical psychology.* Englewood Cliffs, NJ: Prentice-Hall.

Report of the Planning Committee on the Boulder Conference on Graduate Education of Clinical Psychologists. (1949). Shakow Papers, M1383. In *Archives of the History of American Psychology,* University of Akron, Ohio.

Riccio, C. A. (2005). Auditory processing measure: Correlation with neuropsychological measures of attention, memory, and behavior. *Child Neuropsychology, 11,* 363–372.

Rosenberg, G. (2002). Classroom acoustics and personal FM technology in management of auditory processing disorders. *Seminars in Hearing, 23,* 309–318.

Rourke, B. (1995). *Syndrome of nonverbal learning disability: Neurodevelopmental manifestations.* New York, NY: Guilford Press.

Russo, N., Nicol, T., Zecker, S., Hayes, E., & Kraus, N. (2005). Auditory training improves neural timing in the human brainstem. *Behavioral Brain Research, 156,* 95–103.

Scientific Learning Corporation. (1997). *Fast ForWord training program for children. Procedure manual for professionals.* Berkeley, CA: Scientific Learning Corporation.

Stach, B., Loiselle, L., Jerger, J., Mintz, S., & Taylor, C. (1987). Clinical experience with personal FM assistive listening devices. *Hearing Journal, 40,* 24–30.

Tallal, P., Miller, S., Bedi, G., Wang, X., Nagarajan, S. S., Schreiner, C., . . . & Merzenich, M. M. (1996). Language comprehension in language-learning impaired children improved with acoustically modified speech. *Science, 271,* 81–84.

Tillery, K. (2012). Use of medication with auditory processing disorders. In D. Geffner & D. Swain (Eds.), *Auditory processing disorders: Management and treatment* (pp. 719–729). San Diego, CA: Plural.

Tillery, K. L., Katz, J., & Keller, W. (2000). Effects of methylphenidate (Ritalin™) on auditory performance in children with attention and auditory processing disorders. *Journal of Speech, Language, and Hearing Research, 43,* 893–901.

Tillery, K., & Kim, L. (1998). Central auditory processing assessment and therapeutic strategies for children with attention deficit hyperactivity disorder. In G. Masters, N. Stecker, & J. Katz (Eds.), *Central auditory processing disorders: Mostly management* (pp. 175–194). Boston, MA: Allyn & Bacon.

Tremblay, K. (2007). Training-related changes in the brain: Evidence from human auditory evoked potentials. *Seminars in Hearing, 28,* 120–132.

Tremblay, K., & Kraus, N. (2002). Auditory training induces asymmetrical changes in cortical neural activity. *Journal of Speech, Language, and Hearing Research, 45,* 564–572.

Tremblay, K., Kraus, N., Carrell, T., & McGee, T. (1997). Central auditory system plasticity: Generalization to novel stimulation following listening training. *Journal of the Acoustical Society of America, 102,* 3762–3773.

Tremblay, K., Kraus, N., & McGee, T. (1998). The time course of auditory perceptual learning: Neurophysiological changes during speech-sound training. *NeuroReport, 9,* 3557–3560.

Tremblay, K., Kraus, N., McGee, T., Ponton, C., & Otis, B. (2001). Central auditory plasticity: Changes in the N1-P2 complex after speech-sound training. *Ear and Hearing, 22,* 79–90.

Warrier, C. M., Johnson, K. L., Hayes, E. A., Nicol, T., & Kraus, N. (2004). Learning impaired children exhibit timing deficits and training-related improvements in auditory cortical responses to speech in noise. *Experimental Brain Research, 157,* 431–441.

Weihing, J. A., & Musiek, F. E. (2007). Dichotic interaural intensity difference (DIID) training: Principles and procedures. In D. Geffner & D. Ross-Swain (Eds.), *Auditory processing disorders: Assessment, management and treatment* (pp. 281–300). San Diego, CA: Plural.

Williams, A., Chacko, A., Fabiano, G. A., & Pelham, W. E. (2001). Behavioral treatments for children with attention-deficit hyperactivity disorder. *Primary Psychiatry, 8,* 67–72.

CHAPTER 20

DIFFERENTIAL INTERVENTION

for Central Auditory Processing Disorder, Attention Deficit Hyperactivity Disorder, and Learning Disability

JEANANE M. FERRE

The purpose of diagnosis is to determine the presence or absence and describe the nature of a disorder. Once properly diagnosed, appropriate intervention can commence designed to treat directly the disorder and to manage the impact of the disorder on the client's day-to-day life. Resources to minimize the adverse effects of the disorder on the listener's life can be allocated effectively, but only after the nature of the deficit has been diagnosed clearly.

Central auditory processing disorder (CAPD) refers to a deficit in the perceptual processing of auditory stimuli and the neurobiological activity underlying that processing (ASHA, 2005). CAPD is not the result of higher order language, cognitive, or related disorders, but may be associated with difficulties in higher order language, learning, and commu-

nication function. That is to say, CAPD may coexist with, but is not the result of, dysfunction in other modalities (ASHA, 2005). However, many disorders present behavioral characteristics similar to CAPD that can cause the listener to perform poorly on behavioral central auditory function tests and/or exhibit similar functional listening difficulties. There continues to be ongoing debate across disciplines regarding the validity of CAPD as a diagnostic entity due to the considerable shared symptomatology of CAPD as it is currently defined and other sensory, neurocognitive, and language-learning deficits (Dawes & Bishop, 2009; Jerger, 2009; Kamhi, 2011; Richard, 2011). Disorders coexisting with and/or sharing symptoms of CAPD include neurocognitive disorders (e.g., attention deficit hyperactivity disorder [ADHD], executive function disorder), cognitive impairment (e.g., mental retardation), communication disorders (e.g., autistic spectrum disorder, Asperger syndrome, language processing disorders, specific language impairment), social-emotional disturbance (e.g., behavior disorders), learning disability, and other sensory processing impairments (e.g., sensory integration disorder) (ASHA, 2005; Bellis, 2006; Bruder, Schneier, Stewart, McGrath, & Quitkin, 2004; Dlouha, 2003; Ferguson, Hall, Riley, & Moore, 2011; Keller, Tillery, & McFadden, 2006; Sharma, Purdy, & Kelly, 2009; Witton, 2010). Misdiagnosis of these disorders as CAPD, or conversely, misdiagnosis of CAPD as one of these disorders can lead to ineffective use of treatment resources, and thereby compromise intervention. Furthermore, the effects of a CAPD may exacerbate and/or be exacerbated by other sensory, communicative, or neurocognitive difficulties.

To plan effective individualized intervention that avoids misdiagnosis and/or clarifies the nature of an individual's listening or learning challenges, *differential diagnosis* must be undertaken. Differential diagnosis refers to the differentiation among two or more disorders that have similar symptoms and/or manifestations (ASHA, 2005; Bellis, 2006). As Myklebust (1954) eloquently observed, "The practical importance of making a correct diagnosis is that children having different types of problems vary significantly in their needs and unless a differential diagnosis is made, their potentialities are lost" (p. 8). That practical importance has never been more clear or imperative. Over the past 15 years the number of students receiving special education services under IDEA (Individuals with Disabilities in Education Act, 2004) has risen steadily to over six mil-

lion, of whom nearly all present with an auditory or (potentially) auditory related disorder (Figure 20–1). Those six million (plus) students represent nearly 10% of the total population of students nationwide and present with functional limitations that, if left unaddressed or inappropriately addressed, undermine their future and risks increasing the number of adults with communication disabilities significant enough to limit their ability to function in society (U.S. Dept of Education, 2008).

The differential evaluation and diagnosis of CAPD from other similar disorders requires input from a variety of disciplines, including, but not limited to, audiology, speech-language pathology, psychology/neuropsychology, occupational therapy (OT), physical therapy (PT), education, and other related professions. The audiologist administers well controlled tests designed to determine the presence or absence of an auditory disorder and to describe the nature of any specific auditory deficit(s) in the peripheral and/or central auditory systems. Other professionals contribute information regarding the extent to which there exist difficulties in other sensory processing skills and/or in higher order cognitive, linguistic, or learning skills that may confound auditory test results or may coexist with or be exacerbated by a CAPD. By examining intra- and intertest patterns within the central auditory processing test battery and relating these findings to the functional, observed day-to-day difficulties experienced by the listener, the audiologist is able to identify the presence and nature of the CAPD, describe the impact the disorder is likely to have on the listener's life, and determine the relative contribution of nonauditory factors to the listener's functioning (Bellis,

Percentage of school-age students receiving services under IDEA by disability category (adapted from U.S. Department of Education, 2008).

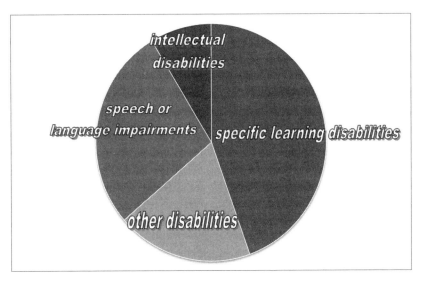

Figure 20–1. Specific learning disabilities: 45%, speech or language impairments: 19%, intellectual disabilities: 9%, other disabilities, includes autism, attention deficit disorder, emotional disturbance, hearing or vision impairment, developmental delay, and multiple disabilities: 27%

2006). This multidisciplinary approach to differential diagnosis leads logically to implementation of timely, deficit-specific intervention that mitigates lost potential, maximizes successful treatment outcomes, minimizes residual functional deficits, and utilizes resources efficiently (ASHA, 2005).

Because CAPD can have varied manifestations, intervention, like diagnosis, should be multidisciplinary in nature. The audiologist works as part of a team of professionals to develop specific, meaningful, and realistic treatment and management strategies designed to improve auditory and related skills, as well as to minimize the day-to-day impact of the disorder on the listener's academic success, communication abilities, and psychological well-being. The audiologist applies neuroscientific principles to assist in developing deficit-specific treatment and management goals, to gauge the success of those strategies, and to extend intervention principles to the variety of environments in which the individual operates in order to maximize benefit. Detailed discussions of differential diagnosis of CAPD can be found in Chapters 18 through 20 of Volume 1 of this Handbook.

This chapter describes the *differential intervention* of CAPD and related disorders (i.e., ADHD and learning disability). Case studies illustrate the shared be-havioral characteristics between/ among disorders and the multidisciplinary assessment process used to explicate characteristics unique to the diagnosis of CAPD. Selection and development of deficit-specific intervention goals by the audiologist and collaboration among professionals in implementation and determination of effectiveness of the intervention plan are described.

Steps in Developing Customized Intervention Programs

Effective intervention for CAPD requires a comprehensive therapeutic treatment and management program designed to reduce or resolve specific impairments and to minimize the adverse impact of the disorder on the listener's life skills. In treatment, deficit-specific procedures are implemented to improve deficient skills and to teach compensatory strategies. In management, efforts are directed toward minimizing the impact of the disorder on the listener's day-to-day life. The development of customized intervention programs for students with CAPD involves four steps: (1) identification of the specific auditory deficit(s), (2) determination of functional impairments as they relate to the disorder, (3) selection of deficit-appropriate treatment and management strategies, and (4) evaluation of treatment effectiveness and management success (Bellis, 2002).

Identifying the Nature of the Auditory Disorder

The evaluation of CAPD is accomplished through the administration of a battery of well-controlled, efficient tests designed to identify impairments in central audi-

tory processing skills. In general, the central auditory skill sets include auditory discrimination, binaural processing and temporal processing. More specifically, these skills include sound localization and lateralization, dependent on discrimination and binaural processing; temporal processing, including temporal discrimination, ordering, integration, and masking; auditory performance in the presence of competing signals (including dichotic listening), binaural tasks that may also tax discrimination (e.g., binaural fusion); auditory performance with degraded acoustic signals (including auditory closure); auditory discrimination; and auditory pattern recognition, associated with temporal and discrimination functions (ASHA, 1996, 2005; Bellis, 2003; Chermak & Musiek, 1997). By including tests designed to assess these skills, the audiologist not only determines the presence or absence of an auditory disorder, but also describes the nature of the disorder and specific auditory skill areas that are deficient. For a detailed discussion of specific central auditory processing tests, the reader is referred to Section 3 of Volume 1 of this Handbook.

Functional Impairments Related to CAPD

Disorder refers to a disruption of, or interference with, normal functions or established systems (Mosby Medical Dictionary, 2002). Disability refers to a physical or mental impairment that substantially limits one or more of the major life activities of an individual (Americans with Disabilities Act, 1990). The term "child with a disability" means a child: (1) with mental retardation, hearing impairments (including deafness), speech or language impairments, visual impairments (including blindness), serious emotional disturbance, orthopedic impairments, autism, traumatic brain injury, other health impairments, or specific learning disabilities; or (2) one who is experiencing developmental delays in physical development, cognitive development, communication development, social or emotional development, or adaptive development; and (3) one who needs special education and related services (Individuals with Disabilities in Education Act, 2004). The Americans with Disabilities Act (ADA) mandates safeguards afforded to and reasonable accommodations that must be provided for all citizens with disabilities; the Individuals with Disabilities in Education Act (IDEA) outlines these protections and services for children with respect to their educational experience. Because neither document specifies a federal category for CAPD, in order to establish the presence of a disability, it is essential that the *impact* of CAPD on the listener's life be described fully. It is not sufficient to identify only the presence of CAPD. Diagnostic test results must be related to educational impact and day-to-day behaviors to qualify a child for services and in order for meaningful intervention to take place. See Chapter 5 for discussion of school policies, processes, and services for children with CAPD.

To this end, the Bellis-Ferre model (1999) outlined five central auditory processing test profiles that describe the nature of the disorder based on key central auditory test findings and measures of cognition, communication, and/or learning, and associated behavioral manifestations. These manifestations include behavioral characteristics that

also may be associated with other disorders. By identifying the nonauditory factors that may affect listening, as well as the auditory factors that may affect other life skills, the multidisciplinary team is able to diagnose differentially CAPD from other related disorders in order to develop individualized intervention programs. The model is a theoretical framework in which individual test scores as well as inter- and intratest patterns of performance are examined in order to relate central auditory test findings to both their presumed underlying neurophysiological bases and functional sequelae (ASHA, 2005; Bellis, 2003, 2006; Bellis & Ferre, 1999; Ferre, 1997, 2006). The model describes three primary central auditory deficit profiles characterized by presumed underlying site of dysfunction. Two secondary profiles yield unique patterns of results on central auditory tests; however, they may be described more appropriately as manifestations of supramodal or cognitive-linguistic disorders. For a comprehensive discussion of these deficit profiles, the reader is referred to Bellis (2003, 2006) and Bellis and Ferre (1999). For the purposes of this discussion, they are described briefly here, as well as in Chapter 13.

Processing Deficit Profiles

Auditory decoding profile is characterized primarily by a deficit in auditory closure and related sound discrimination representing dysfunction in the primary (usually left) central auditory pathways. Auditory discrimination refers to the ability to analyze and extract fine acoustic differences in the speech spectrum. On central auditory tests, this profile is characterized by poor performance on degraded speech tests (e.g., recognition of filtered or time-compressed targets) and measures of temporal discrimination (e.g., temporal gap detection). Binaural and/or right ear deficits may be observed on dichotic listening tests, especially those with relatively substantial linguistic demand (e.g., dichotic words versus dichotic digits). Poor discrimination means the individual's auditory system is having difficulty extracting the fine acoustic changes within the speech spectrum. Difficulty extracting and/or discriminating fine acoustic differences in the speech spectra places the listener at risk for listening difficulties when noise is present, in highly reverberant environments (e.g., playground, cafeteria), when extra visual and/or contextual cues are not available, or when listening to a soft-spoken speaker or one whose dialect or accent differs from the listener's. Even under optimal listening conditions, the auditory system of an individual with this profile presumably is working harder than that of a typical listener to analyze incoming acoustic information. As the acoustic or linguistic conditions deteriorate, more neural energy is expended to process the acoustic portions of the signal, leaving less energy for higher order linguistic-cognitive processing. Processing inefficiency can result in fatigue and reduced listening comprehension. These behavioral listening difficulties are similar to those observed among listeners with peripheral hearing loss as well as those with ADHD. Like the listener with peripheral hearing impairment, secondary psychosocial issues may arise including social withdrawal or depressive disorder. Auditory decoding deficit can create secondary difficulties in communication skills (e.g., vocabulary, syntax, semantics, second language acquisition) and

academic skills (e.g., reading decoding, spelling, note-taking, direction following) (Bellis & Ferre, 1999). Thus, the diagnosis of this CAPD profile may co-occur with diagnoses of specific speech-language impairment or learning disability.

The integration deficit profile deficit is characterized by deficient ability to recognize and utilize unisensory or multisensory gestalt patterns quickly and efficiently. Integration deficit is believed to be the result of inefficient communication across the corpus callosum and is characterized on central auditory tests by excessive left ear suppression on dichotic listening tests combined with poor labelling but good mimicking (i.e., imitation) of tonal patterns (e.g., pitch patterns test). Deficits in skills needed for information integration may adversely affect sound-symbol association skills needed for reading, spelling, writing, and working memory, as well as the ability to complete assignments in a timely fashion and/or to get started on long assignments, direction-following and note-taking. Receptive and expressive language may be affected, especially higher level semantic, symbolic and syntactic skills. Deficits in other integrative skills (e.g., visual-motor, auditory-visual) are common in this profile (Bellis & Ferre, 1999; Ferre, 1997, 2002b, 2006). Students with integration weakness require an alternative strategy for task completion as well as extra time and practice/repetition. As task demands increase, the student may become less able to tolerate extraneous distraction. Fatigue may set in, listening attitude may deteriorate and client may give up if processing demands become overwhelming, often appearing inattentive and/or confused (Ferre, 2006, 2007). In the assessment process, impaired (auditory) integration should be differentiated from ADHD, sensory integration disorder (SI), deficits of executive functioning that may adversely affect sensory regulation, focus, and planning/execution skills; and general anxiety or depression.

When a listener displays difficulty in auditory pattern recognition, regardless of response mode (labeling or imitation) as well as excessive left ear suppression on dichotic listening tests, a prosodic deficit may be inferred. Prosodic deficit profile is characterized by deficiency in using prosodic features of the signal; a predominantly right hemisphere function. Running speech can be conceptualized as a series of acoustic patterns to which specific meaning must be attached for comprehension to occur. Too often, as we speak, word endings are dropped and perceptual timing boundaries are blurred due to failure to enunciate clearly (Picheny, Durlach, & Braida, 1985, 1986). In everyday communication, the listener must *navigate* between and among these rapidly changing acoustic patterns; analyzing, synthesizing, manipulating, and attaching meaning to them quickly and efficiently. A nonimpaired listener is able to perceive the ebb and flow of these changing patterns in the speech stream and make sense of the signals even when they are disrupted. The listener with prosodic deficit has difficulty recognizing the acoustic contours (i.e., patterns) in the rapidly occurring speech stream and perceiving timing cues in running speech (e.g., pacing, segmentation, rhythm cues). Deficient recognition of the acoustic patterns in a speech signal will impair the listener's ability to attach meaning and execute an appropriate response. For many of these listeners, little in the speech stream stands out and

speech may be perceived as a blur of largely unintelligible targets.

Prosodic deficit may manifest as inconsistent processing of rapid speech and/or difficulties listening in highly noisy or reverberant environments, when listening to unfamiliar vocabulary, an unfamiliar speaker, or to someone not speaking clearly. The listener may misperceive the intent of the message or perceive one that is very different from that which was spoken, resulting in miscommunication (Bellis, 2003).

Poor temporal patterning can affect reading, phonological, and spelling skills; direction following; note-taking; sequencing; auditory attention; working memory; and problem solving. Ability to recognize and use other types of sensory patterns (e.g., visual, tactile) may be impaired. Communication problems of the listener with prosodic deficit can include difficulties in syntactic, semantic, pragmatic, and social language skills, including difficulty understanding sarcasm and recognizing and using nonverbal pragmatic language cues such as facial expressions, body language, and gestures. (Bellis, 2006; Bellis & Ferre, 1999; Ferre, 2007). Prosodic deficit may contribute to or be misdiagnosed as pervasive developmental disorder (PDD), Asperger syndrome, nonverbal learning disability (NVLD), or oppositional defiant disorder (ODD).

As noted previously, an important central auditory skill set is binaural processing, including binaural integration and separation. Binaural integration refers to the ability to process multiple incoming auditory targets. Binaural separation refers to the processing of one target when presented with a competing signal. A primary CAPD can impair binaural processing by virtue of impaired discrimination and closure, as in the decoding profile; impaired interhemispheric communication, as in the integration profile, or impaired right hemisphere function, as in the prosodic profile. Additionally, performance on tests of binaural processing may be poor as the result of inefficient intrahemispheric communication; the presumed underlying cause of associative deficit. A secondary central auditory processing test profile, this deficit is characterized by significant auditory-language processing difficulties, believed to be related to dysfunction in the communication between the primary (Heschl's gyrus) and secondary or auditory association (Wernicke's area) cortexes of the dominant (usually left) hemisphere (Bellis & Ferre, 1999; Ferre, 1997). On central auditory tests, ability to recognize degraded speech and temporal patterns is age appropriate. The listener exhibits marked difficulty, typically bilateral or right-ear deficits, on dichotic listening tasks taxing binaural integration and separation skills. Difficulty attaching labels to patterns also may be present. Deficits in these skills impact language processing, as the listener has difficulty attaching linguistic meaning to incoming acoustic signals quickly and efficiently, that is, associating the auditory sound stream with language. As such, the listener has difficulty extracting the key information from within a message. In general, listeners with this auditory-language association deficit don't speak the same language as their peers and do not glean linguistic meaning as easily as nonimpaired listeners. The listener tends to take most statements literally and often sees ambiguity even in seemingly straightforward messages (Bellis, 2003, 2006; Bellis & Ferre, 1999; Ferre, 2006).

The listener with impaired association skills is at risk for listening difficulties in situations where vocabulary is unfamiliar, information is presented without sufficient contextual or visual cues, or when the message is linguistically ambiguous. Reading comprehension, listening comprehension, spelling, note-taking, and following directions can be adversely affected. Receptive and expressive language skills may be impaired including syntactic, semantic, symbolic, and social/pragmatic skills and/or word recall/retrieval and verbal and/or written expression. Even when specific language skills are intact, there can remain deficits in functional communication skills (i.e., using language in everyday situations to learn and communicate) (Bellis, 2003, 2006; Bellis & Ferre, 1999; Ferre, 2006). Disorders having similar symptomatology include behavior disorders, for example, oppositional defiant disorder or anxiety disorder, language-based learning disability (LLD), specific language impairment (SLI), and attention deficit disorder-inattentive type.

When discussing auditory abilities, the focus often is on the ascending auditory nervous system and issues related to signal reception. However, the discussion of the "process" of processing is incomplete without considering the listener's ability to execute a response as evidenced by accurate and appropriate verbal or written expression or successful task completion. Disorders in auditory-verbal receptive skills such as those affecting signal discrimination, analysis, synthesis, and/or meaning attachment can create disability in expression or execution skills. For example, the student who mishears *page 56* as *page 66* risks not being able to complete the assignment and may appear to have impaired direction-following abilities. However, difficulties of a performance nature (e.g., poor direction following or task completion) may exist in the absence of receptive sensory or linguistic dysfunction. In the classroom, these two students exhibit similar behaviors due to different underlying issues. Disruptions associated with impaired expressive skills or difficulty executing a response may manifest on central auditory tests as the output-organization deficit profile. Diagnostically, this secondary central auditory processing test profile is characterized by poor scores on central auditory tests requiring the reporting of multiple or precisely sequenced targets, with normal performance seen on single target and/or free recall tasks. Atypical crossed reflexes or otoacoustic emissions may be seen (Bellis, 2003). Difficulty in skills needed for information organization or recall may adversely affect planning, applied problem solving, listening comprehension, direction following, spelling, writing, expressive speech and language skills, including articulation and word finding and retrieval, and the ability to complete assignments in a timely fashion and/or to get started on long assignments. Behaviorally, the listener may exhibit difficulty hearing in noise, be disorganized, impulsive, or present with issues in executive functioning. Executive functions are the brain processes that regulate temposequential ordering, spatial ordering, attention, and working memory. They underlie the ability to set goals, manage time, organize information, and maintain focus and concentration and an active listening demeanor (Fahy & Richard, 2005). Although no specific neurophysiologic region of dysfunction is implicated by test findings, the central auditory test results and behavioral manifestations

implicate the frontal and prefrontal cortices or efferent (i.e., motor) pathways as possible sites of dysfunction (Bellis, 2006; Bellis & Ferre, 1996; Ferre, 1997; Richard 2001).

Central auditory processing assessment profiles can occur singly or in combination, although one profile typically predominates. In this regard, it is important to note that if the listener exhibits deficits in all auditory processes assessed or test results suggest the presence of more than two of the five functional deficit profiles, consideration should be given to the likelihood of a more global, higher order disorder rather than CAPD as the primary condition creating the day-to-day listening, language, and learning difficulties. Additionally, the secondary profiles described above (associative and output-organization deficit) are best viewed not as true CAPD but rather as the product of some other supramodal or linguistic-cognitive dysfunction. In the differential assessment process, the audiologist, having identified a secondary deficit profile or finding evidence suggesting global auditory processing impairment, would not diagnose a CAPD in these cases as a coexisting or contributing factor, but would provide a different perspective on another disorder, offering insight into the impact of the disorder on the student's ability to use auditory information. In differential intervention, this additional perspective can inform specificity in school or workplace accommodations, compensatory strategies, or treatment options, maximizing effectiveness of the client's overall intervention plan. Finally, it is important to note that any central auditory processing profiling system should not be used as a terminal classification system into which a student's test scores or behaviors must be fit; but rather as a starting point for conceptualizing and clarifying those findings. The students described here represent prototypical cases using the Bellis-Ferre model; their central auditory test results could be described using other conceptualizations or models. Regardless of the model one chooses to interpret assessment findings, it is imperative that a multidisciplinary approach be used in the assessment process, test scores across disciplines be related to functional needs, and management and treatment be collaborative in order to be effective (ASHA, 2005a; Bellis, 2006, 2007; Chermak, 2007; Ferre, 2006). See Chapter 8 in Volume 1 of the Handbook for discussion of the use and limitations of CAPD profiles.

Relationship of CAPD to Other Disorders

As indicated previously, there is overlap among characteristics of CAPD and the symptoms of other disorders. Disorders that share symptoms of CAPD include all types of ADHD, executive function disorder, behavior disorders including depression, anxiety disorder, oppositional defiant disorder, developmental and communication disorders such as autism spectrum disorders, Asperger disorder, and pervasive developmental disorder, specific language impairment, sensory integration disorder, and verbal and nonverbal learning disability. Characteristics associated with CAPD that are shared by other disorders are summarized in Table 20–1.

Symptomalogical overlap is especially evident in the case of ADHD, which shares characteristics with many other disorders, including CAPD. The *Diagnostic Statistical Manual* IV (DSM-IV) criteria for ADHD include difficulty attending

and sustaining attention, poor listening, inability to follow through on instructions and assignments, distractibility, forgetfulness, disorganization, hyperactivity, and impulsivity (APA, 2000). These symptoms also are associated with four of the five central auditory processing deficit profiles outlined above, including auditory decoding, integration, associative, and output-organization profiles. Similarly, executive functions are a complex set of behaviors reflecting metacognitive and control/organizational processes and include attention, working memory, strategy development, monitoring of strategies, and refinement of goals and strategies to meet needs (Hunter, 2005; Luria, 1973; Richard & Fahey, 2005). Deficits in these skills are among the behavioral characteristics of the integration, output-organization and associative profiles.

Also reflecting overlapping symptomatology, the diagnostic criteria for behavior disorders, such as oppositional defiant disorder, include symptoms of active defiance, noncompliance, and frequent arguing with adults (APA, 2000), characteristics that also may be observed among listeners who are unable to perceive message meaning or intent, such as those with prosodic or associative deficit profiles. Impaired ability to discriminate or attach meaning to incoming speech signals can lead to poor focus, fatigue and performance anxiety, characteristics of general anxiety, social phobia, and depressive disorders (APA, 2000).

Pervasive developmental disorders include autistic spectrum disorder (ASD) and Asperger disorder (APA, 2000). ASD is characterized by impaired social interactions and qualitative impairments in communication, including impaired use of nonverbal cues and social and pragmatic language, delayed development of

Table 20–1. Summary of Disorders That Share Symptoms with CAPD

Attention Deficit Disorder

distractible, inattentive, disorganized

Executive Function Disorder

poor working memory and strategy development, loses focus

Behavior Disorders

opposition, perseveration, noncompliance

Asperger's Disorder

poor social language, impaired affect

Autistic Spectrum Disorder

atypical responses to auditory input, impaired communication

Pervasive Developmental Disorder

impaired sensory processing, impaired verbal communication

Nonverbal Learning Disability

impaired prosody, poor use of nonverbal cues, impaired music perception

Verbal Learning Disability

impaired spelling, writing, syntax, semantics, poor direction-following

Speech-Language Impairment

poor phonological awareness, impaired pragmatic language

---

spoken language, and tendency to use stereotyped and/or idiosyncratic language (APA, 2000). These characteristics also may be observed among listeners diagnosed with associative or prosodic deficits. Asperger disorder is characterized by impairments in social interaction including lack of social or emotional reciprocity (e.g., affect) and impaired use of multiple nonverbal cues, such as facial expressions and gestures (APA, 2000), characteristics that are shared by the prosodic deficit profile.

In addition to exhibiting shared symptomatology with other disorders, presence of poor central auditory processing may be among the criteria for diagnosing another disorder or disabling condition. Impairments of auditory processing are included in the checklist of symptoms associated with sensory integration disorder (Ayers, 1994). For many students, presence of poor speech sound discrimination, associated with the decoding profile, poor working memory skills, observed with the associative profile, or poor sound-symbol association and synthesis skills, noted for the integration profile are contributing factors when determining presence of speech-language impairment or specific learning disability (IDEA, 2004). Furthermore, IDEA defines specific learning disability as failure to achieve adequately for age in any of several areas including listening comprehension, a functional skill set often adversely affected by CAPD. Finally, difficulty recognizing and using prosodic cues are among the characteristics of NVLD (Palombo, 2001; Tanguay, 2001; Thompson, 1997).

That symptoms co-occur across disorders and/or that symptoms of CAPD are included in the diagnostic criteria of other disorders does not invalidate the finding of impaired central auditory processing skills. Instead, the central auditory processing evaluation contributes to the clarification of the nature of the disorder underlying these shared symptoms, leading to effective differential intervention of comorbid or coexisting conditions. Inclusion of specific treatment and management of the central auditory processing component of these disorders in the individual's overall intervention plan may minimize or resolve the associated disorder or functional disability.

Selecting Appropriate Intervention Strategies

Once differential diagnosis has been accomplished, appropriate intervention strategies can be selected. To be effective, intervention must be the balanced implementation of treatment and management goals/objectives. In treatment, formal and informal therapy techniques are used to reduce or resolve auditory deficits and to teach functional compensatory strategies. In management, compensatory strategies and environmental accommodations are selected to minimize the impact of the disorder on the listener's day-to-day functioning. Following a brief overview of treatment and management approaches for CAPD, intervention programming customized for individuals presenting with CAPD in

conjunction with other sensory processing, neurocognitive, or language disorders is outlined. The reader is referred to Section 2 of this volume for in-depth coverage of components of intervention for CAPD.

Treatment Options

The inclusion of treatment in the intervention plan is designed to remediate deficient skills and teach compensatory strategies. When choosing a specific therapy, the clinician should consider the extent to which the therapy protocol is: (a) based on sound neuroscientific principles (i.e., should it work?), (b) supported by treatment outcome data (i.e., does it work?), and (c) appropriate for the type of deficit and functional needs of the listener (i.e., does it fit?) (Ferre, 2006). Any treatment program chosen must adhere to currently accepted neuropsychological, neurophysiological, and/or neuroscience principles. Therapy programs that cannot be shown to be founded on these basic principles should not be considered in the intervention plan for the listener with CAPD.

For any program under consideration, the clinician should attempt to locate reports of successful outcomes based on treatment efficacy data, treatment effectiveness data, and/or anecdotal evidence. Treatment efficacy refers to evidence of documented change for a specified population accrued under controlled conditions and provides the clinician with the highest quality evidence that the treatment program is likely to meet the listener's needs (Shapiro & Balthazar, 2004). Treatment effectiveness refers to evidence of positive outcomes for a specified population obtained in everyday conditions and is useful when efficacy data are not available (Shapiro & Balthazar, 2004). So called anecdotal evidence, while having face validity, is not a reliable index of treatment effectiveness or efficacy. Programs supported only by anecdotal reports or *expert* opinion should be used with caution and only after careful consideration of all options. See Chapters 2 and 3 of this volume for discussions of evidence-based practice and treatment efficacy.

Because of the complexity of the central nervous system and the interactive and dynamic nature of the skills it subserves, it can be safely said that there is no *silver bullet* for treating CAPD. A program that may be effective for one listener may be ineffective for another based on the specific auditory skills affected and the impact of the disorder on the listener's life. Before implementing any treatment program, the audiologist should verify the specific needs of the listener with CAPD in the classroom, workplace, and at home. In addition, the nature of the processing deficit should be described as fully as possible, as not all treatment programs may be beneficial for all types of CAPD.

Regardless of type of deficit and functional sequelae, treatment goals for CAPD should include both bottom-up therapy, designed to reduce the deficit, and top-down therapies designed to minimize the residual effects of the disorder (ASHA, 2005; Chermak & Musiek, 1997). The inclusion of bottom-up auditory training is based on neural plasticity/brain organization theory, referring to the brain's ability to reorganize itself in response to internal and/or external changes. An increasing body of work exists documenting the potential of bottom-up training to change auditory behavior (Alonso & Schochat, 2009; Chermak, Musiek, &

Bellis, 2007; Delhommeau, Micheyl, & Jouvent, 2005; Delhommeau, Micheyl, Jouvent, & Collet, 2002; Foxton, Brown, Chambers, & Griffiths, 2004; Kraus, McGee, Carrell, King, Tremblay, & Nicol, 1995; Loo, Bamiou, Campbell, & Luxon, 2008; Moore, Rosenberg, & Coleman, 2005; Musiek, 2004; Tremblay, 2007; Tremblay & Kraus, 2002; Tremblay, Kraus, Carrell & McGee, 1997; Tremblay, Kraus, McGee, Picton, & Otis, 2001). Bottom-up therapy for auditory and related skills may include, but is not limited to, auditory training, including binaural processing training, temporal discrimination and patterning training, interhemispheric transfer training, speech recognition in noise training, and even speechreading training (Bellis, 2003; Chermak & Musiek, 1997, 2002; Ferre, 1997, 2002a; Flowers, 1983; Kelly, 1995; Masters, 1998; Moore et al., 2005; Musiek, 2005; Sloan, 1995; Musiek, Chermak, & Weihing, 2007).

Although intensive bottom-up training exploits plasticity, top-down therapy is considered extensive treatment designed to complement bottom-up training efforts, maximize generalization of skills across settings and minimize functional deficits. By strengthening higher order metalinguistic, metacognitive, and metamemory skills, day-to-day listening, language, and learning problems can be minimized (ASHA, 2005). Top-down therapies include auditory closure training, prosody training, metamemory skills training, metalinguistic skills training, and metacognitive strategies training (Bellis, 2003; Chermak, 1998, 2007; Ellis, 1989; Ferre, 1997).

Management Strategies

The goal of the management plan for the listener with CAPD is to maximize the individual's ability to communicate effectively across a variety of settings (ASHA, 2005). To accomplish this goal, management strategies (summarized in Table 20–2) may include modifications to the environment, adjustments to auditory or academic demands at home, work, or school, or use of support services and/or technology. Environmental modifications include, but are not limited to, noise abatement in school, the workplace, or the home, physical, and architectural changes to the listening environment, preferential seating, increased availability of visual cues, and instruction to talkers to speak more clearly (i.e., clear speech) in order to improve signal access (Ferre, 2002b, 2007).

Improving room acoustics enhances the listening skills of all listeners (ANSI, 2002; Crandell & Smaldino, 2002). Noise abatement techniques may range from simple to extensive, depending upon listener's needs and available resources. Extensive, and often expensive, solutions for improving workplace or classroom acoustics include elimination of open classrooms and/or cubicle-type workspaces; relocation of teaching or work spaces away from areas of outside noise (e.g., playgrounds, train tracks); use of double-paned windows or noise dampening devices on heating, air conditioning, and ventilation systems; lowered ceilings and smaller rooms. Simpler and less expensive noise abatement can be accomplished in the home or at school or work by closing windows and doors, carpeting rooms, using curtains and/or acoustic ceiling tiles, placing baffles

Table 20–2. Management Strategies for Central Auditory Processing Disorder

Bottom-up Management Focus on Signal Access	Top-Down Management Focus on Communication
Clear Speech—Enhances Acoustics • slightly reduced speed/increased loudness • repetition	Clear Language—Clarifies Message • rephrase • minimize/generic nonliteral language
Visual Cues—Supplements Auditory Information • manipulatives, graphs/charts • speechreading	Familiarity & Linguistic Redundancy—Improves Communication Access • preview material • knowledge of "rules" in advance
Noise Abatement—Improves Access • baffles/damping, infrastructure changes • listener located away from noise	Curricular Changes—Minimizes Processing Overload • listening breaks, schedule changes • extended time
Listening Technology—Improves Signal Quality, Reduces Fatigue Speed • FM systems • noise-reducing earplugs	Technology—Compensates for Impaired Auditory Skills • computer use • digital recorder/smart pen

within the listening space, damping highly reflective surfaces, rearranging furniture, and minimizing the number of speakers talking at the same time. For more detailed discussion of acoustics and CAPD management, the reader is referred to Chapter 4 of this volume.

Sitting or standing near and facing the speaker can counteract the adverse effects of distance, noise or poor lighting and enhance the listener's ability to use available relevant visual cues. In clear speech, the focus is on enhancing speech recognition by modifying the speech of the talker. The speaker is trained to speak at a slightly reduced rate and to use a slightly increased volume, thus enhancing spectral boundaries and characteristics, improving signal timing and prosody, and increasing relative consonant-to-vowel intensities (Bradlow et al., 2003; Ferguson & Kewley-Port, 2002; Krause & Braida, 2004; Picheny, Durlach, & Braida, 1985, 1986). By using clear speech in an auditory-visual presentation, speech recognition is enhanced compared with an auditory-only presentation (Helfer, 1997). By using clear speech and clear language, listening comprehension is improved. Clear language includes minimizing generic language and nonspecific references, rephrasing, minimizing ambiguous statements or questions, adding or emphasizing "tag" words such as *first, last, before, after,* using verbal cues and prompts, and limiting the overall amount of information given at one time (Ellis, 1989).

While useful to all listeners, clear language is especially important when considering adjustments to the daily listening and learning demands of the student with CAPD. Other adjustments include preteaching or previewing new material, which enhances familiarity with the target, extended time or reduced workload, course substitutions or waivers, adjusted schedules, multisensory educational or work environment, repetition and rephrasing, and test-taking modifications. Finally, some listeners will require support for information access that takes the form of direct signal enhancement via assistive listening technology, supported learning via computer assistance, use of concrete manipulatives (e.g., number line, beads for learning math concepts), organizers, digital recording devices (e.g., smart pen), or note-taking service or scribe. For detailed discussion of management strategies the reader is referred to Chapters 13 and 14 of this volume.

Relationships Among Intervention Strategies for CAPD and Related Disorders

Because CAPD shares symptomatology with other disorders, it should not be surprising that intervention for CAPD may be, in some cases, similar to the treatment and management strategies recommended for other disorders. Bottom-up therapy to improve speech recognition in noise, indicated for listeners with auditory decoding and, often, output-organization profiles (Ferre, 1997), also may be a useful addition to the behavioral treatment plan for the listener with ADHD or for students on the autistic spectrum. Temporal patterning training and its top-down extension, prosody training, are appropriate treatment options for listeners with the prosodic profile. Language therapy to improve use of prosodic elements (e.g., rhythm, stress, and intonation) is among the treatment recommendations for clients with NVLD (Tanguay, 2001; Thompson, 1997), as well as for students with phonological processing disorders (Tyler, 1997). Interhemispheric transfer training, which often includes whole-body exercises, is an appropriate intervention for the listener with the integration deficit profile and for listeners with autistic spectrum disorder, sensory integration disorder (Ayers, 1994), and NVLD (Thompson, 1997). Finally, treatment options for listeners with ADHD, executive function disorder, NVLD, Asperger's syndrome, language processing disorders, and language-based learning disabilities include some of the same kinds of top-down therapies appropriate for CAPD, including metamemory skills training, metalinguistic skills training, and metacognitive strategies training (Duesenberg, 2006; Gerber, 1993; Ingersoll & Goldstein, 1993; Johnson, 1983; Phillips-Keeley, 2003; Richard, 2001; Richard & Fahey, 2005; Thompson, 1997).

In the classroom, home, or workplace, listeners with auditory decoding deficit profile require modifications and compensations that improve the quality of and access to the acoustic signal and enhance access to nonauditory cues. For listeners with associative deficit profile, management strategies that transform the signal to improve linguistic comprehension are needed. Strategies that adjust the quantity and structure of the signal are indicated for the listener with the integration deficit profile, while listeners with the prosodic deficit profile require improvement to both signal quantity and quality. Finally, students presenting the output-organization deficit profile need enhanced signal salience and assistance in organization of their responses to the signal (Ferre, 2002b). These same management strategies are among the environmental modifications and supports that are recommended for clients with ADHD (Duesenberg, 2006; Ingersoll & Goldstein, 1993), executive function dis-

order (Phillips-Keeley, 2003; Richard & Fahey, 2005), NVLD (Thompson, 1997), learning disability (e.g., dyslexia) (Horn & Horn, 2005), and language processing disorders (Richard, 2001). The degree of overlap among symptoms and intervention options for central auditor processing and other disorders that can impair language, listening, and learning does not invalidate the diagnosis of any or either disorder, but rather necessitates both differential diagnosis to inform our intervention plan and differential intervention to effect positive outcomes for our clients.

Gauging Success

Selection of appropriate treatment and management goals is incomplete without the inclusion of measurable outcomes to determine whether intervention goals and objectives have been achieved (ASHA, 2005). The multidisciplinary team has a variety of methods available to gauge the success of the intervention plan. To document treatment efficacy and/or effectiveness, one must establish that real change has occurred as a result of the treatment and not of some uncontrolled factor or, in the case of a child, maturation (Goldstein, 1990). For treatments designed to improve specific auditory skills, the clinician may rely on auditory test performance, measured pretreatment, at regular intervals during the course of the therapy, and again at a specified posttreatment interval to determine treatment effectiveness and/or efficacy. These data may include documentation from both behavioral and electrophysiological measures (Ferre, 1998; Jirsa, 2002; Kraus, McGee, Ferre, Hoeppner, Carrell, Sharma, & Nicol, 1993; Putter-Katz, Said, Feldman, Miran, Kushnir, Muchnik, & Hildesheimer, 2002; Seats, 1998; Tremblay, 2007).

Because CAPD may lead to or be associated with other disorders, improved central auditory function may contribute to improvement in other skill areas. The overall goal of intervention should be improved auditory performance and improved language, learning, and listening skills. Outcome measures should include both evidence of improvement in performance on tests of auditory function and documented change in related functional skills at home and school (ASHA, 2005; Chermak & Musiek, 1997). Team members may find evidence of positive outcomes by examining changes in performance on academic and language tests following implementation of a customized intervention plan (Chermak, Curtis, & Seikel, 1996; Ferre, 1997; 1998; Shapiro & Mistal, 1985, 1986; Tallal & Merzenich, 1997). Improved values on listening performance checklists such as the CHAPS (Children's Auditory Performance Scale) (Smoski, Brunt, & Tannahill, 1998) or on self-assessment measures (Ferre, 1997; Kelly, 1995) provide outcome data concerning the extent to which overall communication skills across a variety of settings have improved. Finally, observations of the client, teacher, parent, family members, caregivers, or other significant others should not be discounted as real-life, albeit subjective, measures of success or shortcomings of the intervention plan.

Case Studies In Differential Diagnosis and Intervention

The following cases illustrate the application of differential diagnosis and intervention for CAPD and related dis-

orders. For all students, central auditory test results were interpreted using the Bellis-Ferre model (1999), which also characterizes behaviors suggestive of comorbid disorders in other sensory, neurocognitive, and/or language skills. Given the nature of central auditory tests, results cannot rule in or rule out deficits in other sensory processes, linguistic, or neurocognitive skills. Multidisciplinary evaluations are needed to determine definitively primary and, as appropriate, secondary diagnoses. For some cases presented below, evaluations by related professionals preceded the central auditory processing evaluation and in others, followed it. The order in which diagnostic assessments are completed for any listener is dependent on presenting complaints of the client and likely of less importance than the fact that a differential diagnostic assessment is undertaken.

Hannah—CAPD and Visual Processing Disorder

This 9-year-old student, with reported behavior disorder, was referred for evaluation by the classroom teacher following observation of poor outcomes of a classroom behavior management program. The original management plan included verbal and visual cueing by the teacher and classroom aide (e.g., change in tone of voice, use of facial expressions) to assist the student in classroom listening, maintaining focus, remaining on task, and following directions. Neuropsychological evaluation had ruled out presence of ADHD as a contributing factor. Central auditory evaluation was requested to examine CAPD as a potential contributing factor. Central auditory test findings revealed excessive left ear suppression on dichotic listening tasks and inability to label or mimic auditory patterns, indicating prosodic deficit profile, a right hemisphere–based processing deficit.

At the team meeting, the audiologist noted that inability to recognize and use prosodic features of speech might explain the student's inability to benefit from the verbal cueing and facial expressions incorporated in the original management plan. Aural rehabilitation recommendations included implementation of a temporal patterning training protocol that consisted of the following specific stepwise goals: discrimination of same-difference for two-tone and three-tone sequences varying in pitch, loudness, or duration; identification of these pattern types from a closed set, imitation of tonal patterns, labelling of two- and three-tone sequences; discrimination, identification, and recognition of stress in words and sentences, interpretation of stress in sentences, and prosodic interpretation (e.g., determination of message intent) all executed first in a quiet listening environment and again in varying levels of background noise. In addition, recommendation was made for comprehensive evaluation by a developmental vision specialist who subsequently diagnosed deficits in visual tracking and visual pattern recognition. The use of verbal and visual cueing was temporarily suspended in favor of implementation of treatment to improve both auditory and visual pattern recognition skills. Following successful vision therapy, goals to improve lipreading/speechreading and other nonverbal cues were added to the individualized educational plan (IEP).

This case highlights the importance of differential diagnosis and outcome measurement for effective intervention. This student had been misdiagnosed as having a behavior disorder with implementation of an intervention plan judged,

by observation, to be ineffective. In this case, thorough diagnostic testing led to appropriate diagnosis of comorbid sensory processing disorders and effective differential intervention for these related processing issues that subsequently improved social interactions and classroom listening behaviors.

Seth—Suspected CAPD and Language Processing Disorder

This 14-year-old (8th grade) student was referred for central auditory testing by the speech-language pathologist to determine the extent to which apparent language processing difficulties might have resulted from CAPD. Speech-language evaluation indicated age appropriate basic language skills with evidence of higher order language processing deficiency (e.g., deficits in recognizing and using word associations, attributes, multiple meaning words, and ambiguous statements). Additionally, Seth had performed poorly on a screening test of central auditory function, as well as on several measures of related auditory-language function. Following the basic audiologic evaluation indicating normal peripheral hearing function, a central auditory evaluation was completed that indicated normal performance for degraded speech and auditory patterning tasks, but bilaterally poor scores for three tests of dichotic listening. Taken together, auditory and language test results and presence of functional difficulties when asked to apply the rules of language across contexts (e.g., tended to answer *yes* initially to questions such as, *Which do want, A or B?*; displayed poor topic maintenance in conversation; and tended to respond to literal meaning of statements where response to implied meaning was required, such as responding *yes* to questions that began, *Didn't I tell you yesterday . . .*) resulted in diagnoses of comorbid central auditory associative profile and language processing disorder.

This student's IEP included a 30-week therapy program to improve dichotic listening, metalinguistic and metacognitive skills, language processing, and social/pragmatic language skills. Recommended modifications and compensations for this student included: rephrasing using concrete language; clarification and demonstration of abstract concepts; avoidance of ambiguous and/or misleading language by parents and teachers (e.g., *Don't park your bike in the driveway* instead of *How many times have I told you not to park your bike in the driveway?*); preteaching new vocabulary, especially in science classes; waiver of middle school second language requirement; use of books on tape, study guides, and Cliff's Notes™[1]; and academic tests administered by speech-language pathologist with questions read to student and clarified as needed.

The student's family was encouraged to play games at home that could build auditory-language proficiency including Password®, Taboo®, Catch-Phrase®, Scattergories®, Plexers®(word puzzles), and Quizzles® (logic puzzles).[2] Re-evaluation of auditory skills at 10-week intervals during therapy and 12 weeks after termination of therapy indicated steady improvement in dichotic listening skills with age appropriate levels noted at final evaluation (12 weeks posttherapy). Speech-language evaluation conducted at the beginning of 9th grade indicated

significant improvement in language processing and related functional communication skills. Therapy was discontinued and environmental modifications and compensations were maintained as needed through high school to minimize residual effects on day-to-day functioning. In this case, differential diagnosis clarified the nature of the student's functional communication difficulties and differential intervention with a motivated student created successful functional outcomes in a relatively short period of time.

Brooke—CAPD and ADHD

This 10-year-old student was referred for evaluation upon arrival from another school district. Parents reported that previous evaluation had indicated CAPD and the need for computer-assisted auditory perceptual training and classroom use of an assistive listening device; however, no documentation was available. As a new student to the district, the case study team recommended reevaluation prior to the implementation of what was considered an intensive and costly intervention plan.

The student reported difficulty sustaining attention and neuropsychological evaluation could not rule out ADHD as a contributing factor. Parents were reluctant to initiate a medication trial based on available diagnostic information. Central auditory evaluation confirmed presence of deficits in auditory closure and discrimination with poor performance noted on degraded speech and temporal discrimination tasks. Behavioral

---

[1]Cliffs Notes™ is a registered trademark of Hungry Minds, Inc.
[2]Scattergories®, Catch Phrase®, and Taboo® are registered trademarks of Hasbro, Inc; Password® is a registered trademark of Mark Goodson Productions, LLC; Plexers® is a registered trademark of Plexers, Inc.; Quizzles® is a registered trademark of Dale Seymour Publications, Inc.

characteristics exhibited by the student were consistent with an auditory decoding deficit profile, but also could be accounted for by presence of ADHD. Intervention team concurred with the original reported recommendations of trial use of an assistive listening device (personal FM system) and participation in the Fast ForWord auditory perceptual training program.[3]

Use of a personal FM system was terminated after three weeks based upon reports by the teacher of minimal noticeable change in classroom listening behaviors and the student's negative response to the device. Auditory reevaluation 3 months after conclusion of intensive (daily) computer-assisted auditory training revealed normal performance on all tests of central auditory function. However, observational and self-assessment checklists indicated only modest improvement in day-to-day listening skills despite the apparent resolution of the auditory deficits and implementation of a customized classroom management plan. Although treatment outcome was excellent with respect to specific, discrete auditory performance (as measured by central auditory function tests), overall intervention effectiveness was judged to be unsatisfactory. Additional consultation with parents led to trial use of nonstimulant medication to control symptoms of (apparent) ADHD. Student, parents, and teachers noted significant change in listening and day-to-day communication skills within 30 days of addition of medication to the intervention plan.

This case illustrates the importance of diagnosing comorbid conditions and addressing those conditions concurrently.

Although diagnosis of ADHD was inconclusive and parents were reluctant to pursue pharmacological intervention options, limited treatment success led to review and revision of the intervention plan.

Daniel—Subjective and Objective Outcome Evidence Informs Differential Diagnostic Process

This 10-year-old boy was diagnosed with decoding type central auditory processing deficit. Follow-up electrophysiological assessment noted atypical cortical evoked potentials. Neuropsychological assessment could not rule out ADHD. Like Brooke, above, Daniel's parents were reluctant to pursue medication trial, requesting behavioral therapy, instead. Aural rehabilitation was initiated that included activities to improve auditory discrimination and closure, use of visual cues, and active listening. Twenty individual one-hour sessions were provided (over a 20-week period), after which behavioral and electrophysiological central auditory reevaluations were conducted, as well as consultation with a second (different) neuropsychologist. Post-therapy assessments revealed all behavioral central auditory test scores within normal limits for age, brainstem and cortical evoked potentials with normal latencies, amplitudes, and morphologies; and no evidence of ADHD on second neuropsychological consultation. Daniel's short-term auditory therapy was judged to be completely successful not only in resolving the auditory perceptual deficit, as indicated by objective electrophysiological data, but also in eliminating func-

---

[3]Fast ForWord is a registered trademark of Scientific Learning Corporation.

tional behaviors shared by two diagnostic entities, CAPD and ADHD.

Vale—CAPD, Visual Processing Disorder, Language Disorder, and Learning Disability in Two Languages

Vale, age 9 years, 7 months at first visit, was seen following neuropsychological testing. Vale resides in a bilingual home (Spanish-English). Medical history included multiple ear infections beginning during first year of life, insertion of pressure equalization tubes (PE) at one year of age, and diagnosis of attention deficit disorder for which medication was tried with no reported positive outcomes. Prior to central auditory evaluation, Vale had begun receiving bilingual speech-language therapy and computer-assisted auditory training (English targets). Vision evaluation noted binocular teaming issues for which vision therapy was recommended. At the time of her initial evaluation, she attended a bilingual (English-Spanish) school and was struggling to meet the demands of a third grade curriculum, particularly in reading comprehension and expressive language skills. Initial central auditory evaluation revealed age appropriate ability to imitate tonal patterns, but poor auditory discrimination, excessive left-ear suppression on dichotic listening tests and very poor ability to label tonal patterns. The comprehensive intervention program developed among parents and professionals included continued computer-assisted auditory training, dichotic listening and temporal patterning (labeling) training, vision therapy, occupational therapy (OT), continued speech-language therapy and multisensory educational remediation. Vale engaged in intensive auditory and speech-language therapy for 4 weeks in the United States that yielded statistically significant improvement in a relatively short period (Table 20–3, age 9 yrs, 11 mos). Decision was made to home-school Vale with additional daily services from a private bilingual speech-language pathologist. Academic progress after 3 months (age 10 yrs, 2mos) was significant with Vale working at a 4th grade

Table 20–3. Summary of Pre- and Posttherapy Scores for Client Vale

Test/Age	9 yrs. 7 mos.	9 yrs. 11mos.	10 yrs. 2 mos.	10 yrs. 6 mos.	10 yrs. 11mos.	11 yrs. 1 mos.
LPFS	**60/40**	DNT	**60/64**	88/76	DNT	80/84
DD	93/**50**	85/**65**	95/**75**	85/83	88/85	90/88
DR	43/**30**	46/**36**	40/40	DNT	DNT	46/46
CST	93/**25**	95/**20**	95/**35**	95/**35**	95/**60**	95/**65**
PPS-labeled	**20**	**50**	**50**	**60**	85	**80**

LPFS = low-pass filtered speech; *DD* = dichotic digits; *DR* = dichotic rhyme; *CST* = competing sentences test; *PPS* = pitch patterns sequencing–labeled response; *DNT* = did not test.

All scores are percent correct recorded as Right ear/Left ear.

Scores in **bold type** are below normal limits for age.

level in all subjects, in both languages, except math (at 3rd grade level). She continued to receive daily OT and vision therapy in addition to ongoing speech-language and aural rehabilitation with continued modest improvement noted. Rechecks at age 10 years, 6 months and 10 years, 11 months, the latter following repeat 4-week therapy block, noted auditory discrimination, binaural integration and ability to label tonal patterns at age appropriate levels with persistent difficulty in binaural separation skills. Recheck at age 11 years, 1 month indicated auditory closure/discrimination, temporal processing, and binaural integration skills at expected levels for age, but persistent weakness in binaural separation skills. At the time of this writing, Vale is in a regular fifth grade bilingual classroom (predominantly English, some Spanish) with educational support in the form of educational accommodations only. Private educational/speech-language therapy is continuing with emphasis on word retrieval strategies and semantic language. Vision therapy has been reduced to three sessions per week with a maintenance schedule established for implementation following completion of two specific training exercises.

In this case, numerous professionals and parents worked together to identify clearly the sensory, communicative, and educational challenges facing this student. Her intervention program was comprehensive, differential, dynamic, intensive and extensive, and designed to meet her particular individual needs. Deficit-specific therapy, adjustments to the listening and learning environment, and maturation conspired positively to reduce significantly Vale's sensory defi-

cits and coexisting communicative and academic challenges and provide her with the functional skills she will need for future success.

Eli—Auditory Processing Issues: Not CAPD

This 8-year-old boy was referred by his neuropsychologist following comprehensive assessment. That evaluation noted superior performance in visual-related tasks of psychological and achievement tests with below average performance in auditory-related tasks. ADHD was ruled out. Follow-up speech-language evaluation noted difficulties in auditory memory and listening comprehension skills. Parents reported that Eli was beginning to dislike school, limit his participation in class, and complain that he "could not hear." Both the neuropsychologist and the speech-language pathologist requested a comprehensive central auditory processing evaluation to determine the extent to which observed functional auditory weakness was the result of specific central auditory impairment.

Eli exhibited normal peripheral auditory function and scores within normal limits for age across all central auditory tests including recognition of filtered words, time-compressed speech, dichotic listening tests (including dichotic digits dichotic rhyme and competing sentences), temporal resolution, and pitch sequencing task. When asked to repeat single words presented in a background of equal (0 SNR) or louder (−5 SNR) multispeaker babble, scores were judged to be adequate for age. Of particular interest was the finding of a decrease in word recognition ability when words were presented at –5 SNR with visual (lipreading) cues. Eli's score fell from 80% auditory-only to 48% with the auditory-visual (AV) presentation, unexpected given the finding that addition of visual cues tends to enhance word recognition for most listeners (Helfer, 1997). In this case, cumulative results confirmed the presence of poor listening abilities for age that adversely affected Eli's performance on cognitive-linguistic tests, in the classroom, and at home but no evidence of specific central auditory impairment. As Eli was already being seen by a speech-language pathologist (SLP) for work on memory and verbal direction following, the audiologist recommended inclusion of training in the use of visual cues, listening in noise, and ability to identify key elements in a verbal message as additional components of his therapy designed to improve overall active listening skills. At the time of this writing, therapy is ongoing with preliminary reports from the SLP and parents of noticeable improvement in direction following, class participation, and short-term memory. Eli was overheard to remark to friends that he is learning to "listen with my eyes and not just my ears."

Eli's case illustrates two key points. The central auditory assessment examined the integrity of Eli's auditory skills —peripheral, central, and functional— and was not designed simply to diagnose a CAPD. More importantly, true collaboration among professionals in the assessment process uncovered the nature of a problem having symptoms associated with any number of specific issues and in intervention, all professionals provided input to address not simply performance on tests but functional listening, learning, and life skills.

Summary

CAPD can affect adversely academic achievement, communication proficiency, life skills, and sense of self, and can coexist with deficits in attention, learning, language, and listening. The differential diagnosis of CAPD and related, often comorbid disorders leads to differential intervention that is essential to efficacy. In differential diagnosis, parents and members of the multidisciplinary team interpret results of formal assessments and informal observation to clarify the nature of the deficit or deficits that adversely affect a listener's life. In differential intervention, that same team develops recommendations for management and treatment that are deficit- and listener-specific. Management goals should target improved access to and use of auditory-verbal information at home, in the classroom, and/ or at work. Treatment programs should be chosen to target deficient auditory and related skills, and this customized plan must be extended and expanded throughout the day and across listening environments in order to be effective. In so doing, the personal and financial resources available for assessment and intervention are used effectively to create positive outcomes for the listener.

References

Alonso, R., & Schochat, E. (2009). The efficacy of formal auditory training in children with (central) auditory processing disorder: Behavioral and electrophysiological evaluation. *Brazilian Journal of Otorhinolaryngology, 75,* 726–732.

American National Standards Institute. (2002). *ANSI S12.60-2002. Acoustical performance criteria, design requirements and guidelines for schools.* Melville, NY: Author.

American Psychiatric Association. (2000). *Diagnostic criteria from the DSM-IV-TR®.* Arlington, VA: Author.

Americans with Disabilities Act, Public Law 336. (1990). Retrieved from http://www.usdoj.gov/crt/ada/publicat.htm

ASHA (American Speech Language Hearing Association). (1996). Central auditory processing: Current status of research and implications for clinical practice. *American Journal of Audiology, 5,* 41–54.

ASHA. (2005). *Technical report: (Central) auditory processing disorders.* Rockville, MD: Author.

Ayers, M. (1994). *Sensory integration and the child.* Los Angeles, CA: Western Psychological Services.

Bellis, T. (2002). Developing deficit-specific intervention plans for individuals with auditory processing disorders. *Seminars in Hearing, 23,* 287–295.

Bellis, T. (2003). *Assessment and management of central auditory processing disorders in the educational setting* (2nd ed.). Clifton Park, NY: Thomson Delmar Learning.

Bellis, T. (2006). Interpretation of APD test results. In T.K. Parthasarathy (Ed.), *An introduction to auditory processing disorders in children* (pp. 145–160). Mahwah, NJ: Lawrence Erlbaum Associates.

Bellis, T. (2007). Historical foundations and the nature of (central) auditory processing disorder. In F. Musiek & G. Chermak (Eds.), *Handbook of (central) auditory processing disorder: Auditory neuroscience and diagnosis* (Vol. I, pp. 119–136). San Diego, CA: Plural.

Bellis, T., & Ferre, J. (1999). Multidimensional approach to differential diagnosis of central auditory processing disorders in children. *Journal of the American Academy of Audiology, 10,* 319–328.

Bradlow, A., Kraus, N., & Hayes, E. (2003). Speaking clearly for children with learning disabilities: Sentence perception in noise. *Journal of Speech, Language, and Hearing Research, 46,* 80–97.

Bruder, G., Schneier, F., Stewart, J., McGrath, P., & Quitkin, F. (2004). Left hemisphere dysfunction during verbal dichotic listening tests in patients who have social phobia with or without comorbid depressive disorder. *American Journal of Psychiatry, 161,* 72–78.

Carrow-Woodfolk, E. (1999). *Comprehensive Assessment of Spoken Language.* Circle Pines, MN: American Guidance Service.

Chermak, G. D. (1998). Metacognitive approaches to managing central auditory processing disorders. In M. Masters, N. Stecker, & J. Katz. (Eds). *Central auditory processing disorders: Mostly management* (pp. 49–61). Boston, MA: Allyn & Bacon.

Chermak, G. (2007). Central resource training: Cognitive, metacognitive, and metalinguistic skills and strategies. In G. Chermak & F. Musiek (Eds.), *Handbook of (central) auditory processing disorder: Comprehensive intervention* (Vol. II, pp. 107–166). San Diego, CA: Plural.

Chermak, G., Musiek, F., & Bellis, T. (2007). Neurobiology, cognitive science, and intervention. In G. Chermak & F. Musiek (Eds.), *Handbook of (central) auditory processing disorder: Comprehensive intervention* (Vol. II, pp. 3–28). San Diego, CA: Plural.

Chermak, G. D., Curtis, L., & Seikel, J. (1996). The effectiveness of an interactive hearing conservation program for elementary school children. *Language, Speech, and Hearing Services in Schools, 27,* 29–39.

Chermak, G. D., & Musiek, F. E. (1997). *Central auditory processing disorders: New perspectives.* San Diego, CA: Singular.

Chermak, G. D., & Musiek, F. E. (2002). Auditory training principles and approaches for remediating and managing auditory processing disorders. *Seminars in Hearing, 23,* 297–308.

Crandell, C., & Smaldino J. (2002). Room acoustics and auditory rehabilitation technology. In J. Katz (Ed.), *Handbook of clinical audiology* (5th ed., pp. 607–630). Philadelphia, PA: Lippincott Williams & Wilkins.

Dawes, P., & Bishop, D. (2009) Auditory processing disorder in relation to developmental disorders of language, communication, and attention: A review and critique. *International Journal of Language and Communication Disorders, 44*, 440–465.

Delmommeau, K., Micheyl, C., & Jouvent, R. (2005). Generalization of frequency discrimination learning across frequencies and ears: Implications for underlying neural mechanisms in humans. *Journal of the Association for Research in Otolaryngology, 6*, 171–179.

Delmommeau, K., Micheyl, C., Jouvent, R. & Collett, L. (2002). Transfer of learning across durations and ears in auditory frequency discrimination. *Perception and Psychophysics, 64*, 426–436.

Dlouha, O. (2003). Central auditory processing disorder in children with developmental dysphasia. *International Congress Series, 1240*, 231–234.

Duesenberg, D. (2006). ADHD: Diagnosis and current treatment options to improve functional outcomes. In T. Parthasarathy (Ed.), *An introduction to auditory processing disorders in children* (pp. 187–201). Mahwah, NJ: Lawrence Erlbaum Associates.

Ellis, E. (1989). A metacognitive intervention for increasing class participation. *Learning Disabilities Focus, 5*, 36–46.

Fahy, J., & Richard, G. (2005). *The source for development of executive functions.* East Moline, IL: Linguisystems.

Ferguson, M., Hall, R., Riley, A., & Moore, D. (2011). Communication, listening, cognitive, and speech perception skills in children with auditory processing disorder (APD) or specific language impairment (SLI). *Journal of Speech, Language, and Hearing Research, 54*, 211–227.

Ferguson, S., & Kewley-Port, D. (2002). Vowel intelligibility in clear and conversational speech for normal-hearing and hearing-impaired listeners. *Journal of the Acoustical Society of America, 112*, 259–271.

Ferre, J. (1997). *Processing Power: A guide to CAPD assessment and management.* San Antonio, TX: Psychological Corporation.

Ferre, J. (1998). The M3 model for treating central auditory processing disorders. In M. Masters, N. Stecker, & J. Katz (Eds.). *Central auditory processing disorders: Mostly management* (pp. 103–116). Boston, MA: Allyn & Bacon.

Ferre, J. (2002a). Behavioral therapeutic approaches for central auditory problems. In J. Katz. (Ed.), *Handbook of clinical audiology* (5th ed., pp. 525–531). Philadelphia, PA: Lippincott Williams & Wilkins.

Ferre, J. (2002b). Managing children's auditory processing deficits in the real world: What teachers and parents want to know. *Seminars in Hearing, 23*, 319–326.

Ferre, J. (2006). Management strategies for APD. In T. K. Parthasarathy (Ed.), *An introduction to auditory processing disorders in children* (pp. 161–183). Mahwah, NJ: Lawrence Erlbaum Associates.

Ferre, J. (2007). The ABCs of CAP: Practical strategies for enhancing central auditory processing skills. In D. Geffner & D. R. Swain (Eds.), *Auditory processing disorders* (pp. 187–205). San Diego, CA: Plural.

Flowers, A. (1983). *Auditory perception, speech, language, and learning.* Dearborn, MI: Perceptual Learning Systems.

Foxton, J., Brown, A., Chambers, S., & Griffiths, T. (2004). Training improves acoustic pattern perception. *Current Biology, 14*, 322–325.

Gerber, A. (1993). *Language-related learning disabilities: Their nature and treatment.* Baltimore, MD: Paul H. Brookes.

Goldstein, H. (1990). Assessing clinical significance. In L. Olswang, C. Thompson, S. Warren, & N. Minghetti (Eds.), *Treatment efficacy research in communication disorders* (pp. 91– 98). Rockville, MD: ASHA.

Helfer, K. (1997). Auditory and auditory-visual perception of clear and conversational speech. *Journal of Speech, Language, and Hearing Research, 40*, 432–443.

Horn, S., & Horn, D. (2005). *ADHD and dyslexia: Choosing effective interventions.* Paper presented at the annual meeting of the International Dyslexia Association. Denver, CO.

Hunter, S. (2005). *Working memory as an executive function: Implications for education.* Paper presented at the annual meeting of the Illinois Branch of the International Dyslexia Association, Oakbrook Terrace, IL.

Individuals with Disabilities in Education Act of 2004. (2004). Retrieved from http://idea.ed.gov/explore

Ingersoll, B., & Goldstein, S. (1993). *Attention deficit disorder and learning disabilities: Realities, myths, and controversial treatments.* New York, NY: Doubleday Dell.

Jerger, J. (2009). The concept of auditory processing disorder: A brief history. In A. Cacace & D. McFarland (Eds.), *Controversies in auditory processing disorder* (pp. 1–14). San Diego, CA: Plural.

Jirsa, R. (2002). Clinical efficacy of electrophysiologic measures in auditory processing disorders management programs. *Seminars in Hearing, 23,* 349–356.

Johnson, D. (1983). Design for individualization of language intervention programs. In J. Miller, D. Yoder, & R. Schiefelbusch (Eds.), *Contemporary issues in language intervention. ASHA Reports 12* (pp. 165–176). Rockville, MD: ASHA.

Kamhi, A. (2011). What speech-language pathologists need to know about auditory processing disorder. *Language, Speech, and Hearing Services in Schools, 42,* 265–272.

Keller, W., Tillery, K., & McFadden, S. (2006). Auditory processing disorder in children diagnosed with nonverbal learning disability. *American Journal of Audiology, 15,* 108–113.

Kelly, D. (1995). *Central auditory processing disorders: strategies for use with children and adolescents.* San Antonio, TX: Psychological Corporation.

Kraus, N., McGee, T., Carrell, T., King, C., Tremblay, K., & Nicol, T. (1995). Central auditory system plasticity associated with speech discrimination training. *Journal of Cognitive Neuroscience, 7,* 25–32.

Kraus, N., McGee, T., Ferre, J., Hoeppner, J., Carrell, T., Sharma, A., & Nicol, T. (1993). Mismatch negativity in the neurophysi-ologic/behavioral evaluation of auditory processing disorders: A case study. *Ear and Hearing, 14,* 223–234.

Krause, J., & Braida, L. (2004). Acoustic properties of naturally produced clear speech at normal speaking rates. *Journal of the Acoustical Society of America, 115,* 362–378.

Loo, J., Bamiou, D., Campbell, N., & Luxon, L. (2010). Computer-based auditory training (CBAT): Benefits for children with language- and reading-related learning difficulties. *Development Medicine and Child Neurology, 52,* 708–717.

Luria, A. (1973). *The working brain.* London, UK: Penguin Press.

Masters G. (1998). Speech and language management of central auditory processing disorders. In M. Masters, N. Stecker, & J. Katz (Eds), *Central auditory processing disorders: Mostly management* (pp. 117–129). Boston, MA: Allyn & Bacon.

Moore, D., Rosenberg, J., & Coleman, J. (2005). Discrimination training of phonemic contrasts enhances phonological processing in mainstream school children. *Brain and Language, 94,* 72–85.

Mosby's Medical, Nursing, and Allied Health Dictionary (6th ed.). (2002). St. Louis, MO: Mosby.

Musiek, F. (2004). Hearing and the brain: Audiological consequences of neurobiological Disorders. *Journal of the American Academy of Audiology, Special Issue 15.*

Musiek, F. (2005). *Advances in CAPD diagnosis and management.* Seminar presented at the annual meeting of the Massachusetts Speech-Hearing Language Association, Worcester, MA.

Musiek, F., Chermak, G., & Weihing, J. (2007). Auditory training. In G. Chermak & F. Musiek (Eds.). *Handbook of (central) auditory processing disorder: Comprehensive intervention* (Vol. II, pp. 77–106). San Diego, CA: Plural.

Myklebust, H. (1954). *Auditory disorders in children* (p. 8). New York, NY: Grune & Stratton.

Palombo, J. (2001). *Learning disorders and disorders of the self in children and adolescents*. New York, NY: W. W. Norton.

Phillips-Keeley, S. (2003). *The source for executive function disorders*. East Moline, IL: LinguiSystems.

Picheny, M., Durlach, N., & Braida, L. (1985). Speaking clearly for the hard of hearing I: Intelligibility differences between clear and conversational speech. *Journal of Speech and Hearing Research, 28*, 96–103.

Picheny, M., Durlach, N., & Braida, L. (1986). Speaking clearly for the hard of hearing II: Acoustic characteristics of clear and conversational speech. *Journal of Speech and Hearing Research, 29*, 434–446.

Putter-Katz, H., Said, A., Feldman, I., Miran, D., Kushnir, D., Muchnik, C., & Hildesheimer, M. (2002). Treatment and evaluation indices of auditory processing disorders. *Seminars in Hearing, 23*, 357–364.

Richard, G. (2001). *The source for processing disorders*. East Moline, IL: LinguiSystems.

Richard, G. (2011). Prologue: The role of the speech-language pathologist in identifying and treating children with auditory processing disorders. *Language, Speech, and Hearing Services in Schools, 42*, 241–245.

Richard, G., & Fahey, J. (2005). *The source for development of executive function disorders*. East Moline, IL: LinguiSystems.

Richard, G., & Hanner, M. (1995). *The Language Processing Test–Revised*. East Moline, IL: LinguiSystems.

Seats, T. (1998). *Treatment efficacy of temporal exercises in habilitating children with central auditory processing disorders*. Paper presented at annual meeting of the American Speech-Language-Hearing Association, San Antonio, TX.

Shapiro, A., & Mistal, G. (1985). ITE-aid auditory training for reading and spelling-disabled children: Clinical case studies. *Hearing Journal, 38*, 14–16.

Shapiro, A., & Mistal, G. (1986). ITE-aid auditory training for reading and spelling-disabled children: A longitudinal study of matched groups. *Hearing Journal, 39*, 14–16.

Shapiro, H., & Balthazar, C. (2004). *A study of treatment effectiveness for two children learning reading skills*. Paper presented at the annual meeting of the Illinois Speech-Language-Hearing Association. Arlington Heights, IL.

Sharma, M., Purdy, S., & Kelly, A. (2009). Comorbidity of auditory processing, language, and reading disorders. *Journal of Speech, Language, and Hearing Research, 52*, 706–722.

Sloan, C. (1995). *Treating auditory processing difficulties in children*. San Diego, CA: Singular.

Smoski, W., Brunt, M., & Tannahill, C. (1998). *Children's Auditory Performance Scale*. Tampa, FL: Educational Audiology Association.

Tallal, P., & Merzenich, M. (1997). *Fast ForWord training for children with language-learning problems. National field test results*. Paper presented at the annual meeting of the American Speech-Language-Hearing Association, Boston, MA.

Tanguay, P. (2001). *Nonverbal learning disabilities at home: A parent's guide*. London, UK: Jessica Kingsley.

Thompson, S. (1997). *The source for nonverbal learning disorders*. East Moline, IL: LinguiSystems.

Tremblay, K. (2007). Training-related changes in the brain: Evidence from human auditory evoked potentials. *Seminars in Hearing, 28*, 120–132.

Tremblay, K., & Kraus, N. (2002). Auditory training induces asymmetrical changes in cortical activity. *Journal of Speech, Language, and Hearing Research, 45*, 564–572.

Tremblay, K., Kraus, N., Carrell, T., & McGee, T. (1997). Central auditory system plasticity: Generalization to novel stimulation following listening training. *Journal of the Acoustical Society of America, 102*, 3762–3773.

Tremblay, K., Kraus, N., McGee, T., Picton, C., & Otis, B. (2001). Central auditory plasticity: Changes in the N1-P2 complex after speech-sound training. *Ear and Hearing, 22*, 79–90.

Tyler, A. (1997). Evidence of linguistic interactions in intervention. *Topics in Language Disorders, 17*, 23–40.

U.S. Department of Education. (2008). *Thirtieth annual report to Congress on the* implementation of the Individuals with Disabilities Education Act. Retrieved from http://www.ed.gov/about/reports/annual/osep/2008/index.html

Witton, C. (2010). Childhood auditory processing disorder as a developmental disorder: The case for a multi-professional approach to diagnosis and management. *International Journal of Audiology, 49*, 83–87.

SECTION 4

Case Studies

CHAPTER 21

CASE STUDIES: INTERVENTION

ANNETTE E. HURLEY and CASSANDRA BILLIET

In recent years there has been increased demand for services related to the diagnosis and treatment of central auditory processing disorder (CAPD). Audiologists are uniquely qualified to diagnose and assess CAPD, and also play an integral part in the intervention process, including formulating goals, determining appropriate therapeutic approaches, and documenting improvements in central auditory function. The following case studies illustrate positive changes in the central auditory nervous system (CANS) following successful intervention. Several different types of intervention, such as dichotic listening training, speech-in-noise-training, phonemic awareness training, and computer-mediated language interventions, have been included to illustrate the importance of deficit-spe-cific intervention. Following the case presentations, a "debriefing" is provided to foster further reflection and discussion.

Case Study 1 (James)

Background

James is 12-year-old male who was a participant in a study examining pre- and postbehavioral and electrophysiological measures after Fast ForWord training was provided by a local school system. James was delivered without incident following a normal pregnancy. Development was reported as normal until the age of 3. At that time, it was noted by his parents that James' speech and language skills regressed. Initially this decline was attributed to sibling jealousy, as it coincided with the birth of sibling and the family's relocation. James presented a history of otitis media, and a lack of progression in speech and language, which was attributed to his history of ear infections. Normal hearing thresholds were obtained bilaterally. Subsequently, autism and pervasive developmental disorder were erroneously diagnosed. Seizure activity began at the age of 3 to 6 years; a diagnosis of Landau Kleffner syndrome (LKS) was made after a characteristic spiking electroencephalography (EEG) occurring in the left temporal lobe was noted. Nocturnal seizure activity continued until James was 11 years old. James attended speech/language therapy and occupational therapy through early intervention programs in order to address expressive and receptive language delay and verbal apraxia. He sporadically uses sign language as needed when he experiences difficulty with word finding or speech production. He has been in special education classes and is receiving speech/language therapy at school two times per week, 30 minutes per session. A speech-language assessment indicated a moderate to severe receptive and expressive language disorder, characterized by moderately impaired receptive language skills, severely impaired expressive language skills, and severely impaired language memory skills. Expressive language skills were significantly weaker than receptive language skills. Articulation skills also were impaired and consistent with a diagnosis of verbal dyspraxia. Speech intelligibility was fair in known contexts and fair to poor in unknown contexts. James is taking anticonvulsion medication for seizures and is medically managed for ADHD.

Assessment

Normal peripheral hearing was established bilaterally. Because of James' apraxia and speech difficulty, either nonverbal tests or those with low-linguistic loading (e.g., Dichotic Digits Test) were administered. He could not repeat any numbers presented to the right ear (0%), but had a left ear score of 92%. He demonstrated normal temporal resolution (2 msec-gap detection threshold) and scored 100% in the labeling condition on the Frequency Pattern Test and Duration Pattern Test. A normal 500 Hz masking level difference (MLD) of 10 dB HL was obtained. An electrophysiological study yielded the following: normal auditory brainstem response (ABR), bilaterally; abnormal bilateral complex ABR (cABR); and absent P300 responses, bilaterally.

Intervention and Outcomes

James completed an eight-week program of Fast ForWord, provided by his school district. He also received dichotic listening therapy, once per week for fifty minutes, for two semesters, for a total of twenty-two sessions. Additional therapy sessions could not be scheduled due to James' geographical distance from the clinic. James continued to receive speech and language therapy two times per week for 30 minutes per session at his school.

No change in the right dichotic scores was noted following completion of Fast ForWord. Progress was made during dichotic listening therapy, as shown for binaural separation scores for the right ear in Table 21–1. Listed also is the intensity level of the signal to the left ear. (For further discussion of dichotic listening therapy, the reader is referred to Chapter 9.)

A normal ABR was obtained for the right and left ears. Wave latency and amplitude values are recorded in Table 21–2. As expected, there was no difference in the ABR after Fast ForWord or dichotic listening therapy training, as changes are usually reflected in higher CANS recordings (Figure 21–1). The ABR is interpreted as within normal limits.

Pre and post-cABR recordings for the right and left ears are shown in Figure 21–2. The latency values of Waves V

Table 21–1. Dichotic Training Progress Summary for Case Study 1 (James)

	Left Intensity	Right Intensity	Right Binaural Separation Score
Pre Fast ForWord	55	55	0%
Post Fast ForWord	55	55	0%
Post Dichotic Listening Training	55	55	94%

Table 21–2. ABR Latency and Amplitude Recorded Pre- and Post-Therapy for Case 1 (James)

Ear	Wave	Pre-Therapy	Post Fast ForWord	Post Dichotic Training
Latencies in msec				
Left	I	1.62	1.57	1.57
	III	3.95	3.99	3.95
	V	5.74	5.74	5.65
Right	I	1.66	1.62	1.57
	III	3.91	3.99	3.99
	V	5.61	5.53	5.53
Amplitude in μV				
Left	I	.40	.41	.41
	III	.17	.24	.26
	V	.27	.27	.45
Right	I	.30	.30	.31
	III	.22	.22	.22
	V	.26	.26	.36

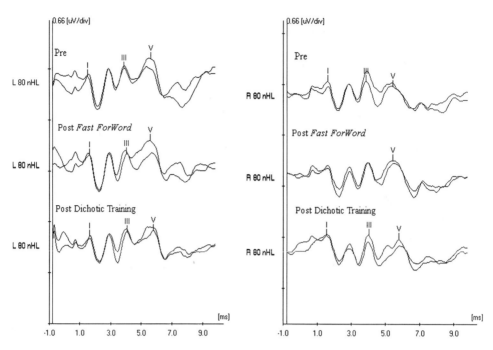

Figure 21–1. This figure shows a normal auditory brainstem response (ABR) recorded pre-Fast ForWord and post-Fast ForWord and Dichotic Listening training for the right and left ears.

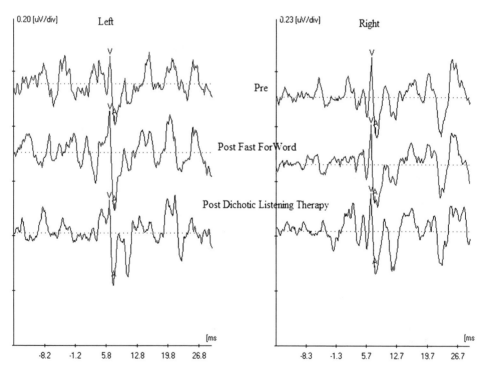

Figure 21–2. Pre- and posttherapy cABR recordings are depicted for the left and right ears.

and A are shown in Table 21–3. A decrease in the latency of Waves V and A are noted after training reflecting the plasticity of the CANS.

There was no discernable P300 response for either the right or left recordings. This might be due to our patient's lack of attention to the rare stimulus. James was instructed to count the deviant stimuli, but his responses were not accurate. Pre- and post-ALER responses for the "standard" tone are shown in Figure 21–3. Pre- and postlatency and amplitude N1–P2 measures are recorded in

Table 21–3. Latency of Waves V and A for the cABR for Case 1 (James)

Measure	Ear	Pre-Therapy	Post Fast ForWord	Post Dichotic Listening Training
Wave V latency (in msec)	Left	6.78	6.62	6.53
Wave A latency (in msec)	Left	7.83	7.70	7.39
Wave V latency (in msec)	Right	6.87	6.70	6.70
Wave A latency (in msec)	Right	8.03	7.70	7.70

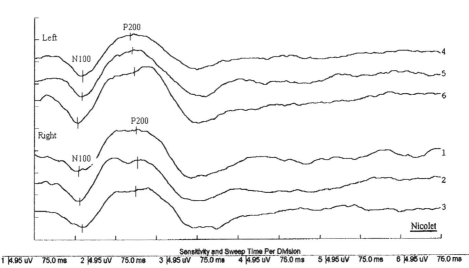

Figure 21–3. Pre- and posttherapy auditory late evoked response (ALER) for the left and right ears are shown. Prerecordings are shown in tracings 4 and 1, post-Fast ForWord recordings are shown in tracings 5 and 2, and postdichotic listening training therapy recordings are depicted in tracings 6 and 3.

Table 21–4. A slight improvement in N1–P2 amplitude is noted for the right ear, but may reflect variability of the response.

Comments

After dichotic listening training, binaural separation scores were within normal limits, but binaural integration was still difficult. Because of the geographical distance from James' home and clinic, therapy was discontinued and dichotic exercises were provided for James to continue at home. In addition to objective evidence of improvement in the central auditory pathway, unsolicited parental reports were positive. Family members, as well as his teachers, reported James' speech was improving and that he was speaking in complete sentences and thoughts, rather than in telegraphic-type speech as he had prior to auditory training. He was also initiating phone conversations, something he had never done in the past. They also reported that he rarely used signs anymore. James has not returned for formal follow-up evaluation; however, his mother reported James completed neurofeedback training, a type of brain wave biofeedback. She also reported that he is no longer taking ADHD medication and is not placed in any special education classes, nor does he qualify for any resource services through the school system at this time.

Debriefing

- What should audiologists and speech-language pathologists (SLPs) know about LKS?

  LKS is a rare neurological disorder that results in the inability to understand or express language and an acquired CAPD. The onset of LKS usually occurs between 3 and 7 years. It is characterized by a sudden or gradual deterioration in the ability to understand or express language. Often, children with LKS are referred to audiologists to rule out hearing impairment. Children with LKS may be misdiagnosed as autistic or hearing impaired (Tharpe, Johnson, & Glasscock, 1991). LKS is characterized by an abnormal electroencephalogram (EEG), typified by abnormal spike activity in the

Table 21–4. Latency and Amplitude of the ALER Recordings for Case 1 (James)

Ear	Measure	Pre-therapy	Post Fast ForWord	Post Dichotic Training
Left	N1 Latency (in msec)	91.5	81	82.5
	P2 Latency (in msec)	172.5	174	169.5
	N1/P2 Amplitude (in μV)	8.61	8.64	8.14
Right	N1 Latency (in msec)	85.5	85.5	79.5
	P2 Latency (in msec)	181.5	182.5	177
	N1/P2 Amplitude (in μV)	9.55	10.57	11.35

temporal and/or parietal regions (Deonna, 1991). The abnormal EEG activity predominately occurs in the left temporal lobe, but may be present in both temporal lobes with nocturnal seizures occurring in over 80% of patients with LKS (Patry, Lyagoubi, & Tassinari, 1971).

■ Discuss the appropriateness of computer-mediated language interventions (Fast ForWord, Earobics, etc.) to treat CAPD.
Computer-mediated programs have many advantages. They are convenient, hold the interest of patients, can provide intensive training, and there is standardization and control of the stimuli. Clinicians must be aware of the specific deficits one is targeting as there is not one computer-mediated program that is appropriate for all deficits associated with CAPD.

Fast ForWord is one popular commercially available software program that purports to capitalize on the plasticity of the auditory system. The Fast ForWord program is designed to develop temporal and acoustic skills to detect rapid transitions of speech. It has been reported that CAPD or auditory-based learning difficulties (language and reading disorders) may be remediated through intensive training provided by the Fast ForWord program (Merzenich et al., 1996; Tallal et al., 1996). The exercises in the Fast ForWord program use five levels of acoustically modified speech. At the beginning of the program, the exercises prolong and emphasize the sounds so that they are easier to distinguish. As the listener progresses,

speech sounds approach normal speech. As the listener improves, the exercises become more challenging, and the participant develops enhanced language awareness and comprehension. See Chapter 11 for comparison of computer-assisted auditory training programs.

■ What is the theory behind dichotic listening therapy?
Kimura (1961) was first to model the contralateral pathway as dominant and composed of more neurons than the ipsilateral pathway. Early work in the 19th century noted that most aphasia is the result of left cerebral hemisphere lesions and contributed to the conclusion that most people are left hemisphere dominant for expressive and receptive language (Webster, 1995). When there is damage or a lesion in the auditory temporal lobe, the ear contralateral to the lesion will be affected in dichotic listening tasks, as the contralateral pathway is the dominant pathway (Berlin, Lowe-Bell, Jannetta, & Kline, 1972). Importantly, in most cases of LKS, the left temporal lobe is the lesioned area; therefore, a right ear deficit on dichotic testing is expected. Dichotic training is an innovative therapy for the remediation of the compromised central auditory pathway (Musiek, Chermak, & Weihing, 2007). During dichotic listening training, the signal intensity presented to the unimpaired pathway is first decreased and then slowly increased over time as the weaker, impaired pathway grows stronger. This specifically targets the deficit ear; thus, activating brain regions that receive auditory sensory

input on the side of the lesion. See Chapter 9 for elaboration of the dichotic training paradigm.

■ Discuss the inclusion of electrophysiological recordings in CAPD diagnosis and treatment.

Behavioral tests and electrophysiological procedures are utilized in the diagnosis of a CAPD. Electrophysiologic recordings of the central and peripheral neural auditory pathway and auditory cortex may reflect neural functions and processes involved in neural coding for speech. Electrophysiological measures are recommended when there is a questionable neurologic disorder (e.g., possible auditory neuropathy spectrum disorder [ANSD]) or in difficult to test children (ASHA, 2005). Electrophysiological procedures also are recommended to corroborate results of the behavioral test battery and/or to provide additional objective insights as to the underlying neurophysiology of the central auditory pathways (Bellis, 2003; Chermak & Musiek, 1997). The use of both electrophysiologic procedures and behavioral tests may provide useful information regarding possible gross site of dysfunction in the CANS. Currently, electrophysiologic measures are not sufficient to replace the behavioral test battery for CAPD; however, in conjunction with behavioral tests, they provide valuable information about the physiology and integrity of the CANS. Moreover, electrophysiological measures can provide an objective means to monitor the progress of an auditory training program and serve as an outcome measure.

Case Study 2 (Jack)

Background

Jack is a 5-year-old male referred for a hearing evaluation and central auditory screening for CAPD. Jack was born five weeks premature and mechanical ventilation was required at birth. Developmental milestones were achieved at appropriate ages. Jack presents a positive history of middle ear infections and three sets of pressure equalization tubes have been placed. Currently, Jack is in the first grade. School performance is described as "poor." He is demonstrating poor phonemic skills, difficulty learning to read, difficulty hearing in group situations, and mispronounces many words. There is a family history of dyslexia.

Assessment

Normal peripheral hearing was established bilaterally, and tympanometry revealed normal middle ear function, bilaterally. He failed the screening portion of the SCAN-3:C, as shown in Table 21–5. A normal ABR was obtained, bilaterally. An abnormal cABR was recorded, bilaterally, and depicted in Figure 21–4.

Recommendations

Jack was referred for a speech-language evaluation. Results of this assessment indicated a phonological disorder. Jack began weekly speech therapy sessions. A computer-mediated software program, Earobics, was begun at home. A list of informal listening activities was provided.

Intervention and Outcomes

Jack returned to the clinic after six months at age 6. Follow-up screening

Table 21–5. SCAN-3:C Screening Results for Case 2 (Jack)

	Auditory Figure Ground		Competing Words Free Recall	
	Raw Score	Outcome	Raw Score	Outcome
Age 5.5	18	Fail	36	Pass
Age 6	35	Pass	40	Pass

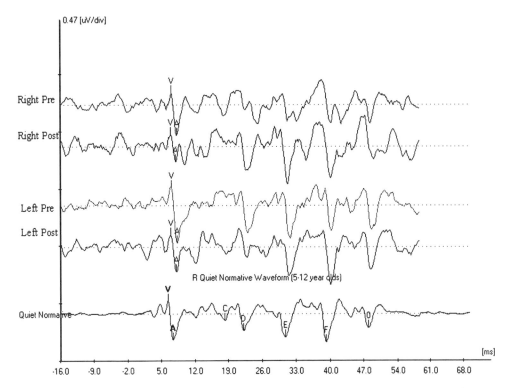

Figure 21–4. Pre- and post-cABR recordings for the right and left ears are shown. Also depicted is a normative waveform.

results are shown in Table 21–5 and are within normal limits. The cABR improved, but remained abnormal as depicted in Figure 21–4. Jack's mother reported significant improvement in his performance at school, which was confirmed by his teachers. Jack has been discharged from speech-language therapy as phonological skills are within normal limits. Jack's

progress will continue to be followed annually.

Debriefing

■ What were the CAPD risk factors and/or comorbid conditions? *Prematurity, mechanical ventilation, history of middle ear infections, poor performance in reading and spelling, and a family history of dyslexia were noted in the case history.*

◼ Would you continue to follow this patient?
Annual comprehensive central auditory assessment, including behavioral and electrophysiological measures, will ensure that Jack is progressing appropriately for his age. After one year of traditional speech-language therapy and working through Earobics, Jack's cABR remained abnormal. The abnormal cABR is not characteristic of a specific type of learning disorder or CAPD; however, it is found in approximately 30% of patients with a language-based learning disability (Johnson, Nicol, & Kraus, 2005; Russo, Nicol, Zecker, Hayes, & Kraus, 2005; Wible, Nicol, & Kraus, 2004).

◼ Why, despite the failure on the SCAN-3:C, was no formal central auditory diagnostic battery administered?
Jack was initially seen at age 5 for central auditory processing screening. There are very few tests with developmental norms for this age. Jack will return at age 7 for further diagnostic testing.

Case 3 (Carrie)

Background

Carrie is a 15-year-old, right-handed female who was referred to clinic by her psychologist after completing a psychoeducational evaluation. The psychoeducational assessment revealed average intelligence, with deficits in reading comprehension, language processing, and auditory processing. Attention deficit disorder was ruled out. Since this assessment, Carrie has begun language and reading therapy with a private speech-language pathologist. She reports difficulty with reading comprehension and has previously completed reading tutoring at a commercial learning center with some success. Carrie is the product of a normal pregnancy. Developmental milestones were achieved at appropriate times. Carrie is entering the 10th grade at a private school. Carrie's mother reports that Carrie is frustrated at school, as she works very hard and struggles to earn B's and C's.

Assessment

Normal peripheral hearing was established, bilaterally. Tests results of the behavioral central auditory test battery are shown in Table 21–6. A diagnosis of CAPD with probable interhemispheric transfer dysfunction was made. Normal ABR and cABR were recorded bilaterally. The ALER, recorded to right and left stimulation, as shown in Figure 21–5, was normal. Amplitude and latencies are shown in Table 21–7.

Recommendations

A list of environmental modifications and compensatory strategies were provided to Carrie. Based on the psychoeducational assessment, documenting language and reading deficits, Carrie will begin Fast ForWord program, provided by her school system, prior to beginning dichotic listening therapy.

Intervention and Outcomes

Carrie returned for follow-up after completing Fast ForWord therapy. Behavioral

Table 21–6. Pre- and Post- Behavioral CAPD Test Results for Case 3 (Carrie)

Filtered Words Standard Score		Auditory Figure Ground Standard Score		Competing Words Standard Score		Competing Sentences Standard Score		Dichotic Digits Left Ear		Dichotic Digits Right Ear		Frequency Pattern Test Left Verbal		Gap Detection Threshold	
Pre	Post	Pre	Post	Pre	Post	Pre	Post	Pre	Post	Pre	Post	Pre	Post	Pre	Post
9	12	10	12	4	10	6	10	38%	98%	100%	100%	40%	90%	*WNL	WNL

*WNL = Within normal limits

Table 21–7. Pre- and Post- ALER Latency and Amplitude Recordings for Case 3 (Carrie)

Ear	Pre N1 Latency (msec)	Post N1 Latency (msec)	Pre P2 Latency (msec)	Post P2 Latency (msec)	Pre N1–P2 Amplitude (µV)	Post N1–P2 Amplitude (µV)
Left	104.34	112.67	160.56	175.13	4.98	6.77
Right	102.26	90.81	168.89	152.23	6.76	8.83

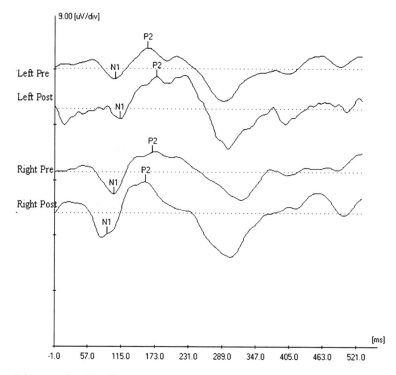

Figure 21–5. Pre- and post-ALER recordings for the right and left ears from Cz to the ipsilateral ear are shown in this figure. A summed response from two individual recordings is depicted.

tests were within normal limits as shown in the "Post" column in Table 21–6. She reported that Fast ForWord "helped her process information quicker." Electrophysiological recordings also were repeated, as shown in Figure 21–5. Improvement of the N1–P2 amplitude was found for the right and left recordings, as shown in Table 21–7. A one-year follow-up showed maintenance of progress. No additional audiological recommendations were made.

Debriefing

■ What were the risk factors for CAPD and/or comorbid conditions?
Poor performance in school and language and reading deficits are reported.

■ Discuss the appropriateness of Fast ForWord to treat interhemispheric dysfunction.
Fast ForWord is a computer-mediated language-to-reading program. Although dichotic listening exercises are not included in this training, dichotic speech scores improved Post-Fast ForWord. Carrie's improvement in dichotic scores may reflect generalization of auditory training or "transfer of learning" (Tremblay, Krause, Carrell, & Magee, 1996).

■ When would you suggest follow-up?
We would like to re-assess central auditory processing in one year in order to ensure progress is maintained.

Case 4 (Edward)

Background

Edward is a 7-year-old, right-handed male who was referred for a central auditory assessment by his speech-language pathologist. Pregnancy and gross motor development were reported as normal; however, speech was reported as delayed. Edward has been receiving speech-language therapy since age 3. He has a diagnosis of a severe receptive and profound expressive language delay. There is a history of otitis media and pressure equalization tubes. Edward is in the second grade; his academic performance is reported as poor to average. He is struggling learning to read. He receives speech services twice weekly at school. A diagnosis of ADHD was made; however, pharmacologic management has not begun.

Assessment

Normal peripheral hearing was established bilaterally. Results of the behavioral central auditory test battery indicated deficits for many processes, as shown in Table 21–8. Normal ABR and cABR were recorded, bilaterally.

Recommendations

Initial test results should be interpreted with caution, given Edward's diagnosis of ADHD and lack of medical management. It is important to note that Edward was impulsive during the assessment and asked to "take a break" several times during each test. Short breaks were given after each test. It is also important to note that Edward is a "young" 7 year old and his auditory system may be immature.

A list of environmental modifications and compensatory strategies were provided. Direct remediation recommendations included: (1) continuation of speech-language therapy to target weak phonemic awareness skills, with listening activities included during therapy; (2) participation in a computer-mediated language-to-reading program, provided by the school; and (3) home-based therapy to include informal listening activities.

Intervention and Outcomes

Edward returned one year after his initial evaluation at age 8. He had completed Earobics Step 1 and Step 2. Improvement of behavioral central auditory test scores was noted as seen in Table 21–8, in column Post 1, Age 8. Edward's mother reported that medication to treat ADHD still had not been initiated. Continuation of speech-language therapy was recommended. Dichotic listening therapy also was recommended; however, Edward's mother could not commit to this therapy, due to the geographical distance from the clinic. Informal dichotic listening training was recommended for home. Edward returned one year later at age 9. Edward's mother reported initiating medication for ADHD after comments from Edward's teachers and reported a significant improvement in his ability to focus. Behavioral central auditory test results were within normal limits bilaterally, as shown in Table 21–8 and listed under the column Post 2, Age 9. Edward is currently doing well (As and Bs) in school and his mother reports he is more confident and less frustrated. Results of a recent speech-language evaluation indicate normal speech-language abilities. Annual central auditory processing evaluations are recommended.

Table 21–8. CAPD Behavioral Test Battery Results for Case 4 (Edward)

	Initial Age 7	Post 1 Age 8	Post 2 Age 9
SCAN: 3C Auditory Figure Ground Standard Score	5	7	10
SCAN: 3C Filtered Words Standard Score	5	7	11
SCAN: 3C Competing Words Standard Score	4	7	10
SCAN: 3C Competing Sentences Standard Score	4	5	11
SCAN: 3C Time-Compressed Speech Standard Score	2	5	9
Dichotic Digits Right Ear	40%	65%	92%
Dichotic Digits Left Ear	40%	60%	90%
Frequency Pattern Test Left Verbal	60%	80%	100%
Gap Detection Threshold	Within Normal Limits	Did Not Test	Did Not Test

Debriefing

■ What were risk factors for CAPD and/or comorbid conditions?
A history of otitis media, poor school performance, and diagnoses of ADHD and language disorder are reported.

■ Would you continue to follow this patient?
We would like to continue to follow Edward's progress at least until he is 12 years of age to ensure he maintains progress and normal maturation of the CANS. Maturation of the CANS pathway continues throughout childhood. Myelination of the corpus callosum and auditory association areas may not be completed until a child is 10 to 12 years or older, and often extends beyond that time (Musiek, Gollegly, & Baran, 1984; Roeser, Valente, & Hosford-Dunn, 2007).

■ What does the change in central auditory test results from age 7 to 9 years suggest?

Positive changes in behavioral scores reflect plasticity of the CANS. These changes may be attributed to developmental maturation course of the CANS and learning related plasticity which occurs due to habilitation efforts.

■ What considerations should be given when testing children age 7 to 8 and younger and with comorbid diagnosis of ADHD?

Clinicians should be aware of inattention, fatigue, and motivation when testing young children for CAPD. Often, numerous breaks may be given. If possible, testing should be done with children on medication. An auditory vigilance test may be useful to test the effectiveness of attention and impulsivity.

Case 5 (Peggy)

Background

Peggy is a 52-year-old female, who experienced a cerebral vascular accident (CVA or stroke) six years prior. She was first seen at this clinic for a speech-language evaluation three years ago and to continue speech-language therapy, as she had been dismissed from private speech-language therapy. She presented with right hemiparesis with no functional use of her right arm or hand. She currently walks with a cane. Results from the initial assessment indicated a nonfluent mixed aphasia characterized by effortful, nonfluent speech, marked by significant word finding difficulty, decreased auditory comprehension skills, and occasional perseveration.

Assessment

Normal peripheral hearing was established, bilaterally. A right ear deficit on dichotic speech tests was found. Peggy performed within normal limits on filtered words and speech-in-noise tests. (Extended response time was provided.) A normal ABR and ALER were recorded and shown in Figures 21–6 and 21–7.

Intervention and Outcomes

Peggy completed 30 one-hour sessions of dichotic listening training over 36 weeks. Results are shown in Table 21–9. A significant improvement in the right ear for binaural separation was noted. Peggy sometimes responded by pointing to numbers, as well as vocalizing the

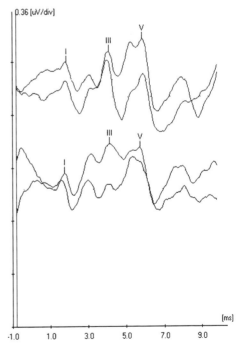

Figure 21–6. A normal ABR was obtained before beginning dichotic listening training.

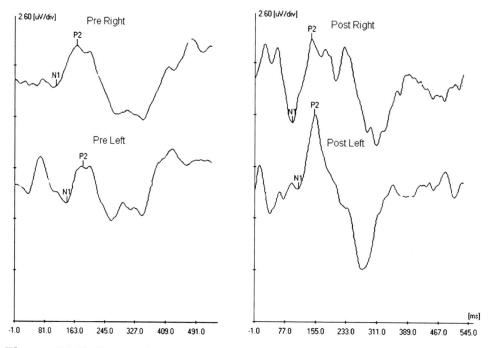

Figure 21–7. Pre- and post-ALER recordings from Cz to the ipsilateral ear are shown for the right and left ears.

Table 21–9. Dichotic Listening Therapy Progress Summary for Case Study 5 (Peggy)

	Left Intensity	Right Intensity	Right Binaural Separation Score
Session 1	0 dB	55 dB	100%
	5 dB	55 dB	65%
	10 dB	55 dB	56%
	10 dB	55 dB	52%
	20 dB	55 dB	56%
Session 10	40 dB	55 dB	80%
	45 dB	55 dB	34%
	45 dB	55 dB	40%
Session 15	50 dB	55 dB	56%
Session 20	52 dB	55dB	68%
	55 dB	55dB	40%
Session 24	55dB	55dB	68%
Session 30	55dB	55dB	84%

response and was given extra time to formulate her responses.

Pre- and post-ALERs are shown in Figure 21–7 and latency and amplitude values are reported in Table 21–10. An increase in the N1–P2 amplitude for left ear stimulation is shown. This may reflect intrasubject variability of the response.

Peggy's diagnosis has improved from a mixed nonfluent aphasia to a severe Broca's aphasia. Progress continues in naming objects, using verbs, expressively identifying descriptors, and using multi-word phrases to describe action pictures. Peggy continues in speech-language therapy with an enthusiastic, motivational outlook. Peggy's family reports improved auditory comprehension, as reflected by her participation in conversations and interest in watching television. Peggy has been dismissed from dichotic listening training, but continues informal dichotic listening training at home (listening to audio books using only the right earphone while background noise plays in the background).

Debriefing

■ Should central auditory processing be assessed in patients with CVA?
Although auditory impairments are associated with aphasia, little information is available regarding current practices of assessing peripheral and central auditory function after the onset of aphasia. A recent investigation reported 86% of stroke patients had auditory complaints and these complaints would have gone undetected unless formally screened (Edwards et al., 2006). Traditional pure-tone assessment is insufficient for identifying acquired CAPD. Central auditory processing assessments are needed to guide the development of a deficit specific auditory training program that may remediate auditory complaints experienced by these individuals.

■ How does dichotic listening training differ from traditional speech-language therapy?
Dichotic listening training specifically targets the patient's deficit ear and activates brain regions that receive auditory sensory input on the side of the lesion. The damaged auditory pathway is forced to work by direct auditory stimulation. This is accomplished via dichotic listening tasks by decreasing the signal intensity of the unimpaired pathway and slowly increasing the intensity level over time, as the weaker, impaired pathway grows stronger. See Chapter 9 for elaboration of this procedure.

Table 21–10. Electrophysiological Data for Case 5 (Peggy)

	Pre-Training			Post-Training		
	N1 msec	P2 msec	N1–P2' Amplitude μV	N1 msec	P2 msec	N1–P2' Amplitude μV
Right	108.51	182.42	1.81	102.26	154.31	1.63
Left	109.55	155.35	0.81	102.66	143.21	2.00

■ Briefly discuss the role of neuroplasticity in remediation of acquired CAPD. *There is a substantial body of literature that supports the plasticity of the CANS and neural reorganization after auditory training. Because the brain retains a lifelong capacity for plasticity and adaptive reorganization, reorganization may be accomplished with a direct and intensive training program. Reorganization is reflected in an increase in the number of synapses, increased neural density, and improvement in auditory electrophysiological recordings and behavioral responses (Elbert, Pantev, Wienbruch, Rockstroh, & Taub, 1995; Merzenich & Jenkins, 1995; Raconzone, Schreiner, & Merzenich, 1993). Compensatory plasticity occurs as other parts of the brain reorganize to assume the specific function of the damaged area (Musiek, Chermak, & Weihing, 2007).*

Improvements in behavioral and electrophysiological responses after auditory training programs have been shown for an adult with traumatic brain injury (Musiek, Baran, & Shinn, 2004), and an adult with a left hemisphere stroke (Weihing, Musiek, Munroe, Swainson, & Cho, 2006), as well as for a patient with Landau Kleffner syndrome (Hurley & Hurley, 2009) after completing dichotic listening therapy.

Case Study 6 (Debbie)

Background

Debbie is a 30-year-old, right-handed female graduate student studying speech-language pathology. She self-referred for a central auditory assessment after an audiological assessment established normal peripheral hearing bilaterally. Debbie is experiencing difficulty transcribing and distinguishing/discriminating phonemes required as part of a phonetics course. She reports normal developmental history. She has never before experienced academic difficulties. Debbie graduated with a bachelor in science in biology with a 3.9 grade point average. Of interest are Debbie's history of protracted middle ear infections and the placement of pressure equalization tubes as a young child.

Assessment

Results of the behavioral central auditory assessment, are shown in Table 21–11 and indicate difficulty listening in degraded acoustic environments.

Recommendations

A list of environmental modifications and compensatory strategies were provided. The Listening and Communication Enhancement (LACE) (Sweetow & Henderson Sabes, 2004) program was recommended for Debbie for home use. Additionally, Debbie will begin dichotic listening training three times per week, 30 minutes per session, for four weeks.

Intervention and Outcomes

Debbie completed 12 sessions of dichotic listening training and the LACE program. Post-testing shows improved scores (see Table 21–11). She reports positive changes following therapy. She reports phonetic transcription exercises are much easier and she is more confident

Table 21–11. Pre- and Post-Behavioral (C)APD Test Results for Case 6 (Debbie)

	Filtered Words		Auditory Figure Ground		Time Compressed Speech		Competing Sentences		Dichotic Digits		Frequency Pattern Test Verbal		Gap Detection Threshold	
	Pre	Post	Pre	Post	Pre	Post	Pre	Post	Pre	Post	Pre	Post	Pre	Post
Right	82%	98%	74%	100%	64%	92%	100%	100%	100%	100%	DNT	DNT	2 msec	DNT
Left	76%	94%	62%	96%	56%	88%	80%	100%	88%	100%	100%	DNT	DNT	DNT

in her responses since she can "hear easier." She also reports moving to the front of the classroom and requesting that a classroom amplification system be used. She also commented that the dichotic listening training and LACE exercises were important for her to complete as they provided her with first-hand knowledge of aural rehabilitation training programs.

Debriefing

- Discuss how intelligence may affect CAPD diagnosis?
  It is always important to consider a patient's mental and cognitive age in administration and interpretation of tests of central auditory processing. The diagnosis of CAPD is not appropriate when there is higher order cognitive deficit (ASHA, 2005). Alternatively, a person with high intelligence may be able to compensate for deficits in everyday life using metacognitive skills.

- What risk factors for CAPD are presented by this case?
  An early childhood history of otitis media is reported. Poor discrimination in phonetics class also is reported.

- Are there differences between hearing and listening?
  Yes. Hearing refers to the basic sensory process of detection and discrimination of acoustic stimuli. Listening requires linguistic and cognitive (e.g., working memory) effort to give meaning to the acoustic signal. Aural rehabilitation programs equip the brain with listening skills. The reader is referred to Sweetow (2005) for additional information about the benefits of LACE and cognitive training.

- Briefly discuss the importance of accurate phonetic transcription for an SLP.
  Accurate phonetic transcription is important for many clinical tasks including analyzing speech production, communicating speech-language production to other professionals, and accurately diagnosing speech disorders (Singh & Singh, 2006). Recent investigations (Moran & Fitch, 2001; Robinson, Mahurin, & Justus 2001) report poor phonological awareness is related to phonetic transcription. Identifying students with poor phonological skills and offering remediation and training may be useful.

Case Study 7 (Liam)

Background

Liam is a 9-year-old male who was referred to our clinic to rule out auditory neuropathy spectrum disorder (ANSD) as a contributing factor to his difficulties. Liam reports his hearing "goes out," even though normal peripheral hearing has previously been established. Normal pregnancy is reported; however, intrauterine growth restriction was noted and as result, Liam was small at birth. Some feeding complications were also reported. He has a positive history of otitis media, had pressure equalization tubes, and suffers from severe allergies. Liam is nearsighted and color blind, wears glasses, and has had vision therapy. Gross motor and fine motor milestones have been delayed. Liam has been diagnosed with ADHD, for which he takes medication. He also has been diagnosed with sensory integration disorder, visual processing disorder, and dyslexia. It is reported that he has received speech therapy since he was two years of age and has previously received occupational therapy. He has completed one Fast ForWord program and is going to continue with the program. He is currently in special education classes. Liam's mother reports that results from a psychoeducational assessment indicated cognitive abilities in the "low-to-average" range. He receives private speech therapy one hour per week.

Assessment

Normal peripheral hearing was established bilaterally, prior to the administration of the central auditory test battery. Results of the behavioral central auditory test battery are shown in Table 21–12. Liam did not perform within the normal range for his age on any of the behavioral tests, possibly reflecting global or pansensory deficits. Normal ABRs were recorded to both condensation and rarefaction clicks for the right and left ears, as shown in Figure 21–8. Normal cABRs were recorded for the right and left ears. Normal ALERs were recorded for right and left ear stimulations and shown in Figure 21–9. Amplitude and latencies of the ALER are shown in Table 21–13.

Recommendations

Liam's parents reported positive improvements after completing one Fast ForWord program and plan to begin another program, which will last approximately six weeks. Dichotic listening training was recommended and proprietary dichotic speech exercises were provided to Liam's speech-language pathologist. Twenty minutes of dichotic listening therapy

will be incorporated into Liam's speech therapy sessions. A list of informal listening activities was provided to Liam's parents for home use. Liam will return to the clinic for follow-up after completing Fast ForWord.

Intervention and Outcomes

Most central auditory tests scores improved following completion of Fast ForWord and dichotic listening training. Test results are shown in Table 21–12 under the column Post 1. Dichotic speech scores had improved, but were still deficient. A slight improvement of the N1–P2 complex of the ALER was seen (shown in Figure 21–9), which might simply reflect variability of the response. Latency and amplitudes for the ALER are shown in Table 21–13. Additional dichotic training was recommended. Liam returned in six months for additional testing. Behavioral tests results are shown in Table 21–12 under the column titled, Post 2. Improvement in dichotic speech tests was noted. Again, continuation of dichotic listening training was recommended. Liam's parents reported improvement in Liam's communication ability. They reported that he seems to actively participate in conversations and is more "tuned in." Electrophysiological testing was not completed during this reassessment due to equipment malfunction. Liam will return for follow-up in six months.

Debriefing

■ What were the risk factors for CAPD and/or comorbid conditions?
Low birth weight, a history of otitis media, ADHD, gross motor delay, and diagnosis of sensory integration disorder and dyslexia are reported.

Table 21–12. Pre- and Post-Behavioral CAPD Test Results for Case 7 (Liam)

	Filtered Words			Auditory Figure Ground			Time-Compressed Speech			Competing Sentences		
	Pre	Post 1	Post 2	Pre	Post 1	Post 2	Pre	Post 1	Post 2	Pre	Post 1	Post 2
Right	82%	92%	90%	74%	100%	98%	44%	76%	78%	60%	80%	84%
Left	76%	94%	94%	62%	96%	94%	26%	66%	74%	40%	50%	70%

	Dichotic Digits			Frequency Pattern Test Left Verbal			Gap Detection Threshold					
	Pre	Post 1	Post 2	Pre	Post 1	Post 2	Pre	Post 1 & 2				
Right	40%	80%	90%	40%	60%	70%	2 ms	DNT				
Left	60%	70%	88%									

*DNT = Did Not Test.

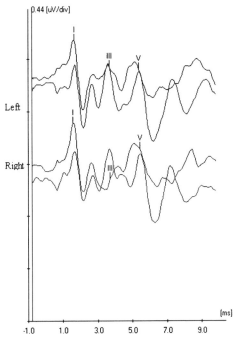

Figure 21–8. A normal ABR is shown for rarefaction and condensation clicks for the right and left ears.

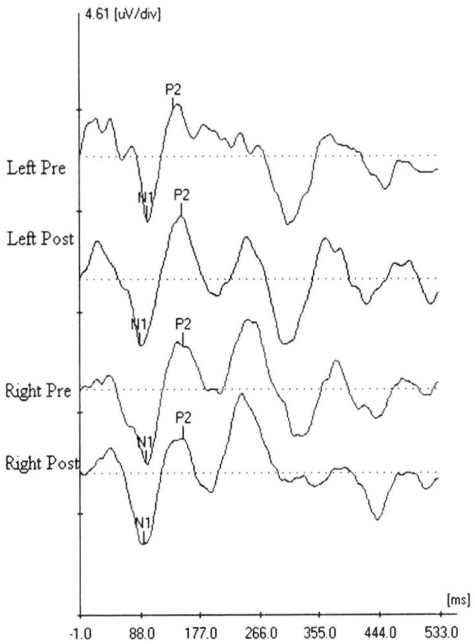

Figure 21–9. Pre and post-ALER recordings for the right and left ears are displayed.

Table 21–13. ALER Latency and Amplitude Recordings for Case 7 (Liam)

Ear	Pre N1 Latency (msec)	Post N1 Latency (msec)	Pre P2 Latency (msec)	Post P2 Latency (msec)	Pre N1–P2 Amplitude (µV)	Post N1–P2 Amplitude (µV)
Left	97.06	87.69	136.61	149.11	4.93	5.86
Right	92.89	96.01	151.19	151.19	4.78	5.36

■ Are there other recommendations? *We were concerned about Liam's self-report of his hearing "going out"? We recommended a hearing assessment should be done immediately at the time that Liam reports his hearing has "gone out" to ensure there is no change in peripheral hearing.*

■ Should dichotic training continue in the absence of limited progress? *Improvement of dichotic speech scores was noted. Liam is participating in dichotic speech exercises for 20 minutes per week. If no additional improvement in dichotic speech scores are seen and/or no positive reports from family members concerning listening abilities are received, dichotic therapy will be discontinued after 8 to 12 weeks. This is the authors' opinions and research to support this position is recommended. Moncrieff and Wertz (2008) reported that some children received optimal success after only a few dichotic listening sessions, whereas other children never showed improvement.*

Case 8 (Brandon)

Background

Brandon is a right-handed 20-year-old male with a long history of speech and language problems, academic difficulties (in particular reading and writing), attention problems, and anxiety. Normal pregnancy and attainment of developmental milestones were reported. There is no history of otitis media. There is a positive family history of ADHD, learning disabilities, and mental illness, including bipolar disorder and depression.

At age 16, Brandon underwent a comprehensive multidisciplinary evaluation and was diagnosed with developmental dyslexia and a receptive and expressive language delay. Despite this diagnoses and severe academic difficulties, Brandon did not meet criteria for special education services, but did qualify for a Section 504 accommodations plan. After graduating high school, Brandon had a psychoeducational assessment in order to gain a better understanding and insight into his abilities and talents so that he might successfully pursue postsecondary education and vocational goals. Average

in-telligence was indicated, along with a diagnosis of ADHD and dyslexia. Brandon is currently medically managed for ADHD. See Chapter 5 for discussion of school policies, processes and services for students with CAPD.

Assessment: Results of the behavioral central auditory test battery, depicted in Table 21–14, indicate bilateral deficits on the low-pass filtered speech and competing sentences tests.

Recommendations

A list of environmental modifications and metacognitive strategies were provided to Brandon. It was also recommended that he work with a vocational and educational counselor for further assessment of career and employment options. Direct remediation also was recommended to include: (1) dichotic listening training in the clinic; and (2) computer-mediated auditory skills training program for home use.

Intervention and Outcomes

In total, Brandon attended 20, fifty minute sessions of therapy, two times per week over 21 weeks. Brandon was reassessed after 10 sessions. As seen in Table 21–14, Post 1, Brandon's performance improved, but a left ear deficit remained for competing sentences. Additional dichotic listening training was recommended to target binaural separation skills. After completion of 10 additional sessions, reassessment (see Post 2, Table 21–14) indicated that Brandon was performing within normal limits. He was dismissed from dichotic listening training. After dichotic listening training, Brandon reported significant improvement in his hearing.

Table 21–14. Initial and Post CAPD Test Scores for Case 8 (Brandon)

| | Low-Pass Filtered Speech | | | Competing Sentences | | | Dichotic Digits | | | Frequency Pattern Test | | Gap Detection Test | |
	Initial	Post 1	Post 2	Initial	Post 1	Post 2	Initial	Post 1	Post 2	Initial	Post testing 1 & 2	Initial	Post Testing 1 & 2
Right	60%	80%	DNT	10%	90%	90%	95%	95%	95%	DNT*	DNT	WNL*	DNT
Left	60%	80%	DNT	15%	62.5%	85%	95%	95%	92%	84%	DNT	WNL	DNT

*DNT = Did Not Test, WNL = Within Normal Limits.

He reported a significant improvement in his ability to "know what is going on" around him. His parents reported a positive change in Brandon's attitude and outlook on his future. Brandon is completing a computer design and drafting program.

Debriefing

▪ What risk factors for CAPD and/or comorbid conditions were present? *Poor academic performance, diagnoses of a learning disorder, dyslexia, and ADHD, and familial history of learning disorders are reported.*

▪ What are the indicators guiding dichotic training focused on binaural separation versus binaural integration? *During dichotic training, it is important to train both binaural separation (directed listening/attending to one ear) and binaural integration (attending to and repeating stimuli from both ears). If a patient shows a greater deficit for either binaural separation or binaural integration, then training may be focused on that process; however, both aspects of dichotic listening should be exercised in therapy. See Chapter 14 in Volume 1 and Chapter 9 in Volume 2 of the Handbook.*

▪ Would you continue to follow this patient? *We recommend follow-up in one year to determine whether progress is maintained. Brandon will be entering college and will receive accommodations.*

References

ASHA (American Speech-Language-Hearing Association). (2005). *Central auditory processing disorders, technical report: Working group on auditory processing disorders.* Rockville, MD: Author.

Bellis, T. (2003). *Assessment and management of central auditory processing disorders in the educational setting: From science to practice.* Clifton Park, NY: Thomson Delmar Learning.

Berlin, C. I., Lowe-Bell, S. S., Jannetta, P. J., & Kline, D. G. (1972). Central auditory deficits after temporal lobectomy. *Archives of Otolaryngology, 96,* 4–10.

Chermak, G. D., & Musiek, F. E. (1997). *Central auditory processing disorders: New perspectives.* San Diego, CA: Singular.

Deonna, T., Beaumanoir, A., Gaillard, F., & Assal, G. (1977). Acquired aphasia in childhood with seizure disorder: A heterogeneous syndrome. *Neuropadiatrie, 8,* 263–273.

Edwards, D. F., Hahn, M. G., Baum, C. M., Perlumutter, M. S., Sheedy, C., & Dromerick, A. W. (2006). Screening patients with stroke for rehabilitation needs: Validation of the post-stroke rehabilitation guidelines. *Neurorehabilitation and Neural Repair, 20,* 42–48.

Elbert, T., Pantev, C., Wienbruch, C., Rockstroh, B., & Taub, E. (1995) Increased cortical representation of the fingers of the left hand in string players. *Science, 270,* 305–307.

Hurley, A., & Hurley, R. M. (2009). Auditory remediation for a patient with Landau-Kleffner syndrome. *Journal of Educational Audiology Association, 15,* 74–83.

Johnson K. L., Nicol, T. G., & Kraus, N. (2005) Brain stem response to speech: A biological marker of auditory processing. *Ear and Hearing, 26,* 424–434.

Kimura, D. (1961). Cerebral dominance and the perception of verbal stimuli. *Canadian Journal of Psychology, 15,* 166–171.

Merzenich, M. M., & Jenkins, W. M. (1995). Cortical plasticity and learning: Some basic principles. In B. Jules & I. Kovacs (Eds.), *Maturational windows and adult cortical plasticity* (Vol. XXII, pp. 247–272). San Francisco, CA: Addison-Wesley.

Merzenich, M. M., Jenkins, W. M., Johnston, P., Schreiner, C. E., Miller, S. L., & Tallal, P. (1996). Temporal processing deficits of language-learning impaired children ameliorated by training. *Science, 271,* 77–80.

Moncrieff, D. W., & Wertz, D. (2008). Auditory rehabilitation for interaural asymmetry: Preliminary evidence of improved dichotic listening performance following intensive training. *International Journal of Audiology, 47,* 84–97.

Moran, M. J., & Fitch, J. L. (2001). Phonological awareness skills of university students: Implications for teaching phonetics. *Contemporary Issues in Communication Science and Disorders, 28,* 85–90.

Musiek, F. E., Baran, J. A., & Shinn, J. (2004). Assessment and remediation of an auditory processing disorder associated with head trauma. *Journal of the American Academy of Audiology, 15,* 117–132.

Musiek, F., Chermak, G., & Weihing, J. (2007). *Auditory training.* In F. E. Musiek & G. D. Chermak (Eds.), *Handbook of (central) auditory processing disorder: Comprehensive intervention* (Vol. I, pp. 77–106). San Diego, CA: Plural.

Musiek, F. M., Gollegly, K. M., & Baran, J. A. (1984). Myelination of the corpus callosum and auditory processing problems in children: Theoretical and clinical correlates. *Seminars in Hearing, 4,* 231–240.

Patry, G., Lyagoubi, S., & Tassinari, C. A. (1971). Subclinical "electrical status epilepticus" induced by sleep in children. A clinical and electroencephalographic study of six cases. *Archives of Neurology, 24,* 241–252.

Robinson, G. C., Mahurin, S. L., & Justis, B. (2001). Predicting difficulties in learning phonetic transcription: Phonemic awareness screening for beginning speech-language pathology students. *Contemporary Issues in Communication Science and Disorders, 38,* 87–95.

Roeser, R., Valente, M., & Hosford-Dunn, H. (2007). *Audiology diagnosis* (2nd ed., p. 59). New York, NY: Thieme.

Russo N., Nicol T., Zecker S., Hayes E., & Kraus N. (2005) Auditory training improves neural timing in the human brainstem. *Behavioural Brain Research, 156,* 95–103.

Recanzone, G. H., Schreiner, C. E., & Merzenich, M. M. (1993). Plasticity in the frequency representation of primary auditory cortex following discrimination training in adult owl monkeys. *Journal of Neuroscience, 13,* 87–103.

Singh, S., & Singh, K. S. (2006). *Phonetics: Principles and practices* (3rd ed.). San Diego, CA: Plural.

Sweetow, R. W. (2005). Training the adult brain to listen. *Hearing Journal, 58,* 10–16.

Sweetow R. W., & Henderson Sabes, J. (2004). The case for LACE: Listening and auditory communication enhancement training. *Hearing Journal, 57,* 32–40.

Tallal, P., Miller, S. L., Bedi, G., Byma, G., Wang, X., Nagarajan, S. S., . . . Merzenich, M. M. (1996). Language comprehension in language-learning impaired children improved with acoustically modified speech. *Science, 271,* 81–84.

Tharpe, A. B., Johnson, G. D., & Glasscock M. E. III. (1991). Diagnostic and management considerations of acquired epileptic aphasia or Landau-Kleffner syndrome. *American Journal of Otology, 12,* 210–214.

Tremblay, K., Kraus, N., Carrell, T. D., & Magee, T. (1996). Central auditory system plasticity: Generalization to novel stimuli following listening training. *Journal of the Acoustical Society of America, 102,* 3762–3773.

Webster, D. B. (1995). *Neuroscience of communication.* San Diego, CA: Singular.

Weihing, J., Musiek, F. E., Munroe, S., Swainson, S., & Cho, Y. (2006). *Dichotic Interaural intensity difference (DIID) training in a case of left hemisphere stroke.* Poster presentation at the convention of the American Academy of Audiology. Minneapolis, MN.

Wible, B., Nicol, T., & Kraus, N. (2004) Aypical brainstem representation of onset and formant structure of speech sounds in children with language-based learning problems. *Biological Psychology, 67,* 299–317.

SECTION 5

Future Directions

CHAPTER 22

CLINICAL AND RESEARCH ISSUES IN CENTRAL AUDITORY PROCESSING DISORDER

JEFFREY WEIHING, TERI JAMES BELLIS,
GAIL D. CHERMAK, and FRANK E. MUSIEK

Introduction

As with any clinical field, the recommended practices for evaluation of and intervention for children with central auditory processing disorder (CAPD) are dynamic, undergoing re-evaluation and improvements as new research emerges. In the process of trying to maintain currency with the new advancements, clinicians should examine some of the more controversial topics that may be encountered in the literature and how these may (or may not) impact clinical practice. These controversies frequently arise from differences in perspective regarding the theoretical conceptualization of CAPD and/or how the disorder should be diagnosed and treated in the clinic. Although the recommended practices

for diagnosing and providing intervention for CAPD have been developed by consensus groups with careful consideration of the merits of various positions surrounding these controversies (e.g., AAA, 2010; ASHA, 2005a, 2005b), it is important that the clinician also appreciate the research underlying the issues, so as to make better informed, evidence-based clinical decisions. To this end, we examine a number of these controversies in the present chapter with a focus on the current state of the evidence base supporting conceptualizations of and guidelines for CAPD treatment and intervention (e.g., AAA, 2010; ASHA, 2005a, 2005b). Specifically, this chapter focuses on three broad topics: (1) the degree to which CAPD should be considered an auditory-modality-specific disorder and the impact of comorbid or confounding supramodal, cognitive, or pansensory deficits on diagnosing CAPD in the pediatric population; (2) which criteria should be used to define and diagnose the disorder; and (3) the efficacy of auditory interventions for CAPD.

Modality-Specificity of CAPD and Impact of Comorbid or Confounding Disorders

CAPD in children frequently coexists with other language, learning, and related disorders (e.g., Banai, Abrams, & Kraus, 2007; Banai, Nicol, Zecker, & Kraus, 2005; Bellis, 2002; Bellis, Billiet, & Ross, 2011; Bellis & Ferre, 1999; Billiet & Bellis, 2011; Hayes, Warrier, Nichol, Zecker, & Kraus, 2003; Sharma, Purdy, & Kelly, 2009). This comorbidity has led some researchers to the following, not necessarily mutually exclusive, conclusions: (1) CAPD is not an auditory disorder but, instead, is most likely one component of a more generalized cognitive and/or developmental disorder (e.g., BSA, 2010; Moore, 2011); and/or (2) for a diagnosis of CAPD to have any clinical utility, it should be viewed as an auditory-modality-specific deficit. These conclusions have led to arguments such as suggesting that performance-based CAPD evaluations be replaced with parent-report cognition related questionnaires (Moore, 2011) and that central auditory tests should be augmented by analogous testing in other, nonauditory modalities to differentiate CAPD from broader, supramodal or pansensory issues (e.g., Cacace & McFarland, 2005). The distinctions made by these arguments hold significant implications for diagnosis and, especially,

treatment of the disorder. That is, if a child is found to have a sensory processing disorder such as CAPD, whether the disorder exists alone or comorbidly with another disorder in another domain, then deficit-specific auditory interventions are indicated. In contrast, interventions for general developmental or cognitive disorders typically do not include direct auditory remediation, and if they do, that remediation is offered within the context of other treatments (e.g., language, memory) more specific to these other disorders. As such, understanding and disentangling the effects of cognition and sensory processing are critical for appropriate, effective, and efficient treatment and management of the individual child.

Is CAPD Primarily an Auditory Deficit or Should It Be Conceptualized as a General Developmental Disorder or as a Cognitive Disorder?

Certainly, any task that requires a behavioral response from the patient is susceptible to the influence of cognition, assuming that the task requires that the patient be cognizant of what is required of him or her and able and willing to comply with instructions. Perhaps, for this reason, the role of patient cognition is an issue that has surfaced in regard to the behavioral assessment of a wide range of disorders. For example, attention has been paid in the literature to the overlap between cognition and speech-language deficits (ASHA, 2004; Rice, 1983; see Ebert & Kohnert, 2011 for a review), visual deficits (Lee, Kwon, Legge, & Gefrohl, 2010; Lee & Vecera, 2005), and psychological disorders (Zdanowicz & Myslinski, 2010). This issue is compounded by the fact that cognitive measures themselves are not infallible, subject to the same confounds as any other behavioral measure (Heinrich & Schneider, 2011; Merikanto, Lahti, Castaneda, Tuulio-Henriksson, Aalto-Setala, Suvisaari, & Partonen, 2011; Yang, Lung, Jong, Hsu, & Chen, 2010). As one illustration, we note the findings of Merikanto et al. (2011) demonstrating the influence of seasonal variation in mood and behavior on cognitive test performance.

Given the nonmodularity of the central nervous system, there is no question that the influence of cognition and related functions on behavioral tests of central auditory processing should be a concern to the extent that it may cast doubt on the validity of these tests' ability to describe the auditory system's contributions to the exhibited listening difficulties. Auditory processing does not occur in isolation from cognition, nor is cognition independent of sensory-perceptual processing (e.g., auditory processing imposes bottom-up environmental constraints on attention as seen in the *cocktail party effect*; noise increases cognitive load and affects the ability to concentrate (Kujala & Brattico, 2009); musical training, which involves intensive auditory-motor training, strengthens cognitive functions (Strait, Kraus, Parbery-Clark, & Ashley, 2010). In this context, a CAPD is one in which the deficit is primarily auditory, even though there may be comorbid issues in cognitive or related functions. However, it has been argued by some that measures of central auditory processing may *solely* reflect on cognitive processing and do not indicate CANS specific functioning (Moore, 2011; Moore, Ferguson, Edmondson-Jones, Ratib, & Riley, 2010). We present here several lines of evidence that demonstrates that mea-

sures of CANS function explain variance that is unique from cognitive measures. As such, these auditory measures provide unique information that would not be obtained through the administration of cognitive tests alone. These lines of evidence include: examining statistically the overlap between cognitive and auditory processing measures, determining the degree to which auditory processing tests emerge as separate factors in factor analyses, exploring the degree to which medications that influence cognition/attention also modulate behavioral central auditory test performance, considering the percentage of children diagnosed with CAPD who also present normal performance on cognitive batteries, and reviewing CAPD diagnostic measures in which attention and memory effects are significantly reduced, such as electrophysiological measures of auditory function.

Overlap Between Cognitive Variables and Central Auditory Processing Measures

The role of cognition in the behavioral assessment of central auditory processing has been examined statistically via correlation analysis in a variety of different cognitive domains (e.g., attention, memory, IQ) and relative to a number of central auditory processes. The rationale behind these investigations is to demonstrate that variability in central auditory processing measures occurs with some degree of independence from cognitive function. Again, as noted above, we do not suggest that auditory processing occurs in isolation from cognitive function, but rather that central auditory processing and cognition are interdependent and may even be seen as co-modulatory systems, and that the shared variance between auditory processing and cognitive measures is rather modest at best. Scores attained on tasks that incorporate frequency discrimination or temporal sequencing have been shown to overlap with cognitive measures, although the degree of shared variance is low. Rosen, Cohen, and Vanniasegaram (2010) noted that tone discrimination ability shared 21% of its variance with nonverbal IQ, but was unrelated to measures of attention. Auditory temporal sequencing tests have a similar degree of variance associated with cognition, although it is divided almost equally between memory and attention measures, roughly 10% each (Sharma et al., 2009).

There also exist auditory processing measures that show no significant correlation with cognitive measures. Included among these are gap detection, masking level difference, and certain speech-in-noise tasks. Both Sharma et al. (2009) and Breier, Fletcher, Foorman, Klaas, and Gray (2003) noted that attention and/or memory variables did not impact performance on gap detection or masking level difference tasks. Additionally, some speech-in-noise tasks, such as those included in certain subtests of the SCAN, have not been shown to be significantly correlated with memory and/or attention skills (Riccio, Cohen, Garrison, & Smith, 2005; Rosen et al., 2010). It should be pointed out that Rosen et al. (2010) observed that children who scored more poorly on central auditory tests had a significantly lower IQ than those who scored better on these measures. However, this significant difference was due in large part to the finding that the control group exhibited IQs that were significantly higher than average, ranging from

109 to 115 depending on the measure. Children in the poorer central auditory test performing group had near-average IQs ranging from 94 through 98.

In a recent paper, Moore et al. (2010) examined the auditory processing ability of a large sample of children (N = ~1,500) ranging in age from 6 to 11 years using a *population-based approach* to understanding the disorder. Consistent with that approach, participants were not recruited on the basis of auditory, cognitive, or speech-language function as the aim, in part, was to obtain findings that the authors argued would have a high degree of external validity. The authors noted that those participants who scored in the top and bottom 5% on auditory measures also tended to score the highest and lowest, respectively, on selected measures of cognition. The authors *inferred* that those children performing in the bottom 5% on the auditory measure were those who had CAPD, arguing that their sample was representative of the population and thus the prevalence of CAPD is on the order of 5%. Based in large part on this observation, the authors suggested that CAPD may be a cognitive-based disorder. However, as we elaborate below, the analysis and the conclusions drawn from this study are compromised.

First, the amount of shared variance between the cognitive measures and auditory processing measures when examined across the entire sample was extremely small, ranging from .01% to 10%, depending on the comparison being made. That many of these correlations were significant likely reflects the extremely large sample size used in the study. Second, the authors' assumption that the bottom 5% of the sample was those who were most likely to have CAPD overlooks what is well known about childhood disorders frequently being comorbid. It is not surprising that those with very poor cognitive ability also have very poor auditory processing ability, and certainly clear conclusions regarding the validity of any one diagnosis cannot be made when the sample under study can have such a wide range of unidentified issues. Finally, and perhaps most significantly, the authors' test battery was atypical: they assumed that the auditory tasks they designed for this study were indeed appropriate for identifying the auditory deficits exhibited by children with CAPD. In fact, the auditory tasks used in this study have no demonstrated sensitivity to CAPD and were not selected from a plethora of verbal and nonverbal central auditory diagnostic tests that have been used internationally for over three decades in the diagnosis of this disorder. Many of these central auditory diagnostic tests have been shown to have considerable construct validity and sensitivity based on a multitude of publications reporting on adults, and less frequently children, with neurological lesions of the central auditory nervous system (CANS) (Bamiou et al., 2012; Chermak & Musiek, 2011; Hurley & Musiek, 1997; Musiek, Chermak, Weihing, Zappulla, & Nagle, 2011; Musiek, Gollegly, Kibbe, & Verkest-Lenz, 1991; Musiek, Shinn, Jirsa, Bamiou, Baran, & Zaidan, 2005). If the aim of the Moore et al. study was to present an alternative perspective on CAPD, it would seem that including auditory measures with documented efficiency for diagnosis of CAPD and that are widely accepted and used tools to diagnose CAPD in children would have aided the authors in offering a more compelling argument.

Perhaps providing the most compelling data regarding the potential influence of cognitive factors on central auditory processing have been studies using brain imaging and dichotic listening tests, arguably the bedrock of central auditory behavioral tests. Based on hemodynamic data, neural regions that are associated with attention and memory are active when individuals perform dichotic binaural separation (i.e., directed attention to one ear or *forced report* of stimuli from one ear) tasks. This contrasts with dichotic binaural integration (i.e., reporting stimuli heard in both ears in any order or *free report*) measures, which appear to be more reflective of true sensory perceptual asymmetries rather than cognitive processes (Hugdahl et al., 2009). This does not imply that binaural separation is driven entirely by attention, as studies in patients with confirmed neurologic involvement have shown that discrete lesions of central auditory regions contribute to reduced competing sentence performance (Musiek, 1983; Musiek et al., 2011). However, binaural separation tasks do appear to recruit areas associated with cognition to a greater degree than binaural integration tasks, as evident by these fMRI studies (Cowell & Hugdahl, 2000; Hugdahl et al., 2009).

In addition to the fMRI studies, several studies have examined the relationship between central auditory processing and cognition using the same binaural separation and binaural integration measures of dichotic listening. Sharma et al. (2009) examined the relationship between binaural integration and cognitive variables (i.e., attention and memory). They observed that the dichotic measure was significantly correlated with auditory and visual continuous performance, albeit with only 20% shared variance, with no correlation seen with memory. Importantly, the lack of a binaural separation test in this study makes it difficult to comment on the *relative* influence of cognition on binaural integration and separation tasks. Riccio et al. (2005) also examined the relationship between cognition and dichotic tasks. They examined both binaural integration (Staggered Spondaic Words [SSW]) and binaural separation (SCAN—Competing Words) tasks. The sentence recognition subtest of the CELF (Clinical Evaluation of Language Fundamentals) was used as the measure of memory, and a visual (but not an auditory) continuous performance test was applied to assess attention. No correlation was seen between the binaural separation task and attention or memory and the only significant relationship noted for the binaural integration measure was between the right noncompeting condition of the SSW and the sentence recognition test, purportedly a measure of memory. Although this was presented by the authors as a correlation between binaural integration and memory, that the effect was noted only in the noncompeting condition and with a nondirect measure of memory makes this finding difficult to interpret.

Clearly, additional studies are needed that investigate the relationship between behavioral performance on measures of dichotic processing and cognitive ability. Nonetheless, two conclusions appear clear from the evidence available at present. First, despite the fact that binaural integration tasks typically require the listener to report a larger number of stimuli than do binaural separation tasks, binaural separation tasks appear to recruit additional brain regions that subserve executive function and attentional strategies. Second, despite this fact, binaural separation (or directed-report) tasks, nonetheless, are a valid measure of central auditory dysfunction. See Chap-

ter 18 of Volume 1 of the Handbook for additional discussion of the relationship between cognition and central auditory processing.

To summarize, although some auditory performance measures correlate with measures of cognitive ability and other supramodal domains, for the majority of the diagnostic measures of central auditory function, this overlap generally represents a small amount of the variance between the two variables (≤20%) (Riccio et al., 2005; Rosen et al., 2010; Sharma et al., 2009). This does not indicate that auditory processing occurs in isolation from cognitive processing, but merely that central auditory processing tests account for variability that is unique from these supramodal abilities. This likely reflects unique contributions of the CANS to processing of these stimuli. Additionally, there are many central auditory measures that demonstrate no significant relationship with cognitive and other supramodal variables (Riccio et al., 2005; Rosen et al., 2010). Moreover, correlation does not imply causation; therefore, we conclude that attention and memory issues do not *cause* CAPD in children who: (a) have been diagnosed with the disorder using central auditory tests with documented sensitivity and specificity to this disorder, and (b) have had their central auditory processing results interpreted in light of any dominating influence of potential comorbid issues (see AAA, 2010; ASHA, 2005). Notwithstanding the foregoing conclusion, it must be recognized that some degree of shared variance between CAPD tests and supramodal measures is not unexpected, given what is known about the nonmodularity of the central nervous system. When one views the anatomical, physiological, and hemodynamic characteristics of the

CANS within the context of research in neuropsychology (Lopez-Aranda, Lopez-Tellez, Navarro-Lobato, Masmudi-Martin, Gutierrez, & Khan, 2009) and cognitive neuroscience (Ciccio, Meulenbroek, & Turkstra, 2009; Gaffan, 2005; Thiebaut de Schotten, Urbanksi, Duffau, Volle, Levy, Dubois, & Bartolomeo, 2005), there is clear evidence that one should not expect memory, attention, and other cognitive functions to dissociate completely from behavioral auditory functions (see Musiek, Bellis, & Chermak, 2005 for a review). Indeed, one might even predict that attention and memory difficulties might be prevalent in the CAPD population given the increased demands placed on these domains when sensory processing is disrupted (see resource allocation and information processing theories [Pichora-Fuller, Schneider, & Daneman, 1995; Sarampalis, Edwards, Kalluri, & Hafter, 2009; Wong, Ettlinger, Sheppard, Gunasekera, & Ghar, 2010]). Elaborating on this rationale as early as 1996, Bellis (Bellis & Ferre, 1999; see Bellis, 2002 for review) argued that relatively predictable patterns of function across sensory and cognitive domains would occur in many children diagnosed with CAPD. This argument is reinforced by the observation that the frequent comorbidity of CAPD and attention deficit hyperactivity disorder (ADHD) (Chermak, Hall, & Musiek, 1999; Riccio, Hynd, Cohen, Hall, & Molt, 1994) and comorbidity between CAPD and dyslexia (Iliadou, Bamiou, Kaprinis, Kandylis, & Kaprinis, 2009) are at least partly explained on the basis of shared neural substrate and synchronized networks that underlie brain organization and processing (Chermak, Bellis, & Musiek, 2007). Brain organization and function suggest that CAPD may be best characterized not as a disorder in which deficits are auditory alone, but where difficulties in the auditory modality are *most pronounced* (Bellis, Billiet, & Ross, 2011).

Factor Analyses of Central Auditory Processing Measures

Factor analyses of central auditory processing test performance provides another means to analyze the independence of auditory processing from cognition. This statistical approach examines interrelationships among large groups of variables. Variables that are related load on the same factor, whereas unrelated variables load on different factors. This analysis lends itself well to the question under consideration by providing two separate predictions for the factor analysis outcome. If different auditory processing tests are all being driven by one construct, such as cognition (e.g., attention or memory), then these tests should load primarily onto a single factor that would represent the variable that is common to all of the tests. If, however, each central auditory test assesses some relatively independent aspect of CANS function, then each measure should emerge as a separate factor. To the extent that this latter scenario is observed, it can be concluded that central auditory processing measures assess disparate (auditory) abilities. Utilizing factor analysis would, therefore, be of use in determining the degree to which tests of central auditory function exhibit independence from common cognitive or psychological variables. Undoubtedly, all behavioral tests (including behavioral tests of central auditory processing) depend to some degree on these psychological variables. However, if auditory measures provide unique information that has some degree independence from psychological function, then these auditory tests should load separately on factors that are related to the type of auditory task or region of the CANS that is recruited.

Several factor analysis studies have provided evidence supporting the independence of auditory processing from psychological variables. Schow and Chermak (1999) administered the SCAN and the Staggered Spondaic Word (SSW) Test (Katz, 1968) to over 300 children with normal peripheral hearing who were referred for central auditory processing assessment due to reduced classroom performance or attention issues. Subject ages ranged from 6 through 17 years, with the majority of subjects falling in the 7 through 9 years age range. The SCAN competing words, speech in noise, and filtered words subtest scoress and the SSW left and right competing condition scores were examined. Results revealed two factors with Eigenvalues greater than 1.0. The first factor accounted for roughly 40% of the variance and all dichotic test measures (SSW right and left competing, and SCAN competing words) loaded significantly (loadings of ~.7 or greater). The second factor accounted for roughly 20% additional variance, and all monaural low-redundancy test scores (speech in noise and filtered words) loaded significantly. That auditory processing tests that assess the same auditory process loaded together, yet separate from other auditory processes, argues against the interpretation that auditory processing performance is driven by cognitive variables.

Domitz and Schow (2000) who also showed that central auditory tests that assess different auditory processes loaded onto separate factors, albeit with a slightly different factor structure than was found

by Schow and Chermak (1999). A total of 81 children with normal peripheral hearing who ranged in age from 8 through 9 years were recruited. Roughly half of the sample presented no developmental issues, while the rest of the subjects demonstrated a learning disability, speech-language disorder, and/or a diagnosed attention issue. Tests used in the factor analysis included dichotic digits and competing sentences tests based on Musiek (1983) and Willeford and Burleigh (1994) respectively, a frequency patterns test based on Musiek and Pinheiro (1987), a monaural low redundancy test (Selective Auditory Attention Test [Cherry, 1980]), and the subtests of the SCAN included in the Schow and Chermak (1999) study. The factor analysis was performed using criteria similar to Schow and Chermak (1999) and revealed that central auditory tests tended to load only with other tests that measured similar auditory processes. Specifically, the dichotic digits and competing sentences/words measures tended to load on a single factor (with left-ear performance loading more heavily than right ear performance); the monaural low-redundancy tests that required listening for words in ipsilateral competition loaded together; and the filtered words and frequency patterns tests each loaded alone on separate factors. Hence, four factors, each uniquely representing dichotic processing, monaural low-redundancy (ipsilateral competition), monaural low-redundancy (filtered speech), and temporal processing were identified. As with the Schow and Chermak (1999) study, the observation that central auditory processing tests load on factors that are process specific argues against a model that interprets central auditory test performance as being primarily cognitively driven. Were central auditory processing measures a reflection of underlying cognition, we would expect the tests to load onto one or two factors that are relatively unrelated to the central auditory process being measured. Additional studies using factor analyses that include specific tests of cognitive and related function along with diagnostic tests of central auditory processing would provide further support to this contention.

Effect of ADHD Medications on Auditory Processing Performance

Measuring central auditory function in children before and after administering medication prescribed to reduce inattention has been one research design used to examine the effect of attention on auditory processing. The logic of these studies is that if auditory processing performance measures are *relatively* uninfluenced by these medications, then these measures must be less susceptible to attention effects. Note that the underlying reasoning does not assume that CAPD tests are completely devoid of the influence attention, as this would be inconsistent with what has been previously stated regarding the nonmodularity of the central nervous system. Rather, these studies suggest that CAPD tests are not *as* affected by experimental manipulations of attention as are tests designed to specifically measure this psychological property.

Studies using this experimental design generally demonstrate that performance on diagnostic tests of central auditory function does not change when attention deficits are treated with medication. Tillery, Katz, and Keller (2000) recruited children with ADHD and normal IQ, approximately 60% of whom were also diagnosed with comorbid CAPD. Patients were administered an auditory continuous performance task (i.e., a measure of attention) and a central auditory test battery on two separate occasions: with no ADHD treatment and while taking Ritalin (methylphenidate). The order of the treatment and control conditions was randomized across subjects to control for potential learning effects in the analysis. Only the auditory continuous performance measure improved significantly while on Ritalin. Furthermore, Sutcliffe, Bishop, Houghton, and Taylor (2006) noted that children diagnosed with ADHD did not perform any differently on frequency modulation tasks when medicated; however, they noted that performance on frequency discrimination tasks changed as a function of medication. As the frequency modulation task always preceded the frequency discrimination task in this study, the latter task may have been more susceptible to subject fatigue. In addition, the longer duration frequency modulation detection stimulus could have afforded the children more time to "tune in," which may have served to minimize between condition differences. In a third study, Keith and Engineer (1991) also noted results that were dependent on the CAPD test utilized: an effect of ADHD medication was seen on dichotic and some auditory closure tests (e.g., filtered words), but not on other auditory closure tests (e.g., speech recognition in speech babble). For more of an elaboration on the effects of medication, the reader is referred to Chapter 19.

Overall, these findings are consistent with the proposition that attention influences performance on psychological measures of this construct more than it influences performance on CAPD measures, supporting the position that these two disorders are different clinical entities. It should be noted that we do not contend here that CAPD measures are completely devoid of attention effects: such a contention would be inconsistent with evidence relating to the nonmodularity of the central nervous system cited in previous sections of this chapter. As stated above, we argue that a CAPD is one in which the deficit is primarily auditory, even though comorbid issues may be present. For this reason, it is generally recommended that children with ADHD who are on medication to control attention-related symptoms be tested in the medicated state for purposes of differential diagnosis of CAPD to reduce any potential negative impact of the attention disorder on auditory processing performance (AAA, 2010).

Poor Auditory Processing Performance in the Presence of Normal Cognition

When examined clinically, there is a notable percentage of patients who demonstrate central auditory processing deficits in the absence of attention, memory, and/or cognitive deficits. Indeed, many clinicians suggest that central auditory diagnostic testing only be conducted after measures of cognition, language, attention, and other possibly confounding factors have been completed (Bellis, 2003; Fandino, Connolly, Usher, Palm, & Kozak, 2011; Whitton, 2010). As these children are generally referred for some type of listening difficulty, it is important to highlight that these listening difficulties would likely be delegated as nonclinical if not for the specific assessment of auditory processing ability. Riccio et al. (1994) observed that 50% of pediatric

patients being evaluated for CAPD and attention disorders showed auditory processing difficulties only. Ricco et al. (2005) found that roughly 30% of their sample was diagnosed with CAPD only, without any comorbid attention or memory disorder. Similarly, Sharma et al. (2009) noted that 30% of their subjects diagnosed with CAPD had no cormorbid attention or memory issues, though some did present with comorbid speech language issues. These findings underscore the need for multidisciplinary input in the differential diagnosis of CAPD, as recommended by current US consensus statements and guidelines (AAA, 2010; ASHA, 2005a, 2005b).

Electrophysiological Findings Are Primarily Sensory Based

Although the influence of cognition on auditory evoked and event-related potentials varies depending on the electrophysiologic measure under consideration, it is generally well accepted that brainstem evoked responses have a very large sensory component. Indeed some of these responses are obtainable while the patient is under sedation with little to no alteration to waveform characteristics. The auditory brainstem response (ABR) can be evoked by clicks, speech, or other complex stimuli, and in a variety of different paradigms. Additionally, the middle-latency response (MLR) and obligatory cortical event-related potentials are also somewhat resistant to general cognitive abilities, although they are potentially more susceptible to nonauditory factors, particularly if proper within-subject indices are not utilized (see below).

Click-evoked ABRs have some, although limited, utility to differentiate children who show characteristics of CAPD from those who do not. Hall and Grose (1993) compared ABRs evoked by clicks in a standard clinical protocol in children who had a significant history of otitis media (OM) but were currently asymptomatic, and those who did not have this history. Results indicated that children with a history of OM showed significantly later waves III and V. As these responses were acquired shortly after the OM episode, the findings do not speak to the persistence of this deficit over time. Research has indicated, however, that OM-driven CAPD deficits tend to persist throughout adolescence and can cause long-term delays in developmental milestones when certain conditions are met (Whitton & Polley, 2011).

Two unique paradigms incorporating click-evoked ABRs have been employed in an attempt to identify children with CAPD. These paradigms are unique in that they go beyond the standard monaural protocol in quiet that is generally performed in the clinic. In the first paradigm, Delb, Strauss, Hohenberg, and Plinkert (2003) computed a binaural interaction component (BIC) in which binaural evoked potentials were evoked at different interaural timing differences (ITD). Using a 400-microsecond ITD and designating absence of the BIC wave as indicating dysfunction, the authors found that the BIC measure had a 76% sensitivity and specificity for predicting those children who also exhibited difficulties on behavioral tests of central auditory function. In the second paradigm, Marler and Champlin (2005) used an ABR backward masking protocol to determine whether children with language-based learning impairment could be differentiated from normally developing controls. They reported that wave V latency did

not differ between groups when the ABR was acquired in quiet; however, when a noise burst immediately followed the ABR stimulus, the wave V latency of the group with language-based learning impairment was significantly longer than the controls. Taken together, these findings suggest that using unconventional ABR protocols as correlates of behavioral auditory processing measures (i.e., binaural hearing and backward masking, respectively) can be useful in identifying children with CAPD, and that because the ABR is a generally thought of as a basic sensory measure, one can conclude that the effect is not heavily influenced by cognition.

In the past decade, the speech-evoked ABR (cABR) has emerged as a relatively reliable and valid means of identifying children with a wide range of deficits who show neural timing issues in the brainstem. Specifically, certain pediatric clinical groups seem to lack the ability to efficiently encode the acoustic characteristics of speech stimuli at the brainstem level (Banai, Abrams, & Kraus, 2007). Evidence for the utility of this measure in objectively identifying auditory contributions to clinical symptoms comes from a variety of different laboratories. For instance, Filippini and Schochat (2009) noted significant differences in cABR indices between children who were diagnosed with CAPD and those who were not. Johnson, Nicol, Zecker, and Kraus (2007) examined the cABRs of two groups of children: one with and without language-based learning based on their performance in a backward masking task. They found that those children with learning difficulties who also showed poor psychoacoustic backward masking ability exhibited significantly delayed cABR latencies relative to those who performed well on the psychoacoustic task. Anderson, Skoe, Chandrasekaran, Zecker, and Kraus (2010) examined cABRs in children with dyslexia, noting a significant relationship between the cABR and behavioral hearing-in-noise ability even after partialing out the effects of memory. Billiet and Bellis (2011) examined performance on behavioral tests of central auditory function in two groups of children diagnosed with dyslexia: those who exhibited normal cABRs and those who did not. They found that the children with normal cABRs tended to exhibit a diagnostic pattern on central auditory tests consistent with a diagnosis of CAPD with a cortical locus of dysfunction. Conversely, those with abnormal cABRs tended not to demonstrate a cortical pattern on the behavioral central auditory tests. Billiet and Bellis concluded that the electrophysiological and behavioral measures tap different aspects of central auditory processing and different neuroanatomical substrates and that only by looking at the results from both measures in tandem can the most sensitive diagnostic battery be determined.

Another electrophysiologic measure that appears to reflect basic sensory processing of auditory stimuli is the middle latency response (MLR). Although the MLR is generally considered to be primarily sensory in nature (Jerger, Johnson, & Loiselle, 1988), it also tends to be more influenced by states of consciousness (i.e., sleep, sedation) than sensory evoked potentials that occur in earlier latency ranges. This influence is generally relatively minor, however, occurring only in specific stages of sleep (McGee, Kraus, Killion, Rosenberg, & King, 1993). Nonetheless, MLR offers some utility as an objective biomarker of CAPD. For

example, children diagnosed with CAPD based on diagnostic behavioral measures have been shown to exhibit significantly smaller MLRs when compared with children who perform well on central auditory test batteries (Schochat, Musiek, Alonso, & Ogata, 2010). Additionally, Purdy, Kelly, and Davies (2002) reported significant differences between children with CAPD and controls on measures of the MLR, specifically a reduction of Nb amplitude and delayed Na latency. As with the MLR, the N1–P2 also tends to be more susceptible to nonauditory factors than brainstem potentials. Nonetheless, it still reflects important contributions from sensory regions of the central nervous system, as evidence by its exogenous nature (Musiek, Froke, & Weihing, 2005). Using this potential, McArthur, Atkinson, and Ellis (2009) reported atypical cortical evoked responses to tones, vowels, and consonant-vowel syllables in 38% of 6- to 12-year-old children with specific language impairment or specific reading disorder.

The clinical utility of both the MLR and the N1–P2 may be enhanced in part by utilizing relative instead of absolute evoked potential indices. An absolute index is one that reflects measurement of an evoked potential under only one set of conditions. For instance, the amplitude of the MLR waveform acquired under left ear stimulation would represent an absolute index. Conversely, a relative index is one that is computed based on two or more absolute indexes (e.g., computing the difference in amplitude between the MLR obtained with right ear stimulation minus that obtained with left ear stimulation). Relative indices offer an advantage in partly controlling for nonauditory individual differences that may be reflected in the evoked potential recordings. For instance, when computing a relative index by subtracting the left ear evoked MLR amplitude from the right ear MLR amplitude, any nonauditory influence can be assumed to be equal for both left and right ear recordings and is subtracted out of the measurement when the relative index is computed. Accordingly, these measures have been shown to significantly reduce the within-group variability of the MLR in normal hearing children from about 7 years of age through the mid-teens (Weihing, Schochat, & Musiek, 2012). Therefore, these relative MLR measures, and their N1–P2 counterparts, could be more likely to indicate central auditory function that is less influenced by nonauditory variables.

Should Cognitive Testing and/or Nonauditory Measures Be Incorporated into Central Auditory Test Batteries to Assist Audiologists in Differential Diagnosis?

Best practice recommendations for the diagnosis of CAPD highlight the importance of incorporating knowledge of the patient's cognitive, speech-language, and related abilities into interpretation of central auditory test battery findings (AAA, 2010; ASHA, 2005a, 2005b). This recommendation is made because auditory processing does not occur separately from psychological processes, and the two can influence each other reciprocally. The goal in evaluation of central auditory processing is to determine if the deficit is primarily (or fundamentally) auditory in nature, so that the most efficient and effective intervention can be applied. Such a determination requires multidisci-

plinary assessments and examination of patterns of brain-behavior relationships. (See Chapters 8, 18, and 20 in Volume 1 of the Handbook.) As noted in these documents, the reasons for multidisciplinary assessment to complement central auditory testing stem from the high prevalence of comorbidity among developmental disorders in pediatric populations and the need to consider functioning across domains for purposes of differential diagnosis and development of the most appropriate, individualized intervention plan. For diagnostic central auditory testing, this means that reducing the impact of these confounds to the greatest extent possible must always be on the clinician's radar if an accurate diagnosis is to be achieved. Some have recommended incorporating cognitive tests in the central auditory evaluation, as well as utilizing visual analogs of central auditory processing tests to rule out supramodal issues. Both these suggestions are considered below.

Incorporation of Cognitive Tests in CAPD Test Batteries

An initially intuitive solution to the issue of teasing out the influence of nonauditory comorbidities would be to incorporate measures of cognition into central auditory assessment, as occurs with some frequency in the United States when screening for CAPD, although there has been no formal protocol established. For example, Bellis (2003) described a screening protocol in which cognitive (e.g., auditory continuous performance testing to rule out attention issues; forward and backward digit span measures to assist in screening for potential memory issues), speech-language, psycho-educational (e.g., intelligence testing to screen general intelligence constructs), and related testing were reviewed to determine candidacy for central auditory evaluation. In the United Kingdom, a more direct approach has been developed by the Institute of Hearing Research Multi-Center Study of Auditory Processing (IMAP) (MRC Institute of Hearing Research). In this protocol, a standardized measure of cognition is administered to all children undergoing evaluation for CAPD to ensure that information relevant to comorbidities is available during the diagnostic session. Several issues arise, however, in either approach, which may not be apparent initially. The largest barrier, at least in the United States, is that administration of cognitive tests beyond a simple screener falls outside the scope of practice of audiologists. Furthermore, many of the more thorough cognitive batteries require a doctoral degree in psychology and/or a clinical psychology license to purchase and administer the tests (Thomas & Hersen, 2010). Failure to follow these guidelines could jeopardize the license of the practicing audiologist.

To overcome this conundrum, the AAA (2010) guidelines for diagnosing and treating CAPD recommends that information relating to cognitive and other comorbid issues should be *available* to the audiologist at the time of CAPD evaluation and/or the CAPD battery must be modified accordingly to account for any known or potential cognitive issues. The implication is that children should be evaluated for CAPD following cognitive and related assessment. Assuming this assessment has been performed, the audiologist should have sufficient information to proceed with the CAPD evaluation, taking into consideration, for example, utilization of tests that limit memory and attention load (see previous section in this chapter). Additionally, if a disor-

der, such as ADHD, has been diagnosed, then appropriate accommodations can be put into place before administering the CAPD battery to reduce the influence of this potential confound (see Chermak, 2007 for discussion).

Given the resources available to the audiologist with this multidisciplinary approach, it would seem unnecessary and, at least in the United States, potentially unethical for audiologists to administer cognitive measures beyond a short screener. Certainly, if such measures were not routinely given by psychologists, these cognitive tests would represent a void in assessment that needed to be filled. However, given that there is already a profession devoted to assessment of cognition and that referrals to these professionals can be made, it would seem unnecessary to incorporate diagnostic cognitive tests into CAPD batteries.

Use of Nonauditory Analogs of CAPD Tests to Rule Out Supramodal Issues

Common to most consensus statements on CAPD (AAA, 2010; ASHA, 2005a, 2005b) is the contention that while CAPD may coexist with dysfunction in other modalities due to shared neuroanatomical substrates, CAPD is not the result of supramodal or global dysfunction but, rather, is a disorder of the CANS. In addition, CAPD should manifest itself primarily, if not solely, in the auditory modality. Coexisting deficits and comorbidities highlight the importance of considering supramodal factors that could influence test results and the symptoms being exhibited by patients. To this end, Cacace and McFarland (2005) have argued for the inclusion of visual analogs of central auditory processing test measures to enhance the diagnostic specificity of CAPD assessment and the clinical utility of the diagnosis. The rationale underlying their approach seems to be that if a child demonstrates difficulties on auditory measures only, then the disorder is likely to be auditory in nature; however, if the child demonstrates difficulties on both auditory and nonauditory (e.g., visual) tests, then it would seem less likely, though not impossible, that the disorder is auditory specific. Although this approach has some merit, logistic pitfalls and issues of compliance with published best practice recommendations render this approach of questionable practical value. Some of these issues are considered below, including: the information gained from the inclusion of nonauditory analogs in central auditory test batteries is redundant with information gained from neuropsychological assessment and intratest measures of CAPD, there exist differences in the way basic sensory elements are processed in the primary auditory and visual cortices, cross-modal test equivalence for behavioral auditory and visual tasks is difficult to achieve, and there is a lack of clinically feasibly visual analogs available to audiologists.

In regard to issues of redundancy in testing, modality specificity encounters many of the same issues identified previously in this chapter. Specifically, the detection of cognitive issues that may cause supramodal deficits is within the purview of the psychologist or neuropsychologist who evaluates the patient prior to CAPD assessment. We can certainly expect that the tools used by these professionals have a sufficiently strong foundation to detect global processing issues that may be contributing to the observed auditory symptoms. If such issues are severe, then their treatment should precede CAPD assessment. Indeed, it could

be that cognitive issues may be the only cause of the patient's listening difficulties and, following treatment for the cognitive issue, the auditory deficit may be resolved. In such a scenario, CAPD assessment is unnecessary.

Also related to redundancy is the finding that intratest analyses of central auditory processing tests can frequently be used to determine if the deficit is primarily auditory or if it is being driven by a supramodal issue, such as ADHD, as demonstrated by Bellis et al., 2011). This study noted that interaural differences on dichotic tests and differences in performance based on response mode on temporal patterning tests were able to correctly differentiate children with CAPD from those with ADHD. Specifically, children with CAPD were shown to perform much better on one ear than the other when given dichotic tests, yielding a large interaural difference, whereas children with ADHD tended to perform poorly on both ears, yielding a small interaural difference. (See Chapter 9 of Volume 2 of this Handbook for elaboration of the mechanisms behind these interaural differences.) For temporal patterning tests, asking children to label a sequence is a significantly more demanding auditory processing task than asking children to simply hum the sequence. In the former, both cerebral hemispheres are recruited as well as the corpus callosum, while in the latter, generally only the right hemisphere is recruited (Musiek, Pinheiro, & Wilson, 1980). The performance difference between these two response modes generally will yield a large difference for children with CAPD. For the child with ADHD, however, the task is equally difficult regardless of response mode, so the performance difference between the two conditions is small or nonexistent. As these intratest comparisons are readily available to audiologists, can be easily calculated, and can differentiate children with CAPD from those with supramodal issues, it is unclear what the audiologist would gain by utilizing visual analogs of CAPD tests.

The differences in which primary auditory and visual cortices process relevant sensory elements is a second barrier to utilizing visual analogs. In a review of the fundamental processing differences between these two systems, King and Nelken (2009) pointed out that the processing that occurs at the first levels of the visual cortex is most similar to the processing that occurs subcortically at the inferior colliculus in the auditory system. Further, the authors highlighted that learning-based plasticity tends to be more dramatic in the auditory system, and that the auditory system has a relatively robust corticofugal pathway that has no equivalent of equal strength in the visual system. Put simply, the auditory system engages in a large degree of subcortical processing that does not occur in the visual system, and appears to demonstrate physiologic properties that are distinct from the latter system. These gross differences between the central auditory and visual systems make it difficult to equate performance on auditory tests and their purported visual analogs.

Perhaps related to this observation, a critical issue in trying to develop visual analogs to auditory processing tasks is to equate stimuli and tasks across the two modalities. There is, for example, no reason to expect that dichotic processing of two digits per ear is of comparable difficulty to dichoptic processing of two digits per visual field. It is entirely possible that the effort and skill required to yield a criterion performance level in one modality could be less than or greater than the effort and skill required

to achieve similar levels in the other modality for a similar task. A recent study by Bellis and Ross (2011) suggests that this is indeed the case, as performance on auditory processing tasks is significantly better than performance on visual analogs of these tasks administered to normal-hearing children and adults. This would seem a shortcoming for an approach that attempts to establish equivalence across two disparate modalities. There are some potential solutions to this issue, however. For instance, psychometric functions could be established for normal hearing subjects that ensure that measures in both modalities are equated for performance.

A final limitation of the analog approach is the feasibility of cross-modal testing in the audiology clinic. Although this approach has been advocated for some time (McFarland & Cacace, 1997), until recently there were no tasks designed for audiologists to perform this testing in the clinic (Bellis & Ross, 2011; Bellis et al., 2011; Lawfield, McFarland, & Cacace, 2011), and it is still unclear how audiologists would go about acquiring these stimulus materials. Further, the research data obtained with these nonauditory analogs does not support feasibility in a clinical setting in their current form.

In summary, inclusion of cognitive measures and/or nonauditory analogs in the diagnosis of CAPD seems inappropriate and of limited utility for one or more of the following reasons: (1) measures are not in audiologists' scope of practice, (2) measures do not generally contribute unique information when compared with central auditory tests already in use in diagnosing CAPD, and (3) difficulties in designing nonauditory analogs to achieve the stated goal. Again, consistent with ASHA (2005a, 2005b) and AAA (2010) recommended practices, it is our view that multidisciplinary testing, which employs standardized, validated, and efficient tests administered by various professionals trained in diagnosis of dysfunction in other sensory modalities and supramodal functions (e.g., executive function, attention, working memory) is a more appropriate approach.

Issues Pertaining to Criteria Used to Diagnose and Define CAPD

In regards to which tests should be used to diagnose and define CAPD, considerable variability in clinical practices and research designs has led to a general misunderstanding of the nature of the disorder. Although the recent AAA (2010) document sought to address many of these issues, this document is still relatively new and many of the issues it was drafted to remedy are still prevalent. Two of the more common issues that have contributed to this variability include: (1) operationally diagnosing CAPD based on self/parent/teacher report of listening difficulties alone, and (2) utilizing tests that have not been validated using the current gold standard in deciding which subject qualifies as having CAPD.

Presence of Listening Difficulties or Parent/Teacher Concern as a Criteria for "Diagnosing" CAPD

Determining (or approximating) the gold standard for CAPD is of considerable consequence for clinical practice, as well as for the conduct of research and the validity of findings. Current recommendations by AAA (2010) and ASHA

(2005a, 2005b) are to utilize subjects with neurological lesions localized mainly to the CANS in determining which tests are most sensitive and specific to the disorder. Proponents of this approach argue that the method provides a clear way to operationally define *pure* forms of the disorder and shows how performance on a measure is affected by very clearly defined CANS involvement (AAA, 2010; ASHA, 2005a, 2005b). Moreover, this brain-behavior approach, which utilizes dissociations and double-dissociations of function, is the bedrock of virtually all diagnostic professions that address neurologic function. Opponents of this approach argue that many individuals who demonstrate behaviors consistent with CAPD, in particular children, do not have clearly defined neurological lesions, and so this method of validation is not satisfactory.

This disagreement has led to a range of methods by which children are determined to present with CAPD when being considered in the research literature. Common to many of these methods, however disparate the methods may be, is an attempt to define central auditory processing ability using *performance-based* measures. Unfortunately, another approach, use of parent and teacher reports of listening difficulties for identification of children *suspected of CAPD*, remains a relatively common practice, especially in classifying research participants. When this approach is used, it is impossible to discern effects that may be attributable to true auditory difficulties versus many unknown variables, as the "suspected of CAPD diagnosis" is based on observation rather than on performance. Illustrative of this issue is a recent study by Ferguson, Hall, Riley, and Moore (2011) in which the communication, listening, cognitive and speech perception skills of children identified as having CAPD on the basis of normal audiometry and *typical* symptoms of CAPD, as reported by parents, were examined. The authors' report of no performance differences between the group *presumed* to have CAPD based on parent report and the group with specific language impairment (who met clinical criteria for this diagnosis), demonstrates that parent report is insufficient to diagnose or differentiate children with CAPD from those with speech-language difficulties.

Moreover, studies that have examined whether screening measures can predict performance on central auditory measures generally have not shown a significant relationship between subjective report of children's listening symptoms and their actual performance on central auditory measures. Since the central auditory measures show a significant degree of construct validity in neurological models of CAPD, this lack of agreement indicates that subjective report of listening difficulties is not predictive of true CAPD. For instance, Wilson et al. (2011) found minimal correlation between questionnaires such as the Children's Auditory Performance Scale (CHAPS) and Screening Instrument for Targeting Educational Risk (SIFTER), Test of Auditory Processing Skills-Revised (TAPS-R), and performance-based diagnostic tests. Specifically, the screening measures shared, at best, only 9% of the variance with diagnostic measures, and the vast majority of the screening subscales demonstrated no significant relationship to diagnostic measures at all. Wilson et al. (2011) concluded that the CHAPS, SIFTER, and TAPS-R do not predict risk for CAPD. They suggested that these questionnaires may be used to highlight concerns about a child, but

not to determine whether a diagnostic central auditory processing assessment is warranted. Similar findings were reported by Drake, Brager, Leyendecker, Preston, Shorten, and Stoos (2006) and Lam and Sanchez (2007), further demonstrating that subjective report of CAPD symptoms is a poor indicator of actual performance-based auditory processing difficulties. It should be noted, however, that Iliadou and Bamiou (2012) observed a much stronger correlation between the CHAPS and diagnostic CAPD measures in a sample in which the age range of the participants was strictly limited to 11 to 12 years. They noted that the reduced variability in this age group relative to younger children may have contributed to the stronger relationship seen between observer-report and performance-based measures.

The serious limitations of the suspected of CAPD diagnosis also is corroborated by the finding that many children referred for CAPD evaluations because of listening difficulties actually perform quite well on central auditory processing measures. One would assume that if parent and teacher reports were good predictors of auditory processing difficulties, then the CAPD hit rate (i.e., true positives) for these referrals would be much higher. For example, Wilson (personal communication) in a forthcoming study used a variety of different diagnostic criteria to determine the percentage of CAPD diagnoses. Using self-reported difficulties as a measure of central auditory dysfunction (per Ferguson et al., 2011), yielded a CAPD hit rate of 100%, whereas using sensitized performance-based measures that followed ASHA (2005a, 2005b) and AAA (2010) diagnostic criteria yielded a smaller hit rate of 71%. The latter percentage is generally consistent with the hit rates reported in other studies utilizing performance-based measures to diagnosis CAPD: Sharma et al. (2009) (72%), Iliadou and Bamiou (2012) (66%), Vanniasegaram, Cohen, and Rosen (2004) (56%), and Rosen et al. (2009) (62%). Clearly, the use of reports of listening difficulties as a diagnostic marker for CAPD leads to over-identification and overuse of the diagnostic label (i.e., higher sensitivity, but at the cost of significantly reduced specificity).

Validity of Diagnostic Tests of Central Auditory Function: The Gold Standard

Proponents of the use of patients with CANS lesions to determine test efficiency for identification of individuals, including children, with CAPD do not argue that all clinical presentations of CAPD involve neurological lesions (for a review of potential causes of CAPD in non-neurological cases, see Chermak & Musiek, 2010 and Musiek & Weihing, 2011). They do contend, however, that when considering the relative merits of a group of central auditory processing tests, we can learn which might be more advantageous for diagnosis than others by administering such measures to individuals who have known neurological involvement of the CANS. All else being equal, if one test differentiates individuals with focal CANS lesions better than another, then that test might be said to be a more valid indicator of difficulties in central auditory processing, since central auditory processing is a reflection of CANS function. Measures that have not been validated in this manner are not considered diagnostic under the guidelines set forth by AAA (2010) and ASHA (2005a, 2005b). Certainly, any measure of central auditory processing could potentially be diag-

nostic, but validation of the test using a clinical *gold standard* group provides a basis on which to make this claim. This requirement applies to both the specific auditory process being tested, as well as to the specific stimuli and paradigm used. That is, it is not sufficient to claim a test is diagnostic because it is dichotic; one must administer the specific dichotic test to a group of individuals with documented CANS dysfunction to determine the relative utility of that specific dichotic test for diagnosis. The sensitivity and specificity of different dichotic tests can vary markedly (Musiek et al., 2011).

The current approach for approximating a gold standard may change with further developments in neuroimaging and other techniques. For example, use of fMRI (Bartel-Friedrich, Broecker, Knoergen, & Koesling, 2010) and transcranial magnetic stimulation (TMS) (Andoh & Zatorre, 2011; At, Spierer, & Clarke, 2011) in normally hearing individuals to determine processing sites for specific central auditory tests might offer one such approach to achieving a gold standard for central auditory tests. Unfortunately, such an approach introduces the risk of inferring how pathology will manifest in the clinic by simulating it in controls. At the present time, there seems to be no better approach to validating clinical tests and determining their sensitivity and specificity than to use patients with confirmed CANS dysfunction.

A recent report by Musiek et al. (2011) demonstrates the benefits of comparing the performance on multiple central auditory tests in the same group of patients with neurological lesions of the CANS. It was noted that, when comparing across individual tests, the Dichotic Digits test (Musiek, 1983) and the Frequency Patterns test (Musiek & Pinheiro,

1987) tended to show the best test efficiency (i.e., balance between sensitivity and specificity). Furthermore, the two-test battery comprised of Dichotic Digits and Frequency Patterns, as well as the Competing Sentences test (Willeford & Burleigh, 1994) and the Frequency Patterns two-test battery tended to show the best test efficiency of all the multiple test batteries compared in the group of adult patients studied. Musiek et al.'s findings should not be interpreted to suggest that these measures and batteries will have the same test efficiency in actual clinical CAPD populations. Their results suggest, however, that these measures and batteries will likely be better at detecting auditory difficulties that originate from the central nervous system in children and adults referred for CAPD testing because individuals with clear CANS dysfunction have difficulty performing these tests. Unfortunately, very few studies have compared performance on central auditory tests in pediatric populations. Jerger (1987) indicated sensitivity and specificity for the Pediatric Sentence Identification Test (Jerger & Jerger, 1984) that approached the efficiency of CAPD tests commonly used in adults with neurological lesions. More recently, several revealing studies have come from Boscariol and colleagues (2009, 2010, 2011), again showing similar central auditory test performance patterns and efficiencies as those typically encountered in adults.

Issues Relating to Intervention for CAPD

Our final section focuses on the efficacy of auditory interventions for children and adults diagnosed with CAPD. This topic is of considerable interest to audiolo-gists and speech-language pathologists, families, and patients, as well as medical professionals who are often point-of-entry service providers for patients who have listening difficulties not explained by their hearing loss. Current research in auditory rehabilitation for patients with CAPD has tended to address how efficacious a given treatment is for individuals diagnosed with the disorder. These clinical studies, along with the basic research upon which the interventions are based, are described below. We restrict our consideration of the literature to auditory interventions that utilize auditory training exercises, where these exercises are defined as behavioral tasks that are auditory-based and aim to strengthen the basic sensory processing of auditory information at the level of the CANS.

Animal Studies

A variety of evidence of the mechanisms underlying benefits obtained from auditory training comes from animal models. Principal among these are reports of structural and/or physiological changes to auditory regions of the central nervous system following participation in an auditory task. For instance, Recanzone, Schreiner, and Merzenich (1993) found tonotopic reorganization of the owl monkey's auditory cortex following intensive training on a frequency discrimination task. The posttraining tonotopic gradient favored the trained frequencies used in the paradigm. Control subjects showed significantly less or no reorganization. Hassmannova, Myslivecek, and Novakova (1981) observed increases in the RNA content of cortical neurons following repetitive stimulation of the auditory cortex via tone pips, suggesting an initiation of processes through which cell division might occur. Similar increases were not seen in a control group. Bao, Chang, Woods, and Merzenich (2004) provided different auditory feedback to rats in a maze depending on their proximity to a food source. They noted that these rats showed an improved neural response to the auditory signal when compared with untrained rats.

These animal models also have been used to examine the question of mechanisms underlying efficacy of auditory training from a somewhat different perspective: How does the CANS adapt beneficially when it is challenged by an environment in which important acoustic cues are degraded. Knudsen (1988) repeatedly assessed localization ability using a behavioral task after unilaterally depriving the barn owl of sound using an ear plug. Initially, performance on this task suffered following insertion of the plug, although a gradual improvement was noted over time. This improvement was attributed to beneficial alterations in CANS organization that reflected a better match between expected object location and the new degraded cues. Removal of the plug again yielded poor performance that gradually improved over time, again reflecting a recalibration of the localization circuitry in response to the change in interaural stimulation. This finding proved to be fairly robust and was replicated in similar studies (Linkenhoker & Knudsen, 2002; Linkenhoker, von der Ohe, & Knudsen, 2005).

Auditory Training in Normally Hearing Human Subjects

One must understand how the normal system works before one can begin to explain the abnormal. A considerable body of auditory training research has been conducted in the normal hearing population, where normal hearing is typically defined as both normal peripheral hearing sensitivity and the absence of any significant disorders. Typically, these investigations examine auditory training within the context of a particular auditory processing task, such as auditory discrimination or temporal processing.

In this regard, the work of Kraus, Tremblay, and colleagues has provided some of the most convincing evidence for the effectiveness of auditory training in normal-hearing subjects. Kraus, McGee, Carrell, King, Tremblay, and Nicol (1995) and Tremblay, Kraus, McGee, Ponton, and Otis (2001) trained subjects on discrimination of consonant-vowel stimuli that varied in their spectral similarity. They indicated that most individuals exhibited behavioral and electrophysiological benefits following one week of training. Tremblay, Kraus, Carrell, and McGee (1997) showed a similar degree of benefit using a CV discrimination training task, and also noted that training effects generalized to stimuli not trained in the experiment. The finding of generalization to stimuli (and tasks) not included in the training protocol has also been reported by Delhommeau and colleagues (Delhommeau, Micheyl, & Jouvent, 2005; Delhommeau, Micheyl, Jouvent, & Collet, 2002), using a frequency discrimination task. Others have reported that improvement typically is greatest on the trained task and may not transfer or generalize between tasks (Hawkey, Amitay, & Moore 2004; Wright & Fitzgerald, 2001). The degree of generalization/transfer seen may be predicted by the subject's initial ability: adult listeners who perform better initially demonstrate greater transfer to untrained stimuli and untrained conditions (Amitay, Hawkey, & Moore, 2005; Roth, Appelbaum, Milo, & Kishon-Rabin,

2008) and the degree of generalization depends on listeners having received a critical amount of exposure to the trained stimulus and task (Delhommeau et al., 2005; Grimault, Micheyl, Carlyon, Bacon, & Collet, 2003; Wright & Sabin, 2007).

Using a nonspeech tonal discrimination task, Jäncke, Gaab, Wustenberg, Scheich, and Heinze (2001) showed that some individuals demonstrated behavioral and electrophysiological benefits from auditory training. Individuals who benefited from training differed from those who did not in that the former group showed a decrease in activity during training in the superior temporal gyrus bilaterally on fMRI. The authors interpreted this hemodymanic finding to be consistent with "fast learning theories," which suggest that fMRI activation decreases as processing becomes more efficient. Foxton, Brown, Chambers, and Griffiths (2004) demonstrated that discriminating differences in auditory contour, or relative changes in frequency over time, relied heavily on frequency discrimination ability. Specifically, subjects who were trained in either frequency or contour discrimination showed an improved ability to discriminate auditory contours. As auditory discrimination and sequencing are thought to be components of language and reading (Wright, Bowen, & Zecker, 2000), this particular finding has obvious implications for the child diagnosed with CAPD.

Auditory Training in Children With CAPD or Auditory-Based Learning Problems

Although animal models and research with normal-hearing individuals demonstrate the mechanisms under which the normal auditory system responds to auditory training, they do not provide direct evidence of the efficacy of interventions used to treat CAPD. We consider here several studies that employ exercises that fall under the strictest definition of auditory training, as defined by ASHA (2005a), and do provide such evidence. As described in the ASHA (2005) report, auditory training includes "bottom-up treatment approaches designed to reduce or resolve the CAPD. Training activities may include but are not limited to procedures targeting intensity, frequency, and duration discrimination; phoneme discrimination and phoneme-to-grapheme skills; temporal gap discrimination; temporal ordering and sequencing; pattern recognition; localization/lateralization; and recognition of auditory information presented within a background noise or competition." Although there exists a variety of evidence for the effectiveness of computer based auditory training (CBAT) paradigms in treating CAPD, we do not consider those in detail here as they cannot be easily categorized under this definition of auditory training. For a review of these CBAT studies, the interested reader should refer to McArthur (2009) and Loo, Bamiou, Campbell, and Luxon (2010).

It has been recommended that auditory training for CAPD follow a processing-specific approach; that is, children with CAPD are given exercises that, generally, target the specific auditory process(es) that have been identified as deficient based on central auditory tests with documented efficiency (AAA, 2010; ASHA, 2005, 205b; Bellis, 2002; Musiek, Weihing, & Chermak, 2007). Most of the published auditory training protocols lead to improved auditory function following a schedule of 15 to 45 minutes of training, two to four times a week, for a period of 1 to 2 months. Several recent studies have provided evidence that auditory training can improve the auditory processing skills of children with CAPD or auditory-based learning problems. McArthur, Ellis, Atkinson, and Coltheart (2008) found that children with language or reading impairments who showed difficulty on frequency discrimination tasks improved on language and reading measures following auditory frequency discrimination training. By contrast, children without similar impairments who were not trained showed no sizable test-retest benefit on the frequency discrimination task. Moncrieff and Wertz (2008) had children diagnosed with significant unilateral or bilateral weakness on dichotic processing tests participate in a dichotic processing task that was similar to the dichotic interaural intensity difference training (DIID) paradigm introduced by Musiek and colleagues (Musiek & Schochat, 1998; Musiek et al., 2008; Musiek & Weihing, 2011; Weihing & Musiek, 2007). Children showed significant improvements in left ear performance on dichotic measures following the termination of training. Cameron and Dillon (2011) trained children with spatial sound separation deficits using a program (i.e., LiSN and Learn) that exercised these skills. Following participation, all children showed a much improved ability in obtaining benefits from spatial separation of speech and competition. Notable was the observation that children did not improve on trials in which spatial separation of speech and competition did not occur, suggesting that the training specifically targeted spatial separation. Schochat et al. (2010) enrolled children in auditory training targeting the difficulties they exhibited, including

intensity discrimination, temporal patterning, dichotic processing, speech in noise recognition, and gap detection. The children also engaged in informal training at home on a daily basis, and this consisted of listening and language exercises. Results confirmed that the trained CAPD group, but not the untrained normal hearing controls, showed improved behavioral performance on CAPD behavioral measures, as well as greater amplitude in middle latency evoked responses following training. Murphy and Schochat (2011) enrolled children with dyslexia in a nonverbal temporal ordering training paradigm. Interestingly, results showed that children who participated in the training improved not only on CAPD measures of temporal sequencing (e.g., frequency patterns), but also on speech-language measures of phonemic awareness. This was in contrast to a second group composed of children with dyslexia who did not receive the training and did not receive similar benefits.

In summary, we are gaining a deeper understanding of how our interventions change the brain, which in turn leads to the development of more efficient and effective interventions. We know that the success of interventions is mediated in part by cognitive (e.g., attention, memory), metacognitive, motivational, and emotional processes (Chermak, Bellis, & Musiek, 2007; Cicerone, 2012). The degree to which these factors influence outcomes of auditory interventions remains unknown. The evidence reviewed here demonstrates that auditory training is an effective treatment for central auditory processing deficits. Although clinicians and researchers might disagree as to the quantity of evidence needed to support the acceptance of scientific results, none should confuse any perceived concern about quantity of evidence with the demonstrated positive outcomes of that evidence. See Chapters 3 and 11 in Volume 2 of this Handbook for additional discussion of the efficacy of auditory training and auditory-language training.

Summary

The chapter provides the authors' perspectives on several issues encountered in the diagnosis and treatment of CAPD, with a particular emphasis on the research and evidence supporting our interpretation. There is considerable interest in the research and clinical communities in explaining the listening difficulties encountered by individuals with normal peripheral hearing. CAPD provides a model that may explain these difficulties in the context of CANS dysfunction. This model is supported by a wide range of studies that have shown that lesions of the CANS inflence listening ability. Further, there is an emerging understanding of what types of dysfunction might lead to compromise of the CANS in cases that do not involve specific neurological issues (see Musiek & Weihing, 2011 for an example).

It is important that audiologists assessing individuals for CAPD understand the role that cognition and related domains play in the listening ability of their patients. As the brain is extremely nonmodular, it is certainly not surprising that CANS function can be influenced by nonauditory regions, or that listening issues can occur in the absence of CANS dysfunction. The present chapter, and the current AAA (2010) best practice document, highlight ways in which audiologists may begin to minimize or rule out the influence of these nonauditory domains by involving multidisciplinary teams, employing cognition screeners and intratest audiological comparisons, selecting tests that do not overly tax cognitive and language systems, and more. Accurate differential diagnosis depends in large part on knowledge of procedures and steps used to differentiate CAPD from confounding or comorbid issues, and the importance of this knowledge cannot be overstated.

References

AAA (American Academy of Audiology). (2010). *Guidelines for the diagnosis, treatment, and management of children and adults with central auditory processing disorder.* Retrieved from http://www.audiology.org/resources/documentlibrary/Documents/CAPD%20Guidelines%208-2010.pdf

Amitay, S., Hawkey, D. J. C., & Moore, D. R. (2005). Auditory frequency discrimination learning is affected by stimulus variability. *Perception and Psychophysics, 67*(4), 691–698.

Anderson, S., Skoe, E., Chandrasekaran, B., Zecker, S., & Kraus, N. (2010). Brainstem correlates of speech-in-noise perception in children. *Hearing Research, 270*(1–2), 151–157.

Andoh, J., & Zatorre, R. J. (2011). Interhemispheric connectivity influences the degree of modulation of TMS-induced effects during auditory processing. *Frontiers in Psychology, 2*(7), 161.

ASHA (American Speech-Language-Hearing Association). (2004). *Preferred practice patterns for the profession of speech language pathology* [Preferred practice patterns]. Retrieved from http://www.asha.org/policy

ASHA. (2005a). *(Central) auditory processing disorders* [Technical report]. Retrieved

from http://www.asha.org/members/desk
ref-journals/deskref/default

ASHA. (2005b). *(Central) auditory processing disorders—the role of the audiologist*
[Position statement]. Retrieved from http://
www.asha.org/members/deskref-journals/
deskref/default

At, A., Spierer, L., & Clarke, S. (2011).
The role of the right parietal cortex in
sound localization: A chronometric single pulse transcranial magnetic stimulation study. *Neuropsychologia, 49*(9),
2794–2797.

Bamiou, D.-E., Werring, D., Cox, K., Stevens,
J., Musiek, F. E., Brown, M. M., & Luxon, L.
M. (2012). Patient-reported auditory functions after stroke of the central auditory
pathway. *Stroke: A Journal of Cerebral Cir-
culation, 43*(5), 1285–1289.

Banai, K., Abrams, D., & Kraus, N. (2007).
Sensory-based learning disability: Insights
from brainstem processing of speech
sounds. *International Journal of Audiology, 46*(9), 524–532.

Banai, K., Nicol, T., Zecker, S. G., & Kraus,
N. (2005). Brainstem timing: implications
for cortical processing and literacy. *Journal of Neuroscience: the Official Journal
of the Society for Neuroscience, 25*(43),
9850–9857.

Bao, S., Chang, E. F., Woods, J., & Merzenich,
M. M. (2004). Temporal plasticity in the
primary auditory cortex induced by operant perceptual learning. *Nature Neuroscience, 7*(9), 974–981.

Bartel-Friedrich, S., Broecker, Y., Knoergen,
M., & Koesling, S. (2010). Development of
fMRI tests for children with central auditory processing disorders. *In Vivo, 24*(2),
201–209.

Bellis, T. J. (2002). *Assessment and management of central auditory processing disorders in the educational setting* (2nd ed.).
Clifton Park, NY: Delmar Learning.

Bellis, T. J., Billiet, C., & Ross, J. (2011). The
utility of visual analogs of central auditory tests in the differential diagnosis of
(central) auditory processing disorder
and attention deficit hyperactivity disor-

der. *Journal of the American Academy of
Audiology, 22*(8), 501–514.

Bellis, T. J., & Ferre, J. M. (1999). Multidimensional approach to the differential diagnosis of central auditory processing disorders in children. *Journal of the American
Academy of Audiology, 10*(6), 319–328.

Bellis, T. J., & Ross, J. (2011). Performance of
normal adults and children on central auditory diagnostic tests and their corresponding visual analogs. *Journal of the American
Academy of Audiology, 22*(8), 491–500.

Billiet, C. R., & Bellis, T. J. (2011). The relationship between brainstem temporal
processing and performance on tests of
central auditory function in children with
reading disorders. *Journal of Speech, Language, and Hearing Research, 54*, 228–
242.

Boscariol, M., André, K. D., & Feniman, M. R.
(2009). Cleft palate children: Performance
in auditory processing tests. *Brazilian
Journal of Otorhinolaryngology, 75*(2),
213–220.

Boscariol, M., Guimarães, C. A., Hage, S. R. de
V., Cendes, F., & Guerreiro, M. M. (2010).
Temporal auditory processing: Correlation
with developmental dyslexia and cortical
malformation. *Pró-fono: Revista de Atual-
ização Científica, 22*(4), 537–542.

Boscariol, M., Guimarães, C. A., Hage, S. R.,
Garcia, V., Schmutzler, K., Cendes, F., &
Guerriero, M (2011). Auditory processing disorder in patients with language-
learning impairment and correlation with
malformation of cortical development.
Brain Development, 33(10), 824–831.

Breier, J. I., Fletcher, J. M., Foorman, B. R.,
Klaas, P., & Gray, L. C. (2003). Auditory
temporal processing in children with specific reading disability with and without
attention deficit/hyperactivity disorder.
*Journal of Speech, Language, and Hear-
ing Research: JSLHR, 46*(1), 31–42.

British Society of Audiology. (2010). *Auditory
processing disorder (APD) steering committee interim position statement on APD.*
Retrieved from http://www.thebsa.org.uk/
apd/Publications.htm

Cacace, A. T., & McFarland, D. J. (2005). The importance of modality specificity in diagnosing central auditory processing disorder. *American Journal of Audiology, 14*(2), 112–123.

Cameron, S., & Dillon, H. (2011). Development and evaluation of the LiSN & learn auditory training software for deficit-specific remediation of binaural processing deficits in children: Preliminary findings. *Journal of the American Academy of Audiology, 22*(10), 678–696.

Chermak, G. (2007). Differential diagnosis of (central) auditory processing disorder and attention deficit hyperactivity disorder. In F. Musiek & G. Chermak (Ed.), *Handbook of (central) auditory processing disorder* (Vol. 1, pp. 365–394). San Diego, CA: Plural.

Chermak, G., Hall, J. W. 3rd, & Musiek, F. E. (1999). Differential diagnosis and management of central auditory processing disorder and attention deficit hyperactivity disorder. *Journal of the American Academy of Audiology, 10*(6), 289–303.

Chermak, G., & Musiek, F. (2011). Neurological substrate of central auditory processing deficits in children. *Current Pediatric Reviews, 7*(3), 241–251.

Ciccia, A., Meulenbroek, P., & Turkstra, L. (2009). Adolescent brain and cognitive developments: Implications for clinical assessment in traumatic brain injury. *Topics in Language Disorders, 29,* 249–265.

Cicerone, K. D. (2012). Facts, theories, values: shaping the course of neurorehabilitation. The 60th John Stanley Coulter memorial lecture. *Archives of Physical Medicine and Rehabilitation, 93*(2), 188–191.

Cowell, P., & Hugdahl, K. (2000). Individual differences in neurobehavioral measures of laterality and interhemispheric function as measured by dichotic listening. *Developmental Neuropsychology, 18*(1), 95–112.

Delb, W., Strauss, D. J., Hohenberg, G., & Plinkert, P. K. (2003). The binaural interaction component (BIC) in children with central auditory processing disorders (CAPD). *International Journal of Audiology, 42*(7), 401–412.

Delhommeau, K., Micheyl, C., & Jouvent, R. (2005). Generalization of frequency discrimination learning across frequencies and ears: Implications for underlying neural mechanisms in humans. *Journal of the Association for Research in Otolaryngology, 6*(2), 171–179.

Delhommeau, K, Micheyl, C., Jouvent, R., & Collet, L. (2002). Transfer of learning across durations and ears in auditory frequency discrimination. *Perception and Psychophysics, 64*(3), 426–436.

Drake, M., Brager, M., Leyendecker, J., Preston, M., Shorten, E., Stoos, M., & De Maio, L. (November 2006). *Comparison of the CHAPPS screening tool and APD diagnosis.* Poster presented at the annual convention of the American Speech-Language-Hearing Association, Miami Beach, FL.

Ebert, K., & Kohnert, K. (2011). Sustained attention in children with primary language impairment: A meta-analysis. *Journal of Speech, Language and Hearing Research, 54*(5), 1372–1384.

Fandiño, M., Connolly, M., Usher, L., Palm, S., & Kozak, F. K. (2011). Landau-Kleffner syndrome: A rare auditory processing disorder series of cases and review of the literature. *International Journal of Pediatric Otorhinolaryngology, 75*(1), 33–38.

Ferguson, M. A., Hall, R. L., Riley, A., & Moore, D. R. (2011). Communication, listening, cognitive and speech perception skills in children with auditory processing disorder (APD) or specific language impairment (SLI). *Journal of Speech, Language, and Hearing Research, 54*(1), 211–227.

Filippini, R., & Schochat, E. (2009). Brainstem evoked auditory potentials with speech stimulus in the auditory processing disorder. *Brazilian Journal of Otorhinolaryngology, 75*(3), 449–455.

Foxton, J. M., Brown, A. C. B., Chambers, S., & Griffiths, T. D. (2004). Training improves acoustic pattern perception. *Current Biology, 14*(4), 322–325.

Gaffan, D. (2005). Neuroscience. Widespread cortical networks underlie memory and attention. *Science, 309*(5744), 2172–2173.

Grimault, N., Micheyl, C., Carlyon, R. P., Bacon, S. P., & Collet, L. (2003). Learning in discrimination of frequency or modulation rate: Generalization to fundamental frequency discrimination. *Hearing Research, 184*(1–2), 41–50.

Hall, J. W., & Grose, J. H. (1993). The effect of otitis media with effusion on the masking-level difference and the auditory brainstem response. *Journal of Speech and Hearing Research, 36*(1), 210–217.

Hassmannova, J., Myslivecek, J., & Novakova, V. (1981). Effects of early auditory stimulation on cortical areas. In J. Syka & L. Aitkin (Eds.), *Neuronal mechanisms of hearing* (pp. 355–359). New York, NY: Plenum Press.

Hawkey, D. J. C., Amitay, S., & Moore, D. R. (2004). Early and rapid perceptual learning. *Nature Neuroscience, 7*(10), 1055–1056.

Hayes, E. A., Warrier, C. M., Nicol, T. G., Zecker, S. G., & Kraus, N. (2003). Neural plasticity following auditory training in children with learning problems. *Clinical Neurophysiology, 114*(4), 673–684.

Heinrich, A., & Schneider, B. A. (2011). The effect of presentation level on memory performance. *Ear and Hearing, 32*(4), 524–532.

Hugdahl, K., Westerhausen, R., Alho, K., Medvedev, S., Laine, M., & Hämäläinen, H. (2009). Attention and cognitive control: Unfolding the dichotic listening story. *Scandinavian Journal of Psychology, 50*(1), 11–22.

Hurley, R. M., & Musiek, F. E. (1997). Effectiveness of three central auditory processing (CAP) tests in identifying cerebral lesions. *Journal of the American Academy of Audiology, 8*(4), 257–262.

Iliadou, V., & Bamiou, D. E. (2012). Psychometric evaluation of children with auditory processing disorder (APD): Comparison to a normal and a clinical non-APD group. *Journal of Speech, Language, and Hearing Research, 55*(3), 791–799.

Iliadou, V., Bamiou, D. E., Kaprinis, S., Kandylis, D., & Kaprinis, G. (2009). Auditory processing disorders in children suspected of learning disabilities—a need for screening? *International Journal of Pediatric Otorhinolaryngology, 73*(7), 1029–1034.

Jäncke, L., Gaab, N., Wüstenberg, T., Scheich, H., & Heinze, H. J. (2001). Short-term functional plasticity in the human auditory cortex: An fMRI study. *Brain Research, 12*(3), 479–485.

Jerger, S, & Jerger, J (1984). *Pediatric Speech Intelligibility Test: Manual for administration.* St. Louis, MO: Auditec.

Jerger, S., Johnson, K., & Loiselle, L. (1988). Pediatric central auditory dysfunction. Comparison of children with confirmed lesions versus suspected processing disorders. *American Journal of Otology, 9*(Suppl.), 63–71.

Johnson, K. L., Nicol, T. G., Zecker, S. G., & Kraus, N. (2007). Auditory brainstem correlates of perceptual timing deficits. *Journal of Cognitive Neuroscience, 19*(3), 376–385.

Katz, J. (1968). The use of staggered spondaic words for assessing the integrity of the central auditory nervous system. *Journal of Auditory Research, 2*, 327–337.

Keith, R. (1986). *SCAN: A screening test for auditory processing disorders in children.* San Antonio, TX: Psychological Corporation.

Keith, R. W., & Engineer, P. (1991). Effects of methylphenidate on the auditory processing abilities of children with attention deficit-hyperactivity disorder. *Journal of Learning Disabilities, 24*(10), 630–636.

King, A. J., & Nelken, I. (2009). Unraveling the principles of auditory cortical processing: Can we learn from the visual system? *Nature Neuroscience, 12*(6), 698–701.

Knudsen, E. I. (1988). Experience shapes sound localization and auditory unit properties during development in the bam owl. In G. M. Edelman, W. E. Gall, & M. W. Cowan (Eds.), *Auditory function: Neurobiological bases of hearing* (pp. 137–149). New York, NY: Wiley.

Kraus, N., McGee, T., Carrell, T., King, C., & Tremblay K. (1995). Central auditory system plasticity associated with speech discrimination training. *Journal of Cognitive Neuroscience, 7*(1), 27–34.

Kujala, T., & Brattico, E. (2009). Detrimental noise effects on brain's speech functions. *Biological Psychology, 81*(2), 135–143.

Lam, E., & Sanchez, L. (2007). Evaluation of screening instruments for auditory processing disorder (APD) in a sample of referred children. *Australian and New Zealand Journal of Audiology, 29*(1), 26–39.

Lawfield, A., McFarland, D. J., & Cacace, A. T. (2011). Dichotic and dichoptic digit perception in normal adults. *Journal of the American Academy of Audiology, 22*(6), 332–341.

Lee, H., & Vecera, S. P. (2005). Visual cognition influences early vision: The role of visual short-term memory in amodal completion. *Psychological Science, 16*(10), 763–768.

Lee, H.-W., Kwon, M., Legge, G. E., & Gefroh, J. J. (2010). Training improves reading speed in peripheral vision: Is it due to attention? *Journal of Vision, 10*(6), 18.

Linkenhoker, B. A., & Knudsen, E. I. (2002). Incremental training increases the plasticity of the auditory space map in adult barn owls. *Nature, 419*(6904), 293–296.

Linkenhoker, B. A., von der Ohe, C. G., & Knudsen, E. I. (2005). Anatomical traces of juvenile learning in the auditory system of adult barn owls. *Nature Neuroscience, 8*(1), 93–98.

Loo, J. H. Y., Bamiou, D. E., Campbell, N., & Luxon, L. M. (2010). Computer-based auditory training (CBAT): Benefits for children with language- and reading-related learning difficulties. *Developmental Medicine and Child Neurology, 52*(8), 708–717.

López-Aranda, M. F., López-Téllez, J. F., Navarro-Lobato, I., Masmudi-Martín, M., Gutiérrez, A., & Khan, Z. U. (2009). Role of layer 6 of V2 visual cortex in object-recognition memory. *Science, 325*(5936), 87–89.

Marler, J. A., & Champlin, C. A. (2005). Sensory processing of backward-masking signals in children with language-learning impairment as assessed with the auditory brainstem response. *Journal of Speech, Language, and Hearing Research, 48*(1), 189–203.

McArthur, G., Atkinson, C., & Ellis, D. (2009). Atypical brain responses to sounds in children with specific language and reading impairments. *Developmental science, 12*(5), 768–783.

McArthur, G. M. (2009). Auditory processing disorders: Can they be treated? *Current Opinion in Neurology, 22*(2), 137–143.

McArthur, G. M., Ellis, D., Atkinson, C. M., & Coltheart, M. (2008). Auditory processing deficits in children with reading and language impairments: Can they (and should they) be treated? *Cognition, 107*(3), 946–977.

McFarland, D. J., & Cacace, A. T. (1997). Modality specificity of auditory and visual pattern recognition: Implications for the assessment of central auditory processing disorders. *Audiology, 36*(5), 249–260.

McGee, T., Kraus, N., Killion, M., Rosenberg, R., & King, C. (1993). Improving the reliability of the auditory middle latency response by monitoring EEG delta activity. *Ear and Hearing, 14*(2), 76–84.

Merikanto, I., Lahti, T., Castaneda, A. E., Tuulio-Henriksson, A., Aalto-Setälä, T., Suvisaari, J., & Partonen, T. (2011). Influence of seasonal variation in mood and behavior on cognitive test performance among young adults. *Nordic Journal of Psychiatry, 66*(5), 303–310.

Moncrieff, D., & Wertz, D. (2008). Auditory rehabilitation for interaural asymmetry: Preliminary evidence of improved dichotic listening performance following intensive training. *International Journal of Audiology, 47*(2), 84–97.

Moore, D. R. (2011). The diagnosis and management of auditory processing disorder. *Language, Speech, and Hearing Services in Schools, 42*(3), 303–308.

Moore, D. R., Ferguson, M. A., Edmondson-Jones, A. M., Ratib, S., & Riley, A. (2010). Nature of auditory processing disorder in children. *Pediatrics, 126*(2), e382–390.

Murphy, C. F. B., & Schochat, E. (2011). Effect of nonlinguistic auditory training on phonological and reading skills. *Folia Phoniatrica et Logopaedica, 63*(3), 147–153.

Musiek, F. E. (1983). Assessment of central auditory dysfunction: The dichotic digit test revisited. *Ear and Hearing, 4*(2), 79–83.

Musiek, F. E., Bellis, T. J., & Chermak, G. D. (2005). Nonmodularity of the central auditory nervous system: Implications for (central) auditory processing disorder. *American journal of Audiology, 14*(2), 128–138.

Musiek, F. E., Chermak, G. D., & Weihing, J. (2007). Auditory training. In G. D. Chermak & F. E. Musiek (Eds.), *Handbook of (central) auditory processing disorder: Vol. II. Comprehensive intervention* (pp. 77–106). San Diego, CA: Plural.

Musiek, F. E., Chermak, G. D., Weihing, J., Zappulla, M., & Nagle, S. (2011). Diagnostic accuracy of established central auditory processing test batteries in patients with documented brain lesions. *Journal of the American Academy of Audiology, 22*(6), 342–358.

Musiek, F. E., Froke, R., & Weihing, J. (2005). The auditory P300 at or near threshold. *Journal of the American Academy of Audiology, 16*(9), 698–707.

Musiek, F. E., Gollegly, K. M., Kibbe, K. S., & Verkest-Lenz, S. B. (1991). Proposed screening test for central auditory disorders: Follow-up on the dichotic digits test. *American Journal of Otology, 12*(2), 109–113.

Musiek, F. E., & Pinheiro, M. L. (1987). Frequency patterns in cochlear, brainstem, and cerebral lesions. *Audiology, 26*(2), 79–88.

Musiek, F. E., Pinheiro, M. L., & Wilson, D. H. (1980). Auditory pattern perception in "split brain" patients. *Archives of Otolaryngology, 106*(10), 610–612.

Musiek, F. E., & Schochat, E. (1998). Auditory training and central auditory processing disorders—a case study. *Seminars in Hearing, 19(4)*, 357–366.

Musiek, F. E., Shinn, J. B., Jirsa, R., Bamiou, D. E., Baran, J. A., & Zaida, E. (2005). GIN (Gaps-In-Noise) test performance in subjects with confirmed central auditory nervous system involvement. *Ear and Hearing, 26*(6), 608–618.

Musiek, F. E., & Weihing, J. (2011). Perspectives on dichotic listening and the corpus callosum. *Brain and Cognition, 76*(2), 225–232.

Pichora-Fuller, M. K., Schneider, B. A., & Daneman, M. (1995). How young and old adults listen to and remember speech in noise. *Journal of the Acoustical Society of America, 97*(1), 593–608.

Purdy, S. C., Kelly, A. S., & Davies, M. G. (2002). Auditory brainstem response, middle latency response, and late cortical evoked potentials in children with learning disabilities. *Journal of the American Academy of Audiology, 13*(7), 367–382.

Recanzone, G. H., Schreiner, C. E., & Merzenich, M. M. (1993). Plasticity in the frequency representation of primary auditory cortex following discrimination training in adult owl monkeys. *Journal of Neuroscience, 13*(1), 87–103.

Riccio, C. A., Cohen, M. J., Garrison, T., & Smith, B. (2005). Auditory processing measures: correlation with neuropsychological measures of attention, memory, and behavior. *Child Neuropsychology, 11*(4), 363–372.

Riccio, C. A., Hynd, G. W., Cohen, M. J., Hall, J., & Molt, L. (1994). Comorbidity of central auditory processing disorder and attention-deficit hyperactivity disorder. *Journal of the American Academy of Child and Adolescent Psychiatry, 33*(6), 849–857.

Rice, M. L. (1983). Contemporary accounts of the cognition/language relationship: Implications for speech-language clinicians. *Journal of Speech and Hearing Disorders, 48*(4), 347–359.

Rosen, S., Cohen, M., & Vanniasegaram, I. (2010). Auditory and cognitive abilities of children suspected of auditory processing disorder (APD). *International Journal of Pediatric Otorhinolaryngology, 74*(6), 594–600.

Roth, D. A. E., Appelbaum, M., Milo, C., & Kishon-Rabin, L. (2008). Generalization to untrained conditions following training with identical stimuli. *Journal of Basic and Clinical Physiology and Pharmacology, 19*(3–4), 223–236.

Sarampalis, A., Kalluri, S., Edwards, B., & Hafter, E. (2009). Objective measures of listening effort: effects of background noise and noise reduction. *Journal of Speech, Language, and Hearing Research, 52*(5), 1230–1240.

Schochat, E., Musiek, F. E., Alonso, R., & Ogata, J. (2010). Effect of auditory training on the middle latency response in children with (central) auditory processing disorder. *Brazilian Journal of Medical and Biological Research, 43*(8), 777–785.

Sharma, M., Purdy, S. C., & Kelly, A. S. (2009). Comorbidity of auditory processing, language, and reading disorders. *Journal of Speech, Language, and Hearing Research, 52*(3), 706–722.

Strait, D. L., Kraus, N., Parbery-Clark, A., & Ashley, R. (2010). Musical experience shapes top-down auditory mechanisms: Evidence from masking and auditory attention performance. *Hearing Research, 261*(1–2), 22–29.

Sutcliffe, P. A., Bishop, D. V. M., Houghton, S., & Taylor, M. (2006). Effect of attentional state on frequency discrimination: A comparison of children with ADHD on and off medication. *Journal of Speech, Language, and Hearing Research, 49*(5), 1072–1084.

Thiebaut de Schotten, M., Urbanski, M., Duffau, H., Volle, E., Lévy, R., Dubois, B., & Bartolomeo, P. (2005). Direct evidence for a parietal-frontal pathway subserving spatial awareness in humans. *Science, 309*(5744), 2226–2228.

Thomas, J. C., & Hersen, M. (Eds.). (2010). *Handbook of clinical psychology competencies. Child assessment and intervention* (Vol. 3). New York, NY: Springer.

Tillery, K. L., Katz, J., & Keller, W. D. (2000). Effects of methylphenidate (Ritalin) on auditory performance in children with attention and auditory processing disorders. *Journal of Speech, Language, and Hearing Research, 43*(4), 893–901.

Tremblay, K., Kraus, N., Carrell, T. D., & McGee, T. (1997). Central auditory system plasticity: Generalization to novel stimuli following listening training. *Journal of the Acoustical Society of America, 102*(6), 3762–3773.

Tremblay, K., Kraus, N., McGee, T., Ponton, C., & Otis, B. (2001). Central auditory plasticity: changes in the N1-P2 complex after speech-sound training. *Ear and Hearing, 22*(2), 79–90.

Vanniasegaram, I., Cohen, M., & Rosen, S. (2004). Evaluation of selected auditory tests in school-age children suspected of auditory processing disorders. *Ear and Hearing, 25*(6), 586–597.

Weihing, J., & Musiek, F. (2007). DIID training. In D. Geffner & D. Ross-Swain (Eds.), *Auditory processing disorders: Assessment, management, and treatment.* San Diego, CA: Plural.

Weihing, J., Schochat, E., & Musiek, F. (2012). Ear and electrode effects reduce within-group variability in middle latency response amplitude measures. *International Journal of Audiology, 51*(5), 405–412.

Whitton, J. P., & Polley, D. B. (2011). Evaluating the perceptual and pathophysiological consequences of auditory deprivation in early postnatal life: A comparison of basic and clinical studies. *Journal of the Association for Research in Otolaryngology, 12*(5), 535–547.

Willeford, J. A., & Burleigh, J. M. (1994). Sentence procedures in central testing. In J. Katz (Ed.), *Handbook of clinical audiology* (4th ed., pp. 256–268). Baltimore, MD: Williams & Wilkins.

Wilson, W. J., Jackson, A., Pender, A., Rose, C., Wilson, J., Heine, C., & Khan, A. (2011). The CHAPS, SIFTER, and TAPS-R as predictors of (C)AP skills and (C)APD. *Jour-*

nal of Speech, Language, and Hearing Research, 54(1), 278–291.

Witton, C. (2010). Childhood auditory processing disorder as a developmental disorder: The case for a multi-professional approach to diagnosis and management. *International Journal of Audiology, 49*(2), 83–87.

Wong, P. C. M., Ettlinger, M., Sheppard, J. P., Gunasekera, G. M., & Dhar, S. (2010). Neuroanatomical characteristics and speech perception in noise in older adults. *Ear and Hearing, 31*(4), 471–479.

Wright, B. A., Bowen, R. W., & Zecker, S. G. (2000). Nonlinguistic perceptual deficits associated with reading and language disorders. *Current Opinion in Neurobiology, 10*(4), 482–486.

Wright, B. A., & Fitzgerald, M. B. (2001). Different patterns of human discrimination learning for two interaural cues to sound-source location. *Proceedings of the National Academy of Sciences of the United States of America, 98*(21), 12307–12312.

Wright, B. A., & Sabin, A. T. (2007). Perceptual learning: How much daily training is enough? *Experimental Brain Research, 180*(4), 727–736.

Yang, P., Lung, F. W., Jong, Y. J., Hsu, H. Y., & Chen, C. C. (2010). Stability and change of cognitive attributes in children with uneven/delayed cognitive development from preschool through childhood. *Research in Developmental Disabilities, 31*(4), 895–902.

Zdanowicz, N., & Myslinski, A. (2010). ADHD and bipolar disorder among adolescents: nosology in question. *Psychiatria Danubina, 22*(Suppl. 1), S139–S142.

CHAPTER 23

EMERGING AND FUTURE DIRECTIONS IN INTERVENTION FOR CENTRAL AUDITORY PROCESSING DISORDER

GAIL D. CHERMAK and FRANK E. MUSIEK

Identification, diagnosis, and intervention for central auditory processing disorder (CAPD) have improved markedly over the last 10 years due in large part to research advances in auditory neuroscience and related fields and their innovative applications to clinical practice. The intense interest in CAPD shown by professional associations over this same time period has encouraged this translation of science into practice. The convening of task forces and consensus conferences, the publication of position papers and technical reports (e.g., AAA, 2010; ASHA, 2005a, 2005b; BSA, 2010), international conferences focused on CAPD exclusively, and conference tracks and featured and keynote sessions at professional conferences have raised the visibility of issues pertaining to CAPD, promoted best clinical practices, and

encouraged research into the various clinical and basic science dimensions of the disorder. Perhaps a watershed event, the first evidence-based clinical practice guidelines for the diagnosis and treatment of children and adults with CAPD were published in 2010 (AAA, 2010). This document built on an earlier consensus report of the American Speech-Language-Hearing Association's (ASHA) task force delineating the status of research and clinical practices in CAPD (ASHA, 1996). Together these documents have heralded a renewed commitment to additional research, expanded professional education, and improved clinical services.

In this final chapter, we focus on emerging and projected behavioral, technological, and pharmacologic treatment strategies and research priorities. Underlying this discussion is the recognition that collaboration between clinicians and scientists—combining the clinician's first-hand knowledge of clinical needs with the researcher's expertise in the scientific method—provides a potent approach to asking the right questions and obtaining enduring answers. It is imperative that we exploit the momentum that has taken us to our current level of understanding and delivery of clinical services, as described in the preceding chapters. We begin our final chapter with a few comments about the neurobiological engine of rehabilitation—neuroplasticity—and the evidence of successful outcomes of intervention—efficacy.

Plasticity

It has become abundantly clear that exposure to auditory enrichment, especially, but not exclusively, during sensitive periods, can result in large functional changes in the central auditory nervous system (CANS) (see Keuroghlian & Knudsen, 2007 for review). We now know that even mature sensory systems retain the potential for extensive plasticity and that stimulation and training induce neural changes that are reflected in behavioral change or learning (Pienkowski & Eggermont, 2011). To exploit the tremendous potential of neuroplasticity to sculpt or remap the brain demands early, aggressive, and intensive intervention.

Measuring Efficacy and Outcomes of Intervention

Establishing the efficacy of our treatments is among the highest research priorities in the intervention arena. Cli-nicians and patients (and third party payers) demand evidence to support the effectiveness (and efficiency) of a particular intervention. Outcome data can be used to evaluate treatment outcomes, inform quality improvement efforts, and conduct cost-benefit analyses. Effective intervention should be evidence-based and individualized. Although studies generating what are considered to be the highest levels of evidence (e.g., randomized controlled trials; meta-analysis of randomized controlled trials) may be few in number (Musiek, Bellis, & Chermak, 2005), there is a solid base of evidence documenting improved auditory and listening behavior following auditory training (see Auditory Training and Technology below).

Clinical evidence is assigned a value denoting its strength; higher values typically are assigned to group research designed as double-blind, prospective, randomized clinical trials. However, several caveats are in order regarding the evidence-base ratings. Group studies reflect average performance, which might not be directly applicable to a particular clinical case. Case studies and retrospective studies (which are classified as lower level evidence) often provide evidence appropriate for a particular individual's profile and intervention (Barlow & Hersen, 1984. Indeed, "practice-based" evidence (PBE), wherein a clinician reports on the particular intervention outcomes of an individual patient, although not intended to replace randomized clinical trials, can provide another source of information to improve clinical practice (Horn & Gassaway, 2007). Although some disagree as to the quantity of evidence supporting the efficacy of CAPD interventions (Bellis, Chermak, Weihing, & Musiek, 2012; Fey et al., 2011), it is important to be clear: Limited evidence does not indicate limited effectiveness and the limitations of the evidence does not mean that the interventions offer no benefit. Regardless of one's view regarding the quantity or the quality of the published evidence, most would likely agree that additional research is needed to demonstrate the effectiveness and efficacy of various CAPD treatment approaches, using both auditory and other behavioral and electrophysiological outcome measures with individuals specifically diagnosed with CAPD (as opposed to individuals "suspected of CAPD" or other diagnoses).

It is our view that sufficient evidence is available today to guide intervention for CAPD using information gained from audiologic diagnosis and multidisciplinary assessment across functional domains (AAA, 2010; Alonso & Schochat, 2009; Delhommeau, Micheyl, & Jouvent, 2005; Foxton, Brown, Chambers, & Griffiths, 2004; Loo, Bamiou, Campbell, & Luxon, 2010; Moncrieff & Wertz, 2008; Murphy & Schochat, 2011; Schochat, Musiek, Alonso, & Ogata, 2010; Pinheiro & Capellini, 2010). Nevertheless, additional carefully designed clinical studies, controlling threats to internal validity and incorporating appropriate outcome measures, are needed to firmly establish the efficacy of a number of treatments currently recommended for CAPD. Research is needed in the area of treatment effectiveness and efficacy to enhance the selection and customization of deficit-focused remediation approaches and to guide recommendations regarding necessary and sufficient frequency, intensiveness, and duration of treatment programs and treatment termination (ASHA, 2005a, 2005b). Controlling subject selection and precisely defining subject characteristics are necessary given the comorbidity and possible linkage among a number of related disorders (e.g., CAPD, attention

deficit hyperactivity disorder, learning disability). Such controls should lead to clarification regarding the relationships among the spectrum of conditions manifesting central auditory processing deficits, and they will enable us to determine how treatment programs affect well-defined CAPD, including which treatment strategies and programs are most efficacious in meeting the needs of clients with particular CAPD subprofiles at particular life stages (Chermak & Musiek, 1997). To ensure treatments and findings can be transferred from lab to clinic, it is imperative that clinical research studies be conducted in real clinical settings in collaboration with clinicians to demonstrate both the effectiveness and ease of implementation of treatments. Too many lab studies have concluded a particular treatment is efficacious or not; however, these results often are not replicated in an actual clinical environment or implementation of the treatment in a clinically demanding environment leads clinicians to abandon or never even adopt the treatment (see Dhar, 2009).

Additional research is needed as well to develop customized, deficit-focused intervention plans to address particular clinical subprofiles. For example, a left-ear deficit related to corpus callosum transfer problems would suggest training using interhemispheric transfer and dichotics exercises (Bellis & Ferre, 1999; Moncrieff & Wertz, 2008; Musiek, Chermak, & Weihing, 2007). In contrast, temporal patterning, pragmatics and prosody training might be more appropriate for a patient with a left-ear deficit that reflects right hemisphere involvement (Bellis & Ferre, 1999). Finally, outcome measures must be carefully selected and sufficiently broad (e.g., improved spoken language comprehension) to demonstrate significant change in central auditory processing as well as listening in functionally relevant contexts (e.g., school, home, work). Outcome measures should include probes of specific central auditory processes previously determined to be deficient (e.g., gap detection or pitch pattern recognition), as well as more expansive measures (e.g., listening comprehension and spoken language processing) if one wishes to examine generalization to associated and comorbid functional deficits and demonstrate treatment outcomes in a more ecologically relevant context. However, one must exercise caution in selecting functional outcome measures. The effectiveness of auditory treatments for central auditory processing deficits should not be judged using these more expansive outcome measures. For example, improvement in reading, language processing, and social skills, may be seen in some cases following intervention for CAPD; however, these other abilities are dependent on a number of nonauditory variables, many of which are far removed from the auditory domain (Musiek et al., 2005). Therefore, the effectiveness and efficacy of interventions for CAPD should be gauged by improvements in auditory function, which then may support improvements in those domains that are dependent upon audition.

The use of auditory brainstem and cortical potentials to document treatment outcomes is especially promising. Electrophysiologic measures may be more sensitive than comparable behavioral indices and are less influenced by extraneous variables (i.e., confounds) (Hendler, Squires, & Emmerich, 1990; Jerger et al., 2002; McPherson & Salamat 2004; Schochat, Musiek, Alonso, & Ogata, 2010; Tremblay, 2007; Tremblay et al., 1998). At the same time, they are more time consuming and more expensive to administer, some are difficult to observe in young children (e.g., middle-latency response), some are highly variable (e.g., P300), and some are difficult to identify and present poor correlation with behavioral measures (e.g., MMN) (Dalebout & Fox, 2001). Recent findings suggesting that the auditory brainstem response to speech may reflect the subcortical source of deficient temporal processing of speech sound onset ultimately may provide for a reliable, objective marker of auditory processing (Banai, Nicol, Zecker, & Kraus, 2005; Russo, Nicol, Zecker, Hayes, & Kraus, 2005). Other applications of this finding include the potential for differentiating among cortical and brainstem sources of CAPD and better customizing intervention, as discussed below in Profiling CAPD and Customizing Intervention.

Auditory Training

Ongoing research continues to reveal the neurobiologic processes underlying auditory processing, the linkages between neural encoding of sound in the CANS and higher level language skills, and learning-associated brain plasticity (e.g., Banai et al., 2005; Cunningham, Nicol, Zecker, Bradlow, & Kraus, 2001; King, Warrier, Hayes, & Kraus, 2002; Kraus, McGee, Carrell, Zecker, Nicol, & Koch, 1996; Purdy, Kelly, & Davies, 2002; Wible, Nicol, & Kraus, 2005). The capability to change auditory behavior through auditory training is perhaps the most exciting development in intervention for CAPD. In addition to considerable evidence of the mechanisms underlying benefits obtained from auditory training obtained from animals (e.g., Bao, Chang,

Woods, & Merzenich, 2004; Hassmannova, Myslivecek, & Novakova, 1981; Knudsen, 1988; Linkenhoker & Knudsen, 2002; Linkenhoker, von der Ohe, & Knudsen, 2005; Recanzone, Schreiner, & Merzenich, 1993), an extensive corpus of research has documented improved psychophysical performance, neurophysiologic representation of acoustic stimuli, and listening and related function in children and adults following targeted auditory training (e.g., Cameron & Dillon, 2011; Delhommeau, Micheyl, & Jouvent, 2005; Hayes, Warrier, Nicol, Zecker, & Kraus, 2003; Jancke, Gaab, Wustenberg, Scheich, & Heinzel, 2001; Jirsa, 1992; Kraus & Disterhoft, 1982; Kraus, McGee, Carrell, King, Tremblay, & Nicol, 1995; Loo, Bamiou, Campbell, & Luxon, 2010; McArthur, Ellis, Atkinson, & Coltheart,2008; Merzenich, Jenkins, Johnston, Schreiner, Miller, & Tallal, 1996; Moncrieff & Wertz, 2008; Musiek, Baran, & Pinheiro, 1992; Musiek, Baran, & Shinn, 2004; Musiek & Schochat, 1998; Russo et al., 2005; Tallal et al., 1996; Schochat, Musiek, Alonso, & Ogata, 2010; Tremblay & Kraus, 2002; Tremblay, Kraus, Carrell, & McGee, 1997; Tremblay, Kraus, & McGee, 1998; Tremblay, Kraus, McGee, Ponton, & Otis, 2001; Warrier, Johnson, Hayes, Nicol, & Kraus, 2004). These studies have not only documented improved performance as a result of auditory training, but some show correlations between those performance gains and underlying neural representations (Temple et al., 2003; Tremblay et al., 1997; Schochat et al., 2010).

Considerable research is underway to determine the degree to which learning transfers and generalizes across stimuli and tasks. Understanding the nature of the relationship between training stimuli and performance following training is of considerable theoretical and clinical interest as it will allow training to be tailored most efficiently and intensively to achieve desired outcomes. For example, the degree to which nonverbal stimuli and/or training in a nonlinguistic context generalizes to a linguistic context will significantly inform auditory treatment approaches. Findings to date are disparate, with some reports demonstrating limited transfer or generalization between tasks (e.g., Amitay et al., 2008; Hawkey et al., 2004; Lakshminarayanan & Tallal, 2007; Wright & Fitzgerald, 2001), and other reports demonstrating transfer to other untrained task or stimulus conditions (Demany, 1985; Delhommeau et al., 2002; Karmarkar & Buonomano, 2003; Wright et al., 1997; Wright & Sabin, 2007). Lakshminarayanan and Tallal (2007), who reported some generalization from nonlinguistic to linguistic contexts, cautioned that the task-specific demands (e.g., features to which attention is actively paid) of training influence the extent of generalization.

Ongoing research examining other factors known to influence training outcomes, including motivation, the frequency, duration, and distribution of training, task difficulty, patient's age and severity of central auditory processing deficit, is providing insights driving improved training paradigms (Amitay, Halliday, Taylor, Sohoglu, & Moore, 2010; Tsodykes & Gilbert, 2004; Musiek, Chermak & Weihing, 2007; Thibbodeau, 2007). For example, Amitay, Irwin, and Moore (2006) Reported reduced learning if the training task is too easy; however, auditory tasks cannot be made too difficult, if sufficient, task-appropriate attention is engaged during learning. Regarding the question of how much training is required to attain performance gains,

Atienza, Cantero, and Dominguez-Marin (2002) and Gottselig, Brandeis, Hofer-Tinguely, Borberly, and Achermann (2004) found enhanced MMN amplitude within a single training session; however, they noted that it might have reflected the participants' increased attention to recently learned auditory material and perhaps not learning per se.

Auditory Training Techniques

Grounded in the neurophysiology of the CANS, a number of new auditory training techniques are gaining widespread clinical use in changing auditory behavior. For example, following training employing the dichotic interaural intensity difference (DIID) paradigm, Musiek and Schochat (1998) reported improved binaural listening and academic performance. Similarly, Musiek et al. (2004) reported markedly improved dichotic listening by a client with mild head trauma following DIID training. Post-DIID training, left ear scores increased and right ear scores decreased for split brain patients and for children with left ear deficits (Musiek, Shinn, & Hare, 2002). Interhemispheric transfer training also has emerged as an important component of auditory training (Moncrieff & Wertz, 2008). Because interhemispheric transfer of information underlies binaural hearing and binaural processing, exercises to train interhemispheric transfer using interaural offsets and intensity differences, as well as other unimodal (e.g., linking prosodic and linguistic acoustic features) and multimodal (e.g., writing to dictation, verbally describing a picture while drawing) exercises lead to improve auditory behavior (Chermak & Musiek, 1997, 2002; Musiek, Baran, & Schochat, 1999).

A number of interactive computer-based auditory/auditory-language training programs are commercially available or in development (Chermak, Weihing, & Musiek, in preparation; Diehl, 1999; Kraus, 2001; Morrison, 1998; Phillips, 2002; Tallal, Merzenich, Miller, & Jenkins, 1998), as well as downloadable auditory training applications for mobile devices and tablet computers (e.g., iPads). (See Chapter 11.) Free, open source, cross-platform software for recording and editing sounds also is available allowing clinicians and scientists to create their own tasks to their own specifications (e.g., Audacity, Adobe Audition). Research is needed to determine the comparative efficacy of various interactive computer-based auditory training programs for individuals presenting different clinical profiles. It is important to determine for whom particular training is most useful, as well as how training alters the neural representation of sound at various levels in the CANS (Kraus, 2001; Phillips, 2002). The few studies that have involved software comparisons have reported little additional benefit for one computerized program over another (Cohen et al., 2005; Gillam, Crofford, Gale, & Hoffman, 2001; Gillam et al., 2008).

Music and Auditory Training

A growing body of research has demonstrated the many advantages music might offer as a vehicle for auditory training. Recognizing the potential that musical experience can aid (or induce) neuroplasticity (Herholz & Zatorre, 2012; Kraus & Chandrasekaran, 2010), Chermak (2010) viewed musical training as a procedure that could enhance auditory function, and in particular central auditory function. Reports over the last decade have demonstrated that musical training alters auditory cortical representations. Trainor, Shahin, and Roberts (2003) measured enhancement of the P2 auditory evoked potential in adult nonmusicians following auditory training. Gabb et al. (2005) concluded that musical training may enhance the brain's efficiency in distinguishing split-second differences between rapidly changing sounds, and thereby improve temporal processing. Other work has demonstrated that musical training enhances pitch pattern recognition and increases verbal memory and that preschool children's phonemic awareness and early reading skill are correlated with their musical training (Anvari, Trainor, Woodside, & Levy, 2002; Chan, Ho, & Cheung, 1998; Kilgour, Jakobson, & Cuddy, 2000; Lamb & Gregory, 1993). Overy (2003) reported that group music lessons, as well more individualized passive and active music listening, may improve timing (i.e., temporal) deficits in children with dyslexia. Music training, including rhythmic games, was shown to improve phonologic and spelling skills. Using functional magnetic resonance imaging (fMRI), Bodner, Muftuler, Nalcioglu, and Shaw (2001) documented the so-called Mozart effect, the short-term enhancement of spatial-temporal reasoning ability following listening to Mozart's Sonata for Two Pianos in D Major (K. 448) (Rauscher, Shaw, & Ky, 1993, 1995). Bodner et al. (2001) reported dramatic, statistically significant activation differences in normal adults listening to the Mozart Sonata in areas of the brain (e.g., dorsolateral prefrontal cortex, occipital cortex, and cerebellum) important to spatial-temporal reasoning.

More recent research has demonstrated the benefits of musical training for neural encoding of speech. Musicians show more robust and efficient neural responses in subcortical and cortical regions that support language (e.g., Elmer, Meyer, & Jancke, 2011; Meyer, Elmer, Ringli, Oechslin, Baumann, & Jancke, 2011; Schon, Magne, & Besson, 2004; Wong, Skoe, Russo, Dees, & Kraus, 2007). Musical training leads to more fine-grained frequency discrimination, enhanced working memory, more robust representation of acoustic stimuli in the presence of noise, and enhanced ability to listen in noise and reverberation (Bidelman & Krishnan, 2010; George & Coch, 2011; Parbey-Clark, Skoe, & Kraus, 2009; Parbery-Clark, Skoe, Lam, & Kraus, 2009). Musical training also seems to strengthen cognitive functions (i.e., attention and memory), functions that are known to buttress if not modulate auditory functions (Strait, Kraus, Parbery-Clark, & Ashley, 2010). Moreover, lifelong musicians experience less age-related decline in central auditory processing (e.g., gap detection, speech in noise) (Zendel & Alain, 2011). Based on brainstem responses acquired in the presence of speech babble, Anderson and Kraus (2011) concluded that musicians tend to experience less distraction from background noise than nonmusicians and suggested that musical training my represent an effective training strategy to improve listening in noise. In describing the benefits of music for auditory training, Chermak (2010) categorized music as one of most enjoyable, engaging, and powerful sources of auditory stimulation. In outlining his OPERA hypothesis, Patel (2011, 2012) proposed that music training drives adaptive plasticity in speech networks due to: (1) O—the anatomical *overlap* of neural networks underlying acoustic processing of speech and music;

(2) P—the *precision* (e.g., semitoncs) required in music compared with speech (which is not significantly impacted by monotonal input), which therefore places greater demands on these shared networks; (3) E—the emotional engagement that music elicits; (4) R—the repetitive engagement of these neural networks associated with musical study and practice; and (5) A—the focusing of attention music elicits. Patel (2011) noted that music is likely to engage participants in intensive training and that music focuses training on specific acoustic dimensions, and does not draw attention to other dimensions (e.g., semantic) as would speech, which could accelerate progress.

A mounting body of evidence suggests that musical experience enhances multiple auditory abilities through cortical, cerebellar, and other pathways, as well as the neural encoding of speech. It is important to note, however, that many of these studies demonstrating the benefits of musical training are based on comparisons of accomplished musicians to nonmusicians. Additional research is needed to document the benefits of music as stimuli for auditory training for individuals with CAPD who are using music as a form of auditory training. The reader is referred to Chapters 7 and 9 for specific examples of how music can be used for auditory training.

Technology

Technology is a prime example of the impact of translational research that translates research findings into tools that improve individuals' lives. Technology to reduce noise and improve the listening environment is of high priority since difficulties understanding speech in backgrounds of noise is perhaps the number one complaint presented by individuals with CAPD. Such technology is crucial for children, since listening activities occupy approximately 75% of a typical elementary school day and poor academic performance is linked to noisy classrooms (Hubble-Dahlquist, 1998). Continuing developments in the application of active noise control technology (i.e., sound cancellation by generation of a sound field that is an exact mirror image [i.e., *anti-noise*] of the disturbing sound) may lead to quieter classrooms and other settings where noise control is desired.

Similarly, assistive listening systems (e.g., personal and sound-field amplification) offer enhanced listening experiences. The benefits of sound-field amplification for listening and learning for children with normal hearing, developmental disabilities, and mild hearing loss are reasonably well documented (Dockrell & Shield, 2012; Eriks-Brophy & Ayukawa, 2000; Flexer, Millin, & Brown, 1990; Neuss, Blair, & Viehweg, 1991; Rosenberg, 1998, 2005; Rosenberg et al., 1999). Accumulating data have demonstrated the efficacy of personal FM amplification for individuals with CAPD (Anderson, Goldstein, Colodzin, & Iglehart, 2005; Bellis, 1996; Blake, Field, Foster, Platt, & Wetz, 1991; Johnston, John, Kreisman, Hall, & Crandell, 2009; Rosenberg, 2002; Sharma, Purdy, & Kelly, 2012; Stach, Loiselle, Jerger, Mintz, & Taylor, 1987). Nonetheless, neither a sound-field nor personal FM systems are valid alternatives to good classroom acoustics. In fact, assistive listening systems and other attempts to reduce noise through furnishings (e.g., carpet) and arrangement of furniture (e.g., reducing distance between teacher and students through circular or rectangular arrangements) are only interim steps. Amplification is not the panacea for all classroom acoustics problems: Amplification increases rather than reduces overall classroom sound levels and has limited benefits in excessively noisy or reverberant classrooms. Moreover, amplification does not address sound leakage caused by poorly isolated or insulated classrooms. Unless classroom walls, ceilings, and floors are acoustically upgraded to improve their sound insulation, amplified sound may be heard in adjacent classrooms, interfering with learning there. The potential benefits of sound-field FM systems are more likely to be realized in classrooms that are more acoustically suited to their use in the first place (Wilson et al., 2011). A recent standard for classroom acoustics (i.e., ANSI S12.60-2002) specifies acoustical performance criteria, design requirements, and guidelines for schools. However, this standard is completely voluntary and must be incorporated into building codes for widespread implementation. In the meantime, school districts should require all school construction and renovation to comply with the new standard by including it in the bidding process.

There have been a number of recent developments in FM technology. Some systems now adjust gain automatically as a function of background noise level. One transmitter can now send two digitized signals for simultaneous transmission to personal FM and sound-field FM systems. Loudspeaker arrays provide better horizontal distribution (and less vertical distribution), requiring less gain to deliver higher signal levels at the back of the classroom. Interestingly, although the advantages of binaural hearing are well known, systematic examination of the benefits of binaural personal FM fittings has not yet been reported. Also needed are studies to determine the efficacy of personal FM systems for listening, learning, and psychosocial function in individuals with a CAPD diagnosis (Johnston et al., 2009).

Hearing aids have been suggested as another possible approach to personal amplification for children with CAPD (Kuk, Jackson, Keenan, & Lau, 2008; Kuk, 2011). Use of mild-gain (~10 dB), mini-BTE, open-ear bilaterally fitted hearing aids with noise reduction circuitry and directional microphones may improve speech recognition in noise in some children with CAPD; however, large variability in outcomes has been reported (Kuk et al., 2008). The benefits of low-gain hearing aids in such cases, especially in comparison to personal FM systems, require additional examination.

Given the importance of temporal cues as well as spectral (frequency-specific) cues for recognition of speech (Shannon, Zeng, Kamath, Wygonski, & Ekelid, 1995; Van Tassell, Soli, Kirby, & Widin, 1987), developments in real-time speech rate conversion technology are encouraging. By reducing the speed of speech delivery, while maintaining pitch and quality, and synchronizing auditory and visual cues, individuals with temporal processing deficits (as well as those with peripheral hearing impairment) may be able to follow ongoing speech (Imai, Takagi, & Takeishi, 2005). This technology incorporates an algorithm that expands speech while contracting pauses and has been shown helpful for older adults (Imai et al., 2005). Speech processing algorithms that increase the salience of the rapidly changing acoustic elements of speech offer promise for enhancing comprehension of spoken language among those with CAPD and language impairment (Tallal et al., 1996).

Perhaps also forthcoming in the near future is software that converts ongoing speech into clear speech, the speech speakers reliably produce when asked to speak more clearly (Picheny, Durlach, & Braida, 1985, 1986, 1989). In contrast to speech produced in casual conversation, clear speech is more intelligible due the marked reduction in speaking rate, increased energy in the 1000 to 3000 Hz range, enhanced temporal and amplitude modulations, and expanded voice pitch range and vowel space. The benefits of clear speech has been demonstrated in diverse populations, including those with learning disabilities, auditory neuropathy, and cochlear implants (Bradlow, Kraus, & Hayes, 2003; Kraus et al., 2000). Of particular interest, Cunningham, Nicol, Zecker, Bradlow, and Kraus (2001) found improved behavioral performance for CVCs with increased stop-gap duration and amplitude of consonant burst (i.e., modifications common in naturally produced clear speech) and increased P2/N2 amplitudes in noise in children with auditory-based learning problems.

In addition to offering new solutions to processing problems, technological enhancements, especially computer technology, have begun to demonstrate the potential of technology to provide more novel instructional formats, which elicit greater attention, motivation, and persistence than more traditional formats (Chermak & Musiek, 1997). Computerized delivery is engaging and offers a number of advantages, including multisensory stimulation, precision of stimulus control, hierarchical sequencing of tasks, and generous feedback and reinforcement, all of which facilitate intensive training needed for successful outcomes (ASHA,

2005a). Moreover, adaptive approaches that alter parameters of subsequent trials based on subject performance improve training efficiency. As discussed above under Auditory Training, a growing number of reports have documented the advantages of computer-assisted therapy for CAPD and associated listening and language processing deficits (e.g., Hayes et al., 2003; Russo et al., 2005; Tallal et al., 1996). Despite the potential of computerized approaches, additional data are needed to demonstrate the effectiveness and efficacy of these approaches (ASHA, 2005b; Phillips, 2002).

Neuropharmacologic Treatment and Neural Repair for CAPD

Knowledge of the plastic changes in the CANS may open new vistas in the pharmacological treatment of CAPD. The essential role of neurotransmitters and molecular mechanisms in facilitating auditory plasticity and central auditory processing has intensified research in pharmacologic interventions that can alter physiologic and behavioral aspects of audition, including selective auditory attention, signal detection in noise, and temporal processing (Aoki & Siekevitz, 1988; Feldman, Brainard, & Knudsen, 1996; Gleich, Hamann, Klump, Kittel, & Strutz, 2003; Gopal, Bishop, & Carney, 2004; Gopal, Daly, Daniloff, & Pennartz, 2000; Morley & Happe, 2000; Musiek & Hoffman, 1990; Sahley, Kalish, Musiek, & Hoffman, 1991; Sahley, Musiek, & Nodar, 1996; Sahley & Nodar, 1994; Syka, 2002; Wenthold, 1991). By altering primarily dopamine metabolism, several drugs have been shown to improve behavioral regulation and vigilance in attention deficit hyperactivity disorder (ADHD), which may lead to improved performance on a number of behaviors, including auditory processing (AAP, 2001). However, no pharmacologic agent has yet been demonstrated effective specifically for CAPD (Chermak & Musiek, 1997; Tillery, Katz, & Keller, 2000).

Pickles and Comis' (1973) early finding that injected atropine sulfate raised noise thresholds more so than quiet thresholds suggested that this drug affects the olivocochlear system, the system posited to improve neural signal-to-noise ratios and enhance the detection of signals in noise (Dewson, 1968; Dolan & Nuttall, 1988; Nieder & Nieder, 1970; Wiederhold, 1986). Other findings have suggested an even broader role for the olivocochlear system, influencing selective auditory attention, improving the clarity of sound, and modulation of auditory nerve activity, as well as signal in noise detection (Art & Fettiplace, 1984; Wiederhold, 1986; although see de Boer, Thornton, & Krumbholz, 2012 and Zhao & Dhar, 2012 for another perspective on the benefits of the olivocochlear system for speech-in-noise processing).

More recent work underscores the potential of pharmacologic intervention to alter the efferent system. Gopal, Bishop, and Carney (2004) demonstrated the potential of pharmacologic intervention to alter central auditory processing by comparing electrophysiologic potentials of unmedicated and medicated patients taking selective serotonin reuptake inhibitors (SSRIs) for treatment of depression. Since the neurotransmitter serotonin modulates the cholinergic-mediated efferent system's inhibitory function, Gopal et al. (2004) explained their findings of shorter latencies of auditory brainstem

and late latency responses in the unmedicated patients as a result of lower serotonin levels that led to reduced efferent system function and reduced inhibition.

Reported decrements in neurotransmitter levels in the auditory areas of the brains of aged animals suggest that central auditory processing deficits among older adults may respond to pharmacologic intervention (Banay-Schwartz, Laztha, & Palkovits, 1989; Caspary, Milbrandt, & Helfert, 1995; Caspary, Raza, Lawhorn-Armour, Pippin, & Arneric, 1990). For example, Gleich, Hamann, Klump, Kittel, and Strutz (2003) demonstrated improved temporal processing in older mice following the administration of gamma-aminobutyric acid (GABA). In another study, clozapine boosted insufficient inhibitory processing in older mice as measured by the P50 auditory evoked potential (Simoski, Stevens, Adler, & Freedman, 2002).

Preliminary reports suggesting some therapeutic efficacy for a number of pharmacologic agents (e.g., adrafinil, aniracetam, modafinil, pentoxifylline, physostigmine, piracetam, propentofylline, vinpocetine) in reducing cognitive, metacognitive, learning, and communication deficits of older adults with organic brain disease and others suffering from a variety of cognitive disorders may presage the development of similar drugs for treatment of similar deficits frequently associated with CAPD (Asthana, 1995; Baranski, Pigeau, Dinich, & Jacobs, 2004; Chai, Li, & Long, 2000; Derouesne et al., 2001; Devasenapathy & Hachinski, 1998; Ferraro et al., 2000; Greener, Enderby, & Whurr, 2010; Hock, 1995; Huber et al., 1993; Ikeda et al., 1992; Kemény, Molnár, Andrejkovics, Makai, & Csiba, 2005; Moller, Maurer, & Saletu, 1994; Muller, Steffenhagen, Regenthal, & Bublak, 2004;

Nicholson, 1990; Parkinson, Rudolphi, & Fredholm, 1994; Saletu, Moller, Grunberger, Deutsch, & Rossner, 1990; Sano et al., 1993; Torigoe et al., 1994; Winblad, 2005). As the neurotransmitters underlying communication in the CANS are identified and quantified (Altschuler & Shore, 2010), the potential for neuropharmacologic treatment of CAPD may soon become an option. It may be possible to prescribe a drug that serves as an agonist to certain excitatory neurons in the CANS to improve central auditory processing.

Restorative neurology or neural repair may offer another approach to intervention and rehabilitation in the future (Tansey, McKay, & Kakulas, 2012). Such repair will likely require individualized interventions matched to a particular patient's unique anatomical and physiological profile following neurological injury. Both neuropharmacologic and neural repair may soon revolutionize the treatment of CAPD and related disorders in children and adults.

Genetic Enhancement

With the completion of the Human Genome Project (HGP) in 2003, interest in genetics has soared both among the public and across the scientific community. The HGP has provided detailed information about the structure, organization and function of the complete set of human genes (approximately 30,000–40,000). The insights provided will likely transform all aspects of health care from disease prevention, to treatment of disease and disorders, and ultimately lead to long sought after cures for the multitude of diseases and disorders that now devastate human beings.

Even prior to the completion of the HGP, researchers suggested that genetic enhancement of cognitive abilities, learning, and intelligence in mammals was feasible (Tang et al., 1999). Much of the research in this area has focused on the role of an enriched environment in promoting biochemical and structural changes in the cortex, the hippocampus, and other brain regions (Kemperman, Kuhn, & Gage, 1997; Rampon et al., 2000). Expression of a large number of genes may serve important roles in modulating learning and memory change in response to enriched environments (Rampon et al., 2000). Since these changes in gene expression can be linked to neuronal structure, synaptic plasticity, and transmission, genetic enhancement may someday serve a role in intervention for CAPD, especially in improving often associated deficits in learning. Demonstrating the specific role of genetics for CAPD, Bamiou and colleagues (2004) reported that PAX6 mutations in humans may affect development of the anterior commissure and possibly the corpus callosum. Individuals with the PAX6 mutation presented dichotic listening deficits linked to callosal dysfunction. If this mutation is an identifiable genetic trait, genetic treatment could possibly minimize or eliminate the callosal dysfunction and the CAPD.

Genetics may also explain a portion of the variation in central auditory processing abilities across individuals (Addis et al., 2010; Peretz, Cummings, & Dube, 2007). For example, 73% of variation in dichotic listening may be due to genetic differences (Morrell et al., 2007). In addition, there is reason to expect that frequently observed comorbidities may stem from common genetic influences (e.g., PAX6 mutation and working memory and interhemispheric transfer deficits) (Bamiou et al., 2007). Animal studies using genetic engineering to induce polymicrogyri in rodents' brains similar to that seen human brains with dyslexia, coupled with the demonstration of auditory processing in these animals, further demonstrate the role of genetics in central auditory processing and its disorders (Szalkowski & Fitch, 2011; Galaburda, Sherman, Rosen, Aboitiz, & Geschwind, 1985).

Profiling CAPD and Customizing Intervention

The varied functional deficits and clinical profiles presented by individuals diagnosed with CAPD reflects variation in the underlying neurophysiologic sources and mechanisms responsible for the flawed auditory processing and behavioral deficits. Documented links, both behavioral and electrophysiological, between inefficient auditory processing and language and learning problems (e.g., Bellis & Ferre, 1999; Kraus et al, 1996; Moncrieff & Musiek, 2002; Wible et al., 2005) may lead to subprofiles of CAPD characterized by patterns or clusters of functional symptoms, central auditory test findings, and associated neurophysiologic bases.

With a firm understanding of CAPD gained from auditory and cognitive neuroscience, it now may be possible to develop functional deficit profiles that reflect patterns of central auditory deficits and functional cognitive, language, learning, and communication sequelae (Bellis, 2002; Bellis & Ferre, 1999). These deficit profiles, which should conform to well-established neuroscience tenets

that demonstrate the presence of brain-behavior relationships across a wide variety of functional areas, could be used to guide development of comprehensive intervention programs that address efficiently and effectively the specific cluster of central auditory and functional symptoms. Such subprofiles should lead to more customized and deficit-focused intervention and, therefore, to more effective intervention (King et al., 2002).

Two examples of subprofiling models are provided by Bellis and Ferre (1999) and Katz (1992). The Bellis and Ferre model is composed of three profiles that are associated with particular behavioral test findings and inferred neuroanatomical dysfunction. For example, they postulate that the corpus callosum is the neurophysiologic source of their integration subprofile. Additional research demonstrating different neurochemical or neurotransmitter responses underlying the presumed CAPD subprofiles would strengthen the position that different neurobiological mechanisms underlie these subprofiles. The Katz, or Buffalo, model includes four profiles based mainly on performance on the Staggered Spondaic Word (SSW) test (Katz, 1962, 1968).

King et al. (2002) demonstrated how subtyping individuals as a function of the neurophysiologic source of auditory dysfunction can lead to specific and customized treatment decisions that might not be as effective for other subgroups. In the King et al. (2002) study, subjects with learning disabilities (LDs) with abnormal brainstem timing benefited more from listening training than did LD subjects not presenting the abnormal brainstem response. Banai et al. (2005) extended these findings demonstrating that LD individuals with abnormal brainstem timing were more likely to show reduced processing of acoustic change at the cortical level and more depressed reading, listening comprehension, and general cognitive ability compared with LD individuals with normal brainstem timing.

Despite the potential of subprofiling to more efficiently treat specific processing deficits, subprofiling models remain theoretical and have not yet been fully validated (AAA, 2010; ASHA, 2005). One recent study clearly demonstrated the limitations of both the Bellis-Ferre and Buffalo models in classifying children with CAPD (Jutras, Loubert, Dupuis, Marcoux, Dumont, & Baril, 2007).

Professional Issues

Recent AAA and ASHA position papers, guidelines, technical reports, and statements of preferred practice patterns affirm the need for a team approach to the diagnosis, assessment, and intervention for children and adults with CAPD (AAA, 2004, 2010; ASHA 2004, 2005a, 2005b). Specifically, the audiologist diagnoses CAPD, while the speech-language pathologist (SLP) is responsible for assessing "aspects of auditory processing involved in language development and use . . . including determining if an auditory-related cognitive-communication and/or language disorder is present" (ASHA, 2004). Professional collaboration also is pivotal to intervention. ASHA (2004, p. 6) states that the audiologist is responsible for the "evaluation and management of children and adults with auditory-related processing disorders," and AAA's scope of practice (2004, p. 3) states that "the audiologist is an integral part of the team within the school system that manages students with hearing impairments and

students with auditory processing disorders." Regarding intervention for CAPD, many audiologists (see below under Professional Education) feel responsible only for enhancing the acoustic signal and the listening environment using assistive technology and noise/reverberation reduction techniques. As noted below, we consider auditory training a primary therapeutic technique for which audiologists should be well prepared to deliver. We agree with ASHA's position that the SLP should provide intervention services for the cognitive-communication and/or language impairments associated with CAPD (ASHA, 2004); however, both professionals should be engaged in auditory training: the audiologist perhaps more so in formal auditory training techniques and the SLP in the more informal approaches to auditory training (Chermak & Musiek, 2002; also see Chapter 7).

Collaboration is consistent with the systems (i.e., ecological) approach to intervention that we have advocated throughout this volume. Individuals cannot be evaluated without an analysis of the contexts in which they interact because environmental factors influence development, learning, and performance (Barkley, 1996; Bartoli & Botel, 1988; Palincsar, Brown, & Campione, 1994; Poplin, 1988a, 1988b; Sameroff, 1983). Although performance deficits noted on a battery of central auditory processing tests may justify a diagnosis of CAPD, comprehensive assessment of CAPD demands evaluation of functional deficits in the variety of contexts in which the individual operates. Information regarding home, school, and employment settings, as well as interactions with family, teachers, peer group, and coworkers should be obtained through case history and/or systematic observation to appropriately evaluate the client and plan effective treatments. The presence of central auditory processing deficits in association with language and/or cognitive deficits (e.g., aphasia, traumatic head injury, learning disabilities) underscores the need for collaboration among audiologists, SLPs, and other professionals responsible for assessment and intervention.

Reimbursement is a professional issue of vital importance to the continued improvement of the quality of clinical services for CAPD. Although recent additions and changes to procedure codes (CPT) improve reimbursement for diagnosis, assessment and treatment services related to CAPD, additional changes are needed to fairly reimburse professionals for their service contributions (ASHA, 2005b). The findings of a recently conducted survey (Emanuel, Ficca, & Korczak, 2011) confirm our earlier findings that audiologists continue to cite poor reimbursement as a major deterrent to becoming involved in either the evaluation or treatment of CAPD (Chermak, Silva, Nye, Hasbrouck, & Musiek, 2007; Chermak, Traynham, Seikel & Musiek, 1998). The Chermak et al. (2007) survey also revealed a continuing shortage of SLPs to whom audiologists can refer clients diagnosed with CAPD for intervention. The shortage of SLPs involved in intervention may be more related to professional education issues than to reimbursement issues, as discussed below.

Professional Education

The quality of clinical services provided by practitioners determines society's valuation of their clinical specialty. Several key studies have demonstrated the underpreparation of both speech-language pathology and audiology graduates in the area of central auditory processing, confirming the urgency to improve graduate education in this area and to develop guidelines for knowledge and skill competencies in diagnosis, assessment, and treatment of CAPD (Chermak et al., 1998, 2007; Henri, 1994). Audiologists providing clinical CAPD services must have a firm understanding of extremely complex brain mechanisms, yet these professionals may be receiving inadequate education and training in this specialty area (Chermak et al., 2007). Emanuel et al. (2011) found that less than 20% of audiologists responding to the survey used any type of electrophysiological measure as part of their CAPD assessment and 32% of the responding audiologists did not offer treatment for CAPD due to lack of training. These findings are of particular concern since half of the audiologists responding in 2011 held doctoral degrees and several clinical practice documents and guidelines have noted the value of electorphysiological measures in the diagnosis of CAPD (AAA, 2010; Jerger & Musiek, 2000). Although nearly 100% of respondents indicated that audiologists should be the professionals to diagnose CAPD; however, these same respondents identified SLPs (74%) and educators (52%) as responsible for providing intervention (Emanuel et al., 2011). While our field has evolved and expanded in numerous directions, including balance and tinnitus diagnosis and treatment, a primary focus has remained on the fitting of hearing aids and other advanced technology, with therapy being deemphasized, including in the area of CAPD. This is in stark contrast with scope of practice documents and guidelines that specifically state that the audiologist is responsible for the diagnosis and treatment/management of children and adults with CAPD (AAA, 2004, 2010; ASHA, 2004, 2005a).

The guidelines should be developed by university educators and clinicians to reflect the demands of the workplace while recognizing the resource constraints of today's graduate education programs. With the move to doctoral level education in audiology, inclusion of appropriate basic science (e.g., anatomy, physiology, and pharmacology of the CANS; psychoacoustics) and applied coursework and clinical experiences in diagnosis, treatment, and management of CAPD is anticipated. Moreover, integration of evidence-based practice (EBP) into undergraduate and graduate audiology curricula will teach students how to incorporate clinical research into clinical decisions. Future graduates will be better prepared to formulate focused clinical questions, efficiently locate and appraise available evidence and apply their findings to improve clinical services for individual patients (Oppenheimer, Self, & Sieff, 2005). (See Chapter 2 in this volume of the Handbook for discussion of EBP.) Perhaps most important, university faculty and clinical supervisors must conceptualize audiological evaluation and rehabilitation more broadly, teaching students that comprehensive evaluation and effective intervention require careful attention to both the peripheral and central auditory systems.

A recent survey offers some encouraging findings. A large majority (80%) of audiologists responding to the survey is customizing test batteries to reflect the patient's age and case history, and customizing management recommendations (75%) based on the findings of diagnostic tests (Emanuel, Ficca, & Korczak, 2011).

Conclusions

CAPD is a dynamic field experiencing rapid advances in research and technology. Accumulating scientific and clinical advances have expanded our understanding of CAPD, resulting in improved diagnostic and intervention services. The neurobiological, genetic, technological, and professional practice frontiers reviewed in this chapter may soon transform clinical practice, perhaps even revolutionizing diagnostic and treatment procedures. Our research priorities are attainable and intertwined: Dramatic improvements in clinical care will continue to unfold rapidly as long as the commitment to the twin engines of basic research and clinical trials that drive these improvements are nourished. More efficient diagnostic test batteries and assessment tools will lead to greater treatment efficacy by more precisely subprofiling and customizing intervention. Technological advances will minimize the impact of CAPD on individuals' lives. Our education and training programs must provide adequate coverage of CAPD, both in the classroom and in the clinic, to ensure that graduates are able to capitalize on scientific and clinical advances throughout their careers and continue to provide the highest quality of patient care. Multidisciplinary collaboration among clinicians, researchers, educators, and families will incite new questions and fuel research that will accelerate the pace of clinical advances. To ensure that we are able to deliver the best clinical services to our patients and their families, we as individuals and the professional organizations that represent us must remain engaged in developing strategic responses to and preparing for the rapidly changing health care landscape, changes that will focus on value-based service delivery, and the convergence of patient-centered outcomes and cost-effectiveness.

References

AAA (American Academy of Audiology). (2010). *Guidelines for the diagnosis, treatment, and management of children and adults with central auditory processing disorder.* Retrieved from http://www.audiology.org/ resources/documentlibrary/Documents/ CAPD%20Guideline %208-2010.pdf

Addis, L., Friederici, A., Kotz, S., Sabbisch, B., Barry, J., Richter, N., . . . Monaco, A. (2010). A locus for an auditory processing deficit and language impairment in an extended pedigree maps to 12p13.31-q14.3. *Genes Brain and Behavior, 9*(6), 545–561.

Alonso, R., & Schochat, E. (2009). The efficacy of formal auditory training in children with (central) auditory processing disorder: Behavioral and electrophysiological evaluation. *Brazilian Journal of Otorhinolaryngology, 75,* 726–732.

American Academy of Audiology. (2004). *Audiology scope of practice.* Retrieved from http://www.audiology.org/resources/doc umentlibrary/Pages/ScopeofPractice.aspx

American Academy of Pediatrics Subcommittee on Attention-Deficit/Hyperactivity Disorder Committee on Quality Improvement. (2001). Clinical practice guideline: Treatment of the school-aged child with attention-deficit/hyperactivity disorder. *Pediatrics, 108*(4), 1033–1044.

American National Standards Institute. (2002). *Acoustical performance criteria, design requirements, and guidelines for schools.* (ANSI Standard S12.60). New York, NY: Author.

American Speech-Language-Hearing Association Task Force on Central Auditory Processing Consensus Development. (1996). Central auditory processing: Current status of research and implications for clinical practice. *American Journal of Audiology, 5*(2), 41–54.

ASHA (American Speech-Language-Hearing Association). (2004). *Scope of practice in audiology* [Scope of practice]. Retrieved from http://www.asha.org/policy

ASHA. (2004). *Speech-language pathology (SLP) preferred practice patterns.* Retrieved from http://www.asha.org/members/desk ref-journals/deskref/default

ASHA. (2005a). *(Central) auditory processing disorders.* Retrieved from http://www .asha.org/members/deskref-journals/desk ref/default

ASHA. (2005b). *(Central) auditory processing disorders—the role of the audiologist* [Position statement]. Retrieved from http://www.asha.org/members/deskref -journals/deskref/default

Amitay, S., Halliday, L., Taylor, J., & Moore, D.R. (2008). Auditory learning is driven by dimension-specific attention. *Association for Research in Otolaryngology Abstracts, 457,* 158.

Amitay, S., Halliday, L., Taylor, J., Sohoglu, E., & Moore, D.R. (2010). Motivation and intelligence drive auditory perceptual learning. *PLoS ONE, 5*(3).

Amitay, S., Irwin, A., & Moore, D. (2006). Discrimination learning induced by training with identical stimuli. *Nature Neuroscience, 9,* 1146–1148.

Anderson, K., Goldstein, H., Colodzin, L., & Iglehart, F. (2005). Benefit of S/N enhancing devices to speech perception of children listening in a typical classroom with hearing aids or cochlear implant. *Journal of Educational Audiology, 12,* 14–28.

Anderson, S., & Kraus, N. (2011). Neural encoding of speech and music—implications for hearing speech in noise. *Seminars in Hearing, 32,* 129–139.

Anvari, S., Trainor, L. J., Woodside, J., & Levy, B. A. (2002). Relations among musical skills, phonological processing, and early reading ability in preschool children. *Journal of Experimental Child Psychology, 83,* 111–130.

Aoki, C., & Siekevitz, P. (1988). Plasticity in brain development. *Scientific American, 259,* 56–64.

Art, J. J., & Fettiplace, R. (1984). Efferent desensitization of auditory nerve fibre responses in the cochlea of the turtle pseudemys scripta elegans. *Journal of Physiology, 356,* 507–523.

Asthana, S., Greig, N. H., Hegedus, L., Holloway, H. H., Raffaele, K. C., Schapiro, M. B., & Soncrant, T. T. (1995). Clinical pharmacokinetics of *physostigmine* in patients with Alzheimer's disease. *Clinical Pharmacology and Therapeutics, 58,* 299–309.

Atienza, M., Cantero, J. L., & Dominguez-Marin, E. (2002). The time course of neural changes in underlying auditory perceptual learning. *Learning and Memory, 9,* 138–150.

Bamiou, D., Free, S. L., Sisodiya, S. M., Chong, W. K., Musiek, F., Williamson, K.A., . . . Luxon, L. M. (2007). Auditory interhemispheric transfer deficits, hearing difficulties, and brain magnetic resonance imaging abnormalities in children with congenital anaridia due to PAX6 mutations. *Archives of Pediatrics and Adolescent Medicine, 161,* 463–469.

Bamiou, D. E., Musiek, F. E., Sisodiya, S. M., Free, S. L., Davies, R. A., Moore, A., . . . Luxon, L. M. (2004). Deficient auditory interhemispheric transfer in patients with PAX6 mutations. *Annals of Neurology, 56,* 503–509.

Banai, K., Nicol,T., Zecker, S., & Kraus, N. (2005). Brainstem timing: Implications for cortical processing and literacy. *The Journal of Neuroscience, 25,* 9850–9857.

Banay-Schwartz, M., Laztha, A., & Palkovits, M.(1989). Changes with aging in the levels of amino acids in rat CNS structural elements: I. Glutamate and related amino acids. *Neurochemical Research, 14,* 555–562.

Bao, S., Chang, E. F., Woods, J., & Merzenich, M. M. (2004). Temporal plasticity in the primary auditory cortex induced by operant perceptual learning. *Nature Neuroscience, 7,* 974–981.

Baranski, J., Pigeau, R., Dinich, P., & Jacobs, I. (2004). Effects of modafinil on cognitive and meta-cognitive performance. *Human Psychopharmacology, 19,* 323–332.

Barkley, R. A. (1996). Linkages between attention and executive functions. In G. R. Lyon & N. A. Krasnegor (Eds.), *Attention, memory, and executive function* (pp. 307–326). Baltimore, MD: Paul H. Brookes.

Barlow, D., & Hersen, M. (1984). *Single case experimental designs: Strategies for studying behavior change.* Oxford, UK: Pergamon Press.

Bartoli, J., & Botel, M. (1988). *Reading/learning disability: An ecological approach.* New York, NY: Teachers College Press.

Bellis, T. (1996). *Assessment and management of central auditory processing disorders in the educational setting: From science to practice.* San Diego, CA: Singular.

Bellis, T. J. (2002). Developing deficit-specific intervention plans for individuals with auditory processing disorders. *Seminars in Hearing, 23,* 287–295.

Bellis, T. J., Chermak, G. D., Weihing, J., & Musiek, F. E. (2012). Efficacy of auditory interventions for central auditory processing disorder: A response to Fey et al. (2011). *Language, Speech, and Hearing Services in Schools, 43,* 381–386.

Bellis, T. J., & Ferre, J. M. (1999). Multidimensional approach to the differential diagnosis of central auditory processing disorders in children. *Journal of the American Academy of Audiology, 10,* 319–328.

Bidelman, G. M. & Krishnan. A. (2010). Effects of reverberation on brainstem representation of speech in musicians and non-musicians. *Brain Research, 1355,* 112–125.

Blake, R., Field, B., Foster, C., Platt, F., & Wertz, P. (1991). Effect of FM auditory trainers on attending behaviors of learning-disabled children. *Language, Speech, and Hearing Services in Schools, 22,* 111–114.

Bodner, M., Muftuler, L., Nalcioglu, O., & Shaw, G. (2001). fMRI study relevant to the Mozart effect: Brain areas involved in spatial-temporal processing. *Neurology Research, 23,* 683–690.

Bradlow, A., Kraus, N., & Hayes, E. (2003). Speaking clearly for children with learning disabilities: Sentence perception in noise. *Journal of Speech, Language, and Hearing Research, 46,* 80–97.

British Society of Audiology. (2010). *Auditory processing disorder (APD) steering committee interim position statement on APD.* Retrieved from http://www.thebsa.org.uk/apd/Publications.htm

Cameron, S., & Dillon, H. (2011). Development and evaluation of the LiSN & learn auditory training software for deficit-specific remediation of binaural processing deficits in children: Preliminary findings. *Journal of the American Academy of Audiology, 22,* 678–696.

Caspary, D. M., Milbrandt, J. C., & Helfert, R. H. (1995). Central auditory aging: GABA changes in the inferior colliculus. *Experimental Gerontology, 30,* 349–360.

Caspary, D. M., Raza, A., Lawhorn-Armour, B., Pippin, J, & Arneric, S. (1990). Immunocytochemical and neurochemical evidence for age-related loss of GABA in the inferior colliclus: Implications for neural presbycusis. *Journal of Neuroscience, 10,* 2363–2372.

Chai, B., Li, J., & Long, J. (2000). Therapeutic effects of aniracetam and piracetam in treatment of hypomnesis. *Chinese Pharmaceutical Journal, 35,* 272–273.

Chan, A. S., Ho, Y. C., & Cheung, M. C. (1998). Music training improves verbal memory. *Nature, 396,* 128.

Chermak, G. D. (2010). Music and auditory training. *Hearing Journal, 63,* 57–58.

Chermak, G., & Musiek, F. (1997). *Central auditory processing disorders: New perspectives.* San Diego, CA: Singular.

Chermak, G. D., & Musiek, F. E. (2002). Auditory training: Principles and approaches for remediating and managing auditory processing disorders. *Seminars in Hearing, 23,* 297–308.

Chermak, G., Silva, M., Nye, J., Hasbrouck, J., & Musiek, F. (2007). An update on professional education and clinical practices in central auditory processing. *Journal of the American Academy of Audiology, 18,* 428–452.

Chermak, G. D., Traynham, W. A., Seikel, J. A., & Musiek, F. E. (1998). Professional education and assessment practices in central auditory processing. *Journal of the American Academy of Audiology, 9,* 452–465.

Chermak, G. D., Weihing, J., & Musiek, F. E. (in preparation). Sound Auditory Training™. San Diego: CA, Plural Publishing.

Cohen, W., Hodson, A., O'Hare, A., Boyle, J., Durrani, T., McCartney, E., . . . Watson, J. (2005). Effects of computer-based intervention through acoustically modified speech (Fast ForWord) in severe mixed receptive-expressive language impairment: Outcomes from a randomized controlled trial. *Journal of Speech, Language, Hearing Research, 48,* 715–729.

Cunningham, J., Nicol, T., Zecker, S. G., Bradlow, A., & Kraus, N. (2001). Neurobiologic responses to speech in noise in children with learning problems: Deficits and strategies for improvement. *Clinical Neurophysiology, 112,* 758–767.

Dalebout, S., & Fox, L. (2001). Reliability of the mismatched negativity in the response of individual listeners. *Journal of the American Academy of Audiology, 12,* 245–253.

de Boer, J., Thornton, A., & Krumbholz, K. (2012). What is the role of the medial olivocochlear system in speech-in-noise processing? *Journal of Neurophysiology, 107,* 1301–1312.

Delhommeau, K., Micheyl, C., & Jouvent, R. (2005). Generalization of frequency discrimination learning across frequencies and ears: Implications for underlying neural mechanisms in humans. *Journal of the Association for Research in Otolaryngology, 6,* 171–179.

Delhommeau, K., Micheyl, C., Jouvent, R., & Collet, L. (2002). Transfer of learning across durations and ears in auditory frequency discrimination. *Perception and Psychophysics, 64,* 426–436.

Demany, L. (1985). Perceptual learning in frequency discrimination. *Journal of the Acoustical Society of America, 78*, 1118–1120.

Derouesne, C., Cailler, I., Kohler, F., Piette, F., Boyer, P., Sauron, B., & Lubin, S. (2001). Effectiveness of adrafinil on the memory complaint in the adult over fifty years of age: Results of a controlled double blind therapeutic trial of adrafinil versus placebo. *Revue de Geriatrie, 26*(10S), 851–858.

Devasenapathy, A., & Hachinski, V. C. (1998). Cognitive impairment poststroke. *Physical Medicine and Rehabilitation, 12*, 543–555.

Dewson, J. H. (1968) Efferent olivocochlear bundle: Some relationship to stimulus discrimination in noise. *Journal of Neurophysiology, 31*, 122–130.

Dhar, S. (2009, November). *Sifting for facts.* Paper presented at the Annual Mayo Clinic Conference, Rochester, MN.

Diehl, S. (1999). Listen learn? A software review of Earobics. *Language, Speech, and Hearing Services in Schools, 30*, 108–116.

Dockrell, J., & Shield, B. (2012). The impact of sound-field systems on learning and attention in elementary school classrooms. *Journal of Speech, Language, and Hearing Research, 55*, 1163–1176.

Dolan, D. F., & Nuttall, A. L. (1988). Masked cochlear whole-nerve response intensity functions altered by electrical stimulation of the crossed olivocochlear bundle. *Journal of the Acoustical Society of America, 83*, 1081–1086.

Elmer, S., Meyer, M., & Jancke, L. (2012). Neurofunctional and behavioral correlates of phonetic and temporal categorization in musically trained and untrained subjects. *Cerebral Cortex, 22*, 650–658.

Emanuel, D., Ficca, K., & Korczak, P. (2011). Survey of the diagnosis and management of auditory processing disorder. *American Journal of Audiology, 20*, 448–460.

Eriks-Brophy, A., & Ayukawa, H. (2000). The benefits of sound field amplification in classrooms of Inuit students of Nunavik: A pilot project. *Language, Speech, and Hearing Services in Schools, 31*, 324–335.

Feldman, D. E., Brainard, M. S., & Knudsen, E. I. (1996). Newly learned auditory responses mediated by NMDA receptors in the owl inferior colliculus. *Science, 271*, 525–528.

Ferraro, L., Fuxe, K., Tanganelli, S., Fernandez, M., Rambert, F., & Antonelli, T. (2000). Amplification of cortical serotonin release: A further neurochemical action of the vigilance-promoting drug modafinil. *Neuropharmacology, 39*, 1974–1983.

Fey, M. E., Richard, G. J., Geffner, D., Kamhi, A. G., Medwetsky, L., Paul, D., . . . Schooling , T. (2011). Auditory processing disorder and auditory/language interventions: An evidence-based systematic review. *Language, Speech, and Hearing Services in Schools, 42*, 246–264.

Flexer, C., Millin, J. P., & Brown, L. (1990). Children with developmental disabilities: The effect of sound field amplification on word identification. *Language, Speech, and Hearing Services in Schools, 21*, 177–182.

Gabb, N., Tallal, P., Kim, H., Lakshminarayanan, K., Archie, J., Glover, G., & J. Gabrieli (2005). Neural correlates of rapid spectrotemporal processing in musicians and non-musicians. *Annals of the New York Academy of Sciences, 1060*, 82–88.

Galaburda, A., Sherman, G., Rosen, G., Aboitiz, F., & Geschwind, N. (1985). Developmental dyslexia. Four consecutive patients with cortical anomalies. *Annals of Neurology, 18*, 222–233.

George, E., & Coch, D. (2011). Music training and working memory: An ERP study. *Neuropsychologia, 49*, 1083–1094.

Gillam R., Crofford, J., Gale, M., & Hoffman, L. (2001). Language change following computer-assisted language instruction with Fast ForWord or Laureate Learning Systems software. *American Journal of Speech-Language Pathology, 10*, 231–247.

Gillam, R., Loeb, D., Hoffman, L., Bohman, T., Champlin, C., Thibodeau, L., . . . Friel-Patti, S. (2008). The efficacy of fast forword language intervention in school-age children with language impairment: A randomized controlled trial. *Journal of Speech, Language, and Hearing Research, 51*, 97–119.

Gleich, O., Hamann, I., Klump, G., Kittel, M., & Strutz, J. (2003). Boosting GABA improves auditory temporal resolution in the gerbil. *NeuroReport, 14,* 1877–1880.

Gopal, K., Bishop, C., & Carney, L. (2004). Auditory measures in clinically depressed individuals. II. Auditory evoked potentials and behavioral speech tests. *International Journal of Audiology, 43,* 499–505.

Gopal, K. V., Daly, D. M., Daniloff, R. G., & Pennartz, L. (2000). Effects of selective serotonin reuptake inhibitors on auditory processing: Case study. *Journal of the American Academy of Audiology, 11,* 454–463.

Gottselig, J. M., Brandeis, D., Hofer-Tinguely, G., Borberly, A. A., & Achermann, P. (2004). Human central auditory plasticity associated with tone sequence learning. *Learning and Memory, 11,* 151–171.

Greener, J., Enderby, P., & Whurr, R. (2010). Pharmacological treatment for aphasia following stroke. *Cochrane Database of Systematic Reviews, 4,* CD000424.

Hassmannova, J., Myslivecek, J., & Novakova, V. (1981). Effects of early auditory stimulation on cortical areas. In J. Syka & L. Aitkin (Eds.), *Neuronal mechanisms of hearing* (pp. 355–359). New York, NY: Plenum Press.

Hawkey, D. J. C., Amitay, S., & Moore, D. R. (2004). Early and rapid perceptual learning. *Nature Neuroscience, 7,* 1055–1056.

Hayes, E. A., Warrier, C. M., Nichol, T. G., Zecker, S. G., & Kraus, N. (2003). Neural plasticity following auditory training in children with learning problems. *Clinical Neurophysiology, 114,* 673–684.

Hendler, T., Squires, N., & Emmerich, D. (1990). Psychophysical measures of central auditory dysfunction in multiple sclerosis: Neurophysiological and neuroanatomical correlates. *Ear and Hearing, 11,* 403-416.

Henri, B. P. (1994). Graduate student preparation: Tomorrow's challenge. *Asha, 36,* 43–46.

Herholz, S., & Zatorre, R. (2012). Musical training as a framework for brain plasticity: Behavior, function, and structure. *Neuron, 76,* 486–502.

Hock, F. J. (1995). Therapeutic approaches for memory impairments. *Behavioral Brain Research, 66,* 143–150.

Horn, S. D., & Gassaway, J. (2007). Practice-based evidence study design for comparative effectiveness research. *Medical Care, 45,* S50–S57.

Hubble-Dahlquist, L. (1998). *Classroom amplification: Not just for the hearing impaired anymore.* CSUN '98 Papers [online]. Retrieved from http://www.dimf.ne.jp/doc/english/Us_Eu/conf/csun_98/csun98_124.htm

Huber, M., Kittner, B., Hojer, C., Fink, G. R., Neveling, M., & Heiss, W. D. (1993). Effect of propentofylline on regional cerebral glucose metabolism in acute ischemic stroke. *Journal of Cerebral Blood Flow and Metabolism, 13,* 526–530.

Ikeda, T., Yamamoto, K., Takahashi, K., Kahu, Y.,Uchiyama, M., Sugiyama, K., & Yamada, M. (1992). Treatment of Alzheimer-type dementia with intravenous mecobalamin. *Clinical Therapeutics, 14,* 426–427.

Imai, A., Takagi, T., & Takeishi, H. (2005). Development of radio and television receiver with functions to assist hearing of elderly people. *IEEE Transactions on Consumer Electronics, 51,* 268–272.

Jäncke, L., Gaab, N., Wüstenberg, T., Scheich, H., & Heinze, H. J. (2001). Short-term functional plasticity in the human auditory cortex: An fMRI study. *Brain Research, 12,* 479–485.

Jerger, J., & Musiek, F. (2000). Report of the consensus conference on the diagnosis of auditory processing disorders in school-aged children. *Journal of the American Academy of Audiology, 11,* 467–474

Jerger, J., Thibodeau, L., Martin, J., Mehta, J., Tillman, G., Greenwald, R., . . . Scott, J., & Overson, G. (2002). Behavioral and electrophysiologic evidence of auditory processing disorder: A twin study. *Journal of the American Academy of Audiology, 13,* 438–460.

Jirsa, R. E. (1992). The clinical utility of the P3 AERP in children with auditory processing disorders. *Journal of Speech and Hearing Research, 35,* 903–912.

Johnston, K. N., John, A. B., Kreisman, N. V., Hall, J. W., & Crandell, C. C. (2009). Multiple benefits of personal FM system use by children with auditory processing disorder (APD). *International Journal of Audiology, 48,* 371–383.

Jutras, B., Loubert, M., Dupuis, J., Marcoux, C., Dumont, V., & Baril, M. (2007). Applicability of central auditory processing disorder models. *American Journal of Audiology, 16,* 100–106

Karmarkar, U., & Buonomano, D. (2003). Temporal specificity of perceptual learning in an auditory discrimination task. *Learning and Memory, 10,* 141–147.

Kemény, V., Molnár, S., Andrejkovics, M., Makai, A., & Csiba, L. (2005). Acute and chronic effects of vinpocetine on cerebral hemodynamics and neuropsychological performance in multi-infarct patients. *Journal of Clinical Pharmacology, 45,* 1048–1054

Kemperman, G., Kuhn, H., & Gage, F. (1997). More hippocampal neurons in adult mice living in an enriched environment. *Nature, 386,* 493–495.

Keuroghlian, A. S., & Knudsen, E. I. (2007). Adaptive auditory plasticity in developing and adult animals. *Progress in Neurobiology, 82,* 109–121.

Kilgour, A. R., Jakobson, L. S., & Cuddy, L. L. (2000). Music training and rate of presentation as mediators of text and song recall. *Memory and Cognition, 28,* 700–710.

King, C., Warrier, C. M., Hayes, E., & Kraus, N. (2002). Deficits in auditory brainstem encoding of speech sounds in children with learning problems. *Neuroscience Letters, 319,* 111–115.

Knudsen, E. I. (1988). Experience shapes sound localization and auditory unit properties during development in the bam owl. In G. M. Edelman, W. E. Gall, & M. W. Cowan (Eds.), *Auditory function: Neurobiological bases of hearing* (pp. 137–149). New York, NY: Wiley.

Kraus, N. (2001). Auditory pathway encoding and neural plasticity in children with learning problems. *Audiology Neurootology, 6,* 221–227.

Kraus, N., Bradlow, A., Cheatham. M., Cunningham, J., King, C., Koch, D., . . . Wright, B. (2000). Consequences of neural asynchrony: A case of auditory neuropathy. *Journal of the Association for Research in Otolaryngology, 1,* 33–45.

Kraus, N., & Chandrasekaran, B. (2010). Music training for the development of auditory skills. *Nature Reviews Neuroscience, 11,* 599–605.

Kraus, N., & Disterhoff, J.F. (1982). Response plasticity of single neurons in rabbit auditory association cortex during tone-signalled learning. *Brain Research, 246,* 205–215.

Kraus, N., McGee, T., Carrell, T., King, C., Tremblay, K., & Nicol, T. (1995). Central auditory system plasticity associated with speech discrimination training. *Journal of Cognitive Neuroscience, 7,* 25–32.

Kraus, N., McGee, T. J., Carrell, T. D., Zecker, S.G., Nicol, T. G., & Koch, D. B. (1996). Auditory neurophysiologic responses and discrimination deficits in children with learning problems. *Science, 273,* 971–973.

Kuk, F. (2011). Hearing aids for children with auditory processing disorders? *Seminars in Hearing, 32,* 189–195.

Kuk, F., Jackson A., Keenan, D., & Lau, C. (2008). Personal amplification for school-aged children with auditory processing disorders. *Journal of the American Academy of Audiology, 19,* 465–480.

Lakshimnarayanan, K., & Tallal, P. (2007). Generalization of non-linguistic auditory perceptual training to syllable discrimination. *Restorative Neurology and Neuroscience, 25,* 263–272.

Lamb, S. J., & Gregory, A. H. (1993). The relationship between music and reading in beginning readers. *Journal of Educational Psychology, 13,* 13–27.

Linkenhoker, B. A., & Knudsen, E. I. (2002). Incremental training increases the plasticity of the auditory space map in adult barn owls. *Nature, 419,* 293–296.

Linkenhoker, B. A., von der Ohe, C. G., & Knudsen, E. I. (2005). Anatomical traces of juvenile learning in the auditory system of adult barn owls. *Nature Neuroscience, 8*(1), 93–98.

Loo, J. H. Y., Bamiou, D.-E., Campbell, N., & Luxon, L. M. (2010). Computer-based auditory training (CBAT): benefits for children with language- and reading-related learning difficulties. *Developmental medicine and child neurology, 52*, 708–717.

McArthur, G. M., Ellis, D., Atkinson, C. M., & Coltheart, M. (2008). Auditory processing deficits in children with reading and language impairments: Can they (and should they) be treated? *Cognition, 107*, 946–977.

McPherson, D. L., & Salamat, M. T. (2004). Interactions among variables in the P_{300} response to a continuous performance task in normal and ADHD adults. *Journal of the American Academy of Audiology, 15*, 666–677.

Merzenich, M., Jenkins, W. M., Johnston, P., Schreiner, C., Miller, S. L., & Tallal, P. (1996). Temporal processing deficits of language-learning impaired children ameliorated by training. *Science, 271*, 77–80.

Meyer, M., Elmer, S., Ringli, M., Oechslin, M., Baumann, S., & Jancke, L. (2011). Long-term exposure to music enhances the sensitivity of the auditory system in children. *European Journal Neuroscience, 34*, 755–765.

Moller, H. J., Maurer, I., & Saletu, B. (1994). Placebo controlled trial of the xanthine derivative propentofylline in dementia. *Psychopharmacology, 101*, 147–159.

Moncrieff, D., & Musiek, F. (2002). Interaural asymmetries revealed by dichotic listening tests in normal and dyslexic children. *Journal of the American Academy of Audiology, 13*, 428–437.

Moncrieff, D., & Wertz, D. (2008). Auditory rehabilitation for interaural asymmetry: Preliminary evidence of improved dichotic listening performance following intensive training. *International Journal of Audiology, 47*, 484-497.

Morell., R., Brewer, C., Ge, D., Snieder, H., Zalewski, C., King, K., Drayna, D., & Friedman, T. (2007). A twin study of auditory processing indicates that dichotic listening ability is a strongly heritable trait. *Human Genetics, 122*, 103–111.

Morley, B. J., & Happe, H. K. (2000). Cholinergic receptors: Dual roles in transduction and plasticity. *Hearing Research, 147*, 104–112.

Morrison, S. (1998). Computer applications: Earobics. *Child language teaching and therapy*. London, UK: Arnold.

Muller, U., Steffenhagen, N., Regenthal, R., & Bublak, P. (2004). Effects of modafinil on working memory processes in humans. *Psychopharmacology, 177*, 161–169.

Murphy, C., & Schochat, E. (2011). Effect of nonlinguistic auditory training on phonological and reading skills. *Folia phoniatrica et logopaedica, 63*, 147–153.

Musiek, F. E., Baran, J. A., & Shinn, J. (2004). Assessment and Remediation of an auditory processing disorder associated with head trauma. *Journal of the American Academy of Audiology, 15*, 117–132.

Musiek, F. E., Baran, J. A., & Pinheiro, M. L. (1992). P300 results in patients with lesions of the auditory areas of the cerebrum. *Journal of the American Academy of Audiology, 3*, 5–15.

Musiek, F. E., Baran, J., & Schochat, E. (1999). Selected management approaches to central auditory processing disorders. *Scandinavian Audiology, 51*, 63–76.

Musiek, F. E., Bellis, T. J., & Chermak, G. D. (2005). Nonmodularity of the CANS: Implications for (central) auditory processing disorder: A critique of Cacace and McFarland's "The importance of modality specificity in diagnosing central auditory processing disorder (CAPD)." *American Journal of Audiology, 14*, 128–138.

Musiek, F. E., Chermak, G. D., & Weihing, J. (2007). Auditory training. In G. D. Chermak & F. E. Musiek (Eds.), *Handbook of (central) auditory processing disorder: Vol. II. Comprehensive intervention* (pp. 77–106). San Diego, CA: Plural.

Musiek, F. E., & Hoffman, D. W. (1990). An introduction to the functional neurochemistry of the auditory system. *Ear and Hearing, 11*, 395–402.

Musiek, F. E., & Schochat, E. (1998). Auditory training and central auditory processing disorders—a case study. *Seminars in Hearing, 19*, 357–366.

Musiek, F. E., Shinn, J., & Hare, C. (2002). Plasticity, auditory training, and auditory processing disorders. *Seminars in Hearing, 23,* 263–275.

Neuss, D., Blair, J., & Viehweg, S. (1991). Sound field amplification: Does it improve word recognition in a background of noise for students with minimal hearing impairments? *Educational Audiology Monograph, 2,* 43–52.

Nicholson, C. D. (1990). Pharmacology of nootropics and metabolically active comounds in relation to their use in dementia. *Psychopharmacology, 101,* 147–159.

Nieder, P. C., & Nieder, I. (1970). Antimasking effect of crossed olivocochlear bundle stimulation with loud clicks in guinea pigs. *Experimental Neurology, 28,* 179–188.

Oppenheimer, B., Self, T., & Sieff, S. (2005). *Integration of clinical practice and research: Successful curriculum models.* Rockville, MD: American Speech-Language-Hearing Association.

Overy, K. (2003). Dyslexia and music: From timing deficits to musical intervention. *Annals of the New York Academy of Sciences, 999,* 497–505.

Palincsar, A. S., Brown, A. L., & Campione, J. C. (1994). Models and practices of dynamic assessment. In G. P. Wallach & K. G. Butler (Eds.), *Language learning disabilities in school-age children and adolescents* (pp. 132–144). New York, NY: Charles E. Merrill.

Parbery-Clark, A., Skoe, E., & Kraus, N. (2009). Musical experience limits the degradative effects of background noise on the neural processing of sound. *Journal of Neuroscience, 29,* 14100–14107.

Parbery-Clark, A., Skoe, E., Lam, C., & Kraus, N. (2009). Musician enhancement for speech-in-noise. *Ear and Hearing, 30,* 653–661.

Parkinson, F. E., Rudolphi, K. A., & Fredholm, B. B. (1994). Propentofylline: A nucleoside transport inhibitor with neuroprotective effects in cerebral ischemia. *General Pharmacology, 25,* 1053–1058.

Patel, A. (2011). Why would musical training benefit the neural encoding of speech? The OPERA hypothesis. *Frontiers in Psychology, 2,* 1–12.

Patel, A. (2012). The OPERA hypothesis: Assumptions and clarifications. *Annals of the New York Academy of Sciences, 1252,* 124–128.

Peretz, I., Cummings, S., & Dube, M-P. (2007). The genetics of congenital amusia (tone deafness): A family-aggregation study. *American Journal Human Genetics, 81,* 582–588.

Phillips, D. P. (2002). Central auditory system and central auditory processing disorders: Some conceptual issues. *Seminars in Hearing, 23,* 251–261.

Pichney, M. A., Durlach, N. I., & Braida, L. D. (1985). Speaking clearly for the hard of hearing. I: Intelligibility differences between clear and conversational speech. *Journal of Speech and Hearing Research, 28,* 96–103.

Pichney, M. A., Durlach, N. I., & Braida, L. D. (1986). Speaking clearly for the hard of hearing. II: Acoustic characteristics of clear and conversational speech. *Journal of Speech and Hearing Research, 29,* 434–446.

Picheny, M. A., Durlach, N. I., & Braida, L. D. (1989). Speaking clearly for the hard of hearing: III. An attempt to determine the contribution of speaking rates to differences in intelligibility between clear and conversational speech. *Journal of Speech and Hearing Research, 32,* 600–603.

Pickles, J. O., & Comis, S. D. (1973). Role of centrifugal pathways to cochlear nucleus in detection of signals in noise. *Journal of Neurophysiology, 36,* 1131–1137.

Pienkowski, M., & Eggermont, J. (2011). Cortical tonotopic map plasticity and behavior. *Neuroscience and Biobehavioral Reviews, 35,* 2117–2128.

Pinheiro, F., & Capellini, S. (2010). Auditory training in students with learning disabilities. *Pro Fono, 22,* 49–54.

Poplin, M. S. (1988a). Holistic/constructivist principles of the teaching/learning process: Implications for the field of learning disabilities. *Journal of Learning Disabilities, 21*, 401–416.

Poplin, M. S. (1988b). The reductionist fallacy in learning disabilities: Replicating the past by reducing the present. *Journal of Learning Disabilities, 21*, 389–400.

Purdy, S., Kelly, A., & Davies, M. (2002). Auditory brainstem response, middle latency response, and late cortical evoked potentials in children with learning disabilities. *Journal of the American Academy of Audiology, 13*, 367–382.

Rampon, C., Jiang, C., Dong, H., Tang, Y., Lockhart, D., Schultz, P., . . . Hu, Y. (2000). Effects of environmental enrichment on gene expression in the brain. *Proceedings of the National Academy of Sciences, 97*, 12880–12884.

Rauscher, F. H., Shaw, G. L., Ky, K. N. (1993). Music and spatial task performance. *Nature, 365*, 611.

Rauscher, F. H., Shaw, G. L., & Ky, K. N. (1995). Listening to Mozart enhances spatial-temporal reasoning: Towards a neurophysiological basis. *Neuroscience Letters, 185*, 44–47.

Recanzone, G. H., Schreiner, C. E., & Merzenich, M. M. (1993). Plasticity in the frequency representation of primary auditory cortex following discrimination training in adult owl monkeys. *Journal of Neuroscience, 13*, 87–103.

Rosenberg, G., (1998). FM sounds field research identifies benefits for students and teachers. *Educational Audiology Review, 3*, 6–8.

Rosenberg, G. (2002). Classroom acoustics and personal FM technology in management of auditory processing disorder. *Seminars in Hearing, 23*, 309–318.

Rosenberg, G. G. (2005). Sound field amplification: A comprehensive literature review. In C. Crandall, J. Smaldino, & C. Flexer (Eds.), *Sound field amplification: Applications to speech perception and classroom acoustics* (2nd ed., pp. 72–111). New York, NY: Thomson Delmar Learning.

Rosenberg, G., Blake-Rahter, P., Heavner, J., Allen, L., Redmond, B., Phillips, J., & Stigers, K. (1999). Improving classroom acoustics (ICA): A three-year FM sound-field classroom amplification study. *Journal of Educational Audiology, 7*, 8–28.

Russo, N., Nicol, T., Zecker, S., Hayes, E., & Kraus, N. (2005). Auditory training improves neural timing in the human brainstem. *Behavioural Brain Research, 156*, 95–103.

Sahley, T. L., Kalish, R. B., Musiek, F. E., & Hoffman, D. (1991). Effects of opioid drugs on auditory evoked potentials suggest a role of lateral efferent olivocochlear dynorphins in auditory function. *Hearing Research, 55*, 133–142.

Sahley, T. L., Musiek, F. E., & Nodar, R. H. (1996). Naloxone blockage of (–)pentazocine-induced changes in auditory function. *Ear and Hearing, 17*, 341–353.

Sahley, T. L., & Nodar, R. H. (1994). Improvement in auditory function following pentazocine suggests a role for dynorphins in auditory sensitivity. *Ear and Hearing, 15*, 422–431.

Saletu, B., Moller, H. J., Grunberger, J., Deutsch, H., & Rossner, M. (1990). Propentofylline in adult-onset cognitive disorders: Double-blind, placebo-controlled, clinical, psychometric and brain mapping studies. *Neuropsychobiology, 24*, 173–184.

Sameroff, A. J. (1983). Developmental systems: Contexts and evolution. In W. Kessen (Ed.), *History, theory, and methods* (Vol. 1). In P. H. Mussen (Ed.), *Handbook of child psychology*, (4th ed., pp. 237–294). New York, NY: John Wiley.

Sano, M., Bell, K., Marder, K., Stricks, L., Stern, Y., & Mayeux, R. (1993). Safety and efficacy of oral physostigmine in the treatment of Alzheimer disease. *Clinical Neuropharmacology, 16*, 61–69.

Schochat, E., Musiek, F. E., Alonso, R., & Ogata, J. (2010). Effect of auditory training on the middle latency response in children with (central) auditory processing disorder. *Brazilian Journal of Medical and Biological Research, 43*, 777–785.

Schon, D., Magne, C., & Besson, M. (2004). The music of speech: Music training facilitates pitch processing in both music and language. *Psychophysiology, 41*, 341–349.

Shannon, R. V., Zeng, F. G., Kamath, V., Wygonski, J., & Ekelid, M. (1995). Speech recognition with primarily temporal cues. *Science, 270*, 303–304.

Sharma, M., Purdy, S., & Kelly, A. (2012). A randomized control trial of interventions in school-aged children with auditory processing disorders. *International Journal of Audiology, 51*, 506–518.

Simoski, J., Stevens, K., Adler, L., & Freedman, P. (2002). Clozapine improves deficient inhibitory auditory processing in DBA/2 mice, via a nicotinic cholinergic mechanism. *Psychopharmacology, 165*, 386–396.

Stach, B. A., Loiselle, L. H., Jerger, J. F., Mintz, S. L., & Taylor, C. D. (1987). Clinical experience with personal FM assistive listening devices. *Hearing Journal, 10*, 24–30.

Strait. D.L., Kraus, N., Parbery-Clark, A., & Ashley, R. (2010). Musical experience shapes top-down auditory mechanisms: Evidence from masking and auditory attention performance. *Hearing Research, 261*, 22–29.

Syka, J. (2002). Plastic changes in the central auditory system after hearing loss, restoration of function, and duration learning. *Physiological Reviews, 82*, 601–636.

Szalkowski, C. E., & Fitch, R. H. (2011). Candidate dyslexia susceptibility genes and disorders of neuronal migration: Behavioral effects of cortical dysgenesis in a rodent model. In A. Girard & L. Moreau (Eds.), *Neuronal migration* (pp. 1–23). New York, NY: Nova Science.

Tallal, P., Merzenich, M., Miller, S., & Jenkins, W. (1998). Language learning impairment: Integrating basic science, technology, and remediation. *Experimental Brain Research, 123*, 210–219.

Tallal, P., Miller, S., Bedi, G., Byma, G., Wang, X., Nagarajan, S. S., . . . Merzenich, M. M. (1996). Language comprehension in language-learning impaired children improved with acoustically modified speech. *Science, 271*, 81–84.

Tang, Y., Shimizu, E., Dube, G., Rampon, C., Kerchner, G., Zhuo, M., . . . Tsien, J. (1999). Genetic enhancement of learning and memory in mice. *Nature, 401*, 63–69.

Tansey, K., McKay, W., & Kakulas, B. (2012). Resotrative neurology: Consideration of the new anatomy and physiology of the injured nervous system. *Clinical Neurology and Neurosurgery, 114*, 436–440.

Temple, E., Deutsch, G. K., Poldrack, R. A., Miller, S. L., Tallal, P., Merzenich, M. M., & Gabrieli, J. D. (2003). Neural deficits in children with dyslexia ameliorated by behavioral remediation: Evidence from functional MRI. *Proceedings of the National Academy of Sciences USA, 100*, 2860–2865.

Thibodeau, L. M. (2007). Computer-based auditory training for (central) auditory processing disorder. In G. D. Chermak & F. E. Musiek (Eds.), *Handbook of (central) auditory processing disorder: Comprehensive intervention* (Vol. II, pp. 167–206). San Diego, CA: Plural.

Tillery, K. L., Katz, J., & Keller, W. D. (2000). Effects of methylphenidate (Ritalin) on auditory performance in children with attention and auditory processing disorders. *Journal of Speech, Language, and Hearing Research, 43*, 893–901.

Torigoe, R., Hayashi, T., Anegawa, S., Harada, K., Toda, K., Maeda, K., & Katsuragi, M. (1994). The effect of propentofylline and pentoxifylline on cerebral blood flow using ^{123}I-IMP SPECT in patients with cerebral arteriosclerosis. *Clinical Therapeutics, 16*, 65–73.

Tsodyks, M., & Gilbert, C. (2004). Neural networks and perceptual learning. *Nature, 431*, 775–781.

Trainor, L., Shahin, A., & Roberts, L. (2003). Effects of musical training on the auditory cortex in children. *Annals of the New York Academy of Sciences, 999*, 506–513.

Tremblay, K. (2007). Training-related changes in the brain: Evidence from human auditory evoked potentials. *Seminars in Hearing, 28*, 120–132.

Tremblay, K., & Kraus, N. (2002). Auditory training induces asymmetrical changes in cortical neural activity. *Journal of Speech, Language, and Hearing Research, 45*, 564–572.

Tremblay, K., Kraus, N., Carrell, T., & McGee, T. (1997). Central auditory system plasticity: Generalization to novel stimulation following listening training. *Journal of the Acoustical Society of America, 102*, 3762–3773.

Tremblay, K., Kraus, N., & McGee, T. (1998). The time course of auditory perceptual learning: Neurophysiological changes during speech-sound training. *NeuroReport, 9*, 3557–3560.

Tremblay, K., Kraus, N., McGee, T., Ponton, C., & Otis, B. (2001). Central auditory plasticity: Changes in the N1-P2 complex after speech-sound training. *Ear and Hearing, 22*, 79–90.

Tsodyks, M., & Gilbert, C. (2004). Neural networks and perceptual learning. *Nature, 431*, 775–81.

Van Tasell, D. J., Soli, S. D., Kirby, V. M., & Widin, G. P. (1987). Speech waveform envelope cues for consonant recognition. *Journal of the Acoustical Society of America, 82*, 1152–1161.

Warrier, C.M., Johnson, K.L., Hayes, E.A., Nicol, T., & Kraus, N. (2004). Learning impaired children exhibit timing deficits and training-related improvements in auditory cortical responses to speech in noise. *Experimental Brain Research, 157*, 431–441.

Wenthold, R. (1991). Neurotransmitters of brainstem auditory nuclei. In R. A. Altshuler, B. M. Clopton, R. P. Bobbin, & D. W. Hoffman (Eds.), *Neurobiology of hearing: The central auditory system* (pp. 121–139). New York, NY: Raven Press.

Wible, B., Nicol, T., & Kraus, N. (2005). Correlation between brainstem and cortical auditory processes in normal and language-impaired children. *Brain, 128*, 417–423.

Wiederhold, M. L. (1986). Physiology of the olivocochlear system. In R. A. Altschuler, D. W. Hoffman, & R. P. Bobbin (Eds.), *Neurobiology of hearing: The cochlea* (pp. 349–370). New York, NY: Raven Press.

Wilson, W., Marinac, J., Pitty, K., & Burrows, C. (2011). The use of sound-field amplification devices in different types of classrooms. *Language, Speech, and Hearing Services in Schools, 42*, 395–407.

Winblad, B. (2005). Piracetam: A review of pharmacological properties and clinical uses. *CNS Drug Reviews, 11*, 169–182.

Wong, P. Skoe, E., Russo, N., Dees, T., & Kraus, N. (2007). Musical experience shapes human brainstem encoding of linguistic pitch patterns. *Nature Neuroscience, 10*, 420–422.

Wright, B. A., & Fitzgerald, M. B. (2001). Different patterns of human discrimination learning for two interaural cues to sound-source location. *Proceedings of the National Academy of Sciences USA, 98*, 12307–12312.

Wright, B. A., Lombardino, L. J., King, W. M., Puranik, C. S., Leonard, C. M., & Merzenich, M. M. (1997). Deficits in auditory temporal and spectral resolution in language-impaired children. *Nature, 387*, 176–178.

Wright B. A., & Sabin A. T. (2007). Perceptual learning: How much daily training is enough? *Experimental Brain Research, 180*, 727–736.

Zendel, B., & Alain, C. (2012). Musicians experience less age-related decline in central auditory processing, *Psychology and Aging, 27*, 410–417.

Zhao, W., & Dhar, S. (2012). Frequency tuning of the contralateral medialolivocochlear reflex in humans. *Journal of Neurophysiology, 108*, 25–30.

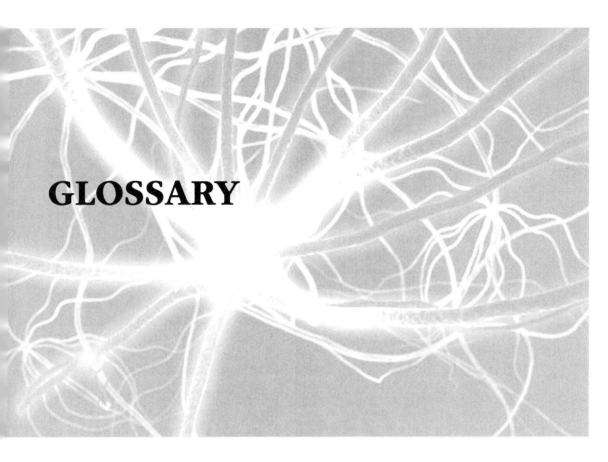

GLOSSARY

Absorption. Property of a material or an object whereby sound energy is converted into heat by propagation in a medium or when sound strikes the boundary between two media. It is determined for a specified frequency or for a stated frequency band.

Accommodation. Making facilities and programs accessible to and usable by persons with disabilities through appropriate changes, including policy adjustments, task restructuring, adjusted schedules, equipment acquisition or alteration, training, or provision of qualified readers or interpreters, and other similar accommodations.

Acoustic access. Access through the auditory channel, either unaided or aided, to acoustic information.

Acoustic saliency. An acoustically salient phoneme (speech sound) or word is one that is obvious and prominent in an utterance. In a sentence context, acoustically nonsalient morphemes are shorter in duration and softer than louder phonemes in adjacent portions of the utterance.

Adaptive training. Training in which stimulus parameters vary on the basis of the participant's performance on preceding trials.

Afferent. Used to refer to neurons carrying information to the brain, such as those in the ascending auditory pathways.

Amplitude modulation (AM). Variation in the envelope of a sound over time.

Analog. Refers to a signal that varies continuously over time.

Assessment. Formal and informal procedures to collect data and gather evidence; delineation of functional areas of strength or weakness and/or determination of ability or capacity in associated areas.

Assistive listening system. A device that delivers sound to individuals with peripheral or central auditory deficits to mitigate listening problems (e.g., frequency modulated [FM] systems, personal amplifiers, infrared systems).

Association area. Areas of the cerebral cortex not believed to receive direct sensory inputs or send outputs to motor neurons, but to communicate with other cerebrocortical areas.

Attention. Gateway to conscious experience; maintains primacy of certain information in ongoing information processing.

    Divided attention. Ability to attend to multiple stimuli simultaneously.

    Selective (focused) attention. Ability to focus on relevant stimuli while ignoring simultaneously presented, but irrelevant stimuli (i.e., distractors).

    Sustained attention (vigilance). Ability to inhibit interference; requires sustained focus for a period of time while awaiting the occurrence of a target stimulus.

Attention deficit hyperactivity disorder (ADHD). Persistent pattern of inattention and/or hyperactivity-impulsivity that is more frequent and severe than is typically observed in individuals at a comparable level of development; manifested in multiple settings; interferes with developmentally appropriate social, academic, or occupational functions; and has been present prior to age 12 years.

    Combined type. Attention deficit characterized by hyperactivity-impulsivity and inattention.

    Predominantly inattentive type. Presents primary symptoms of inattention.

    Predominantly hyperactive-impulsive type. Behavioral regulation disorder.

Attenuation. Reduction in magnitude of a physical quantity such as sound, either by electronic means (e.g., by an attenuator), or by a physical barrier, including various absorptive materials. It is usually measured in decibels.

Auditory brainstem response (ABR). A sequence of synchronous electrical activity in the auditory brainstem (i.e., auditory [eighth nerve] nerve, cochlear nuclei, superior olivary complex, trapezoid body, lateral lemniscus, inferior colliculus, and possibly the medial geniculate body) in response to an auditory or acoustic stimulus.

Auditory cortex. Area of the cerebral cortex that is the final destination of auditory inputs; located in the floor of the lateral sulcus in the superior temporal gyrus; see also primary auditory area.

Auditory discrimination. Differentiating similar acoustic stimuli that differ in frequency, intensity, and/or temporal parameters.

Auditory evoked response/auditory evoked potential (AEP). Synchronous electrical activity (potentials) within the auditory nerve or auditory regions of the brain evoked by auditory or acoustic stimuli.

Auditory late latency response (ALLR). Synchronous electrical activity (N1–P2–N2 complex) occurring in the range of approximately 60 to 250 msec arising from thalamo-cortical regions (i.e., superior temporal plane, lateral temporal lobe, and adjacent parietal regions).

Auditory middle latency response (AMLR). Synchronous electrical activity (potential) arising from the midbrain (i.e., Na component) and the superior temporal gyrus (i.e., Pa) within the auditory cortex.

Auditory neuropathy spectrum disorder (ANSD). A *peripheral* neural disorder, thought to arise from spiral ganglion cells, their processes, and/or the eighth (auditory) cranial nerve, characterized by normal otoacoustic emissions (OAEs), a recordable cochlear microphonic (CM), and an absent or grossly abnormal auditory brainstem response (ABR). The primary complaint of a person diagnosed with ANSD is difficulty understanding speech, especially in background noise.

Auditory training. Direct auditory skills remediation to maximize processing (use) of acoustic signals; set of acoustic conditions and/or repetitive tasks designed to activate auditory and related systems, change their neural base, and improve the ability to perceive auditory events.

Aural rehabilitation. An ecological, interactive process that facilitates one's ability to minimize or prevent the limitations and restrictions that auditory dysfunctions can impose on well-being and communication, including interpersonal, psychosocial, educational, and vocational functioning.

Backward masking. The presence of one sound renders a previously presented sound less detectable.

Binaural fusion. The fusion (merging) of signals from the two ears into a single coherent sound image at the level of the brainstem.

Binaural interaction. Central auditory processing of intensity or time differences of acoustic stimuli presented diotically to the two ears.

Binaural interference. A phenomenon whereby the performance of the poorer ear interferes with that of the better ear resulting in poorer binaural performance than monaural performance of the better ear.

Binaural masking level difference. A measure of the advantage in signal detection that can result from the use of binaural cues; the difference in signal threshold between a situation in which the masker and signal have the same interaural time difference and interaural level difference, and a situation in which the interaural time and/or level differences for the masker and the signal differ.

Binaural summation. A summation of the acoustic energy that is presented to the two ears simultaneously, which affects thresholds and supra-threshold loudness.

Brain imaging. Procedures used to map the structure and metabolic and electrophysiological properties of the brain; includes computed tomography, magnetic resonance imaging, positron emission topography, regional cerebral blood flow, and brain electrical activity mapping.

Bottom-up processing. Information processing that is data driven; properties of the data are primary determinants of higher level representations and constructions.

Central auditory nervous system (CANS). The auditory brainstem, subcortical pathways, auditory cortex, and corpus callosum.

Central auditory processes. Auditory system mechanisms and processes that underlie the following abilities or skills: sound localization and lateralization; auditory discrimination; auditory pattern recognition; temporal aspects of audition including, temporal integration, temporal discrimination (e.g., temporal gap detection), temporal ordering, and temporal masking; auditory performance with competing acoustic signals (including dichotic listening); and auditory performance with degraded acoustic signals.

Central auditory processing disorder (CAPD). Difficulties in the perceptual processing of auditory information in the central nervous system, that cannot be *attributed to* higher order language, cognitive, or related supramodal confounds, and manifests as poor performance in one or more of the central auditory processes, with associated changes in the neurobiologic activity underlying those processes that give rise to the auditory evoked potentials.

Characteristic frequency. The pure tone frequency to which a given place on the basilar membrane, or a given neuron in the auditory system, is most sensitive at low stimulation levels.

Classroom audio distribution system (CADS). A system whose primary design goal is to electroacoustically distribute the audio portion of spoken communications and curricular content throughout the learning space or listening area.

Clear speech. Speech produced by a speaker who has been instructed to speak as clearly as possible, as if trying to communicate in a noisy background.

Clinical decision analysis (CDA). A quantitative, systematic approach to clinical decision making derived from signal detection theory.

Closure. The ability to subjectively complete and make whole an incomplete form. Listeners use language knowledge and inductive and deductive reasoning, as well as auditory and grammatic closure to derive the meaning of words and messages.

> **Auditory closure.** The ability to recognize a whole word despite the absence of certain elements.

> **Grammatic closure.** The ability to complete phrases or sentences despite missing words or morphemes (e.g., filling in the verb form *are* versus *is* to conjugate with the subject *they*).

> **Verbal auditory closure.** The ability to use spoken contextual information to facilitate speech recognition.

Cochlear microphonic (CM). An alternating current potential that follows the waveform of the stimulus and the vibrations of the basilar membrane. One of two potentials comprising the ECochG. See Electrocochleography.

Cognition. Activity of knowing, encompassing the acquisition, organization, and use of knowledge; automatic and unconscious processes that transform, reduce, elaborate, store, recover, and use sensory input; processes involved in knowing, including perceiving, recognizing, conceiving, judging, sensing, and reasoning; primary phase in the development of knowledge.

Cognitive style. An individual's approach to processing information, problem solving, and cognitive tasks (e.g., bottom-up/top-down, impulsive/reflective, field dependent/field independent).

Commissure. A group of axons of neurons passing from one side of the brain, usually, to a similar structure on the opposite side of the brain.

Commissurotomy. The medical term for surgical sectioning of a brain commissure, usually the corpus callosum.

Comorbidity. Existence of two or more disorders, diseases, or pathologic processes in an individual that are not necessarily related.

Compensation. Rehabilitative approach directed toward reducing the negative impact of a disorder or disease not amenable to complete recovery through treatment.

Consonant-vowel (CV). Nonsense syllable comprised of a consonant followed by a vowel (e.g., ba, da, ga).

Corpus callosum. Principal commissure of the cerebral hemispheres.

Critical distance. Distance from a sound source at which direct sound level and reverberant sound level are equal.

Damping. Dissipation of energy with time or distance; loss of energy in a system resulting from friction (internal or external) or other resistance.

Desktop sound-field FM system. A self-contained system designed for personal or small group listening in which the FM signal transmitted over a wireless microphone is presented to the listener(s) via a speaker which is placed on the user's desk.

Deductive inferencing. Reasoning from the general to the specific.

Depolarization. An increase in the electric potential of a hair cell or neuron from a negative resting potential.

Diagnosis. Identification and categorization of impairment/dysfunction; determination of presence and nature of a disorder.

Dichotic. Simultaneous presentation of two different acoustic events, one to each ear.

Difference limen. Just noticeable difference or smallest detectable change in a stimulus, usually pertaining to frequency, intensity, or duration; the difference in a quantity that a listener can just detect at some criterion level of performance.

Differential diagnosis. Distinguishing between two or more conditions presenting with similar symptoms or attributes.

Diffraction. Bending of sound waves around obstacles whose dimensions are smaller than the wavelength of the sound; the spreading out of waves beyond openings that are smaller than the wavelength of the sound. Diffraction involves a change in direction of a wave as it passes through a small opening or around a barrier in its path.

Diffusion. Process of spreading or dispersing radiated energy so that it is less direct or coherent. In acoustics, diffusion is caused by sound waves reflected from an uneven surface.

Distortion. Undesired change of a waveform resulting in the presence of some frequency components in the output signal that are not present in the input signal.

Dynamic assessment. Approach to evaluation focused on the different ways by which an individual achieves a score rather than the score achieved; approach is characterized by guided learning to determine an individual's potential for change.

Effect size. Calculated measure used to determine the extent of practical significance for particular research results.

Effectiveness. Effects of treatment; how well a treatment works in real-world settings.

Efferent system. The portion of the auditory system, also called the descending system, that courses from the brain down to the cochlea following a similar pathway as the afferent system.

Efficacy. Effects of treatment; how well a treatment can work under ideal circumstances and adequate control; documenting treatment efficacy requires demonstrating that a particular treatment produces the desired outcomes or behavior change in an efficient manner (e.g., cost effective) as a result of the treatment.

Efficiency. A measure of a test's combined sensitivity and specificity; ability of a test to identify correctly those individuals who have the dysfunction/disorder and correctly identify those individuals who do not have the dysfunction.

Electroacoustic measures. Recordings of acoustic signals from within the ear canal that are generated spontaneously or in response to acoustic stimuli (e.g., otoacoustic emissions, acoustic reflexes).

Electrocochleography (ECochG). An auditory evoked response that arises from the cochlea and eight (auditory) cranial nerve within the first 2 to 3 msec. following an abrupt stimulus. See Cochlear microphonic.

Electrophysiologic measures. Recordings of electrical potentials that reflect synchronous activity generated by the central nervous system in response to a wide variety of acoustic events (e.g., auditory brainstem response, steady-state evoked potentials, auditory middle-latency response, frequency following response, cortical auditory event-related potentials [P1, N1, P2, P300]).

Endogenous. Refers to evoked potentials (e.g., P300) that are relatively invariant to changes in the eliciting physical stimulus, but are highly influenced by subject state and require an internal or mental activity (e.g., perceptual or cognitive process) to generate the potential.

Evaluation. Interpretation of assessment data, evidence, and related information.

Evidence-based practice. Explicit and judicious use of current best evidence in making decisions about the care of individual patients by integrating individual clinical expertise with the best available external clinical evidence from systematic research; a systematic method to evaluate and implement best practices for assessment and treatment in clinical fields.

Executive function. Component of metacognition; set of general control processes that coordinate knowledge (i.e., cognition) and metacognitive knowledge, transforming such knowledge into behavioral strategies, which ensure that an individual's behavior is adaptive, consistent with some goal, and beneficial to the individual; self-directed actions of an individual that are used to self-regulate so as to accomplish self-control, goal-directed behavior, and maximize future outcomes.

Exogenous. Refers to evoked potentials that are highly dependent on acoustic features of the stimulus.

Extra-axial. Lesions of the brainstem that do not arise from within the brainstem, but from near structures that encroach upon the brainstem.

Forward masking. The presence of one sound renders a subsequent sound less detectable.

Free field. A sound environment in which there are no significant effects on sound propagation from boundaries and the medium (air) is homogeneous and motionless; under free-field conditions, the loss of energy with distance may be predicted by the inverse square law.

Gyrus (pl. gyri). Bulge on the surface of the cerebral cortex consisting of gray matter with an inner core of white matter.

Hearing assistive technology. See Assistive Listening System.

Impedance. Quotient of a dynamic field quantity (e.g., sound pressure) by a kinematic field quantity (e.g., particle velocity), at a specified frequency; total opposition to energy flow expressed in ohms.

Incidence. Number of individuals who contract a disease during a particular period of time.

Individuals with Disabilities Education Act (IDEA)/Individuals with Disabilities Education Improvement Act (IDEIA). Federal education acts that guarantee special education and related services to children with disabilities.

Induction learning. Discovery learning; a three-step process through which a learner recognizes a pattern or relationship, explains the pattern or relationship, and hypothesizes the rule governing the pattern or relationship.

Inductive inferencing. Reasoning from the particular facts to a general conclusion.

Inferencing. Reaching a conclusion on the basis of facts or evidence.

Information processing. Assigning meaning to sensory input based on the extraction of cues or constraints through various processes or stages of cognition, including encoding, organizing, storing, retrieving, comparing, and generating or reconstructing information; these stages involve the interaction between sensory (e.g., auditory processes) and central processes (e.g., cognitive and linguistic processes) through feedback and feedforward loops.

Interaural timing. Refers to a behavioral task requiring the subject to determine the order of two acoustic events presented to each ear separately at slightly different times.

Intervention. Comprehensive, therapeutic treatment and management of a disorder.

Intra-axial. Refers to lesions of the brainstem that evolve from the brainstem tissue itself, as opposed to extra-axial lesions that arise from nonbrainstem tissue. Extra-axial lesions often are in contact with the brainstem.

Inverse square law. Principle whereby under free field conditions, sound intensity varies inversely with the square of the distance from the source; sound intensity I (in W/m^2) measured at distance r (in m) from the source producing the power P (in W) is described as $I = P/(4\pi r^2)$. Thus, if distance is doubled, sound intensity decreases by a factor of four. When expressed in decibels, level decreases by 6 dB for each doubling of the distance from the source to the point of measurement.

Isolation point. A real-time word recognition processing event, which occurs at the gate when the listener initially identifies the target word.

Latency. The time between occurrence of a physiologic event, usually a spike or evoked potential, and a stimulus.

Lateralization. Process of determining the location of a sound inside the head (i.e., intracranial) within the plane between the two ears.

Learning disabilities. A heterogeneous group of disorders, presumed to be due to central nervous system dysfunction, manifested by significant difficulties in the acquisition and use of listening, speaking, reading, writing, reasoning, or mathematical abilities.

Learning style. An individual's characteristic cognitive, affective, modality, and physiological behaviors and preferences employed in perceiving, interacting with, and respond to the learning environment.

Lexical access. A spoken language processing event in which a percept comes in contact with various features of stored lexical representations.

Lexical activation. Some change in status of a subset of word candidates contained in the mental lexicon.

Linguistic-contextual information. Anything that influences the a priori probability of an uncoming utterance or the post hoc, retroactive recognition of an ongoing utterance.

Localization. Process of determining the location of a sound in the environment.

Management. Procedures (e.g., compensatory strategies, environmental modifications) targeted toward reducing the effects of a disorder and minimizing the impact of the deficits that are resistant to remediation.

Masking. Process by which the threshold of one sound is raised by the presence of another (masking) sound; presence of one sound renders a subsequent sound less detectable.

Memory. Capacity to encode, process, and retrieve events, knowledge, feelings, and decisions of the past.

Short-term memory. Brief storage of limited capacity with minimal processing requirements.

Working memory. Temporary storage of information used during reasoning and planning; involves both storage and executive processing and manipulation of information.

Long-term memory. Declarative or explicit memory and procedural or implicit memory; long-term storage of unlimited capacity; involves both storage and processing of information.

Declarative or explicit memory. Conscious awareness or recollection of previously acquired information, retrieved on demand.

Procedural or implicit memory. Use of previous experience or knowledge, in the absence of conscious awareness or recollection, to support learning and guide performance.

Mesencephalic. Referring to the midbrain, just rostral to the pons.

Meta-analysis. Synthesis of treatment efficacy literature (randomized controlled trials) on a given topic using mathematical procedures to integrate results from multiple studies.

Metacognition. Awareness and appropriate use of knowledge; awareness of the task and strategy variables that affect performance and the use of that knowledge to plan, monitor, and regulate performance, including attention, learning, and the use of language; second phase (following cognition) in the development of knowledge which is active and involves conscious control over knowledge.

Metalinguistics. Aspects of language competence that extend beyond unconscious usage for comprehension and production; involves ability to think about language in its abstract form—to reflect on aspects of language apart from its content, analyze it, and make judgments about it; metalinguistic knowledge underlies performance on a number of tasks, including phonological awareness (e.g., segmentation, rhyming), organization and storage of words (e.g., multiple meaning words), and figurative language (e.g., metaphor, idiom, humor); may be considered a subset of metacognition since using language is one of the goals of metacognitive processes.

Metamemory. Knowledge and awareness of one's own memory systems and strategies.

Minimum audible angle. The smallest detectable angular separation between two sound sources relative to the head.

Mismatch negativity (MMN) response. A negative wave (electrical response), generated from a broad region extending from the frontal lobes to the auditory regions of the temporal lobes, to an unattended, rare (or deviant) auditory stimulus resulting from the subtraction of the waveform to the standard (attended) stimulus from the waveform to the deviant stimulus (i.e., difference wave).

Mnemonics. Artificial or contrived memory aids for organizing information (e.g., acronyms, rhymes, verbal mediators, visual imagery, drawing).

Myogenic. A response that is generated by muscle contractions.

Neural synchrony. Pattern of neural activity in which large populations of neurons fire simultaneously; this type of neural activity generates the electric activity giving rise to auditory evoked potentials. Neural synchrony facilitates transmission of activity across central synapses and becomes more important downstream the auditory pathway.

Neuroaudiology. Study of the auditory nervous system as it relates to hearing.

Neurobiology. Encompasses neuroanatomy, physiology, neurochemistry, and neuropharmacology.

Neuropharmacology. Effects of drugs on neuronal tissue.

Neurotransmitter. Chemical agent released by vesicles of a nerve cell that permits synaptic transmission between neurons, between sensory cells and neurons, and between neurons and muscle cells.

No Child Left Behind Act (NCLB). A federally mandated statute enacted in 2002 designed to improve student achievement in the public schools.

Otoacoustic emissions. Subaudible sounds generated by the outer hair cells in the cochlea either spontaneously or evoked by sound stimulation.

P300. A cognitive/sensory response to auditory (or other sensory modality stimulation) reflecting attention and sensory processing to a stimulus thought to arise from neural generators in the medial temporal lobes, temporal-parietal region, and prefrontal cortex.

Pansensory. Referring to higher level mechanisms that are common to and that support processing across all modalities.

Perceptual training. Regimens in which basic perceptual attributes (e.g., sound frequency or duration) are trained through repeated exposure to a task (typically discrimination or identification).

Personal FM system. A system consisting of a wireless microphone transmitter used by the speaker and a receiver used by the listener which is coupled to the listener's ears via headphones, ear buds, or through personal hearing aids (using direct audio input, induction neckloop, or Bluetooth).

Phase. Proportion of a period through which the waveform of a sound has advanced relative to a given time.

Phase-locking. Tendency of an auditory neuron to fire at a particular time (or phase) during each cycle of vibration on the basilar membrane; more generally, as seen in central neurons, the firing at roughly the same phase of the stimulus frequency cycle, but generally not for every cycle (this happens only for frequencies well below 1 kHz).

Pharmacology. Sources, chemistry, actions, and uses of drugs.

Phonemic analysis. Separating words or syllables into a sequence of phonemes.

Phonemic synthesis. Blending of discrete phonemes into the correctly sequenced, coarticulated sound patterns.

Phonological awareness. Explicit awareness of the sound structure of language, including the recognition that words are comprised of syllables and phonemes.

Plasticity. Reorganization of the cortex by experience, often reflected in behavioral change (i.e., learning); alteration of neurons to conform better to immediate environmental influences, often associated with a change in behavior; changes in the properties of individual neurons or neuronal assemblies following specific use, pattern of stimulation, injury or during development; neural reorganization may be possible to some extent across the life span, as well as following injury (compensatory plasticity), and in response to learning.

Posterior probabilities. The probability that a patient actually has a disease given a positive test result, the probability that a patient does not have a disease given a negative result, and the probability of being incorrect given a test result (i.e., the patient does not have disease despite a positive test result or the patient has the disease despite a negative test result). Posterior probabilities reflect the probability of an outcome given the known prevalence of the disorder in the population.

Precedence effect. Refers to the dominance of information from the leading sound (as opposed to delayed or reflected versions of that sound) for the purpose of sound localization; the effect occurs for stimulus time delays varying from fractions of a millisecond to the upper limit for auditory fusion, after which separate sounds are perceived.

Presbycusis. Age-related hearing loss; the gradual, progressive loss of hearing that occurs as people age.

Prevalence. Total number of cases of a specific disease or disorder existing in a given population at a certain time.

Prevention. Procedures targeted toward reducing the likelihood that impairment will develop.

Primary auditory area (or cortex). The main auditory area of the brain, typically considered to be Heschl's gyrus.

Problem solving. Generating a variety of potentially effective responses to a situation and recognizing and implementing the most effective response.

Prosody. Suprasegmental aspects of spoken language; the dynamic melody, timing, rhythm, and amplitude fluctuations of fluent speech.

Psychoacoustics. The study of the relation between sound (i.e., physical parameters) and perception (i.e., psychological correlates) using behavioral measurement techniques.

Real-time speech. The transitory, ephemeral nature of an ongoing speech signal; when speech is presented in a real-time manner, listeners must quickly recognize phonemes, syllables, and words based on preceding linguistic-contextual cues and ongoing acoustic-phonetic information.

Reasoning. Evaluation of arguments, drawing of inferences and conclusions, and generation and testing of hypotheses.

Receiver operating characteristic (ROC) curve. A plot of the effects of sensitivity (d') and a subject's response criterion on the probability of hits (i.e., subject's correct detection of a signal) and false alarms (i.e., subject's detection of a signal when it is not present). A plot used in clinical decision analysis (CDA) to examine how sensitivity and specificity change as a function of different test cutoff scores.

Reciprocal teaching. Alternating roles between the client and clinician, allowing the client to assume the role of teacher as well as learner.

Reflection. Acoustical phenomenon that occurs whenever sound strikes a surface; reflected sound is the portion of the sound energy striking the surface that bounces off the surface.

Reliability. The consistency, dependability, reproducibility, or stability of a measure.

Remediation (or treatment). Procedures targeted toward resolving an impairment.

Reverberation. Persistence or prolongation of sound in an enclosed space, resulting from multiple reflections of sound waves off hard surfaces after the source of the sound has ceased. Reverberation time (RT_{60}) refers to the time required for a steady-state sound to decay 60 dB from its initial peak amplitude offset.

Schema. Structured cluster of concepts and expectations; an abstract and generic knowledge structure stored in memory that preserves the relations among constituent concepts and generalized knowledge about a text, event, message, situation, or object.

> **Content or contextual schema.** Provides a generalized interpretation of the content of experience; organizes facts and establishes a framework that imposes certain structures on events, precepts, situations, and objects and facilitates interpretation.

> **Formal schema.** Linguistic form that organizes, integrates, and predicts relationships across propositions (e.g., additives [*and, furthermore*], adversative [*although, nevertheless, however*], causal [*because, therefore, accordingly*], disjunctive [*but, instead, on the contrary*], and temporal connectives [*before, after, subsequently*], as well as patterns of parallelism and correlative pairs [*not only/but also*; *neither/nor*]).

Screening. Procedures used to identify individuals who are at risk for an impairment.

Segmentation. Parsing spoken language into its constituent and successive segments; parsing sentences, words, or syllables into their constituent phonetic units; the manner in which listeners demarcate the ongoing spoken utterance into units of lexical access.

Self-regulation. Encompasses metacognitive knowledge and skills, as well as affective/emotional, motivational, and behavioral monitoring and self-control processes.

Semantic network. Construct representing a mental system of nodes and links connecting lexical units; vocabulary building in such a network involves adding new nodes and links, as well as changing activation values of the links between nodes (e.g., building synonymy by strengthening the relationships between nodes).

Sensitivity. The ability of a test to yield positive findings when the person tested truly has the dysfunction/disorder; ability of a test to identify correctly those individuals who have the dysfunction/disorder.

Signal-to-noise ratio. Relationship between the sound levels of the signal and the noise at the listener's ear, commonly reported as the difference in decibels between the intensity of the signal and the intensity of the background noise (e.g., if the speech signal is measured at 70 dB and the noise is 64 dB, the signal-to-noise ratio is +6 dB).

Sound field. The area and/or pattern of air pressure disturbance caused by the compression and rarefaction of energy in the audio frequency range.

Specificity. Ability of a test to identify correctly those individuals who do not have the dysfunction/disorder.

Spectrum level. Level of sound contained in a 1-Hz-wide band; a measure of spectral density.

Speech intelligibility. Percentage of words, sentences or phonemes correctly received out of those transmitted; an important measure of the effectiveness or adequacy of a communication system or of the ability of people to communicate in noisy environments.

Spoken language processing. An interactive system of peripheral and central functions used to recognize and understand real-world transitory utterances as meaningful speech.

Standing wave. Phenomenon resulting from the interference of sound waves of the same frequency and kind traveling in opposite directions; characterized by the absence of propagation and the existence of nodes and antinodes that are fixed in space.

Sulcus. Infolding on the cerebral surface separating gyri.

Synapse. Junction where information is transmitted between two neurons.

Synaptic transmission. Passage of an electrical impulse across a synapse through transduction to a chemical neurotransmitter presynaptically and transduction back to an electrical signal postsynaptically.

Systems theory. Study of systems as an entity rather than a conglomeration of parts; provides a conceptual framework for understanding the organization, interaction, and dynamicity of elements comprising systems.

Temporal integration. Refers to the relationship between stimulus duration and intensity within a time frame of less than one-half second; integration of energy sampled within a time frame of approximately 200 milliseconds; sensitivity improves as signal duration increases up to approximately 200 to 300 milliseconds, after which thresholds remain essentially constant; also known as temporal summation.

Temporal masking. Masking that occurs when the signal and the masker do not overlap in time; also known as nonsimultaneous masking.

Temporal ordering. See Temporal sequencing.

Temporal processing. Auditory mechanisms and processes responsible for temporal patterning (e.g., phase locking, synchronization) of neural discharges and the following behavioral phenomena: temporal resolution (i.e., detection of changes in durations of auditory stimuli and time intervals between auditory stimuli over time), temporal ordering (i.e., detection of sequence of sounds over time), temporal integration (i.e., summation of power over durations less than 200 milliseconds), and temporal masking (i.e., obscuring of probe by pre- or poststimulatory presentation of masker).

Temporal resolution. Refers to the shortest time period over which the ear can discriminate two signals; also known as temporal discrimination.

Temporal sequencing. The ability to discern the correct order of rapid acoustic events as they occur over time.

Tonotopic. Organization of auditory neurons in a particular structure according to their responsiveness to specific frequencies; a system of sound frequency representation in which the frequency determines the place (for example, in a neural array) of activation.

Top-down processing. Information processing that is knowledge or concept driven such that higher level constraints guide data processing, leading to data interpretation consistent with these constraints.

TORCH+S complex. A group of perinatal medical problems often linked to hearing loss. T = toxoplasmosis; O = other (e.g., associated ophthalmologic disease); R = rubella; C = cytomegalovirus; H = herpes; S = syphilis.

Total acceptance point. A late event in the real-time word recognition process when a listener recognizes the target word with a high level of confidence.

Treatment (remediation). Procedures targeted toward resolving an impairment.

Treatment outcomes. General term to denote change on measurements from pre to post intervention.

Tuning curve. A graph depicting the response of a neuron at a given percentage (e.g., 10%) above spontaneous activity, plotted as a function of stimulus intensity and frequency. The lowest sound level to which the neuron responds is represented by the tip of the tuning curve (i.e., characteristic frequency).

Two-alternative forced choice method (2AFC). A psychophysical method in which the participant is asked to decide which of two successive intervals contains a signal.

Validity. The degree to which a test measures what it is intended to measure.

Wernicke's area. The receptive auditory-language associational area of the cortex that may include part of the planum temporale and the posterosuperior temporal gyrus.

Word predictability. Amount of *fill-in-the blank* meaningfulness in a preceding spoken context. In predictability-high (PH) sentences, preceding semantic-contextual information is presented in the form of clue words; no such clue words are available in predictability-low (PL) sentences.

Word recognition. A spoken language processing event marking the conclusion of the word selection phase; also refers to a listener's ability to perceive and correctly identify a set of words usually presented at suprathreshold hearing level.

Working memory. Holding information in mind, simultaneously manipulating or transforming that information.

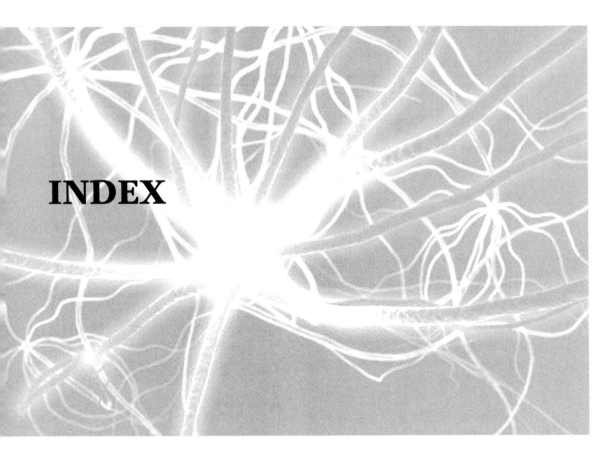

INDEX

Note: Page numbers in **bold** reference non-text material.